Top Nutrients A to Z

ISBN: 978-0-615-93023-7

Pure Source Publishing, LLC
P.O.Box 395 Oceanside, CA 92056.

Design and layout by Bissell Design Studios Inc.

DEDICATION

I would like to dedicate this book to my daughters, Sadie & Sierra and to my husband Garreth, I love you.

INTRODUCTION

This book is intended to identify foods which may be higher or lower in nutrients compared to the foods you are currently eating. It allows a means for estimating how well your current nutrient intake is tracking with the daily amounts recommended by the Institute of Medicine. And by doing so, may help in identifying dietary patterns which potentially could lead to nutrient deficient or toxic levels in the future or may currently exist.

The place to start is with a dietary investigation of the foods you are currently eating on a daily basis, since we are creatures of habit. At the end of each chapter you will find a nutrient data collection form. For two days you will log what you eat on the nutrient collection form. Next estimate a dietary analysis of the nutrients consumed in your current diet by recording the information in this book on the column titled "Book Numbers" on the nutrient data collection form. As you go through the chapters compare your estimated daily intake you have calculated with the recommended daily amounts for each nutrient you are analyzing.

Your goal is to get as close as you can to the recommended amounts, without limiting your variety of foods. Consider the following example of potassium intake. The example below shows a dinner consisting of salmon, white rice, and a mixed vegetable salad with dressing. From this dinner the individuals intake of potassium was 47% of the amount recommended for the day.

Sample Nutrient Data Collection Form

Food Eaten	Amount	Book Numbers	Multiply By	Estimated Nutrient Intake
Salmon	6 oz	347 mg / 3 oz	2	694
White Rice, cooked	1 cup	55 mg cup	1	55
Salad				
Bellpeppers, chopped	1/2 cup	314 mg / cup	1/2	79
Cucumbers	1/2 cup	153 mg / cup	1/2	77
Fresh Spinach, chopped	3 cups	167 mg / cup	3	501
Tomatoes, cherry	1/2 cup	353 mg / cup	1/2	177
Raisins	1/4 cup	1086 mg / cup	1/4	272
Almonds	1/4 cup	252 mg / 1/4 cup	1	252
Ranch Dressing	2 tbsp	9 mg / tbsp	2	18
Nutrient: Potassium	**RDA:** 4500	**Estimated:** 2124	**% of RDA:** 47%	**Total Estimated:** 2124 mg

Daily Values vs Recommended Dietary Allowance

When viewing a product label on any food, one would logically expect that when a product label says 25% of the Daily Value (DV) of a vitamin or mineral, it also means, that it supplies 25% of the daily amount that is recommended you consume. But it does not; DV and the Recommended Dietary Allowance (RDA) recommended by the Institute of Medicine are not interchangeable terms or concepts and must not be confused with each other.

The foundational basis for Daily Values is dependent on averages of populations that did not take into account the different nutritional needs for males, females, infants, children, adults, and the elderly. Daily values can meet the needs of only 50% of the population with some below the RDA and others above.

As an illustration, the product label on a box of the ready-to-eat cereal, Go Lean Crunch, shows a potassium intake of 290 mg per serving and lists this at 8% of the Daily Value (DV). The RDA for potassium intake is 3000 mg for young children and 4700 mg for adults, and 8% of these two numbers are 240 and 376, and not 290. Eight percent of the DV is not equal to 8% of the RDA.

In contrast, the RDA, which is the actual amount of a particular nutrient recommended for daily ingestion is based on sex and age differences and meets the dietary needs of 98% of the population.

Although the Daily Values found on product labels may have some nutritional information about a food product relative to another product or overall diet, the committee responsible for the establishment of the daily values specifically states that the product label is not to be used for planning diets.

Relying on the Daily Values will systematically over or underestimate the actual nutrient intake from a serving, making many foods appear to be more nutritional than they actually are.

A product that contains 100% of the DV will still have only a 50% probability of meeting the recommended daily intake amounts for the general population. It is the RDA that is intended to be used as the targeted goal for individual daily intake of vitamins and minerals and not daily values.

THINGS TO CONSIDER

The macronutrient food values on the breakfast cereals, chili, soups, salad dressings, and yogurts were taken directly from product labels found on shelves in local grocery stores. Additional nutrient information not available on product labels as well as the nutrient values of all other foods is published numerical data taken from the U.S. Department of Agriculture's National Nutrient Database. The USDA nutrient data base is the primary data source used in America for nutritional planning in schools, hospitals, and the military, because it is regularly updated with research, food testing, and nutrient contents. The nutrient content of all foods is given as the mean nutritional value for a given common house hold food portion and is based on the edible portion.

In order to allow an accurate comparison of the nutrient content between foods, serving sizes have been standardized to common household measurements and usage. As an illustration, the product labels on ready-to-eat breakfast cereals lists serving sizes that range between 1/4 to 1-1/3 cups.

Consider the following example of product labels:

Cereals	Serving Size	Sugar / Serving
Corn Chex	1 cup	10g
Apple Cinnamon Cherrios	3/4 cup	10 g
Date & Almond Granola	2/3 cup	10 g

If you were to grab these three boxes of cereals while standing in the aisle of a grocery store, a quick glance would leave an impression of similar amounts of sugar. However, after converting the Cherrios and Granola serving sizes to match the one cup serving size of Corn-Chex, the comparable amounts of sugar actually consumed is significantly different.

Cereals	Serving Size	Sugar / Serving
Corn Chex	1 cup	10 g
Apple Cinnamon Cherrios	1 cup	13 g
Date & Almond Granola	1 cup	15 g

All ready-to-eat cereal serving sizes have been converted to a one cup serving size to allow an accurate comparison of the nutrient content between different cereal brands and different flavors.

ACKNOWLEDGMENTS

We are gratefully indebted to Robert Miskinis, an organic chemist trained at U.C.L.A. It was Robert's nutritional research that made this book possible. A special thank you goes to his nutritional analyst Arlene Pingarron for her encouragement, spirt, and secretarial skills.

And finally, we must recognize and thank all authors of the reference material and all their astute clinical nutritionists, chemist, and physicians whose dedication to research made the information in this book reliable.

DISCLAIMER

TABLE OF CONTENTS

Calcium 1

Calories 55

Carbohydrates 91

Cholesterol 117

Copper 143

Essential Fatty Acids 191

FAT Total 281

FAT Saturated 315

FAT Monounsaturated 351

FAT Polyunsaturated 369

Fiber 381

Iron 405

Magnesium 431

Phosphorus 457

Potassium 521

Protein 547

Sodium 623

Sugar 685

Vitamin A 725

Vitamin B1 751

Vitamin B3 775

Vitamin B6 799

Vitamin B12 823

Vitamin C 839

Vitamin D 857

Vitamin E 877

Vitamin K 901

Zinc 925

References 951

CALCIUM

Calcium and its reactions with phosphorus and vitamin D are involved with the formation, repair and maintenance of bones throughout an entire lifetime.

In humans, science has proven that calcium metabolism is regulated by vitamin D. In fact, the extent of calcium absorption in the intestines is totally dependent on the presence of vitamin D. I'm not just saying vitamin D helps calcium absorption I am saying it dominates it. If vitamin D levels are low in the intestines only 15% of dietary calcium may be absorbed, and most will pass through the body unused.

When the amount of calcium circulating in blood becomes low, the body responds by elevating the levels of its calcium-regulating hormones. This hormone, known as the parathyroid hormone, is the most powerful hormone regulator of healthy bones and is the guardian of calcium concentrations in blood. Once summoned, as genetically programed, it will draw calcium from bone to replace any lost calcium circulating in blood.

This is a natural response, but the loss of calcium in bones will continue as long as the parathyroid hormones are held at elevated levels. The parathyroid hormone plays a dominant role in maintaining blood calcium concentrations strictly within a very narrow range, but it does so at the expense of bone loss.

Therefore, controlling the parathyroid hormones is important to reduce the risk of weakened and fragile bones. This is done, in part, by balancing the dietary intake of calcium with the intake of phosphorus represented by the calcium to phosphorus ratio, (Ca / P).

One of the most important relationships between two essential nutrients, and their effect on human health, is that between calcium and phosphorus. In both animal and human experiments, a high intake of phosphorus relative to intake of calcium increased the parathyroid hormones to above normal levels and destroyed calcium metabolism.

Consider the following summaries of a few studies:

1990 In America, a common dietary pattern in young adult women contains enough phosphorus to cause persistent changes in the parathyroid hormones and could adversely influence bone formation.

1993 The low calcium / phosphorus dietary pattern of American women results in persistent changes in the parathyroid hormones that are neither conducive to peak bone mass nor to slowing the rate of bone loss.

1996 A mechanism that contributes to low bone mass in the United States involves a low calcium / phosphorus dietary ratio.

1999 Healthy women were found to have a positive association between a calcium / phosphorus dietary ratio and bone density.

2010 In healthy women, even when calcium intake is adequate, diets with a low calcium / phosphorus ratio increases the loss of calcium from bones.

Each case above involves elevation of the parathyroid hormone because it is the dominating hormone regulator of bone loss at any stage of the human life cycle and is controlled by diet. Any dietary pattern contributing phosphorus above the RDA will potentially contribute to an abnormally low calcium / phosphorus dietary ratio, which will trigger the body to produce elevated parathyroid hormone levels, and this in turn, will leach calcium from bone and contribute to the loss of bone mass and bone strength. This will take place within hours after each phosphorus rich meal. Thus, daily and meal-to-meal phosphorus rich meals will result in persistent elevated levels of the parathyroid hormones and slow erosion of the human bone.

Symptoms of a calcium deficiency are very difficult to identify during early stages since they vary in both the number and types of underlying causes and exhibit no noticeable symptoms until they surface later in life as weak and fractured bones. Because blood levels of calcium normally do not reflect the body's total nutritional status of calcium a severe deficiency must occur before any clinical symptoms can be recognized. Thus, during the time the bones are being depleted of calcium, there will be no symptoms or pain; blood levels of calcium and intake of calcium may appear normal even though the bones are being depleted of calcium.

The parathyroid hormones must remain within the lower range of what is considered to be a normal range rather than in the upper range. To suppress persistent elevations of the parathyroid hormones, the dietary intake of calcium / phosphorus must be balanced to some degree. The preferred method for balancing is to reduce the intake of phosphorus rather than increasing the intake of calcium. In a large population based study of 9,000 subjects, calcium intake was associated with bone density only among women who had low levels of vitamin D. In all other groups there was no relationship between calcium intake and bone density.

This could explain in part why, although Americans have higher calcium intake than people in other countries, we still have high incidences of osteoporosis.

This brings us to the theoretical optimal dietary calcium / phosphorus ratio for humans. Dividing the RDA for calcium by the RDA for phosphorus equates to a calcium / phosphorus dietary ratio of 1.4 by weight for adults. In infants and children, a calcium / phosphorus ratio of 1.5 is considered to be ideal for optimal growth. In fact, federal law requires the ratio of calcium / phosphorus in infant formulas between 1.1 and 2.0.

Of course you can eat foods above and below these numbers, but the literature shows that, in one experiment, daily intakes of a calcium / phosphorus dietary ratio at .23 resulted in a 26% increase in the parathyroid hormone levels, but a ratio of .8 did not.

In summary, assembled data from many studies indicates that phosphorus intakes above the recommended amounts and a low calcium / phosphorus dietary intake ratio are negatively associated with lower amounts of bone mass later in life. And elevated levels of the parathyroid hormones are indicators of a vitamin D insufficiency and a sign of impaired calcium metabolism. In America, phosphorus is consumed in amounts that are too high for optimal bone health in women. It is strongly recommended that a variety of foods be consumed, to avoid consuming only phosphorus rich foods.

For a discussion on the severe type of a calcium deficiency known as hypocalcemia see the chapter on phosphorus. This chapter lists the amounts of calcium in milligrams (mg) and the calcium / phosphorus ratios for food and beverages commonly consumed by Americans.

The recommended intake for calcium is in milligram, mg, quantities.

Recommend Daily Intakes Levels for Calcium

Children	Calcium, mg
1 to 3 year olds	700
4 to 8 year olds	1000

Males	
9 to 13 year olds	1300
14 to 18 year olds	1300
19 to 30 years	1000
31 to 50 years	1000
51 to 70 years	1000
Over 70	1200

Females	
9 to 13 year olds	1300
14 to 18 year olds	1300
19 to 30 years	1000
31 to 50 years	1000
51 to 70 years	1200
Over 70	1200

Pregnancy	
14 to 18 years	1300
19 to 30 years	1000
31 to 50 years	1000

CALCIUM

Lactation

14 to 18 years	1300
19 to 30 years	1000
31 to 50 years	1000

CALCIUM REFERENCES

1969 Importance of dietary calcium / phosphorus ratios on skeletal, calcium, magnesium, and phosphorus metabolism. Irwin Clark. American Journal of Physiology. September 1969, Vol. 217, No. 3, 865-80.

1986 Relationships between unusual nutrient intake and bone-mineral content of women 35-65 years of age: longitudinal and cross-sectional analysis. Jo. L. Freudenheim, MS., Nancy E. Johnson, PhD., Everett L. Smith, PhD. American Journal of Clinical Nutrition. December 1986, Vol. 44, No. 6, 863-876.

1987 Influence of nutritional factors on calcium-regulating hormones and bone loss. Luket BP, Carey M, McCarty B, Tiemann S, Goodnight L, Helm M, Hassanein R, Stevenson C, Stoskopf M, Doolan L. Calcified Tissues International. March 1987, Vol. 4, No. 3, 119-125.

1987 The problem of calcium requirement. BE Chrostopher Nordin, M.D., DSc, Karen J. Polly, BSc, Allan G. Need, Howard A Morris, PhD., David Marshal PhD. American Journal of Clinical Nutrition. May 1987, Vol. 45, No.5, 1295-1304.

1988 Elevated secretion and action of parathyroid hormones in young women assembled from ordinary foods. Calvo MS, Kumar R, Heath H 3rd. Journal of Clinical Endocrinology & Metabolism. April 1988, Vol. 66, No. 4, 823-829.

CALCIUM

1990 Persistently elevated parathyroid hormone secretion and action in young women after four weeks of ingesting high phosphorus, low calcium diets. Mona S. Calvco, Rajiv Kumar, Hunter Heath . Journal of Clinical Endocrinology & Metabolism. May 1990, Vol. 70, 1334-1340.

1991 Effect of calcium / phosphorus ratio on mineral retention in parenterally fed premature infants. Pelegano JF, Rowe JC, Carey DE, LaBarre DJ, Edgren KW, Lazar AM, Horak E. J. Pediat Gastroenterol Nutr. April 1991, Vol. 12, No. 3, 351-355.

1992 Effects of a short course of oral phosphate treatment on serum parathyroid hormone and biochemical markers of bone turnover: A Dose-Response Study. Kim Brixan, Henning K. Nielsen, Peder Charles, Leif Mosekilde. Calcified Tissues International. 1992, Vol.51, 276-281.

1993 Dietary phosphorus, calcium metabolism, and bone. Mona Schiess Calvo. Journal of Nutrition. 1993, Vol.123, 1627-1633.

1993 Intakes of calcium, phosphorus, protein, and physical activity level are related to radial bone mass in young adult women. Jill A Metz, John JB Andersen, Philip N Gallagher Jr. American Journal of Clinical Nutrition. October 1993, Vol.58, No.4, 537-542.

1996 Changing phosphorus content of the U.S. diet: potential for adverse effects on bone. Mona S. Calvo, Youngmee K. Park. Journal of Nutrition. April 1996, Vol. 126(4Supp), 1168s-1180s.

1996 Calcium, Phosphorus and Human Bone Development. John J.B. Anderson. Journal of Nutrition. 1996, Vol. 126(4Supp), 1153s-1158s.

1998 Dietary calcium, protein, and phosphorus are related to bone mineral density and content in young women. Dorothy Teegarden, Roseann M Lyle, George P McCabe, Linda D Mcabe, William R Proulx, Kathryn Michon, Ada P Knight, C Conrad Johnson, and Connie M Weaver. American Journal of Clinical Nutrition. September 1998, Vol.68, No.3, 749-754.

1999 Relationship between bone mineral density, serum vitamin D metabolites and calcium / phosphorus intake in healthy perimenopausal women. C. Brot, N. Jorgensen, O.R. Madsen, L.B. Jensen, O.H. Sorensen. Journal of Internal Medicine. May 1999, Vol. 245, Issue 5, 509-516.

2001 The Institute of Medicine's Dietary Reference Intake for Phosphorus: A Critical Perspective. Leonard Sax, MD, PhD Journal of the American College of Nutrition. August 2001, Vol. 20, No. 4, 271-278.

2004 Positive association between 25-hydroxyvitamin D levels and bone mineral density: a population based study of young and older adults. Bischoff-Ferrari H.A., Dietrich T., Orav E.J. Dawson-Hughes B., American Journal of Medicine. 2004, Vol. 116, 634-639.

2006 High phosphorus intakes acutely and negatively affect calcium and bone metabolism in a dose-dependent manner in healthy young females. Kemi VE, Karkkainen MU, Lamberg-Allardt CJ. British Journal of Nutrition. 2006, Vol. 96, 545-552.

2009 Dietary calcium and serum 25-hydroxyvitamin D status in relation to BMD among U.S. adults. Bischoff-Ferrari H.A., Kiel D.P., Dawson-Hughes B. Journal Bone Mineral Research. 2009, Vol. 24, 935-942.

2010 Calcium in chronic kidney disease: myths and realities. Craig B. Langman, Jorge B. Cannata-Andia. Clinical Journal of the American Society of Nephrology. January 2010, Vol. 5, s1-s2.

2010 Low calcium / phosphorus ratio in habitual diets affects serum parathyroid hormone concentration and calcium metabolism in healthy women with adequate calcium intake. Virpi E. Kemi, Merja U.M. Karkkainen, Hannu J. Rita, Marika M.L. Laaksonen, Terhi A. Outila, Christel J.E. Lamberg-Allardt. British Journal of Nutrition. 2010, Vol. 103, 561-568.

2013 Effect of calcium plus vitamin D supplementation during pregnancy in Brazilian adolescent mothers: a randomized placebo-controlled trial. Maria Eduarda L. Diogenes, Flavia F. Bezerra, Elaine P. Rezende, Marcia Fernanda Taveria, Isabel Pinhal, Carmen M. Donangelo. American Journal of Clinical Nutrition. July 2013, Vol. 98, No. 1, 82-91.

2013 Unexpected long-term effects of calcium supplementation in pregnancy on material bone outcomes in women with a low calcium intake: A follow-up study. Landing M.A. Jarjou, Yankuba Sawo, Gail R. Goldberg, M. Ann Lasky, Tim J. Cole, Ann Prentice. American Journal of Clinical Nutrition. September 2013, Vol. 98, No. 3, 723-730.

CALCIUM

Alcohol	Amount	Calcium (mg)
Light Beer	1 bottle	14
Regular Beer	1 bottle	14
White Wine	1 glass	13
Red Wine	1 glass	12
Gin, Rum, Vodka, or Whisky	1 shot	0

Beans, Canned	Amount	Calcium (mg)
White beans	1 cup	191
Great Northern	1 cup	139
Navy beans	1 cup	123
Pinto beans	1 cup	113
Cranberry beans	1 cup	88
Baked beans, plain	1 cup	86
Garbanzo beans	1 cup	84
Refried beans	1 cup	79
Kidney beans	1 cup	74
Fava beans	1 cup	67
Green beans	1 cup	58
Lima beans, large	1 cup	51
Black-eyed peas	1 cup	48
Yellow beans	1 cup	40

Beans, Cooked	Amount	Calcium (mg)
Natto	1 cup	380
Soybeans, green	1 cup	261
Winged beans	1 cup	244
Soybeans, matured	1 cup	175
White beans, mature	1 cup	161
White beans, small	1 cup	131
Soybeans, matured, dry roasted	1 cup	130
Navy beans	1 cup	126
Great Northern	1 cup	120
Black Turtle beans, mature	1 cup	102
Edamame	1 cup	98
Cranberry beans	1 cup	88
Lupini beans	1 cup	85
Garbanzo beans, chickpeas	1 cup	80
Pinto beans	1 cup	79
Hyacinath beans	1 cup	78
Pigeon peas	1 cup	72
Yardlong beans, mature	1 cup	72
Adzuki	1 cup	64
Fava beans	1 cup	61

RDA is 1000 mg for adults

CALCIUM

Continued

Yellow beans	1 cup	58
Green beans	1 cup	55
Mung beans, mature seeds	1 cup	55
Kidney beans	1 cup	50
Black beans	1 cup	46
Black-eyed peas	1 cup	41
Lentils	1 cup	38
Lima beans	1 cup	32
Split peas	1 cup	27
Mothbeans	1 cup	5

Beef, Cooked	Amount	Calcium (mg)
Ground beef, 75%	3 oz	26
Ground beef, 80%	3 oz	20
Top sirloin, trimmed to 1/8" fat	3 oz	16
Flank steak, lean, trimmed to 0" fat	3 oz	15
Ground beef, 85%	3 oz	15
Brisket, lean, trimmed to 0" fat	3 oz	14
Chuck roast, trimmed to 1/8" fat	3 oz	11
Filet Mignon, trimmed to 0" fat	3 oz	11
Ground beef, 90%,	3 oz	11
Tri Tip steak	3 oz	10
Beef ribs, trimmed to 1/8" fat	3 oz	9
Skirt Steak, trimmed to 0" fat	3 oz	9
Ground beef, 95%	3 oz	6
Porterhouse steak, trimmed to 0" fat	3 oz	6
Ribeye steak, trimmed to 0" fat	3 oz	6
T-Bone steak, trimmed 0" fat	3 oz	4

Beef, Cooked	Amount	Calcium (mg)
Top Sirloin, trimmed to 1/8" fat	1 lb cooked	91
Flank steak, lean, trimmed to 0" fat	1 lb cooked	82
Brisket, lean, trimmed to 0" fat	1 lb cooked	73
Flank steak, lean, trimmed to 0" fat	1 steak	69
Chuck roast, trimmed to 1/8" fat	1 lb cooked	59
Tri Tip steak, lean, trimmed to 0" fat	1 lb cooked	54
Beef ribs, trimmed to 1/8" fat	1 lb cooked	50
Skirt steak, trimmed to 0" fat	1 lb cooked	50
Porterhouse steak, trimmed to 0" fat	1 lb cooked	32
T-bone steak, trimmed to 0" fat	1 lb cooked	23
Ribeye steak, boneless, trimmed to 0" fat	1 steak	15
Filet Mignon, tenderloin, trimmed to 0" fat	1 steak	13
Ribeye filet, lean, trimmed to 0" fat	1 filet	8
Top Sirloin, choice filet, trimmed to 0" fat	1 filet	7

RDA is 1000 mg for adults

CALCIUM

Beef, Cooked	Amount	Calcium (mg)
Ground beef, 75%	1/4 lb patty	21
Ground beef, 80%	1/4 lb patty	18
Ground beef, 85%	1/4 lb patty	14
Ground beef, 90%	1/4 lb patty	11
Ground beef, 95%	1/4 lb patty	6

Bread	Amount	Calcium (mg)
English Muffin, plain	1 muffin	93
Bagel, plain	4" bagel	79
Indian bread, Naan, plain	1 piece	76
Indian bread, Naan, whole wheat	1 piece	63
Potato bread	1 slice	60
Hamburger & Hot dog buns, plain	1 bun	59
Kaiser rolls	1 roll	54
Pita, white	6" pita	52
Dinner Rolls, brown & serve	1 roll	50
Cornbread, dry mix	1 piece	44
Tortillas, flour	1 tortilla	41
Mexican roll, bolillo	1 roll	40
White bread	1 slice	38
Egg bread	1 slice	37
Wheat	1 slice	36
Whole-Wheat	1 slice	30
Multigrain or Whole grain	1 slice	27
Rye bread	1 slice	23
Pumpernickel	1 slice	22
Reduced calorie white	1 slice	22
Croissants, butter	1 medium	21
Tortillas, corn	1 tortilla	21
Bagel, wheat	4" bagel	20
Oatmeal bread	1 slice	18
Reduced calorie wheat	1 slice	18
Bagel, cinnamon & raisins	4" bagel	17
Raisin bread	1 slice	17
Reduced calorie rye	1 slice	17
Italian	1 slice	16
Bagel, oat bran	4" bagel	13
Bagel, egg	4" bagel	12
Cracked Wheat	1 slice	11
French and Sourdough	1 slice	11

CALCIUM

Cereal, General Mills®	Amount	Calcium (mg)
Total Whole Grain	1 cup	1333
Total Raisin Bran	1 cup	1000
Total Cranberry Crunch	1 cup	800
Basic 4	1 cup	250
Lucky Charms	1 cup	156
Chocolate Chex	1 cup	142
Kix	1 cup	137
Golden Grahams	1 cup	134
Honey Nut Chex	1 cup	134
Cinnamon Chex	1 cup	133
Cocoa Puffs	1 cup	133
Cookie Crisp	1 cup	133
Dora The Explorer	1 cup	133
Multi-Bran CHEX	1 cup	133
Reese's Puffs	1 cup	133
Wheat Chex	1 cup	133
Berry Berry Kix	1 cup	120
Cinnamon Toast Crunch	1 cup	118
Corn Chex	1 cup	100
Rice Chex	1 cup	100
Trix	1 cup	100
KABOOM	1 cup	80
Raisin Nut Bran	1 cup	27
Wheaties	1 cup	27
Oatmeal Crisp, Hearty Raisin	1 cup	20
Honey Nut Clusters	1 cup	19
Oatmeal Crisp, Crunchy Almond	1 cup	18

Cereal, General Mill's Cheerios®	Amount	Calcium (mg)
Frosted	1 cup	138
Apple Cinnamon	1 cup	133
Banana Nut	1 cup	133
Berry Burst	1 cup	133
Dulce De Leche Cheerios	1 cup	133
Chocolate	1 cup	133
Fruity	1 cup	133
Honey Nut	1 cup	133
Yogurt Burst, Strawberry	1 cup	133
Original	1 cup	112
Oat Cluster Cheerios Crunch	1 cup	107
Cinnamon Burst	1 cup	100
Multi-Grain	1 cup	100

RDA is 1000 mg for adults

CALCIUM

Cereal, General Mill's Fiber One®	Amount	Calcium (mg)
80 Calorie Chocolate Squares	1 cup	533
80 Calorie Honey Squares	1 cup	533
Original	1 cup	200
Caramel Delight	1 cup	100
Honey Clusters	1 cup	100
Nutty Clusters & almonds	1 cup	100
Raisin Bran Clusters	1 cup	100
Frosted Shreaded Wheat	1 cup	0

Cereal, Kashi®	Amount	Calcium (mg)
Go Lean Crisp, Cinnamon Crumble	1 cup	107
Go Lean	1 cup	73
Go Lean Crisp, Toasted Berry Crumble	1 cup	69
Go Lean Crunch	1 cup	53
7-Whole Grain Nuggets	1 cup	48
Go Lean Crunch, Honey Almond Flax	1 cup	46
Heart to Heart, Oat Flakes & Blueberry Clusters	1 cup	25
Heart to Heart, Warm Cinnamon	1 cup	21
Island Vanilla	27 biscuits	20
Heart to Heart, Honey Toasted Oat	1 cup	18
Berry Blossom	1 cup	16
Berry Fruitful	29 biscuits	16
7-Whole Grain Flakes	1 cup	14
Good Friends, Original	1 cup	14
Honey Sunshine	1 cup	14
7-Whole Grain Honey Puffs	1 cup	13
Strawberry Fields	1 cup	8
7-Whole Grain Puffs	1 cup	7
Autumn Wheat	29 biscuits	0
Blackberry Hills	1 cup	0
Cinnamon Harvest	28 biscuits	0
Go Lean Vanilla Graham	1 cup	x
Heart to Heart, Nutty Chia Flax	1 cup	x
Indigo Morning	1 cup	x
Simply Maize	1 cup	x

Cereal, Kellogg's®	Amount	Calcium (mg)
All-Bran Original	1 cup	241
All-Bran Bran Buds	1 cup	57
Cocoa Krispies	1 cup	52
MUESLIX	1 cup	48
Cracklin Oat Bran	1 cup	39
Krave Chocolate	1 cup	25

CALCIUM

Raisin Bran	1 cup	25
All-Bran Complete Wheat Flakes	1 cup	20
Fiberplus Cinnamon Oat Crunch	1 cup	19
Frosted MINI-Wheat's, Bite-Size	1 cup	18
Frosted MINI Wheat's, Big-Bite	1 cup	17
Raisin Bran Crunch	1 cup	17
Fiberplus Berry Yogurt Crunch	1 cup	16
Smart Start, Strong Heart Antioxidants	1 cup	12
Crunchy Nut Roasted Nut & Honey O's	1 cup	11
Honey Crunch Corn Flakes	1 cup	9
Honey Smacks	1 cup	9
CINNABON	1 cup	8
Crunchy Nut Golden Honey Nut Flakes	1 cup	8
Smorz	1 cup	7
Product 19	1 cup	5
Rice Krispies Treats	1 cup	4
Apple Jacks	1 cup	3
Crispix	1 cup	3
Froot Loops	1 cup	3
Frosted Rice Krispies	1 cup	3
Corn Flakes	1 cup	2
Corn Pops	1 cup	2
Frosted Flakes	1 cup	1
Rice Krispies	1 cup	1

Cereal, Kellogg's Special-K®	Amount	Calcium (mg)
Low Fat Granola	1 cup	42
Protein Plus	1 cup	34
Vanilla Almond	1 cup	13
Cinnamon Pecan	1 cup	12
Fruit & Yogurt	1 cup	12
Original	1 cup	11
Multigrain Oats & Honey	1 cup	8
Blueberry	1 cup	7
Chocolately Delight	1 cup	7
Red Berries	1 cup	6

Cereal, Post®	Amount	Calcium (mg)
Grape-Nuts Cereal	1 cup	50
Raisin Bran	1 cup	30
Great Grains, Raisin, Date & Pecan	1 cup	29
Shredded Wheat, Original, spoon-size	1 cup	28
Great Grains, Crunchy Pecan	1 cup	27
Great Grains, Cranberry Almond Crunch	1 cup	26
Great Grains, Banana Nut Crunch	1 cup	24

RDA is 1000 mg for adults

CALCIUM

Continued

Bran Flakes	1 cup	22
Honey Nut Shredded Wheat	1 cup	22
Shredded Wheat n' Bran, spoon-size	1 cup	21
Blueberry Morning	1 cup	18
Grape-Nuts Flakes	1 cup	14
Shredded Wheat, Original, big-biscuit	1 biscuit	12
Cocoa Pebbles	1 cup	9
Alpha-Bits	1 cup	7
Fruity Pebbles	1 cup	7
Shredded Wheat, frosted, spoon-size	1 cup	7
Golden Crisp	1 cup	5
Honeycomb Cereal	1 cup	2

Post®Honey Bunches of Oats®	Amount	Calcium (mg)
Just Bunches Honey Roasted	1 cup	36
With Vanilla Bunches	1 cup	18
With Almonds	1 cup	15
With Cinnamon Bunches	1 cup	14
With Strawberries	1 cup	11
Honey Roasted	1 cup	9
Pecan Bunches	1 cup	8

Cereal, Quaker®	Amount	Calcium (mg)
LIFE Cereal, Maple & Brown Sugar	1 cup	149
LIFE Cereal, Cinnamon	1 cup	148
LIFE Cereal, Original	1 cup	147
Oatmeal Squares, Cinnamon	1 cup	119
Oatmeal Squares	1 cup	114
Granola Apple Cranberry Almond	1 cup	96
Toasted Multigrain Crisp	1 cup	87
Oatmeal Squares, Golden Maple	1 cup	86
Corn Bran Crunch	1 cup	26
CAP'N Crunch	1 cup	4
CAP'N Crunch & Crunch Berries	1 cup	4
CAP'N Crunch's OOPs! All Berries	1 cup	4
Honey Graham OH'S	1 cup	4
Puffed Wheat	1 cup	4
CAP'N Crunch's Peanut Butter Crunch	1 cup	3
Puffed Rice	1 cup	2

Cereal, Cooked	Amount	Calcium (mg)
Farina™	1 cup	232
CREAM OF WHEAT™, regular	1 cup	218
WHEATENA®	1 cup	194

RDA is 1000 mg for adults

CALCIUM

Continued

Oats, instant, fortified, plain	1 cup	187
Malt-o-Meal, plain	1 serving	163
Oats, regular, unenriched	1 cup	21
White corn grits	1 cup	2
Yellow corn grits	1 cup	2

Cheese	Amount	Calcium (mg)
Ricotta, part skim milk	1 cup	669
Ricotta, whole milk	1 cup	509
Cottage cheese, low fat, 2 %	1 cup	206
Cottage cheese, creamed, small curd	1 cup	187
Cottage cheese, low fat, 1 %	1 cup	138
Cottage cheese, non fat & uncreamed	1 cup	125

Cheese	Amount	Calcium (mg)
Parmesan, grated	1 oz	314
Romano	1 oz	302
American, pasteurized process, fortified	1 oz	296
Gruyere	1 oz	287
Mozzarella, non fat	1 oz	272
Swiss, low fat	1 oz	269
Goat cheese, hard type	1 oz	254
Swiss	1 oz	224
Provolone	1 oz	214
Provolone, reduced fat	1 oz	212
Monterey	1 oz	211
Mozzarella, skim milk, low moisture	1 oz	207
Cheddar	1 oz	204
Muenster	1 oz	203
Gouda	1 oz	198
Monterey, low fat	1 oz	197
Colby	1 oz	194
American, pasteurized process, low fat	1 oz	192
Roquefort	1 oz	188
American, pasteurized process, imitation	1 oz	184
Fontina	1 oz	156
Blue cheese	1 oz	150
Muenster, low fat	1 oz	148
Mozzarella, whole milk	1 oz	143
Feta	1 oz	140
Velveeta, pasteurized process	1 oz	130
Cheddar, low-fat	1 oz	118
Cheez Whiz, pasteurized process	1 oz	101
Cream cheese, fat free	1 oz	100
Goat cheese, semisoft	1 oz	84

RDA is 1000 mg for adults

CALCIUM

Continued

Ricotta, part skim milk	1 oz	77
Ricotta, whole milk	1 oz	59
Brie	1 oz	52
Goat cheese, soft type	1 oz	40
Cream cheese	1 oz	28

Chicken, Cooked	Amount	Calcium (mg)
Breast, with skin, fried in flour	1/2 breast	16
Breast, with skin, roasted	1/2 breast	14
Breast, no skin, roasted	1/2 breast	13
Wing with skin, fried in batter	1 wing	10
Thigh, with skin, fried in flour	1 thigh	9
Drumstick, with skin, fried in flour	1 drumstick	6
Thigh, no skin, roasted	1 thigh	6
Drumstick, no skin, roasted	1 drumstick	5
Wing with skin, roasted	1 wing	5

Chicken, Cooked	Amount	Calcium (mg)
Breast with skin, fried in flour	3 oz	14
Cornish game hens, meat only	3 oz	14
Wing meat only, no skin, roasted	3 oz	14
Breast meat only, no skin, roasted	3 oz	13
Wing with skin, fried in flour	3 oz	13
Wing with skin, roasted	3 oz	13
Breast with skin, roasted	3 oz	12
Thigh with skin, fried in flour	3 oz	12
Drumstick meat only, no skin, roasted	3 oz	10
Drumstick with skin, fried in flour	3 oz	10
Drumstick with skin, roasted	3 oz	10
Thigh meat only, no skin, roasted	3 oz	8
Thigh with skin, roasted	3 oz	8

Cream	Amount	Calcium (mg)
Half & Half	1 tbsp	16
Sour Cream, reduced fat	1 tbsp	16
Light Coffee Cream	1 tbsp	14
Sour Cream, cultured	1 tbsp	13
Heavy Cream	1 tbsp	10
Whipped Topping, pressurized	1 tbsp	3

Eggs	Amount	Calcium (mg)
Egg substitute, liquid, fat free	1/4 cup	44
Egg whole, scrambled	1 large	40
Egg whole, fried	1 large	29

RDA is 1000 mg for adults

CALCIUM

Continued

Egg whole, poached	1 large	28
Egg whole, hard-boiled	1 large	25
Egg yolk	1 large	21
Egg whites, dried	1 tbsp	18
Egg whites, dried powder, stabilized	1 tbsp	6
Egg whites	1 large	2

Fish, Canned	Amount	Calcium (mg)
Atlantic Sardines, in oil	3 oz	325
Light tuna, in oil	3 oz	14
Light tuna, in water	3 oz	14
White (albacore) tuna, in water	3 oz	12
White (albacore) tuna, in oil	3 oz	3

Fish, Cooked	Amount	Calcium (mg)
Walleye pike	3 oz	120
Freshwater bass	3 oz	88
Rainbow trout, wild	3 oz	73
Atlantic herring, pickeled	3 oz	65
Atlantic pollock	3 oz	65
Northern pike	3 oz	62
Walleye pollock	3 oz	61
Whiting	3 oz	53
Carp	3 oz	44
Coho salmon, wild	3 oz	38
Cat fish, breaded & fried	3 oz	37
Florida pompano	3 oz	37
King mackerel	3 oz	34
Snapper	3 oz	34
Skipjack (aku) tuna	3 oz	31
Atlantic perch	3 oz	29
Alaskan halibut	3 oz	28
Atlantic croaker	3 oz	27
Rainbow trout, farmed	3 oz	26
Striped mullet	3 oz	26
Pacific & Jack mackerel	3 oz	25
Yellowtail	3 oz	25
King, chinook salmon	3 oz	24
Flounder & sole	3 oz	21
Atlantic cod	3 oz	18
Grouper	3 oz	18
Sea bass	3 oz	16
Pacific rockfish	3 oz	14
Atlantic mackerel	3 oz	13
Atlantic salmon, farmed	3 oz	13

RDA is 1000 mg for adults

CALCIUM

Atlantic salmon, wild	3 oz	13
Haddock	3 oz	12
Keta, (chum) salmon	3 oz	12
Tilapia	3 oz	12
Spanish mackerel	3 oz	11
Striped bass	3 oz	11
Coho salmon, farmed	3 oz	10
Sockeye salmon	3 oz	10
Catfish, wild	3 oz	9
King, chinook salmon, smoked	3 oz	9
Orange roughy	3 oz	9
Salmon, Lox	3 oz	9
Atlantic & Pacific halibut	3 oz	8
Bluefin tuna	3 oz	8
Catfish, farmed	3 oz	8
Pacific cod	3 oz	8
Surimi	3 oz	8
Pink salmon	3 oz	7
Swordfish	3 oz	5
Greenland halibut	3 oz	3
Yellowfin tuna	3 oz	3

Fish, Shellfish, Cooked	Amount	Calcium (mg)
Shrimp, canned	3 oz	123
Octopus	3 oz	90
Blue crab cakes	3 oz	89
Northern lobster	3 oz	82
Eastern oysters, wild	3 oz	78
Blue crab	3 oz	77
Blue crab, canned	3 oz	77
Shrimp	3 oz	77
Shrimp, breaded & fried	3 oz	57
Clams, canned	3 oz	55
Clams, breaded & fried	3 oz	54
Oysters, breaded & fried	3 oz	53
Crayfish	3 oz	51
Alaskan King Crab	3 oz	50
Eastern oysters, farmed	3 oz	48
Scallops, breaded & fried	3 oz	36
Squid, fried	3 oz	33
Abalone	3 oz	31
Queen crab	3 oz	28
Alaskan King Crab, imitation	3 oz	11

CALCIUM

Fruit, Canned	Amount	Calcium (mg)
Pineapple	1 cup	36
Apricots	1 cup	23
Plums	1 cup	23
Olives, black	5 large	19
Pears	1 cup	13
Applesauce, unsweetened	1 cup	10
Applesauce, sweetened	1 cup	8
Peaches	1 cup	8
Olives, green	5 large	7

Fruit, Dried	Amount	Calcium (mg)
Figs	1 cup	241
Currants	1 cup	124
Apricots	1 cup	72
Pears	1 cup	61
Peaches	1 cup	45
Apples	1 cup	12
Cranberries	1 cup	12

Fruit, Frozen	Amount	Calcium (mg)
Blackberries, unsweetened	1 cup	44
Raspberries	1 cup	38
Strawberries	1 cup	28
Blueberries	1 cup	14
Peaches	1 cup	8

Fruit, Raw	Amount	Calcium (mg)
Florida Oranges, sections	1 cup	80
Raisins	1 cup	72
Tangerine	1 cup	72
Valencias Oranges, sections	1 cup	72
Black currants	1 cup	62
Kiwi	1 cup	61
Naval Oranges	1 cup	60
Dates	1 cup	57
Elderberries	1 cup	55
Grapefruit, pink or red, sections	1 cup	51
Stewed prunes	1 cup	47
Prunes, uncooked	1 cup	43
Blackberries	1 cup	42
Raspberries	1 cup	31
Avocado, California	1 cup	30
Papayas	1 cup	29

RDA is 1000 mg for adults

CALCIUM

Continued

Strawberries	1 cup	27
Avocado, Florida	1 cup	23
Chayote, 1" pieces	1 cup	22
Pineapple	1 cup	21
Apricots	1 cup	20
Cherries	1 cup	20
Pomegrenates	1 cup	17
Grapes, red or green	1 cup	16
Jicama	1 cup	16
Cantaloupe	1 cup	14
Honeydew	1 cup	14
Pears	1 cup	13
Water mellon	1 cup	11
Peaches, slices	1 cup	10
Plums	1 cup	10
Blueberries	1 cup	9
Nectarine	1 cup	9
Apples	1 cup	8
Cranberries	1 cup	8
Pummelo	1 cup	8
Plantains	1 cup	4

Fruit, Raw	Amount	Calcium (mg)
Figs, dried	5 fruit	70
Florida Oranges	1 fruit	61
Naval Oranges	1 fruit	60
Valencias Oranges	1 fruit	48
Mango	1 fruit	37
Chayote	1 fruit	35
Papayas, small size	1 fruit	31
Tangerine	1 fruit	31
Avocado, Florida	1 fruit	30
Pomegranates	1 fruit	28
Grapefruit, pink or red	1/2 fruit	27
Kiwi	1 fruit	26
Cantaloupe	1/2 fruit	25
Cherimoya	1 fruit	24
Pummelo	1 fruit	24
Raisins	1 small box	22
Avocado, California	1 fruit	18
Prunes, uncooked	5 fruit	18
Pears	1 fruit	15
Dates	5 fruit	14
Persimmons, Japanese	1 fruit	13
Kumquats	1 fruit	12

CALCIUM

Continued

Cherries	10 fruit	11
Strawberries	5 fruit	10
Apples	1 fruit	8
Nectarine	1 fruit	8
Persimmons, small native	1 fruit	7
Banana	1 fruit	6
Peaches	1 fruit	6
Pineapple, slices	1/2" x 3"	6
Apricots	1 fruit	5
Plantains	1 fruit	5
Plums	1 fruit	4
Pineapple guava, Feijoa	1 fruit	3
Star fruit, Carambola	1 fruit	3
Passion fruit	1 fruit	2

Game Meat, Cooked	Amount	Calcium (mg)
Caribou	3 oz	19
Rabbit	3 oz	15
Wild boar	3 oz	14
Venison, ground	3 oz	12
Bison, ground	3 oz	11
Duck	3 oz	10
Elk, ground	3 oz	8
Elk, roasted	3 oz	4
Antelope	3 oz	3
Buffalo, steak, free range	3 oz	3
Squirrel	3 oz	3

Grains, Cooked	Amount	Calcium (mg)
Amaranth	1 cup	116
Spaghetti, spinach	1 cup	42
White rice, long-grain, enriched	1 cup	33
Quinoa	1 cup	31
Egg & Spinach noodles	1 cup	30
Oat bran	1 cup	22
Macaroni, Whole-Wheat	1 cup	21
Oats, regular, unenriched	1 cup	21
Spaghetti, Whole-Wheat	1 cup	21
Brown rice	1 cup	20
Egg noodles	1 cup	19
Spelt	1 cup	19
Bulgur	1 cup	18
Barley, pearled	1 cup	17
Kamut	1 cup	17
White rice, long-grain, regular	1 cup	16

RDA is 1000 mg for adults

CALCIUM

Couscous	1 cup	13
White rice, long-grain, instant	1 cup	13
Buckwheat	1 cup	12
Macaroni	1 cup	10
Spaghetti, enriched	1 cup	10
Rice noodles	1 cup	7
Millet	1 cup	5
Soba noodles	1 cup	5
Wild rice	1 cup	5

Herbs & Spices	Amount	Calcium (mg)
Celery seeds	1 tsp	35
Basil, dried & ground	1 tsp	31
Oregano, dried, ground	1 tsp	29
Cinnamon powder	1 tsp	26
Fennel seed	1 tsp	24
Thyme, dried, ground	1 tsp	23
Thyme, dried, leaves	1 tsp	19
Dill weed, dried	1 tsp	18
Tarragon, dried, ground	1 tsp	18
Basil, dried leaves	1 tsp	16
Oregano, dried, leaves	1 tsp	16
Rosemary, dried	1 tsp	15
Anise seed	1 tsp	14
Caraway seeds	1 tsp	14
All-spice, ground	1 tsp	13
Cloves, ground	1 tsp	13
Coriander, seeds	1 tsp	13
Pepper, black, whole	1 tsp	13
Marjoram, dried	1 tsp	12
Sage, ground	1 tsp	12
Curry powder	1 tsp	10
Chili powder	1 tsp	9
Onion powder	1 tsp	9
Pepper, black, ground	1 tsp	9
Chervil, dried	1 tsp	8
Coriander, dried leafs	1 tsp	7
Spearmint, dried	1 tsp	7
Tarragon, dried, leaves	1 tsp	7
Parsley, dried	1 tsp	6
Bay leaf, crumbled	1 tsp	5
Dill weed, fresh	1/4 cup	5
Paprika	1 tsp	5
Mace, ground	1 tsp	4
Nutmeg, ground	1 tsp	4

CALCIUM

Continued

Spearmint, fresh	1 tsp	4
Turmeric, ground	1 tsp	4
Cilantro	1/4 cup	3
Thyme, fresh	1 tsp	3
Basil, fresh	1 tsp	2
Garlic powder	1 tsp	2
Ginger, ground	1 tsp	2
Rosemary, fresh	1 tsp	2
Capers	1 tsp	1
Chives, raw	1 tsp	1
Saffron	1 tsp	1

Juice	Amount	Calcium (mg)
Carrot	1 cup	57
Prune	1 cup	47
Pineapple	1 cup	33
Grape	1 cup	28
Orange, raw	1 cup	27
Pomegranate	1 cup	27
Vegetable, cocktail	1 cup	27
Tomato	1 cup	24
Apple	1 cup	20
Grapefruit juice, raw	1 cup	20
Lemon, raw	1 cup	15
Cranberry, cocktail	1 cup	8

Lamb, Cooked	Amount	Calcium (mg)
Ground	3 oz	19
Chops, loin, lean, trimmed to 1/4" fat	3 oz	17
Foreshank, trimmed to 1/8" fat	3 oz	17
Rib, lean, trimmed to 1/4" fat	3 oz	14
Cubed, for stew or kabob	3 oz	11
Leg, whole, trimmed to 1/4" fat	3 oz	9

Milk	Amount	Calcium (mg)
Canned, condensed, sweetened	1 cup	869
Canned, evaporated, non fat	1 cup	742
Canned, evaporated	1 cup	658
Sheep milk	1 cup	473
Almond Milk, sweetened, Vanilla flavor	1 cup	451
Goat milk	1 cup	327
Low fat,1%	1 cup	305
Non fat, fat free or skim milk	1 cup	299
Reduced fat, 2%	1 cup	293

RDA is 1000 mg for adults

CALCIUM

Whole milk, dry powder	1/4 cup	292
Buttermilk, low fat	1 cup	284
Dry, instant, non fat	1/3 cup	283
Buttermilk, whole milk	1 cup	282
Whole milk, liquid, 3.25%	1 cup	276
Human milk	1 cup	79
Soymilk, original, unfortified	1 cup	61
Coconut milk, canned	1 cup	41

Nuts & Seeds	Amount	Calcium (mg)
Sesame seeds	1 oz	276
Chia seeds	1 oz	179
Tahini	1 oz	121
Almonds	1 oz	75
Flaxseeds	1 oz	72
Brazilnuts	1 oz	45
Hazelnuts	1 oz	32
Trail mix, regular with chocolate chips	1 oz	31
Pistachio	1 oz	30
English walnuts	1 oz	28
Peanuts	1 oz	26
Macadamia	1 oz	24
Mixed nuts, roasted with peanuts, no salt	1 oz	24
Sunflower seeds	1 oz	22
Trail mix, regular, salted	1 oz	22
Pecans	1 oz	20
Black walnuts	1 oz	17
Trail mix, tropical	1 oz	16
Pumpkin seeds	1 oz	13
Peanut butter, smooth style	1 oz	12
Cashews	1 oz	10
Pine nuts	1 oz	5
Coconut, raw meat	1 oz	4

Nuts & Seeds	Amount	Calcium (mg)
Sesame seeds	1/4 cup	351
Flaxseeds	1/4 cup	107
Almonds	1/4 cup	94
Sesame seeds	1 tbsp	88
Brazilnuts, whole	1/4 cup	53
Trail mix, regular with chocolate chips	1/4 cup	40
Peanuts	1/4 cup	34
Hazelnuts	1/4 cup	33
Pistachio	1/4 cup	32
Trail mix, regular, salted	1/4 cup	29

RDA is 1000 mg for adults

CALCIUM

Macadamia	1/4 cup	28
Peanut butter, smooth	1/4 cup	28
Sunflower seeds	1/4 cup	27
Flaxseeds	1 tbsp	26
English walnuts, chopped	1/4 cup	24
Mixed nuts, roasted, peanuts, no salt	1/4 cup	24
Trail mix, tropical	1/4 cup	20
Black walnuts, chopped	1/4 cup	19
Pecans, halves	1/4 cup	17
Pumpkin seeds	1/4 cup	15
Pine nuts	1/4 cup	5
Coconut meat, shredded	1/4 cup	3
Cashews	1/4 cup	x
Chia seeds	1/4 cup	x

Pork, Cooked	Amount	Calcium (mg)
Chops, pan-fried	3 oz	45
Chops, lean, pan-fried	3 oz	43
Spareribs	3 oz	40
Backribs	3 oz	39
Bratwurst	3 oz	24
Center loin pork chops	3 oz	20
Chops, broiled	3 oz	20
Italian sausage	3 oz	18
Liverwurst spread	1/4 cup	12
Sausage	3 oz	11
Polish sausage	3 oz	10
Bacon, pan-fried	3 oz	9
Braunschweiger	3 oz	9
Sirloin pork chops	3 oz	9
Canadian-style bacon	3 oz	8
Cured ham	3 oz	6
Cured ham, lean	3 oz	6
Tenderloin	3 oz	5

Tofu	Amount	Calcium (mg)
House Foods Premium Firm	3 oz	125
House Foods Premium Soft	3 oz	66
Mori-Nu, Silken, Lite Extra Firm	3 oz	36
Mori-Nu, Silken, Lite Firm	3 oz	30
Mori-Nu, Silken, Firm	3 oz	27
Mori-Nu, Silken, Extra Firm	3 oz	26
Mori-Nu, Silken, Soft	3 oz	26

RDA is 1000 mg for adults

CALCIUM

Turkey, Cooked	Amount	Calcium (mg)
Ground turkey, 85% lean	3 oz	41
Breast meat	3 oz	37
Ground turkey, 93% lean	3 oz	25
Liver	3 oz	16
Turkey sausage, reduced fat	3 oz	16
Dark meat	3 oz	14
Light meat	3 oz	8
Turkey bacon	3 oz	8
Ground turkey, fat free	3 oz	5

Veal, Cooked	Amount	Calcium (mg)
Foreshank	3 oz	28
Loin	3 oz	16
Cubed, for stew	3 oz	14
Ground	3 oz	14
Sirloin	3 oz	11
Rib	3 oz	9
Breast	3 oz	8
Leg, top round	3 oz	7

Vegetables, Canned	Amount	Calcium (mg)
Spinach	1 cup	272
Tomato paste	1 cup	94
Stewed tomatoes	1 cup	87
Tomatoes	1 cup	74
Sauerkraut	1 cup	71
Pumpkin	1 cup	64
Green beans	1 cup	51
Tomato pure	1 cup	45
Asparagus	1 cup	39
Green peas	1 cup	39
Carrots	1 cup	37
Sweet potato	1 cup	33
Tomato sauce	1 cup	32
Beets	1 cup	26
Mushrooms	1 cup	17
Corn	1 cup	11

Vegetables, Cooked	Amount	Calcium (mg)
Lambsquarters, chopped	1 cup	464
Mustard Spinach	1 cup	284
Collard greens	1 cup	268
Spinach	1 cup	245

RDA is 1000 mg for adults

CALCIUM

Continued

Cactus pads, nopales	1 cup	244
Turnip greens	1 cup	197
Beet greens	1 cup	164
Bok-Choy, chinese cabbage	1 cup	158
Dandelion greens	1 cup	147
Okra	1 cup	123
Mustard greens	1 cup	104
Swiss chard	1 cup	102
Broccoli raab	1 cup	100
Kale	1 cup	94
Acorn squash, cubes	1 cup	90
Purslane	1 cup	90
Sweet potato, mashed	1 cup	89
Broccolini	1 cup	88
Butternut squash	1 cup	84
Rutabagas	1 cup	82
Cabbage	1 cup	72
Snow peas	1 cup	67
Cabbage, Red	1 cup	63
Celery	1 cup	63
Broccoli	1 cup	62
Parsnips	1 cup	58
Brussels sprouts	1 cup	56
Green beans	1 cup	55
Turnips	1 cup	51
Potatoes, mashed with whole milk	1 cup	50
Summer squash	1 cup	49
Carrots	1 cup	47
Onions	1 cup	46
Winter squash	1 cup	45
Cabbage, Savoy	1 cup	44
Asparagus	1 cup	41
Kohlrabi	1 cup	41
Crookneck or Straighneck Squash, slices	1 cup	40
Pumpkin	1 cup	37
Artichokes	1 cup	35
Hubbard squash	1 cup	35
Spaghetti winter squash	1 cup	33
Cabbage, Napa	1 cup	32
Zucchini	1 cup	32
Leeks	1 cup	31
Beets	1 cup	27
Scallop or Pattypan Squash, slices	1 cup	27
Split peas	1 cup	27
Tomatoes, red	1 cup	26

RDA is 1000 mg for adults

CALCIUM

Continued

Taro	1 cup	24
Cauliflower	1 cup	20
Yams, cubes	1 cup	19
White mushrooms	1 cup	9
Eggplant	1 cup	6
Potatoes, flesh, baked	1 cup	6
Corn, yellow	1 cup	4
Shitake mushrooms	1 cup	4

Vegetables, Frozen	Amount	Calcium (mg)
Collard greens	1 cup	357
Rhubarb	1 cup	348
Spinach	1 cup	291
Turnip greens	1 cup	249
Kale	1 cup	179
Okra	1 cup	136
Broccoli	1 cup	61
Green beans	1 cup	57
Carrots	1 cup	51
Butternut squash	1 cup	46
Brussels sprouts	1 cup	40
Green peas	1 cup	38
Asparagus	1 cup	32
Cauliflower	1 cup	31
Corn	1 cup	5

Vegetables, Raw	Amount	Calcium (mg)
Mustard Spinach, chopped	1 cup	315
Cactus pads, Nopales	1 cup	141
Dandelion greens, chopped	1 cup	103
Kale, chopped	1 cup	90
Bok-choy, chinese cabbage	1 cup	74
Green onions & scallions	1 cup	72
Butternut squash	1 cup	67
Celery	1 cup	48
Broccoli	1 cup	43
Raab broccoli, chopped	1 cup	43
Snow peas, chopped	1 cup	42
Watercress, chopped	1 cup	41
Carrots, slices	1 cup	40
Onions	1 cup	37
Arugula	1 cup	32
Red cabbage, shredded	1 cup	32
Spinach	1 cup	30

CALCIUM

Chicory greens, chopped	1 cup	29
Cabbage, shredded	1 cup	28
Morel mushrooms	1 cup	28
Purslane	1 cup	28
Endive, chopped	1 cup	26
Cauliflower, chopped	1 cup	24
Savoy cabbage, shredded	1 cup	24
Green leaf lettuce	1 cup	20
Butterhead, boston, and bibb lettuce	1 cup	19
Romaine lettuce	1 cup	18
Swiss chard	1 cup	18
Tomatoes	1 cup	18
Zucchini	1 cup	18
Belgian endive	1 cup	17
Cucumbers, slices	1 cup	17
Summer squash, sliced	1 cup	17
Yellow bell peppers	1 cup	16
Green bell peppers, chopped	1 cup	15
Tomatoes, cherry	1 cup	15
Crimini mushrooms, sliced	1 cup	13
Iceberg lettuce	1 cup	10
Red bell peppers	1 cup	10
Red leaf lettuce	1 cup	9
Tomatillos, chopped	1 cup	9
Radicchio	1 cup	8
Spirulina, dried	1 tbsp	8
Oyster mushrooms, sliced	1 cup	3
Portabella mushrooms	1 cup	3
Tomatillos, chopped	1 each	2
White mushrooms, sliced	1 cup	2
Enoki mushrooms	1 cup	0
Shiitake mushrooms	1 whole	0
Shiitake mushrooms, dried	1 each	0

RDA is 1000 mg for adults

Nutrient Data Collection Form

Food	Amount	Book Numbers	Multiply By	Estimated Nutrient Intake
Nutrient::	RDA:	Estimated:	% of RDA:	Total Estimated:

To download additional forms for free, go to www.TopNutrients4U.com

NOTES

CALCIUM / PHOSPHORUS RATIO

Alcohol	Amount	Calcium / Phosphorus
White Table Wine	1 glass	0.50
Red Table Wine	1 glass	0.35
Light Beer	1 bottle	0.33
Regular Beer	1 bottle	0.28
Gin, Rum, Vodka, or Whisky	1 shot	0

Beans, Canned	Amount	Calcium / Phosphorus
Green beans	1 cup	1.81
Yellow beans	1 cup	1.38
White beans, mature	1 cup	0.80
Pinto beans	1 cup	0.51
Baked beans, plain	1 cup	0.46
Garbanzo beans	1 cup	0.44
Cranberry beans	1 cup	0.39
Great Northern	1 cup	0.39
Navy beans	1 cup	0.35
Fava beans	1 cup	0.33
Refried beans	1 cup	0.30
Lima beans, large	1 cup	0.29
Black-eyed peas	1 cup	0.29
Red kidney beans	1 cup	0.27

Beans, Cooked	Amount	Calcium / Phosphorus
Green beans	1 cup	1.53
Natto	1 cup	1.25
Yellow beans	1 cup	1.18
Winged beans	1 cup	0.93
Soybeans, green	1 cup	0.92
Yardlong beans, chinese long beans	1 cup	0.90
White beans, mature	1 cup	0.80
Navy beans	1 cup	0.48
White beans, small	1 cup	0.43
Soybeans, matured	1 cup	0.42
Great Northern	1 cup	0.41
Lupini beans	1 cup	0.40
Edamame	1 cup	0.37
Cranberry beans	1 cup	0.37
Black Turtle beans	1 cup	0.36
Pigeon peas	1 cup	0.36
Hyacinath beans	1 cup	0.33
Pinto beans	1 cup	0.31
Garbanzo beans, chickpeas	1 cup	0.29
Fava beans	1 cup	0.29

CALCIUM / PHOSPHORUS RATIO

Continued

Mung beans	1 cup	0.28
Soybeans, matured, dry roasted	1 cup	0.22
Kidney beans	1 cup	0.20
Black beans	1 cup	0.19
Adzuki	1 cup	0.17
Lima beans	1 cup	0.15
Black-eyed peas	1 cup	0.15
Split peas	1 cup	0.14
Lentils	1 cup	0.11
Moth beans	1 cup	0.02

Beef, Cooked	Amount	Calcium / Phosphrus
Ground beef, 75%	3 oz	0.16
Ground beef, 80%	3 oz	0.12
Filet Mignon, trimmed to 0" fat	3 oz	0.09
Ground beef, 85%	3 oz	0.09
Flank steak, lean, trimmed to 0" fat	3 oz	0.08
Top sirloin, trimmed to 1/8" fat"	3 oz	0.08
Brisket, lean, trimmed to 0" fat	3 oz	0.08
Chuck roast, trimmed to 1/8" fat"	3 oz	0.07
Ground beef, 90%,	3 oz	0.06
Beef ribs, trimmed to 1/8" fat"	3 oz	0.06
Skirt Steak, trimmed to 0" fat"	3 oz	0.05
Porterhouse steak, trimmed to 0" fat"	3 oz	0.04
Ground beef, 95%	3 oz	0.03
Ribeye steak, trimmed to 0" fat	3 oz	0.03
T-Bone steak, trimmed 0" fat"	3 oz	0.02

Bread	Amount	Calcium / Phosphorus
English Muffin, plain	1 muffin	1.79
Dinner Rolls, brown & serve	1 roll	1.47
Hamburger & Hotdog buns, plain	1 bun	1.28
Bagel, plain	4" bagel	1.03
Tortillas, flour	1 tortilla	1.03
Kaiser rolls	1 roll	0.95
Wheat	1 slice	0.92
Pita, white	6" pita"	0.90
Egg bread	1 slice	0.88
White bread	1 slice	0.84
Italian	1 slice	0.76
Raisin bread	1 slice	0.61
Rye bread	1 slice	0.58
Oatmeal bread	1 slice	0.53
Whole-Wheat	1 slice	0.53
Potato bread	1 slice	0.51

CALCIUM / PHOSPHORUS RATIO

Continued

Multigrain or Whole grain	1 slice	0.46
Pumpernickel	1 slice	0.39
French and Sourdough	1 slice	0.38
Croissants, butter	1 medium	0.35
Cracked Wheat	1 slice	0.29
Tortillas, corn	1 tortilla	0.26
Cornbread, dry mix	1 piece	0.19
Bagel, cinnamon & raisins	4" bagel	0.19
Bagel, egg	4" bagel	0.16
Bagel, wheat	4" bagel	0.14
Bagel, oat bran	4" bagel	0.11

Cereal, General Mills®	Amount	Calcium / Phosphorus
Total Whole Grain	1 cup	12.5
Total Cranberry Crunch	1 cup	10.0
Total Raisin Bran	1 cup	10.0
Cinnamon Chex	1 cup	4.9
Honey Nut Chex	1 cup	4.9
Kix	1 cup	3.0
Chocolate Chex	1 cup	2.5
Golden Grahams	1 cup	2.5
Cookie Crisp	1 cup	2.5
Basic 4	1 cup	2.5
Corn Chex	1 cup	2.5
Rice Chex	1 cup	2.5
Berry Berry Kix	1 cup	1.80
Cinnamon Toast Crunch	1 cup	1.70
Reese's Puffs	1 cup	1.66
Cocoa Puffs	1 cup	1.60
Dora The Explorer	1 cup	1.60
Trix	1 cup	1.57
Lucky Charms	1 cup	1.50
Wheat Chex	1 cup	0.67
Multi-Bran CHEX	1 cup	0.66
Wheaties	1 cup	0.25
Raisin Nut Bran	1 cup	0.24
Honey Nut Clusters	1 cup	0.23
Oatmeal Crisp, Hearty Raisin	1 cup	0.20
Oatmeal Crisp, Crunchy Almond	1 cup	0.20

Cereal, General Mill's® Cheerios®	Amount	Calcium / Phosphorus
Apple Cinnamon	1 cup	1.66
Berry Burst	1 cup	1.66
Frosted	1 cup	1.66
Fruity	1 cup	1.66

CALCIUM / PHOSPHORUS RATIO

Continued

Yogurt Burst, Strawberry	1 cup	1.66
Banana Nut	1 cup	1.66
Chocolate	1 cup	1.66
Oat Clusters Cheerios Crunch	1 cup	1.33
Multi-Grain	1 cup	1.25
Honey Nut	1 cup	1.24
Original	1 cup	0.82
Cinnamon Burst	1 cup	x

Cereal, General Mill's Fiber One®	Amount	Calcium / Phosphorus
Frosted Shreaded Wheat	1 cup	x
80 Calorie Chocolate Squares	1 cup	4.9
80 Calorie Honey Squares	1 cup	4.9
Original	1 cup	1.6
Honey Clusters	1 cup	1.5
Raisin Bran Clusters	1 cup	1.2
Caramel Delight	1 cup	1.0
Nutty Clusters & almonds	1 cup	1.0

Cereal, Kashi®	Amount	Calcium / Phorphorus
Heart to Heart, Honey Toasted Oat	1 cup	1.00
Go Lean Crisp, Cinnamon Crumble	1 cup	0.80
Heart to Heart, Warm Cinnamon	1 cup	0.48
Go Lean Crunch	1 cup	0.34
Go Lean Crisp, Toasted Berry Crumble	1 cup	0.31
Honey Sunshine	1 cup	0.31
Go Lean	1 cup	0.30
Berry Blossom	1 cup	0.27
Go Lean Crunch, Honey Almond Flax	1 cup	0.27
Heart to Heart, Oat Flakes & Blueberry Clusters	1 cup	0.24
7-Whole Grain Honey Puffs	1 cup	0.16
7-Whole Grain Flakes	1 cup	0.16
7-Whole Grain Puffs	1 cup	0.15
7-Whole Grain Nuggets	1 cup	0.15
Strawberry Fields	1 cup	0.14
Island Vanilla	27 biscuits	0.13
Berry Fruitful	29 biscuits	0.12
Good Friends, Original	1 cup	0.11
Autum Wheat	29 biscuits	x
Blackberry Hills	1 cup	x
Cinnamon Harvest	28 biscuits	x
Heart to Heart, Nutty Chia Flax	1 cup	x
Indigo Morning	1 cup	x
Simply Maize	1 cup	x

CALCIUM / PHOSPHORUS RATIO

Cereal, Kellogg's®	Amount	Calcium / Phosphorus
Fiberplus Cinnamon Oat Crunch	1 cup	3.80
Raisin Bran	1 cup	1.39
Cocoa Krispies	1 cup	1.24
Crunchy Nut, Roasted Nut & Honey O's	1 cup	0.73
Krave Chocolate	1 cup	0.60
CINNABON	1 cup	0.47
Honey Crunch Corn Flakes	1 cup	0.38
Smorz	1 cup	0.35
All-Bran Original	1 cup	0.34
MUESLIX	1 cup	0.32
Crunchy Nut, Golden Honey Nut Flakes	1 cup	0.31
Cracklin Oat Bran	1 cup	0.21
Product 19	1 cup	0.19
Smart Start, Strong Heart Antioxidants	1 cup	0.18
Fiberplus Berry Yogurt Crunch	1 cup	0.16
Apple Jacks	1 cup	0.15
Froot Loops	1 cup	0.14
Raisin Bran Crunch	1 cup	0.14
All-Bran Bran Buds	1 cup	0.13
Corn Pops	1 cup	0.13
Rice Krispies Treats	1 cup	0.13
Crispix	1 cup	0.12
Honey Smacks	1 cup	0.12
Frosted MINI Wheat's, Big-Bite	1 cup	0.11
Frosted MINI-Wheat's, Bite-Size	1 cup	0.11
All-Bran Complete Wheat Flakes	1 cup	0.10
Frosted Rice Krispies	1 cup	0.09
Corn Flakes	1 cup	0.07
Frosted Flakes	1 cup	0.05
Rice Krispies	1 cup	0.03

Cereal, Kellogg's Special-K®	Amount	Calcium / Phosphorus
Original	1 cup	0.47
Protein Plus	1 cup	0.22
Fruit & Yogurt	1 cup	0.18
Low Fat Granola	1 cup	0.17
Vanilla Almond	1 cup	0.16
Cinnamon Pecan	1 cup	0.16
Red Berries	1 cup	0.12
Blueberry	1 cup	0.10
Chocolately Delight	1 cup	0.09
Multigrain Oats & Honey	1 cup	0.08

CALCIUM / PHOSPHORUS RATIO

Cereal, Post®	Amount	Calcium / Phosphorus
Fruity Pebbles	1 cup	0.27
Blueberry Morning	1 cup	0.25
Cocoa Pebbles	1 cup	0.24
Great Grains, Cranberry Almond Crunch	1 cup	0.16
Great Grains, Raisin, Date & Pecan	1 cup	0.16
Shredded Wheat, Original, spoon-size	1 cup	0.15
Great Grains, Banana Nut Crunch	1 cup	0.14
Honey Nut Shredded Wheat	1 cup	0.14
Grape-Nuts Cereal	1 cup	0.13
Grape-Nuts Flakes	1 cup	0.13
Great Grains, Crunchy Pecan	1 cup	0.13
Raisin Bran	1 cup	0.13
Shredded Wheat, Original, big-biscuit	1 biscuit	0.13
Alpha-Bits	1 cup	0.11
Shredded Wheat n' Bran, spoon-size	1 cup	0.11
Bran Flakes	1 cup	0.10
Golden Crisp	1 cup	0.06
Honeycomb Cereal	1 cup	0.06
Shredded Wheat, frosted, spoon-size	1 cup	0.05

Post®Honey Bunches of Oats®	Amount	Calcium / Phosphorus
Honey Roasted	1 cup	0.58
With Cinnamon Bunches	1 cup	0.23
With Almonds	1 cup	0.21
With Strawberries	1 cup	0.19
Just Bunches Honey Roasted	1 cup	0.18
Pecan Bunches	1 cup	0.14
With Vanilla Bunches	1 cup	0.14
Just Bunches Cinnamon	1 cup	x
Raisin Medley	1 cup	x

Cereal, Quaker®	Amount	Calcium / Phosphorus
LIFE Cereal, Cinnamon	1 cup	0.90
LIFE Cereal, Maple & Brown Sugar	1 cup .	0.90
LIFE Cereal, Original	1 cup	0.83
Oatmeal Squares, Cinnamon	1 cup	0.57
Oatmeal Squares	1 cup	0.55
Oatmeal Squares, Golden Maple	1 cup	0.41
Corn Bran Crunch	1 cup	0.39
Toasted Multigrain Crisp	1 cup	0.37
Granola Apple Cranberry Almond	1 cup	0.29
Puffed Rice	1 cup	0.09
Honey Graham OH'S	1 cup	0.08

CALCIUM / PHOSPHORUS RATIO

Continued

Puffed Wheat	1 cup	0.08
CAP'N Crunch	1 cup	0.07
CAP'N Crunch & Crunch Berries	1 cup	0.07
CAP'N Crunch's OOPs! All Berries	1 cup	0.07
CAP'N Crunch's Peanut Butter Crunch	1 cup	0.04

Cereal, Cooked	Amount	Calcium / Phosphorus
CREAM OF WHEAT, regular	1 cup	5.74
Farina®	1 cup	2.64
Malt-o-Meal, plain	1 serving	2.43
WHEATENA®	1 cup	1.33
Oats, regular, unenriched	1 cup	0.11
Yellow corn grits	1 cup	0.06
White corn grits	1 cup	0.04

Cheese	Amount	Calcium / Phosphorus
Ricotta, part skim milk	1 cup	1.49
Ricotta, whole milk	1 cup	1.31
Cottage cheese, low fat, 2 %	1 cup	0.58
Cottage cheese, creamed, small curd	1 cup	0.51
Cottage cheese, low fat, 1 %	1 cup	0.46
Cottage cheese, non fat & uncreamed	1 cup	0.45

Cheese	Amount	Calcium / Phosphorus
Roquefort	1 oz	1.7
Monterey	1 oz	1.7
Gruyere	1 oz	1.7
American, pasteurized process, fortified	1 oz	1.6
Fontina	1 oz	1.6
Swiss, low fat	1 oz	1.6
Monterey, low fat	1 oz	1.6
Muenster	1 oz	1.5
Provolone, reduced fat	1 oz	1.5
Provolone	1 oz	1.5
Parmesan, grated	1 oz	1.5
Colby	1 oz	1.5
Ricotta, part skim milk	1 oz	1.5
Mozzarella, non fat	1 oz	1.5
Feta	1 oz	1.5
Mozzarella, whole milk	1 oz	1.4
Cheddar	1 oz	1.4
Romano	1 oz	1.4
Swiss	1 oz	1.4
Mozzarella, skim milk, low moisture	1 oz	1.4

CALCIUM / PHOSPHORUS RATIO

Continued

Blue cheese	1 oz	1.4
Ricotta, whole milk	1 oz	1.3
Gouda	1 oz	1.3
Goat cheese, hard type	1 oz	1.2
Muenster, low fat	1 oz	1.1
American, pasturized, imitation	1 oz	1.1
Brie	1 oz	1.0
Cream cheese	1 oz	0.9
Cheddar, low-fat	1 oz	0.9
American, pasturized, low fat	1 oz	0.8
Goat cheese, semisoft	1 oz	0.8
Cream cheese, fat free	1 oz	0.7
Goat cheese, soft type	1 oz	0.5
Velveeta, pasteurized process	1 oz	0.5
Cheez Whiz, pasteurized process	1 oz	0.4

Chicken, Cooked	Amount	Calcium / Phosphorus
Wing with skin, fried in batter	1 wing	0.17
Wing with skin, roasted	1 wing	0.10
Breast, with skin, fried in flour	1/2 breast	0.08
Drumstick, with skin, fried in flour	1 drumstick	0.07
Thigh, with skin, fried in flour	1 thigh	0.07
Thigh, no skin, roasted	1 thigh	0.06
Breast, no skin, roasted	1/2 breast	0.06
Drumstick, no skin, roasted	1 drumstick	0.06
Breast, with skin, roasted	1/2 breast	0.06

Chicken, Cooked	Amount	Calcium / Phosphorus
Cornish game hens, meat only	3 oz	0.11
Wing with skin, fried in flour	3 oz	0.10
Wing with skin, roasted	3 oz	0.10
Wing meat only, no skin, roasted	3 oz	0.10
Thigh with skin, fried in flour	3 oz	0.08
Breast with skin, fried in flour	3 oz	0.07
Breast meat only, no skin, roasted	3 oz	0.07
Drumstick with skin, fried in flour	3 oz	0.07
Breast with skin, roasted	3 oz	0.07
Drumstick with skin, roasted	3 oz	0.06
Drumstick meat only, no skin, roasted	3 oz	0.06
Thigh with skin, roasted	3 oz	0.05
Thigh meat only, no skin, roasted	3 oz	0.04
Liver	3 oz	0.03

CALCIUM / PHOSPHORUS RATIO

Cream	Amount	Calcium / Phosphorus
Light Coffee Cream	1 tbsp	1.17
Half & Half	1 tbsp	1.14
Sour Cream, reduced fat	1 tbsp	1.14
Heavy Cream	1 tbsp	1.11
Whipped Topping, pressurized	1 tbsp	1.00
Sour Cream, cultured	1 tbsp	0.93

Eggs	Amount	Calcium / Phosphorus
Egg substitute, liquid, fat free	1/4 cup	1.02
Egg whites, dried powder, stabilized	1 tbsp	1.00
Egg whites, dried	1 tbsp	0.58
Egg whites	1 large	0.40
Egg whole, scrambled	1 large	0.40
Egg yolk	1 large	0.32
Egg whole, fried	1 large	0.29
Egg whole, hard-boiled	1 large	0.29
Egg whole, poached	1 large	0.28

Fish, Canned	Amount	Calcium / Phosphorus
Atlantic Sardines, in oil	3 oz	0.78
Light tuna, in water	3 oz	0.12
White (albacore) tuna, in water	3 oz	0.07
Light tuna, in oil	3 oz	0.05
White (albacore) tuna, in oil	3 oz	0.01

Fish, Cooked	Amount	Calcium / Phosphorus
Atlantic herring, pickeled	3 oz	0.86
Walleye pike	3 oz	0.52
Freshwater bass	3 oz	0.40
Rainbow trout, wild	3 oz	0.32
Atlantic pollock	3 oz	0.27
Walleye pollock	3 oz	0.27
Northern pike	3 oz	0.26
Whiting	3 oz	0.22
Cat fish, breaded & fried	3 oz	0.20
Snapper	3 oz	0.20
Pacific & Jack mackerel	3 oz	0.18
Atlantic cod	3 oz	0.15
Grouper	3 oz	0.15
Atlantic croaker	3 oz	0.15
Yellowtail	3 oz	0.15
Coho salmon, wild	3 oz	0.14
Skipjack (aku) tuna	3 oz	0.13

CALCIUM / PHOSPHORUS RATIO

Continued

Florida pompano	3 oz	0.13
King mackerel	3 oz	0.13
Striped mullet	3 oz	0.13
Alaskan halibut	3 oz	0.12
Atlantic perch	3 oz	0.11
Rainbow trout, farmed	3 oz	0.11
Orange roughy	3 oz	0.10
Carp	3 oz	0.10
Flounder & sole	3 oz	0.08
King, chinook salmon	3 oz	0.08
Sea bass	3 oz	0.08
Tilapia	3 oz	0.07
Pacific rockfish	3 oz	0.07
King, chinook salmon, smoked	3 oz	0.06
Salmon, Lox	3 oz	0.06
Atlantic salmon, farmed	3 oz	0.06
Atlantic salmon, wild	3 oz	0.06
Atlantic mackerel	3 oz	0.06
Striped bass	3 oz	0.05
Haddock	3 oz	0.05
Spanish mackerel	3 oz	0.05
Keta, (chum) salmon	3 oz	0.04
Catfish, farmed	3 oz	0.04
Sockeye salmon	3 oz	0.04
Coho salmon, farmed	3 oz	0.04
Catfish, wild	3 oz	0.03
Surimi	3 oz	0.03
Atlantic & Pacific halibut	3 oz	0.03
Bluefin tuna	3 oz	0.03
Pacific cod	3 oz	0.03
Pink salmon	3 oz	0.03
Swordfish	3 oz	0.02
Greenland halibut	3 oz	0.02
Yellowfin tuna	3 oz	0.01

Fish, Shellfish, Cooked	Amount	Calcium / Phosphorus
Eastern oysters, wild	3 oz	0.61
Northern lobster	3 oz	0.52
Blue crab cakes	3 oz	0.49
Eastern oysters, farmed	3 oz	0.49
Shrimp, canned	3 oz	0.47
Shrimp	3 oz	0.42
Oysters, breaded & fried	3 oz	0.39
Blue crab	3 oz	0.39

CALCIUM / PHOSPHORUS RATIO

Continued

Blue crab, canned	3 oz	0.39
Octopus	3 oz	0.38
Shrimp, breaded & fried	3 oz	0.34
Clams, breaded & fried	3 oz	0.34
Queen crab	3 oz	0.26
Crayfish	3 oz	0.22
Alaskan King Crab	3 oz	0.21
Clams, canned	3 oz	0.20
Scallops, breaded & fried	3 oz	0.18
Abalone	3 oz	0.17
Squid, fried	3 oz	0.15
Alaskan King Crab, imitation	3 oz	0.05

Fruit, Canned	Amount	Calcium / Phosphorus
Olives, black	5 large	19.00
Olives, green	5 large	7.00
Pineapple	1 cup	2.00
Apricots	1 cup	0.74
Pears	1 cup	0.68
Plums	1 cup	0.68
Applesauce, sweetened	1 cup	0.67
Applesauce, unsweetened	1 cup	0.67
Peaches	1 cup	0.28

Fruit, Dried	Amount	Calcium / Phosphorus
Figs	1 cup	2.41
Cranberries	1 cup	1.20
Apricots	1 cup	0.78
Currants	1 cup	0.69
Pears	1 cup	0.58
Apples	1 cup	0.36
Peaches	1 cup	0.24

Fruit, Frozen	Amount	Calcium / Phosphorus
Blackberries, unsweetened	1 cup	0.98
Raspberries	1 cup	0.90
Blueberries	1 cup	0.88
Strawberries	1 cup	0.85
Peaches	1 cup	0.29

CALCIUM / PHOSPHORUS RATIO

Fruit, Raw	Amount	Calcium / Phosphorus
Florida Oranges, sections	1 cup	3.64
Kiwi	1 cup	2.65
Valencias Oranges, sections	1 cup	2.32
Papayas	1 cup	2.07
Tangerine	1 cup	1.85
Naval Oranges	1 cup	1.62
Pineapple	1 cup	1.62
Blackberries	1 cup	1.31
Grapefruit, pink or red, sections	1 cup	1.24
Chayote, 1" pieces"	1 cup	1.00
Elderberries	1 cup	0.96
Black currants	1 cup	0.94
Raspberries	1 cup	0.86
Honeydew	1 cup	0.74
Pears	1 cup	0.72
Strawberries	1 cup	0.68
Water mellon	1 cup	0.65
Stewed prunes	1 cup	0.64
Dates	1 cup	0.63
Cherries	1 cup	0.63
Cranberries	1 cup	0.62
Cantaloupe	1 cup	0.58
Apples	1 cup	0.57
Blueberries	1 cup	0.53
Apricots	1 cup	0.53
Grapes, red or green	1 cup	0.50
Raisins	1 cup	0.49
Plums	1 cup	0.38
Nectarine	1 cup	0.36
Prunes, uncooked	1 cup	0.36
Peaches, slices	1 cup	0.32
Pomegrenates	1 cup	0.27
Jicama	1 cup	0.26
Avocado, Florida	1 cup	0.25
Pummelo	1 cup	0.25
Avocado, California	1 cup	0.24
Plantains	1 cup	0.08

Fruit, Raw	Amount	Calcium / Phosphorus
Florida Oranges	1 fruit	3.59
Kumquats	1 fruit	3.00
Figs, dried	1 fruit	2.33
Valencias Oranges	1 fruit	2.29
Naval Oranges	1 fruit	1.88

CALCIUM / PHOSPHORUS RATIO

Continued

Tangerine	1 fruit	1.82
Raisins	1 small box	1.57
Pineapple	1/2" x 3" slice"	1.50
Grapefruit, pink or red	1/2 fruit	1.23
Kiwi	1 fruit	1.00
Pomegranates	1 fruit	1.00
Chayote	1 fruit	0.95
Pears	1 fruit	0.83
Strawberries	5 strawberries	0.71
Cherries	10 cherries	0.65
Apricots	1 fruit	0.63
Prunes, uncooked	5 prunes	0.62
Cantaloupe	1/2 fruit	0.61
Avocado, Florida	1 fruit	0.55
Dates	5 dates	0.54
Apples	1 fruit	0.53
Plums	1 fruit	0.36
Peaches	1 fruit	0.30
Avocado, California	1 fruit	0.24
Banana	1 fruit	0.23
Nectarine	1 fruit	0.23
Plantains	1 fruit	0.08

Game Meat, Cooked	Amount	Calcium / Phosphorus
Wild boar	3 oz	0.12
Caribou	3 oz	0.10
Rabbit	3 oz	0.07
Bison, ground	3 oz	0.06
Deer, ground	3 oz	0.06
Duck	3 oz	0.06
Elk, ground	3 oz	0.05
Elk, roasted	3 oz	0.02
Antelope	3 oz	0.02
Squirrel	3 oz	0.02
Buffalo, steak, free range	3 oz	0.01

Grains, Cooked	Amount	Calcium / Phosphorus
Couscous	1 cup	0.37
White rice, long-grain, enriched	1 cup	0.34
Egg & Spinach noodles	1 cup	0.33
Amaranth	1 cup	0.32
Spaghetti, spinach	1 cup	0.28
White rice, long-grain, regular	1 cup	0.24
Bulgur	1 cup	0.23
White rice, long-grain, instant	1 cup	0.21

CALCIUM / PHOSPHORUS RATIO

Continued

Barley, pearled	1 cup	0.20
Rice noodles	1 cup	0.20
Soba noodles	1 cup	0.17
Macaroni, Whole-Wheat	1 cup	0.17
Spaghetti, Whole-Wheat	1 cup	0.17
Egg noodles	1 cup	0.16
Brown rice	1 cup	0.12
Macaroni	1 cup	0.12
Spaghetti, enriched	1 cup	0.12
Oats, regular, unenriched	1 cup	0.12
Quinoa	1 cup	0.11
Buckwheat	1 cup	0.10
Oat bran	1 cup	0.08
Spelt	1 cup	0.07
Kamut	1 cup	0.06
Wild rice	1 cup	0.04
Millet	1 cup	0.03

Herbs & Spices	Amount	Calcium / Phosphorus
Rosemary, dried	1 tsp	15.0
Sage, ground	1 tsp	12.0
Cinnamon powder	1 tsp	11.5
Oregano, dried, ground	1 tsp	9.7
Basil, dried & ground	1 tsp	7.8
Thyme, dried, ground	1 tsp	7.7
All-spice, ground	1 tsp	6.5
Cloves, dried	1 tsp	6.5
Bay leaf, crumbled	1 tsp	5.0
Dill weed, dried	1 tsp	3.6
Tarragon, dried, ground	1 tsp	3.4
Capers	1 tsp	3.3
Celery seeds	1 tsp	3.2
Parsley, dried	1 tsp	3.0
Thyme, fresh	1 tsp	3.0
Chervil, dried	1 tsp	2.7
Coriander, dried	1 tsp	2.3
Pepper, black	1 tsp	2.3
Basil, fresh	1 tsp	2.0
Rosemary, fresh	1 tsp	2.0
Coriander, seeds	1 tsp	1.9
Anise seed	1 tsp	1.6
Curry powder	1 tsp	1.4
Caraway seeds	1 tsp	1.2
Chili powder	1 tsp	1.1
Chives, raw	1 tsp	1.0

CALCIUM / PHOSPHORUS RATIO

Continued

Onion powder	1 tsp	1.0
Paprika	1 tsp	0.7
Ginger, ground	1 tsp	0.7
Turmeric, ground	1 tsp	0.7
Saffron	1 tsp	0.5
Garlic powder	1 tsp	0.2

Juice	Amount	Calcium / Phosphorus
Cranberry, cocktail	1 cup	2.7
Pineapple	1 cup	1.7
Apple	1 cup	1.2
Pomegranate	1 cup	1.0
Grape	1 cup	0.8
Lemon, raw	1 cup	0.8
Prune	1 cup	0.7
Vegetable, cocktail	1 cup	0.7
Orange, raw	1 cup	0.6
Carrot	1 cup	0.6
Tomato	1 cup	0.5
Grapefruit juice, raw	1 cup	0.5

Lamb, Cooked	Amount	Calcium / Phosphorus
Foreshank, trimmed to 1/8" fat	3 oz	0.12
Ground	3 oz	0.11
Chops, loin, lean, trimmed to 1/4" fat"	3 oz	0.10
Rib, lean, trimmed to 1/4" fat"	3 oz	0.08
Cubed, for stew or kabob	3 oz	0.06
Leg, whole, trimmed to 1/4" fat"	3 oz	0.06

Milk	Amount	Calcium / Phosphorus
Human milk	1 cup	2.32
Canned, evaporated, non fat	1 cup	1.49
Buttermilk, whole milk	1 cup	1.36
Whole milk, liquid, 3.25% fat	1 cup	1.35
Low fat, 1%	1 cup	1.31
Reduced fat, 2%	1 cup	1.31
Buttermilk, low fat	1 cup	1.30
Canned, evaporated	1 cup	1.29
Dry, instant, non fat	1/3 cup	1.25
Sheep milk	1 cup	1.22
Non fat, fat free or skim milk	1 cup	1.21
Goat milk	1 cup	1.21
Whole milk, dry powder	1 cup	1.17
Canned, condensed, sweetened	1 cup	1.12

CALCIUM / PHOSPHORUS RATIO

Continued

Soymilk, original, unfortified	1 cup	0.48
Coconut milk, canned	1 cup	0.19
Almond Milk	1 cup	X

Nuts & Seeds	Amount	Calcium / Phosphorus
Sesame seeds	1 oz	1.55
Chia seeds	1 oz	0.73
Tahini	1 oz	0.58
Almonds	1 oz	0.55
Macadamia	1 oz	0.45
Flaxseeds	1 oz	0.40
Hazelnuts	1 oz	0.39
English walnuts	1 oz	0.29
Pecans	1 oz	0.25
Peanuts	1 oz	0.24
Brazilnuts	1 oz	0.22
Pistachio	1 oz	0.22
Coconut, raw meat	1 oz	0.13
Peanut butter, smooth	1 oz	0.12
Sunflower seeds	1 oz	0.12
Black walnuts	1 oz	0.12
Cashews	1 oz	0.06
Pumpkin seeds	1 oz	0.04
Pine nuts	1 oz	0.03

Pork, Cooked	Amount	Calcium / Phosphorus
Backribs	3 oz	0.28
Chops, pan-fried	3 oz	0.21
Chops, lean, pan-fried	3 oz	0.19
Spareribs	3 oz	0.18
Bratwurst	3 oz	0.14
Italian sausage	3 oz	0.13
Center loin pork chops	3 oz	0.11
Chops, broiled	3 oz	0.11
Liverwurst spread	1/4 cup	0.10
Polish sausage	3 oz	0.09
Sausage	3 oz	0.08
Braunschweiger	3 oz	0.06
Sirloin pork chops	3 oz	0.04
Cured ham	3 oz	0.03
Canadian-style bacon	3 oz	0.03
Cured ham, lean	3 oz	0.03
Tenderloin	3 oz	0.02
Bacon, pan-fried	3 oz	0.02

CALCIUM / PHOSPHORUS RATIO

Turkey, Cooked	Amount	Calcium / Phosphorus
Ground turkey, 85% lean	3 oz	0.21
Breast meat	3 oz	0.19
Ground turkey, 93% lean	3 oz	0.14
Turkey sausage, reduced fat	3 oz	0.12
Dark meat	3 oz	0.08
Liver	3 oz	0.06
Light meat	3 oz	0.04
Ground turkey, fat free	3 oz	0.02
Turkey bacon	3 oz	0.02

Veal, Cooked	Amount	Calcium / Phosphorus
Foreshank	3 oz	0.1
Loin	3 oz	0.1
Cubed, for stew	3 oz	0.1
Ground	3 oz	0.1
Sirloin	3 oz	0.1
Rib	3 oz	0.1
Breast	3 oz	0.05
Leg, top round	3 oz	0.03

Vegetables, Canned	Amount	Calcium / Phosphorus
Spinach	1 cup	2.9
Green beans	1 cup	1.8
Stewed tomatoes	1 cup	1.7
Tomatoes	1 cup	1.6
Sauerkraut	1 cup	1.5
Carrots	1 cup	1.1
Beets	1 cup	0.9
Pumpkin	1 cup	0.7
Sweet potato	1 cup	0.7
Tomato sauce	1 cup	0.5
Tomato paste	1 cup	0.4
Asparagus	1 cup	0.4
Green peas	1 cup	0.3
Tomato pure	1 cup	0.3
Mushrooms	1 cup	0.2
Corn	1 cup	0.1

Vegetables, Cooked	Amount	Calcium / Phosphorus
Spaghetti squash	1 cup	33.0
Cactus pad, nopales	1 cup	10.2
Turnip greens	1 cup	4.7
Collard greens	1 cup	4.7

CALCIUM / PHOSPHORUS RATIO

Continued

Dandelion greens	1 cup	3.3
Bok-Choy	1 cup	3.2
Beet greens	1 cup	2.8
Kale	1 cup	2.6
Broccolini	1 cup	2.4
Spinach	1 cup	2.4
Okra	1 cup	2.4
Mustard greens	1 cup	1.8
Swiss chard	1 cup	1.8
Leeks	1 cup	1.7
Celery	1 cup	1.7
Green beans	1 cup	1.5
Butternut squash	1 cup	1.5
Napa cabbage	1 cup	1.5
Cabbage	1 cup	1.4
Broccoli raab	1 cup	1.4
Turnips	1 cup	1.2
Winter squash	1 cup	1.2
Carrots	1 cup	1.0
Acorn squash	1 cup	1.0
Rutabagas	1 cup	0.9
Sweet potato, mashed	1 cup	0.8
Snow peas	1 cup	0.8
Summer squash	1 cup	0.7
Brussels sprouts	1 cup	0.6
Onions	1 cup	0.6
Broccoli	1 cup	0.6
Kohlrabi	1 cup	0.6
Parsnips	1 cup	0.5
Potatoes, mashed with whole milk	1 cup	0.5
Cauliflower	1 cup	0.5
Pumpkin, mashed	1 cup	0.5
Zucchini	1 cup	0.5
Asparagus	1 cup	0.4
Beets	1 cup	0.4
Eggplant	1 cup	0.4
Tomatoes, ripe, red	1 cup	0.4
Artichokes	1 cup	0.3
Yams, cubes	1 cup	0.3
Taro	1 cup	0.2
Split peas	1 cup	0.1
Potatoes, flesh, baked	1 cup	0.1
Shitake mushrooms	1 cup	0.1
White mushrooms	1 cup	0.1
Corn	1 cup	0.03

CALCIUM / PHOSPHORUS RATIO

Continued

Vegetables, Frozen	Amount	Calcium / Phosphorus
Rhubarb	1 cup	18.3
Collard greens	1 cup	7.8
Kale	1 cup	5.0
Turnip greens	1 cup	4.4
Spinach	1 cup	3.1
Okra	1 cup	2.0
Green beans	1 cup	1.5
Butternut squash	1 cup	1.4
Carrots	1 cup	1.1
Cauliflower	1 cup	0.7
Broccoli	1 cup	0.7
Brussels sprouts	1 cup	0.5
Asparagus	1 cup	0.4
Green peas	1 cup	0.3
Corn	1 cup	0.04

Vegetables, Raw	Amount	Calcium / Phosphorus
Cactus pads, Nopales	1 cup	10.1
Mustard spinach	1 cup	8.0
Arugula	1 cup	3.2
Dandelion greens, chopped	1 cup	2.9
Bok-choy, chinese cabbage	1 cup	2.8
Kale, chopped	1 cup	2.4
Chicory greens, chopped	1 cup	2.1
Watercress, chopped	1 cup	2.1
Spinach	1 cup	2.0
Green onions & scallions	1 cup	1.9
Endive, chopped	1 cup	1.9
Celery	1 cup	1.7
Cabbage, shredded	1 cup	1.6
Red cabbage, shredded	1 cup	1.5
Raab broccoli, chopped	1 cup	1.5
Butternut squash	1 cup	1.5
Green leaf lettuce	1 cup	1.3
Red leaf lettuce	1 cup	1.1
Romaine lettuce	1 cup	1.1
Swiss chard	1 cup	1.1
Butterhead, boston, and bibb lettuce	1 cup	1.1
Carrots, slices	1 cup	1.0
Spirulina, dried	1 tbsp	1.0
Iceberg lettuce	1 cup	0.9
Savoy cabbage, shredded	1 cup	0.8
Snow peas, chopped	1 cup	0.8
Onions	1 cup	0.8

CALCIUM / PHOSPHORUS RATIO

Broccoli	1 cup	0.7
Belgian endive	1 cup	0.7
Cucumbers, slices	1 cup	0.7
Cauliflower, chopped	1 cup	0.5
Green bell peppers, chopped	1 cup	0.5
Radicchio	1 cup	0.5
Tomatoes	1 cup	0.4
Zucchini	1 cup	0.4
Tomatoes, cherry	1 cup	0.4
Summer squash, sliced	1 cup	0.4
Yellow bell peppers	1 cup	0.4
Red bell peppers	1 cup	0.3
Tomatillos, chopped	1 cup	0.2
Crimini mushrooms, sliced	1 cup	0.2
White mushrooms, sliced	1 cup	0
Portabella mushrooms	1 cup	0
Oyster mushrooms, sliced	1 cup	0
Enoki mushrooms	1 cup	0
Shiitake mushrooms	1 whole	0
Shiitake mushrooms, dried	1 each	0

CALCIUM / PHOSPHORUS RATIO

A calorie is, by definition, a unit of energy. When you eat food you are transferring the energy stored in the food molecules to your body. The total amount of energy stored in food is represented by the calorie.

Body weight is directly dependent on how many calories you consume and how much your body needs. If you consume more calories than your body needs, the extra calories will be stored as fat. There are only two ways you can lose body fat: either burn more calories than you are eating or consume less calories in your diet.

One pound of your body fat is made up of roughly 3500 calories. So you must burn 3500 calories or eat 3500 fewer calories to lose one pound of fat. If you consume 500 calories less each day, this will equate to losing one pound of body fat per week.

Consider the following table:

Calories Cut per day	Time needed to lose one pound	Pounds lost per year
100	30 days	12
200	18 days	20
300	12 days	30
400	9 days	40
500	7 days	52

This is simpler than you might think. To cut 100 calories per day is less than 3/4 of a cup of milk a day, or 2 slices of white bread, or 1 tablespoon of mayonnaise. If you cut back on all three foods you will be eating 300 fewer calories per day and loosing 1 pound of fat every twelve days for a total of 30 pounds in one year. Of course everybody's metabolism is different. Some people will lose more than 12 pounds and some will lose less, but everyone will benefit to a measurable degree.

Health officials repeatedly state it is unhealthy to lose more than two pounds a week, so don't. Take your time, pay attention to your body, record and study what you're eating. Take responsibility for your health, and in the future, your health and vigor will give others inspiration to strive for a better life. After all it's impossible to be happy without being healthy and it's impossible to be healthy without controlling what you eat.

CALORIES

Alcohol	Amount	Calories
Regular Beer	1 bottle	153
Red Wine	1 glass	125
White Wine	1 glass	121
Light Beer	1 bottle	103
Gin, Rum, Vodka, Whisky	1 shot	97

Beans, Canned	Amount	Calories
Great Northern	1 cup	299
White beans, mature	1 cup	299
Navy beans	1 cup	296
Baked beans, plain	1 cup	239
Refried beans	1 cup	217
Cranberry beans	1 cup	216
Garbanzo beans	1 cup	211
Kidney beans	1 cup	207
Pinto beans	1 cup	197
Lima beans	1 cup	190
Black-eyed peas	1 cup	185
Fava beans,	1 cup	182
Green beans	1 cup	38
Yellow beans	1 cup	31

Beans, Cooked	Amount	Calories
Soybeans, dry roasted	1 cup	419
Natto	1 cup	371
Soybeans, mature	1 cup	297
Adzuki	1 cup	294
Garbanzo beans	1 cup	268
Navy beans	1 cup	254
Soybeans, green	1 cup	254
White beans, small	1 cup	254
Winged beans	1 cup	253
White beans, mature	1 cup	249
Pinto beans	1 cup	244
Cranberry beans	1 cup	241
Black Turtle beans, mature	1 cup	240
Split peas	1 cup	231
Lentils	1 cup	230
Black beans	1 cup	227
Hyacinth beans	1 cup	227
Kidney beans	1 cup	224
Lima beans	1 cup	216
Mung beans, mature seeds	1 cup	212

CALORIES

Continued

Great Northern beans	1 cup	209
Mothbeans	1 cup	207
Pigeon peas	1 cup	203
Black-eyed peas	1 cup	199
Lupini beans	1 cup	198
Edamame	1 cup	189
Fava beans	1 cup	187
Yardlong beans, Chinese long beans	1 cup	49
Yellow beans	1 cup	44
Green beans	1 cup	43

Beef, Cooked	Amount	Calories
Chuck roast, trimmed to 1/8" fat	3 oz	305
Beef ribs, trimmed to 1/8" fat	3 oz	298
Ground beef, 75%	3 oz	236
Porterhouse steak, trimmed to 0" fat	3 oz	235
Ground beef, 80%	3 oz	230
Tri Tip steak, lean, trimmed to 0" fat	3 oz	225
Ground beef, 85%	3 oz	212
T-bone steak, trimmed to 0" fat	3 oz	210
Ribeye steak, boneless, trim to 0" fat	3 oz	209
Top sirloin, trimmed to 1/8" fat	3 oz	207
Flat Iron steak	3 oz	194
Ground beef, 90%	3 oz	184
Skirt steak, trimmed to 0" fat	3 oz	181
Filet Mignon, tenderloin, trimmed to 0" fat	3 oz	179
Brisket, lean, trimmed to 0" fat	3 oz	174
London Broil, top round, trim to 0" fat	3 oz	169
Flank steak, lean, trimmed to 0" fat	3 oz	158
Top Sirloin, choice filet, trimmed to 0" fat	3 oz	148
Ground beef, 95%	3 oz	145

Beef, Cooked	Amount	Calories
Chuck roast, trimmed to 1/8" fat	1 lb	1630
Beef ribs, trimmed to 1/8" fat	1 lb	1594
Porterhouse steak, trimmed to 0" fat	1 lb	1252
Tri Tip steak, lean, trimmed to 0" fat	1 lb	1134
T-bone steak, trimmed to 0" fat	1 lb	1120
Top Sirloin, trimmed to 1/8" fat	1 lb	1103
Skirt steak, trimmed to 0" fat	1 lb	966
Brisket, lean, trimmed to 0" fat	1 lb	931
Flank steak, lean, trimmed to 0" fat	1 steak	712
Ribeye steak, boneless, trim to 0" fat	1 steak	514

CALORIES

Continued

Filet Mignon, tenderloin, trimmed to 0" fat	1 steak	247
Ribeye filet, lean, trimmed to 0" fat	1 filet	240
Top Sirloin, choice filet, trimmed to 0" fat	1 filet	216

Beef, Cooked	Amount	Calories
Ground beef, 80%	1/4 lb patty	209
Ground beef, 75%	1/4 lb patty	195
Ground beef, 85%	1/4 lb patty	192
Ground beef, 90%	1/4 lb patty	178
Ground beef, 95%	1/4 lb patty	140

Bread	Amount	Calories
Mexican roll, bollilo	1 roll	312
Indian bread, Naan, whole wheat	1 piece	303
Bagel, oat bran	4" bagel	268
Indian bread, Naan, plain	1 piece	262
Bagel, egg	4" bagel	247
Bagel, wheat	4" bagel	245
Bagel, cinnamon & raisin	4" bagel	242
Croissants, butter	1 each	231
Bagel, plain	4" bagel	228
Cornbread, dry mix, prepared, cooked	1 piece	188
Kaiser rolls	1 roll	167
Pita, white	6 inch pita	165
English Muffin, plain	1 muffin	129
Hamburger or Hotdog buns, plain	1 bun	119
Egg bread	1 slice	113
Tortillas, flour	1 tortilla	100
Dinner Rolls, brown & serve	1 roll	86
Potato bread	1 slice	85
Rye bread	1 slice	82
Italian bread, Oroweat Premium	1 slice	80
Pumpernickel	1 slice	80
French, Sourdough and Vienna	1 slice	72
Oatmeal bread	1 slice	72
Raisin bread	1 slice	71
Multigrain bread	1 slice	69
Whole-Wheat bread	1 slice	69
Wheat bread	1 slice	66
White bread	1 slice	66
Cracked wheat	1 slice	65
Tortillas, corn	1 tortillas	56

CALORIES

Cereal, Arrowhead Mills®	Amount	Calories
Sweetened Shredded Wheat	1 cup	200
Shredded Wheat, Bite-Size	1 cup	190
Sweetened Rice Flakes	1 cup	180
Maple Buckwheat Flakes	1 cup	170
Amaranth Flakes	1 cup	140
Oat Bran Flakes	1 cup	140
Kamut Flakes	1 cup	120
Spelt Flakes	1 cup	120
Sprouted Multigrain Flakes	1 cup	120

Cereal, Barbara's™	Amount	Calories
Shredded Oats Cinnamon Crunch	1 cup	230
Shredded Minis Blueberry Burst	1 cup	220
Shredded Oats Vanilla Almond	1 cup	220
High Fiber Flax & Granola	1 cup	200
High Fiber Cranberry	1 cup	190
High Fiber Original	1 cup	180
Shredded Oats Original	1 cup	176
Brown Rice Crisps	1 cup	160
Hole 'n Oats Honey Nut	1 cup	160
Hole 'n Oats: Fruit & Juice Sweetened	1 cup	160
Puffins Honey Rice	1 cup	160
Puffins Puffs Crunchy Cocoa	1 cup	160
Puffins Puffs Fruit Medley	1 cup	160
Shredded Spoonfuls Multigrain	1 cup	160
Corn Flakes	1 cup	147
Puffins Multigrain	1 cup	147
Puffins Peanut Butter	1 cup	147
Puffins Peanut Butter & Chocolate	1 cup	147
Shredded Wheat	1 cup	140
Puffins Cinnamon	1 cup	135
Puffins Original	1 cup	120

Cereal, Bear Naked®	Amount	Calories
Banana Nut Granola	1 cup	560
Fruit & Nut Ganola	1 cup	560
Peak Protein, Original Granola	1 cup	560
Vanila Almond Crunch Granola	1 cup	480
Nut Cluster Crunch Cereal	1 cup	210

Cereal, Cascadian Farm™	Amount	Calories
Oats & Honey Granola	1 cup	348
Maple Brown Sugar Granola	1 cup	333

CALORIES

Continued

Cinnamon Raisin Granola	1 cup	318
Dark Chocolate Almond Granola	1 cup	280
French Vanilla Almond Granola	1 cup	280
Fruit & Nut Granola	1 cup	280
Hearty Morning	1 cup	253
Raisin bran	1 cup	190
Multi Gain Squares	1 cup	147
Fruit Ful O's	1 cup	146
Chocolate O's	1 cup	133
Cinnamon Crunch	1 cup	110
Honey Nut O's	1 cup	110
Purel O's	1 cup	110

Cereal, Erewhon®	Amount	Calories
Cocoa Crispy Brown Rice, Gluten Free	1 cup	200
Corn Flakes, Gluten Free	1 cup	173
Raisin Bran	1 cup	170
Crispy Brown Rice, Strawberry Crisp	1 cup	160
Rice Twice, Gluten Free	1 cup	160
Crispy Brown Rice, Mixed Berries	1 cup	120
Crispy Brown Rice, Gluten Free	1 cup	110
Crispy Brown Rice, No Salt Added	1 cup	110
Crispy Brown Rice, Original	1 cup	110

Cereal, Ezekiel	Amount	Calories
Sprouted Grain Almond, 4:9	1 cup	400
Sprouted Grain Original, 4:9	1 cup	380
Sprouted Grain Cinnamon Flax, 4:9	1 cup	380
Sprouted Grain Golden Flax, 4:9	1 cup	360

Cereal, General Mills®	Amount	Calories
Oatmeal Crisp, Hearty raisin	1 cup	230
Oatmeal Crisp, Crunchy Almond	1 cup	216
Multi-Bran CHEX	1 cup	213
Wheat Chex	1 cup	213
Honey Nut Clusters	1 cup	210
Basic 4	1 cup	200
Raisin Nut Bran	1 cup	200
Chocolate Chex	1 cup	173
Cinnamon Toast Crunch	1 cup	171
Total Raisin Bran	1 cup	169
Reese's Puffs	1 cup	167
Cinnamon Chex	1 cup	161
Golden Grams	1 cup	160

CALORIES

Continued

Honey Nut Chex	1 cup	160
Total Cranberry Crunch	1 cup	152
Cocoa Puffs	1 cup	133
Cookie Crisp	1 cup	133
Total Whole Grain	1 cup	133
Dora The Explorer	1 cup	131
Lucky Charms	1 cup	122
Corn Chex	1 cup	120
Trix	1 cup	115
Wheaties	1 cup	104
Rice Chex	1 cup	100
Berry Berry Kix	1 cup	96
KABOOM	1 cup	96
Kix	1 cup	88

General Mills Cheerios®	Amount	Calories
Apple Cinnamon	1 cup	160
Honey Nut Medly Crunch	1 cup	160
Yogurt Burst, Strawberry	1 cup	160
Multi Grain Peanut Butter	1 cup	147
Crunch, Oat Clusters	1 cup	135
Banana Nut	1 cup	133
Berry Burst	1 cup	133
Chocolate	1 cup	133
Dulce de leche	1 cup	133
Frosted	1 cup	133
Fruity	1 cup	133
Honey Nut	1 cup	133
Original	1 cup	133
Cinnamon Burst	1 cup	110
Multi Grain	1 cup	110

General Mill's Fiber One®	Amount	Calories
Frosted Shredded Wheat	1 cup	193
Nuty Clusters & Almond	1 cup	180
Caramel Delight	1 cup	172
Raisin Bran Clusters	1 cup	172
Honey Clusters	1 cup	157
Original Bran	1 cup	120
80 Calorie Honey Squares	1 cup	107

CALORIES

Cereal, Glutino® Gluten Free	Amount	Calories
Honey Nut Cereal	1 cup	240
Apple & Cinnamon Rings	1 cup	240
Corn Rice Flakes	1 cup	120
Berry Sensible Beginning	1 cup	120
Frosted Corn & Rice Flakes	1 cup	120
Corn Rice Flakes with Strawberries	1 cup	120

Cereal, Health Valley®	Amount	Calories
Oat Bran Almond Crunch	1 cup	400
Low Fat Date & Almond Flavored Granola	1 cup	288
Low Fat Raisin Cinnamon Granola	1 cup	288
Cranberry Crunch	1 cup	253
Oat Bran Flakes & Raisins	1 cup	200
Heart Wise	1 cup	200
Oat Bran Flakes	1 cup	190
Golden Flax	1 cup	190
Amaranth Flakes	1 cup	168
Multigrain Apple Cinnamon Squares	1 cup	168
Fiber 7	1 cup	160
Multigrain Maple, Honey, Nut Squares	1 cup	160
Corn Crunch-EMS	1 cup	110
Rice Crunch-EMS	1 cup	88

Cereal, Kashi®	Amount	Calories
7-Whole Grain Nuggets	1 cup	420
Go Lean Crisp, Cinnamon Crumble	1 cup	253
Go Lean Crisp, Toasted Berry Crumble	1 cup	240
Go Lean Crunch	1 cup	200
Go Lean Crunch, Honey Almond Flax	1 cup	200
Heart to Heart, Oat Flakes & Blueberry Clusters	1 cup	200
Strawberry Fields	1 cup	200
Island Vanilla	27 biscuits	190
Autum Wheat	29 biscuits	180
Blackberry Hills	1 cup	180
Cinnamon Harvest	28 biscuits	180
7-Whole Grain Flakes	1 cup	170
Berry Fruitful	29 biscuits	170
Go Lean Vanilla Graham	1 cup	170
Go Lean	1 cup	160
Good Friends	1 cup	160
Heart to Heart, Honey Toasted Oat	1 cup	160
Heart to Heart, Warm Cinnamon	1 cup	160
Heart to Heart, Nutty Chia Flax	1 cup	146

CALORIES

Continued

Berry Blossom	1 cup	133
Honey Sunshine	1 cup	133
Indigo Morning	1 cup	133
Simply Maize	1 cup	133
7-Whole Grain Honey Puffs	1 cup	120
7-Whole Grain Puffs	1 cup	70

Kellogg's®	Amount	Calories
MUESLIX	1 cup	293
Cracklin' Oat Bran	1 cup	266
All-Bran Bran Buds	1 cup	240
Mini Wheats, Crunch	1 cup	200
Mini Wheats, Original	1 cup	200
Raisin Bran	1 cup	190
Raisin Bran Crunch	1 cup	190
Smart Start, Strong Heart, Antioxidants	1 cup	182
Raisin Bran with Flaxseeds	1 cup	180
All-Bran Strawberry Medley	1 cup	175
Frosted MINI-Wheat's, Big-Bite	1 cup	174
Fiberplus Berry Yogurt Crunch	1 cup	167
All-Bran Original	1 cup	160
Cocoa Krispies	1 cup	160
Crunchy Nut Golden Honey Nut Flakes	1 cup	160
Frosted Krispies	1 cup	160
Krave Chocolate	1 cup	160
Raisin Bran Cinnamon Almond	1 cup	160
Rice Krispies Treats	1 cup	160
Honey Crunch Corn Flakes	1 cup	154
Fiberplus Cinnamon Oat Crunch	1 cup	148
Frosted Flakes	1 cup	146
Crunchy Nut Roasted Nut & Honey O's	1 cup	134
Honey Smacks	1 cup	133
All-Bran Complete Wheat Flakes	1 cup	123
Smorz	1 cup	122
Cinnabon	1 cup	120
Corn Pops	1 cup	120
Simply Cinnamon Corn Flakes	1 cup	117
Apple Jacks	1 cup	110
Froot Loops	1 cup	110
Product 19	1 cup	110
Crispix	1 cup	109
Rice Krispies	1 cup	104
Corn Flakes	1 cup	100

CALORIES

Kellogg's Special-K®	Amount	Calories
Low Fat Granola	1 cup	380
Chocolately Delight	1 cup	160
Protein	1 cup	160
Fruit & Yogurt	1 cup	159
Multigrain Oats & Honey	1 cup	158
Cinnamon Pecan	1 cup	146
Vanilla Almond	1 cup	146
Blueberry	1 cup	145
Original	1 cup	120
Red Berries	1 cup	110

Mom's Best Naturals™	Amount	Calories
Raisin Bran	1 cup	230
Blue Pom Wheat Fuls	1 cup	210
Sweetened Wheat Fuls	1 cup	210
Toasted Wheat Fuls	1 cup	200
Honey Graham	1 cup	173
Toasted Cinnamon Squares	1 cup	173
Crispy Cocoa Rice	1 cup	160
Oats & Honey Blend	1 cup	160
Honey Ful Wheats	1 cup	147
Honey Nut Toastey O's	1 cup	120
Mallow Oats	1 cup	120

Nature's Path™	Amount	Calories
Hemp Plus Granola	1 cup	347
Peanut Butter Granola	1 cup	347
Flax Plus Pumpkin Flax Granola	1 cup	347
Pomegran Plus Granola	1 cup	333
Flax Plus Vanilla Almond Granola	1 cup	333
Pomegran Cherry Granola	1 cup	333
AGAVE Plus Granola	1 cup	333
Acai Apple Granola	1 cup	320
Heritage Crunch	1 cup	307
Flax Plus Maple Pecan Crunch	1 cup	293
Flax Plus Redberry Crunch	1 cup	280
Flax Plus Pumpkin Raisin Crunch	1 cup	280
Optimum Power Blueberry Cinnamon	1 cup	267
Optimum Cranberry Ginger	1 cup	253
Optimum Banana Almond	1 cup	253
Flax Plus Raisin Bran Flakes	1 cup	253
Optimum Slim Low Fat Vanilla	1 cup	200
Whole O's	1 cup	182

CALORIES

Continued

Crunchy Maple Sunrise, Gluten Free	1 cup	167
Crunchy Vanilla Sunrise	1 cup	167
Heritage Flakes	1 cup	160
Mesa Sunrise, Gluten Free	1 cup	160
Honeyed Corn Flakes, Gluten Free	1 cup	160
Organic Millet Rice	1 cup	160
Smart Bran	1 cup	160
OATY BITES Whole Grain	1 cup	147
Heritage Heirloom Whole Grain	1 cup	147
Flax Plus Multibran Flakes	1 cup	147
Multigrain Oat bran	1 cup	147

Peace™ All Natural	Amount	Calories
Wild Berry Clusters & Flakes	1 cup	364
Cherry Almond Clusters & Flakes	1 cup	364
Golden Honey Granola	1 cup	364
Walnut Spice Clusters & Flakes	1 cup	348
Vanilla Almond Clusters & Flakes	1 cup	240
Maple Pecan	1 cup	240
Mango Peach Passion Clusters & Flakes	1 cup	230

Post®	Amount	Calories
Grape-Nuts Cereal	1 cup	400
Great Grains, Crunchy Pecan Cereal	1 cup	280
Great Grains, Raisins, Date & Pecan	1 cup	280
Great Grains, Cranberry Almond Crunch	1 cup	264
100% Bran Cereal	1 cup	250
Great Grains, Bannana Nut Crunch	1 cup	240
Honey Nut Shreaded Wheat	1 cup	220
Raisin Bran	1 cup	189
Shredded Wheat, frosted, spoon-size	1 cup	183
Blueberry Morning	1 cup	176
Shredded Wheat, Original, spoon-size	1 cup	170
Shredded Wheat, Wheat n' Bran, spoon size	1 cup	162
Fruity Pebbles	1 cup	160
Cocoa Pebbles	1 cup	159
Shredded Wheat, Sugar and Salt Free	1 cup	155
OREO O's Cereal	1 cup	149
Grape-Nuts Flakes	1 cup	143
Golden Crisp	1 cup	140
Honeycomb Cereal	1 cup	84

CALORIES

Post, Honey Bunches of Oats®	Amount	Calories
Just Bunches Cinnamon	1 cup	379
Just Bunches Honey Roasted	1 cup	379
Vanilla Bunches	1 cup	220
Raisin Medley	1 cup	200
With Almonds	1 cup	173
Cinnamon Bunches	1 cup	160
Fruit Blends	1 cup	160
Honey Roasted	1 cup	160
Pecan Bunches	1 cup	160
With Strawberries	1 cup	160

Quaker®	Amount	Calories
Granola, Oats, Honey, & Almonds	1 cup	429
Granola, Oats, Honey, Raisins, & Almonds	1 cup	420
Granola, Apple, Cranberry, & Almonds	1 cup	410
Oatmeal Squares, Golden Maple	1 cup	213
Oatmeal Squares, Brown Sugar	1 cup	212
Oatmeal Squares, Cinnamon	1 cup	212
Toasted Multigrain Crisp	1 cup	188
LIFE Cereal, Original	1 cup	160
LIFE Cereal, Cinnamon	1 cup	159
LIFE Cereal, Maple & Brown Sugar	1 cup	159
CAP'N Crunch's Peanut Butter Crunch	1 cup	150
Honey Graham OH'S	1 cup	147
LIFE Cereal, Crunchtime Strawberry	1 cup	147
Whole Hearts	1 cup	147
CAP'N Crunch	1 cup	143
CAP'N Crunch with Crunchberries	1 cup	138
CAP'N Crunch's OOPS! All Berries	1 cup	126
Corn Bran Crunch	1 cup	120
Puffed Rice	1 cup	50
Puffed Wheat	1 cup	50

Uncle Sam™	Amount	Calories
Wheat Berry Flakes, Flaxseed, & Strawberry	1 cup	320
Wheat Berry Flakes, Flaxseed, Honey Almond	1 cup	307
Wheat Berry Flakes & Flaxseed, Original	1 cup	253
Skinners Raisin Bran	1 cup	190

Cereal, Wild Harvest™	Amount	Calories
Blueberry Flax Granola	1 cup	379
Golden Honey & Flax Granola	1 cup	364
Crunchy Vanilla Almond Granola	1 cup	348

CALORIES

Continued

Cherry Vanilla Granola	1 cup	320
Maple Pecan Flakes & Clusters	1 cup	240
Mango Crisp	1 cup	230
Cranberry Almond	1 cup	210
Wholesome Raisin Bran	1 cup	180
Wild Berry Crisp	1 cup	160

Cereal, Cooked	Amount	Calories
White corn grits	1 cup	172
Oats, regular, unenriched	1 cup	166
Yellow corn grits	1 cup	157
WHEATENA®	1 cup	136
Farina®	1 cup	131
CREAM OF WHEAT, regular	1 cup	125
Malt-o-Meal™, plain	1 serving	112

Cheese	Amount	Calories
Goat cheese, hard	1 oz	128
Parmesan, grated	1 oz	122
Gruyere	1 oz	117
Cheddar	1 oz	114
Colby	1 oz	110
Dubliner	1 oz	110
Pepper Jack, Red & Green Jalapenos	1 oz	110
Romano	1 oz	110
Fontina	1 oz	108
Swiss	1 oz	107
Monterey	1 oz	106
Roquefort	1 oz	105
American, pasteurized process, fortified	1 oz	104
Muenster	1 oz	104
Goat cheese, semisoft	1 oz	103
Blue cheese	1 oz	100
Gouda	1 oz	100
Provolone	1 oz	100
Cream cheese	1 oz	97
Brie cheese	1 oz	95
Monterey, low fat	1 oz	87
Mozzarella, part skim milk, low moisture	1 oz	85
Mozzarella, whole milk	1 oz	85
Velveeta, pasteurized process	1 oz	85
Cheez Whiz, pasteurized process	1 oz	77

CALORIES

Continued

Provolone, reduced fat	1 oz	77
Goat cheese, soft	1 oz	76
Muenster, low fat	1 oz	76
Feta cheese	1 oz	75
American, pasteurized process, imitation	1 oz	73
American, pasteurized process, low fat	1 oz	50
Cheddar, low fat	1 oz	49
Ricotta cheese whole milk	1 oz	49
Swiss, low fat	1 oz	49
Mozzarella, non fat	1 oz	40
Ricotta cheese, part skim milk	1 oz	39
Cream cheese, fat free	1 oz	30
Cottage cheese, creamed, large & small curd	1 oz	28
Cottage cheese, low fat, 2 %	1 oz	24
Cottage cheese, low fat, 1 %	1 oz	20
Cottage cheese, non fat	1 oz	20

Chicken, Cooked	Amount	Calories
Breast, with skin, fried in flour	1/2 breast	217
Breast, with skin, roasted	1/2 breast	193
Thigh, with skin, fried in flour	1 thigh	162
Wing with skin, fried in batter	1 wing	159
Breast, no skin, roasted	1/2 breast	142
Drumstick with skin, fried in flour	1 drumstick	120
Wing with skin, roasted	1 wing	99
Thigh, meat only, roasted	1 thigh	92
Drumstick, no skin, meat only, roasted	1 drumstick	75

Chicken, Cooked	Amount	Calories
Wing with skin, fried in flour	3 oz	273
Wing with skin, roasted	3 oz	246
Thigh with skin, fried in flour	3 oz	223
Breast with skin, fried in batter	3 oz	221
Drumstick with skin, fried in flour	3 oz	208
Thigh with skin, roasted	3 oz	195
Breast with skin, fried in flour	3 oz	189
Wing meat only, no skin, roasted	3 oz	173
Breast with skin, roasted	3 oz	167
Drumstick with skin, roasted	3 oz	158
Thigh meat only, no skin, roasted	3 oz	150
Breast meat only, no skin, roasted	3 oz	140
Drumstick meat only, no skin, roasted	3 oz	127
Cornish game hens, meat only	3 oz	114

CALORIES

Cream	Amount	Calories
Heavy Cream	1 tbsp	52
Light Coffee Cream	1 tbsp	29
Sour Cream, cultured	1 tbsp	23
Half & Half	1 tbsp	20
Sour Cream, reduced fat, cultured	1 tbsp	20
Whipped Topping, pressurized	1 tbsp	8

Eggs	Amount	Calories
Egg whites, dried	1 ounce	108
Egg whole, fried	1 large	90
Egg whole, scrambled	1 large	90
Egg whole, hard cooked	1 large	77
Egg whole, poached	1 large	69
Egg yolk	1 large	53
Egg substitute, liquid, fat free	1/4 cup	29
Egg whites, dried powder, stabilized	1 tbsp	26
Egg whites	1 large	17

Fish, Canned	Amount	Calories
Light tuna, in oil	3 oz	168
White (albacore) tuna, in oil	3 oz	158
White (albacore) tuna, in water	3 oz	108
Light tuna, in water	3 oz	73

Fish, Cooked	Amount	Calories
Atlantic mackerel	3 oz	223
Atlantic herring	3 oz	222
Greenland halibut	3 oz	203
King, chinook salmon	3 oz	196
Catfish, breaded & fried	3 oz	195
Atlantic croaker	3 oz	188
Florida pompano	3 oz	179
Atlantic salmon, farmed	3 oz	175
Pacific & Jack mackerel	3 oz	171
Yellowtail	3 oz	159
Bluefin tuna, fresh	3 oz	156
Atlantic salmon, wild	3 oz	155
Coho salmon, farmed	3 oz	151
Sockeye salmon	3 oz	150
Swordfish	3 oz	146
Rainbow trout, farmed	3 oz	143
Carp	3 oz	138
Spanish mackerel	3 oz	134

CALORIES

Continued

	Amount	Calories
Keta (chum) salmon	3 oz	131
Pink salmon	3 oz	130
Rainbow trout, wild	3 oz	128
Freshwater bass	3 oz	124
Catfish, farmed	3 oz	122
Coho salmon, wild	3 oz	118
King mackerel	3 oz	114
Skipjack, (aku) tuna	3 oz	112
Yellowfin tuna	3 oz	110
Snapper	3 oz	109
Tilapia	3 oz	109
Sea bass	3 oz	105
Striped bass	3 oz	105
Walleye pike	3 oz	101
Atlantic pollock	3 oz	100
Grouper	3 oz	100
Chinook salmon, smoked	3 oz	99
Lox	3 oz	99
Whiting	3 oz	99
Alaskan halibut	3 oz	96
Northern pike	3 oz	96
Atlantic & Pacific halibut	3 oz	94
Walleye pollock	3 oz	94
Atlantic cod	3 oz	89
Catfish, wild	3 oz	89
Orange roughy	3 oz	89
Atlantic perch	3 oz	82
Haddock	3 oz	76
Mahi Mahi	3 oz	75
Flounder & Sole	3 oz	73
Pacific cod	3 oz	72

Fish, Shellfish, Cooked	Amount	Calories
Shrimp, breaded & fried	3 oz	206
Scallops, breaded & fried	3 oz	184
Clams, breaded & fried	3 oz	172
Oysters, breaded & fried	3 oz	169
Abalone	3 oz	161
Squid, fried	3 oz	149
Octopus	3 oz	139
Blue crab cakes	3 oz	132
Clams, canned	3 oz	120
Shrimp	3 oz	101
Queen crabs	3 oz	98
Scallops, bay & sea, steamed	3 oz	94

CALORIES

Shrimp, canned	3 oz	86
Alaskan king crab	3 oz	82
Alaskan king crab, imitation	3 oz	80
Northern lobster	3 oz	76
Blue crab	3 oz	71
Crayfish	3 oz	70
Eastern oysters, farmed	3 oz	67
Eastern oysters, wild	3 oz	67

Fruit, Canned	Amount	Calories
Plums	1 cup	230
Apricots	1 cup	214
Pineapple	1 cup	198
Pears	1 cup	197
Peaches	1 cup	194
Applesauce, sweetened	1 cup	173
Applesauce, unsweetened	1 cup	102
Olives, black	5 large	25
Olives, green	5 large	20

Fruit, Dried	Amount	Calories
Pears	1 cup	472
Currants	1 cup	408
Peaches	1 cup	382
Cranberries	1 cup	373
Figs	1 cup	371
Apricots	1 cup	313
Apples	1 cup	209

Fruit, Frozen	Amount	Calories
Raspberries	1 cup	258
Strawberries	1 cup	244
Peaches	1 cup	235
Blueberries	1 cup	196
Blackberries, unsweetened	1 cup	97

Fruit, Raw	Amount	Calories
Raisins	1 cup	433
Prunes, uncooked	1 cup	418
Dates	1 cup	415
Avocado, California, pureed	1 cup	384
Avocado, Florida, pureed	1 cup	276
Stewed prunes	1 cup	265
Plantains	1 cup	181

CALORIES

Continued

Pomegranates	1 cup	144
Grapes, red or green	1 cup	110
Kiwi	1 cup	110
Elderberries	1 cup	106
Tangerines	1 cup	103
Mango	1 cup	99
Cherries	1 cup	97
Grapefruit, pink & red, sections	1 cup	97
Pears	1 cup	93
Valencias Oranges	1 cup	88
Sweet cheeries	1 cup	87
Florida Oranges	1 cup	85
Blueberries	1 cup	82
Pineapple	1 cup	82
Naval Oranges	1 cup	81
Apricots	1 cup	79
Plums⁻	1 cup	76
Pummelo, sections	1 cup	72
Black currants	1 cup	71
Peaches	1 cup	66
Apples	1 cup	65
Raspberries	1 cup	64
Nectarines	1 cup	63
Blackberries	1 cup	62
Papayas	1 cup	62
Honeydew	1 cup	61
Mulberries	1 cup	60
Cantaloupe	1 cup	54
Strawberries	1 cup	53
Jicama	1 cup	49
Cranberries, whole	1 cup	46
Water mellon	1 cup	46
Chayote, 1" pieces	1 cup	25

Fruit, Raw	Amount	Calories
Avocado, Florida	1 fruit	365
Pomegranates	1 fruit	234
Pummelo	1 fruit	231
Avocado, California	1 fruit	227
Plantains	1 fruit	218
Mango	1 fruit	202
Cherimoya	1 fruit	176
Raisins	1 small box	129
Persimmons, Japanese	1 fruit	118
Prunes, uncooked	5 fruit	114

CALORIES

Continued

Bananas	1 fruit	105
Figs, dried	5 fruit	105
Dates	5 fruit	100
Pears	1 fruit	96
Cantaloupe	1/2 fruit	94
Apples	1 fruit	72
Naval Oranges	1 fruit	69
Papayas	1 fruit	68
Florida Oranges	1 fruit	65
Nectarine	1 fruit	60
Valencias Oranges	1 fruit	59
Cheeries	10 fruit	52
Grapefruit, pink or red	1/2 fruit	52
Kiwi	1 fruit	46
Tangerine	1 fruit	45
Chayote	1 fruit	39
Peaches	1 small	38
Olives, Black	5 large	34
Persimmons, small native	1 fruit	32
Plums	1 fruit	30
Star fruit, Carambola	1 medium	28
Pineapple, slices	1/2" x 3"	25
Pineapple guava, Feijoa	1 medium	23
Olives, Green	5 large	20
Strawberries	5 fruit	19
Apricots	1 fruit	17
Kumquats	1 fruit	13

Game Meat, Cooked	Amount	Calories
Bison, ground	3 oz	202
Duck	3 oz	171
Elk, ground	3 oz	164
Venison, ground	3 oz	159
Rabbit, wild	3 oz	147
Squirrel	3 oz	147
Caribou	3 oz	142
Wild boar	3 oz	136
Deer	3 oz	134
Antelope	3 oz	128
Buffalo, steak, free range	3 oz	124
Elk	3 oz	124

CALORIES

Grains, cooked	Amount	Calories
Amaranth	1 cup	251
Kamut	1 cup	251
Spelt	1 cup	246
Quinoa	1 cup	222
Egg noodles	1 cup	221
Macaroni	1 cup	221
Spaghetti	1 cup	220
Brown rice	1 cup	216
Egg & Spinach noodles	1 cup	211
Millet	1 cup	207
White rice, regular	1 cup	205
White rice, enriched	1 cup	194
Barley, pearled	1 cup	193
White rice, instant	1 cup	193
Rice noodles	1 cup	192
Spaghetti, Spinach	1 cup	182
Couscous	1 cup	176
Macaroni, Whole-Wheat	1 cup	174
Spaghetti, Whole-Wheat	1 cup	174
Wild Rice	1 cup	166
Buckwheat	1 cup	155
Bulgur	1 cup	151
Soba noodles	1 cup	113
Oat bran	1 cup	88

Juice	Amount	Calories
Prune	1 cup	182
Grape	1 cup	151
Pineapple	1 cup	149
Cranberry	1 cup	137
Pomegranate	1 cup	134
Grapefruit juice, raw	1 cup	115
Apple	1 cup	114
Orange juice, raw	1 cup	111
Carrot	1 cup	94
Lemon juice, raw	1 cup	54
Vegetable	1 cup	46
Tomato	1 cup	41

Lamb, Cooked	Amount	Calories
Chops, loin, lean, trimmed to 1/4" fat	3 oz	269
Ground, broiled	3 oz	241
Leg, whole, trimmed to 1/4" fat	3 oz	219

CALORIES

Foreshank, trimmed to 1/8" fat	3 oz	207
Rib, lean, trimmed to 1/4" fat	3 oz	200
Cubed, for stew or kabob	3 oz	158

Milk	Amount	Calories
Canned, condensed, sweetened	1 cup	982
Coconut milk, canned	1 cup	445
Canned, evaporated	1 cup	338
Sheep milk	1 cup	265
Canned, evaporated, non fat	1 cup	200
Human milk	1 cup	172
Goat milk	1 cup	168
Whole milk, Dry	1/4 cup	159
Whole milk, liquid, 3.25%	1 cup	150
Soymilk, original and vanilla, unfortified	1 cup	131
Reduced fat, 2%	1 cup	122
Low fat, 1%	1 cup	102
Buttermilk, low fat	1 cup	98
Nonfat, fat free or skim milk	1 cup	83
Dry, instant, non fat	1/3 cup	82

Nuts & Seeds	Amount	Calories
Macadamia	1 oz	204
Pecans	1 oz	196
Pine nuts	1 oz	191
Brazil nuts	1 oz	186
English walnuts	1 oz	185
Hazelnuts	1 oz	178
Black walnuts	1 oz	175
Tahini	1 oz	169
Peanut butter, smooth style	1 oz	167
Sunflower seeds	1 oz	166
Almonds	1 oz	163
Sesame seeds	1 oz	162
Peanuts	1 oz	161
Pistachio	1 oz	159
Pumpkin seeds	1 oz	158
Cashews	1 oz	157
Flaxseeds	1 oz	151
Chia seeds	1 oz	138
Coconut, raw meat	1 oz	100

CALORIES

Pork, Cooked	Amount	Calories
Bacon	3 oz	460
Spareribs	3 oz	337
Italian sausage	3 oz	292
Sausage	3 oz	288
Bratwurst	3 oz	283
Braunschweiger	3 oz	278
Polish sausage	3 oz	277
Backribs	3 oz	243
Cured ham	3 oz	207
Chops, pan-fried	3 oz	202
Center loin chops	3 oz	178
Chops, broiled	3 oz	178
Liverwurst spread	1/4 cup	168
Chops, lean, pan-fried	3 oz	166
Canadian-style bacon	3 oz	157
Sirloin chops	3 oz	144
Cured ham, lean	3 oz	133
Tenderloin	3 oz	125

Annies's Organic Dressing	Amount	Calories
Redwine & Olive Oil	2 tbsp	140
Goddnes	2 tbsp	120
Shiitake Sesame	2 tbsp	120
Asian Sesame	2 tbsp	120
Oil & Vinegar	2 tbsp	120
Caesar Dressing	2 tbsp	110
Cowgirl Ranch Dressing	2 tbsp	110
French Dressing	2 tbsp	110
Green Goddness Dressing	2 tbsp	110
Roasted Garlic Vinaigrette	2 tbsp	110
Balsamic Vinaigrette	2 tbsp	100
Papaya Poppy Seed	2 tbsp	90
Sesame Ginger Vinaigrette	2 tbsp	90
Thousand Island	2 tbsp	90
Creamy Asiago Cheese	2 tbsp	80
Green Garlic	2 tbsp	80
Pomegranate Vinaigrette	2 tbsp	70
Buttermilk Dressing	2 tbsp	70

Bernstein's Dressing	Amount	Calories
Herb Garden French	2 tbsp	130
Sweet Herb Italian	2 tbsp	130
Chunky Blue Chees	2 tbsp	120

CALORIES

Continued

Balsamic Italian	2 tbsp	110
Redwine & Garlic Italian	2 tbsp	110
Basil Parmesan	2 tbsp	100
Cheese Fantastico	2 tbsp	100
Restaurant Recipe Italian	2 tbsp	100
Creamy Caesar	2 tbsp	90
Italian & Marinade	2 tbsp	90
Cheese & Garlic Italian	2 tbsp	80
Light Parmesan Garlic Ranch	2 tbsp	50
Light Fantastic Roasted Garlic Balsamic	2 tbsp	45
Light Fantastic Cheese Fantastico	2 tbsp	25

Best Food Mayonnaise Dressing	Amount	Calories
Real Mayonnaise	2 tbsp	180
Mayonesa Con Jugo De Lemon	2 tbsp	180
Mayonnaise with Olive Oil	2 tbsp	80
Canola Cholesterol Free Mayonnaise	2 tbsp	80
Light Mayonnaise	2 tbsp	70
Low Fat Mayonnaise	2 tbsp	30

Bob's Big Boy® Dressing	Amount	Calories
Ranch	2 tbsp	150
Blue Cheese	2 tbsp	140
Roquefort	2 tbsp	140
Thousand Island	2 tbsp	140

Bolthouse Farms Dresssing	Amount	Calories
Caesar Parmigino Yogurt Dressing	2 tbsp	45
Chunky Blue Cheese & Olive Oil	2 tbsp	45
Classic Ranch Yogurt Dressing	2 tbsp	45
Honey Mustard Yogurt Dressing	2 tbsp	45
Salsa Ranch Yogurt Dressing	2 tbsp	45
Zesty French Yogurt	2 tbsp	45
Thousand Island Yogurt Dressing	2 tbsp	40
Asian Ginger & Olive Oil Vinaigrettes	2 tbsp	35
Chunky Bluecheese Yogurt Dressing	2 tbsp	35
Classic Balsamic & Olive Oil	2 tbsp	30
Raspberry Merlot & Olive Oil	2 tbsp	30

Brianna's Dressing	Amount	Calories
The New American	2 tbsp	160
Rich Poppy Seed	2 tbsp	160
Champagne Caper Vinaigrette	2 tbsp	160
Classic Buttermilk Ranch	2 tbsp	160

CALORIES

Continued

	Amount	Calories
Dijon Honey Mustard	2 tbsp	150
Ginger Mandarin	2 tbsp	150
Zesty French	2 tbsp	150
Asiago Caesar	2 tbsp	150
Real French Vinaigrette	2 tbsp	130
True Blue Cheese	2 tbsp	120
Blush Wine Vinaigrette	2 tbsp	120
Chipotle Cheddar	2 tbsp	110
Lively Lemon Tarragon	2 tbsp	35
Rich Santa Fe Blend	2 tbsp	25

Cardini's Dressing	Amount	Calories
Aged Parmesan Ranch	2 tbsp	150
Balsamic Vinaigrette	2 tbsp	100
Honey Mustard	2 tbsp	140
Italian	2 tbsp	100
Original Caesar	2 tbsp	160
Pear Vinaigrette	2 tbsp	100
Raspberry Pomegranate	2 tbsp	100
Roasted Asian Sesame	2 tbsp	120

Drew's Dressing	Amount	Calories
Thai Sesame Lime	2 tbsp	180
Rosemary Balsamic	2 tbsp	160
Shiitake Ginger	2 tbsp	160
Poppy Seed	2 tbsp	160
Sesame Orange	2 tbsp	150
Organic Peppercorn Ranch	2 tbsp	150
Lemon Goddess	2 tbsp	140
Classic Italian	2 tbsp	140
Roasted Garlic & Peppercorn	2 tbsp	140
Honey Dijon	2 tbsp	140
Buttermilk Ranch	2 tbsp	130
Organic Classic Ceasar	2 tbsp	130
Organic Asian Ginger	2 tbsp	130
Organic Harvest Ranch	2 tbsp	130
Greek Olive	2 tbsp	120
Smoked Tomato	2 tbsp	100
Organic Aged Balsamic	2 tbsp	100

Girard's Dressing	Amount	Calories
Champagne	2 tbsp	150
Caesar Dressing	2 tbsp	120
Chinese Chicken Salad	2 tbsp	120

CALORIES

Continued

Original French	2 tbsp	120
Old Venice Italian	2 tbsp	120
Romano Cheese Italian	2 tbsp	120
Apple Poppy Seed	2 tbsp	110
White Balsamic Vinaigrette	2 tbsp	110
Creamy Balsamic Vinaigrette	2 tbsp	100
Greek Feta Vinaigrette	2 tbsp	100
Peach Mimosa Vinaigrette	2 tbsp	100
Blue Cheee Vinaigrette	2 tbsp	90
Light Caesar Dressing	2 tbsp	80
Spinach Salad Dressing	2 tbsp	70
Light Champagne Dressing	2 tbsp	60

Hidden Valley® Creamy Dressing	Amount	Calories
Coleslaw	2 tbsp	150
Spicy Ranch	2 tbsp	150
Bacon Ranch	2 tbsp	140
Original Ranch Dressing	2 tbsp	140
Classic Cheese Ranch	2 tbsp	130
Garden Vegetable Ranch	2 tbsp	130
Old Fashioned Buttermilk Ranch	2 tbsp	130
Cracked Peppercorn Ranch	2 tbsp	120
Original Ranch Light	2 tbsp	80
Buttermilk Ranch Light	2 tbsp	70
Original Ranch Fat Free	2 tbsp	30

Hidden Valley® Farm House Dressing	Amount	Calories
Creamy Parmesan	2 tbsp	130
Garden Tomato & Bacon	2 tbsp	130
Original Caesar	2 tbsp	120
Roasted Onion Parmesan	2 tbsp	120
Savory Bleu Cheese	2 tbsp	120
Hickory Bacon & Onion	2 tbsp	110
Creamy Balsamic with Herb	2 tbsp	100
Dijon Mustard Vinaigrette	2 tbsp	100
Homestyle Italian	2 tbsp	100
Southwest Chipotle	2 tbsp	100
Original Italian with Herb	2 tbsp	80
Pomegranate Vinaigrette	2 tbsp	60

Ken's® Steak House Dressing	Amount	Calories
Buttermilk Ranch Dressing	2 tbsp	180
Pepper Corn Ranch	2 tbsp	180
Caesar Dressing	2 tbsp	170

CALORIES

Continued

	Amount	Calories
Creamy Caesar	2 tbsp	170
Italian Marinade	2 tbsp	160
Chunky Bluecheese	2 tbsp	150
Russian Dressing	2 tbsp	150
Ranch Dressing	2 tbsp	140
Thousand Island	2 tbsp	140
Creamy Italian	2 tbsp	130
Honey Mustard	2 tbsp	130
Italian & Aged Romano	2 tbsp	120
Red Wine Vinegar Oil	2 tbsp	120
3 Cheese Italian	2 tbsp	120
Greek & Olive Oil	2 tbsp	100
Balsamic Vinaigrete	2 tbsp	100
Zesty Italian	2 tbsp	90
Italian with Olive Oil	2 tbsp	90
Balsamic & Honey	2 tbsp	90
Sweet Vidalia Onion	2 tbsp	80
Northern Italian Basil & Romano	2 tbsp	45

Kens® Lite Dressing	Amount	Calories
Creamy Caesar	2 tbsp	90
Blue Cheese	2 tbsp	80
Chunky Blue Cheese	2 tbsp	80
Ranch Dressing	2 tbsp	80
Raspberry & Walnut Vinaigrette	2 tbsp	80
Sweet Vidalia Onion	2 tbsp	80
Asian Sesame Ginger & Soy	2 tbsp	70
Caesar	2 tbsp	70
Thousand Island	2 tbsp	70
Zesty Italian	2 tbsp	45

Kraft® Dressing	Amount	Calories
Ranch with Backon	2 tbsp	150
Creamy French Dressing	2 tbsp	140
Classic Caesar Dressing	2 tbsp	130
Green Goddnes	2 tbsp	130
Thousand Island	2 tbsp	130
Buttermilk Ranch	2 tbsp	120
Creamy Poppyseed	2 tbsp	120
Cucumber Ranch	2 tbsp	120
Peppercorn Ranch	2 tbsp	120
Roka Blue Cheese	2 tbsp	120
Coleslaw Dressing	2 tbsp	110
Ranch	2 tbsp	110
Sweet Honey Catalina	2 tbsp	110

CALORIES

Creamy Italian	2 tbsp	100
Classic Catalina	2 tbsp	90
Sweet Balsamic Vinaigrette Dressing	2 tbsp	80
Lite Ranch	2 tbsp	70
Zesty Italian Anything Dressing	2 tbsp	70
Zesty Italian Dressing & Marinad	2 tbsp	70
Light Thousand Island	2 tbsp	60
Catalina Fat Free	2 tbsp	50
Fat Free Ranch	2 tbsp	50
Free Thousand Island	2 tbsp	45
Light Zesty Italian	2 tbsp	25

Litehouse® Dressing	Amount	Calories
Big Bleu Dressing	2 tbsp	160
Chunky Bleu Cheese	2 tbsp	150
Chunky Garlic Caesar	2 tbsp	150
Original Bleu Cheese	2 tbsp	150
Ceaser-Caesar Dressing	2 tbsp	140
Ceaser Dressing	2 tbsp	130
Honey Mustard	2 tbsp	130
Organic Ranch	2 tbsp	130
Buttermilk Ranch	2 tbsp	120
Homestyle Ranch	2 tbsp	120
Jalapeno Ranch	2 tbsp	120
Original Thousand Island	2 tbsp	120
Ranch Dressing	2 tbsp	120
Barbecue Ranch	2 tbsp	110
Coleslaw Dressing	2 tbsp	110
Creamy Cilantro	2 tbsp	110
Coleslaw with Pinapple	2 tbsp	100
Parmesan Caesar	2 tbsp	100
Sweet French	2 tbsp	90
Yogurt Bleu Cheese with Kefir	2 tbsp	80
Spinach	2 tbsp	70
Yogurt Ranch with Kefir	2 tbsp	60
Pear Gorzonzola Dressing	2 tbsp	50
Sesame Ginger	2 tbsp	40
Harvest Cranberry Greek	2 tbsp	25

Litehouse Lite Dressing	Amount	Calories
Bleu Cheese Dressing	2 tbsp	80
1000 Island Dressing	2 tbsp	70
Caesar Dressing	2 tbsp	70
Coleslaw Dressing	2 tbsp	70
Creamy Ranch Dressing	2 tbsp	70

CALORIES

Continued

Honey Dijon Vinaigrette	2 tbsp	70
Jalapeno Ranch Dressing	2 tbsp	70
Ranch Dressing	2 tbsp	60

Litehouse Vinaigrette Dressing	Amount	Calories
Balsamic Vinaigrette	2 tbsp	100
Raspberry Walnut Vinaigrette	2 tbsp	100
Fuji Apple Vinaigrette	2 tbsp	90
Red Wine Olive Oil Vinaigrette	2 tbsp	90
White Balsamic Vinaigrette	2 tbsp	90
Bleu Cheese Vinaigrette	2 tbsp	80
Organic Balsamic Vinaigrette	2 tbsp	80
Cherry Vinaigrette	2 tbsp	70
Zesty Italian Vinaigrette	2 tbsp	60
Greek Vinaigrette	2 tbsp	50
Harvest Cranberry Vinaigrette	2 tbsp	25
Huckleberry Vinaigrette	2 tbsp	25
Pomegranate Blueberry Vinaigrette	2 tbsp	25

Maries Dressing	Amount	Calories
Creamy Italian Garlic	2 tbsp	180
Caesar	2 tbsp	170
Creamy Chipotle Ranch	2 tbsp	170
Creamy Ranch	2 tbsp	170
Asiago Peppercorn	2 tbsp	160
Chunky Blue Cheese	2 tbsp	160
Jalapeno Ranch	2 tbsp	160
Super Blue Cheese	2 tbsp	160
Buttermilk Ranch	2 tbsp	150
Poppy Seed	2 tbsp	150
Thousand Island	2 tbsp	150
Coleslaw	2 tbsp	140
Honey Mustard	2 tbsp	140
Honey Dijon	2 tbsp	130
Blue Cheese Vinaigrette	2 tbsp	120
Creamy Caesar	2 tbsp	120
Greek Vinaigrette	2 tbsp	110
Sesame Ginger	2 tbsp	100
Yogurt Coleslaw	2 tbsp	90
Italian Vinaigrette	2 tbsp	80
Yogurt Thousand Island	2 tbsp	80
Lite Chunky Blue Cheese	2 tbsp	70
Yogurt Blue Cheese	2 tbsp	70
Yogurt Ranch	2 tbsp	70
Lite Creamy Ranch	2 tbsp	60

CALORIES

Continued

Red Wine Vinaigrette	2 tbsp	60
Spinach Salad with Bacon	2 tbsp	60
Balsamic Vinaigrette	2 tbsp	50
Raspberry Vinaigrette	2 tbsp	50

Newman's® Own Dressing	Amount	Calories
Creamy Ceasar	2 tbsp	170
Ranch Dressing	2 tbsp	150
Caesar Dressing	2 tbsp	150
Olive Oil & Vinegar	2 tbsp	150
Poppy Seed	2 tbsp	140
Family Italian	2 tbsp	130
Honey French	2 tbsp	130
Creamy Balsamic	2 tbsp	110
Parmesan & Garlic	2 tbsp	110
3 Cheese Balsamic	2 tbsp	110
Greek Vinaigrette	2 tbsp	100
Balsamic Vinaigrette	2 tbsp	90
Orange Ginger	2 tbsp	80

Organic Ville Dressing	Amount	Calories
Non Dairy Ranch	2 tbsp	110
Olive Oil & Balsamic Vinaigrette	2 tbsp	100
Miso Ginger Vinaigrette	2 tbsp	100
Herbs De Provence Vinaigrette	2 tbsp	100
Orange Cranberry Vinaigrette	2 tbsp	100
Sesame Tamari Vinaigrette	2 tbsp	90
Non Dairy Thousand island	2 tbsp	80
French	2 tbsp	80
Non Dairy Coleslaw	2 tbsp	70
Sun Dried Tomato Garlic Vinaigrette	2 tbsp	70
Pomegranate Vinaigrette	2 tbsp	70
Non Dairy Caesar	2 tbsp	60
Dijon Vinaigrette	2 tbsp	60

Walden Farm's Dressing	Amount	Calories
Asian	2 tbsp	0
Bacon Ranch	2 tbsp	0
Balsamic Vinaigrette	2 tbsp	0
Bleu Cheese Dressing	2 tbsp	0
Buttermilk Ranch Dressing	2 tbsp	0
Caesar Dressing	2 tbsp	0
Chipotle Ranch Dressing	2 tbsp	0
Colesaw	2 tbsp	0

CALORIES

Continued

Creamy Bacon	2 tbsp	0
Creamy Italian	2 tbsp	0
French Dressing	2 tbsp	0
Honey Dijon Dressing	2 tbsp	0
Italian	2 tbsp	0
Italian Sun Dried Tomato	2 tbsp	0
Jersey Sweet Onion	2 tbsp	0
Ranch	2 tbsp	0
Raspberry Vinaigrette	2 tbsp	0
Russian	2 tbsp	0
Sesame Ginger Dressing	2 tbsp	0
Sweet Onion	2 tbsp	0
Thousand Island Dressing	2 tbsp	0
Zesty Italian	2 tbsp	0

Wish Bone® Creamy Dressing	Amount	Calories
Creamy Caesar	2 tbsp	180
Chunky Blue Cheese	2 tbsp	150
Sweet & Spicy French	2 tbsp	140
Ranch Dressing	2 tbsp	130
Thousand Island Dressing	2 tbsp	130
Delux French	2 tbsp	120
Creamy Italian Dressing	2 tbsp	110
Russian	2 tbsp	110
Light Blue Cheese	2 tbsp	70
Light Creamy Caesar	2 tbsp	70
Light Delux French	2 tbsp	70
Light Ranch Dressing	2 tbsp	70
Light Parmesan Peppercorn Ranch	2 tbsp	60
Light Sweet & Spicy French	2 tbsp	60
Light Thousand Island	2 tbsp	60
Fat Free Chunky Blue Cheese	2 tbsp	30
Fat Free Ranch Dressing	2 tbsp	30

Wish Bone® Oil & Vinegar Dressing	Amount	Calories
House Italian Dressing	2 tbsp	110
Italian Dressing	2 tbsp	80
Light Raspberry Walnut	2 tbsp	80
Raspberrt Hazelnut Vinaigrette	2 tbsp	80
Raspberrt Walnut Vinaigrette	2 tbsp	80
Robusto Italian	2 tbsp	80
Balsamic Italian Vinaigrette	2 tbsp	70
Light Asian Sesame & Ginger	2 tbsp	70
Light Honey Dijon	2 tbsp	70
Red Wine Vinaigrette	2 tbsp	70

CALORIES

Continued

Superfruit Vinaigrette	2 tbsp	70
Balsamic Vinaigrette	2 tbsp	60
Bruschetta Italian	2 tbsp	60
Greek Vinaigrette	2 tbsp	60
Light Balsamic & Basil Vinaigrette	2 tbsp	60
Mediterranean Italian	2 tbsp	60
Olive Oil Vinaigrette	2 tbsp	60
Romano Basil Vinaigrette	2 tbsp	60
Fat Free Red Wine Vinaigrette	2 tbsp	35
Light Italian Dressing	2 tbsp	35
Fat Free Italian Dressing	2 tbsp	15

Turkey, Cooked	Amount	Calories
Turkey bacon	3 oz	325
Ground turkey, 85% lean	3 oz	212
Ground turkey, 93% lean	3 oz	176
Ground turkey	3 oz	173
Turkey sausage, reduced fat	3 oz	173
Turkey liver	3 ox	161
Dark meat	3 oz	147
Light meat	3 oz	125
Ground turkey, fat free	3 oz	117
Breast meat	3 oz	115

Veal, Cooked	Amount	Calories
Rib	3 oz	194
Breast	3 oz	185
Loin	3 oz	184
Leg, top round	3 oz	179
Sirloin	3 oz	172
Foreshank	3 oz	162
Ground	3 oz	146

Vegetables, Canned	Amount	Calories
Tomato paste	1 cup	215
Sweet potato	1 cup	211
Yellow sweet corn	1 cup	165
Green peas, drained	1 cup	117
Tomato pure	1 cup	95
Pumpkin	1 cup	83
Stewed tomatoes	1 cup	66
Spinach, Del Monte	1 cup	60
Tomato sauce	1 cup	59
Beets	1 cup	53

CALORIES

Spinach, drained	1 cup	49
Asparagus	1 cup	46
Sauerkraut	1 cup	45
Tomatoes	1 cup	41
Mushrooms	1 cup	39
Carrots	1 cup	37
Green beans	1 cup	31

Vegetables, Cooked	Amount	Calories
Sweet potato, mashed	1 cup	249
Potatoes, mashed with whole milk & butter	1 cup	237
Split peas	1 cup	231
Taro	1 cup	187
Yams, cubed	1 cup	158
Corn	1 cup	143
Acorn squash	1 cup	115
Potatoes, flesh, baked	1 cup	113
Parsnips	1 cup	110
Hubbard squash	1 cup	102
Onions	1 cup	92
Artichokes	1 cup	89
Butternut squash	1 cup	82
Shitake mushrooms	1 cup	81
Winter squash	1 cup	76
Beets	1 cup	75
Snow peas	1 cup	67
Rutabagas, cubes	1 cup	66
Brussels sprouts	1 cup	56
Broccoli	1 cup	55
Carrots, sliced	1 cup	55
Collard greens	1 cup	49
Pumpkin, mashed	1 cup	49
Kohlrabi	1 cup	48
Green beans	1 cup	44
White mushrooms	1 cup	44
Tomatoes, red, ripe	1 cup	43
Spaghetti winter squash	1 cup	42
Spinach	1 cup	41
Asparagus	1 cup	40
Beet greens	1 cup	39
Kale	1 cup	36
Summer squash	1 cup	36
Dandelion greens	1 cup	35
Eggplant	1 cup	35
Okra	1 cup	35

CALORIES

Swiss chard	1 cup	35
Cabbage, shredded	1 cup	34
Crookneck or Straighneck Squash, slices	1 cup	34
Turnips, cubes	1 cup	34
Leeks, chopped	1 cup	32
Scallop or Pattypan Squash, slices	1 cup	29
Turnip greens	1 cup	29
Broccoli, raab	1 cup	28
Cauliflower	1 cup	28
Celery, diced	1 cup	27
Zucchini	1 cup	27
Cactus pad, nopales	1 cup	22
Mustard greens	1 cup	21
Cabbage, Chinese Bok-Choy	1 cup	20
Broccolini	1 cup	19
Cabbage, Napa	1 cup	13

Vegetables, Frozen	Amount	Calories
Rhubarb	1 cup	278
Yellow sweet corn	1 cup	132
Green peas	1 cup	125
Brussels sprouts	1 cup	65
Spinach	1 cup	65
Collard greens	1 cup	61
Carrots	1 cup	54
Okra	1 cup	53
Broccoli	1 cup	52
Turnip greens	1 cup	47
Kale	1 cup	39
Green beans	1 cup	38
Cauliflower	1 cup	34
Asparagus	1 cup	32

Vegetables, Raw	Amount	Calories
Onions, chopped	1 cup	64
Butternut squash, cubes	1 cup	63
Carrots, sliced	1 cup	50
Red bell peppers, chopped	1 cup	46
Tomatillos, chopped	1 cup	42
Snow peas, chopped	1 cup	42
Yellow bell peppers	1 cup	41
Kale, chopped	1 cup	40
Mustard spinach	1 cup	34
Green onions & scallions, chopped	1 cup	33
Tomatoes, chopped	1 cup	32

CALORIES

Broccoli, chopped	1 cup	30
Green bell peppers, chopped	1 cup	30
Oyster mushrooms, sliced	1 cup	28
Cauliflower, chopped	1 cup	27
Tomatoes, cherry	1 cup	27
Dandelion greens	1 cup	25
Enoki mushrooms, sliced	1 cup	24
Cabbage, Red	1 cup	22
Spirulina, dried	1 tbsp	20
Cabbage, Savoy	1 cup	19
Celery, chopped	1 cup	19
Portabella mushrooms, diced	1 cup	19
Zucchini, sliced	1 cup	19
Cabbage, shredded	1 cup	18
Summer squash, sliced	1 cup	18
Crimini mushrooms, sliced	1 cup	16
Cucumbers, slices	1 cup	16
Belgian endive	1 cup	15
White mushrooms, sliced	1 cup	15
Cactus pads, nopales	1 cup	14
Shiitake mushrooms, dried	1 each	11
Romaine lettuce	1 cup	10
Broccoli, Raab	1 cup	9
Cabbage, Chinese Bok-Choy	1 cup	9
Radicchio	1 cup	9
Endive	1 cup	8
Green leaf lettuce	1 cup	8
Iceberg lettuce	1 cup	8
Butterhead, bibb or boston lettuce	1 cup	7
Chicory greens, chopped	1 cup	7
Spinach	1 cup	7
Swiss chard	1 cup	7
Shiitake mushrooms	1 whole	6
Arugula	1 cup	5
Red leaf lettuce	1 cup	4
Watercress	1 cup	4

Nutrient Data Collection Form

Food	Amount	Book Numbers	Multiply By	Estimated Nutrient Intake
Nutrient::	RDA:	Estimated:	% of RDA:	Total Estimated:

To download additional forms for free, go to www.TopNutrients4U.com

CARBOHYDRATES

Current trends in health emphasize controlling intake of carbohydrates. A high and refined carbohydrate diet is associated with type 2 diabetes, heart disease, kidney disease, cataracts, cancer, and a fatty liver.

Carbohydrates are well recognized as the primary macronutrient responsible for creating a rapid rise in blood glucose after a meal. This rise in blood glucose evokes an equally intensive rise in insulin levels. High insulin levels leads to hypoglycemia, increased hunger, a craving for more carbohydrates, a clinically relevant weight gain, and type 2 diabetes.

To minimize the elevated spikes in blood glucose, restricting intake of carbohydrates is a must for most individuals. In one experiment, two groups consumed different amounts of carbohydrates but equal amounts vegetables, calories, fat, and fiber. When bread, rice, pasta, and cereals were replaced with meats, eggs, dairy, and nuts the group consuming 30% of calories from carbohydrates compared to 55% did experience lower levels of blood glucose after a meal and an improvement in insulin metabolism. Many studies confirm reducing the calorie intake from carbohydrates improves the metabolism of glucose and insulin.

The glycemic index and glycemic load commonly discussed in many well-written books does represent the quantity and quality of a particular food's carbohydrate content and is successful at helping individuals lose weight and body fat. Fortunately, since the index and load are dependent on carbohydrate concentrations, an overall carbohydrate restricted diet will automatically tend to have a lower glycemic load and index effect.

In summary, consuming a low intake of carbohydrates is associated with increases in the body's ability to burn body fat while maintaining muscle, reduces a craving for more carbohydrates, reduces hunger, lowers blood triglycerides, minimizes elevated spikes of blood sugar and insulin after a meal, and reduces the risk of developing type-2 diabetes. This chapter lists carbohydrate intake in grams (g).

CARBOHYDRATES

Alcohol	Amount	Carbohydrate (g)
Regular Beer	1 bottle	12.6
Light Beer	1 bottle	5.8
Red Wine	1 glass	3.8
White Wine	1 glass	3.8
Gin, Rum, Vodka, Whisky	1 shot	0

Beans, Canned	Amount	Carbohydrate (g)
White beans	1 cup	56
Great Northern	1 cup	55
Baked beans, plain	1 cup	54
Navy beans	1 cup	54
Cranberry beans	1 cup	39
Kidney beans	1 cup	38
Lima beans	1 cup	36
Pinto beans	1 cup	36
Refried beans	1 cup	36
Blackeyed peas	1 cup	33
Fava beans	1 cup	32
Garbanzo beans	1 cup	32
Green beans	1 cup	7
Yellow beans	1 cup	7

Beans, Cooked	Amount	Carbohydrate (g)
Adzuki	1 cup	57
Navy beans	1 cup	47
White beans, small	1 cup	46
Yardlong beans, Chinese long beans	1 cup	46
Black Turtle beans, mature	1 cup	45
Garbanzo beans	1 cup	45
Pinto beans	1 cup	45
White beans, mature	1 cup	45
Cranberry beans	1 cup	43
Black beans	1 cup	41
Split peas	1 cup	41
Hyacinth beans	1 cup	40
Kidney beans	1 cup	40
Lentils	1 cup	40
Lima beans	1 cup	39
Mung beans, mature seeds	1 cup	39
Pigeon peas	1 cup	39
Great Northern	1 cup	37
Mothbeans	1 cup	37
Black-eyed peas	1 cup	36

CARBOHYDRATES

Continued

Fava beans	1 cup	33
Soybeans, dry roasted	1 cup	30
Winged beans	1 cup	26
Natto	1 cup	25
Soybeans, green	1 cup	20
Soybeans, mature	1 cup	17
Lupins	1 cup	16
Edamame	1 cup	15
Green beans	1 cup	10
Yellow beans	1 cup	10

Beef	Amount	Carbohydrate (g)
All types	3 oz	0

Bread	Amount	Carbohydrate (g)
Bagel, oat bran	4" bagel	56
Mexican roll, billilo	1 roll	55
Bagel, cinnamon-raisin	4" bagel	49
Indian bread, Naan, whole wheat	1 piece	49
Bagel, wheat	4" bagel	48
Bagel, egg	4" bagel	47
Bagel, plain	4" bagel	45
Indian bread, Naan, plain	1 piece	45
Pita, white	6 inch pita	33
Kaiser rolls	1 roll	30
Cornbread, dry mix, prepared	1 piece	29
Croissants, butter	1 each	26
English Muffin, plain	1 muffin	25
Hamburger & Hotdog buns, plain	1 bun	21
Egg bread	1 slice	19
Tortillas, flour	1 tortillas	16
Italian bread, Oroweat Premium	1 slice	15
Potato bread	1 slice	15
Pumpernickle	1 slice	15
Rye bread	1 slice	15
Dinner Rolls, brown & serve	1 roll	14
French, sourdough	1 slice	14
White bread	1 slice	14
Oatmeal bread	1 slice	13
Raisen bread	1 slice	13
Cracked wheat	1 slice	12
Wheat bread	1 slice	12
Whole-Wheat	1 slice	12
Multi-Grain, includes Whole-Grain	1 slice	11
Tortillas, corn	1 tortillas	11

CARBOHYDRATES

Cereal, Albertsons® Brand	Amount	Carbohydrate (g)
Nutty Nuggets	1 cup	96
Low Fat Granola, Raisin & Almond	1 cup	68
Low Fat Granola & Almonds	1 cup	67
Muesli, Raisin, Dates, Almond	1 cup	62
Raisin Bran	1 cup	46
Raisin Bran Crunch Granola	1 cup	44
Frosted Flakes	1 cup	36
Honey Oats & Flakes with Strawberry	1 cup	35
Cocoa Comets	1 cup	34
Cocoa Crispy Rice	1 cup	34
Crunchy Oat Squares	1 cup	34
Honey Gram Crunch	1 cup	33
Honey Oats & Flakes	1 cup	33
Cinni-Mini Crunches	1 cup	32
Golden Wheat Puffs	1 cup	32
Wheat Bran Flakes	1 cup	32
Apple Crunchies	1 cup	30
Honey Nut Toasted Oats	1 cup	29
Corn Flakes	1 cup	28
Frosted Fruit O's	1 cup	28
Golden Corn Nuggets	1 cup	28
Good Day with Strawberry	1 cup	27
Crispy Crunchy Berry	1 cup	26
Crispy Rice	1 cup	23
Crunch Rice Squares	1 cup	23
Multigrain	1 cup	23
Toasted Oats	1 cup	21

Arrowhead Mills®	Amount	Carbohydrate (g)
Sweetened Shredded Wheat	1 cup	43
Sweetened Rice Flakes	1 cup	40
Shredded Wheat, Bite-Size	1 cup	38
Maple Buckwheat Flakes	1 cup	35
Amaranth Flakes	1 cup	26
Sprouted Multigrain Flakes	1 cup	26
Kamut Flakes	1 cup	25
Sprouted Corn Flakes	1 cup	25
Oat Bran Flakes	1 cup	24
Spelt Flakes	1 cup	24
Sprouted Wheat Bran & Quinoa	1 cup	22

CARBOHYDRATES

Barbara's™	Amount	Carbohydrate (g)
High Fiber Original	1 cup	43
Shredded Minis Blueberry Burst	1 cup	43
Shredded Oats Cinnamon Crunch	1 cup	43
High Fiber Cranberry	1 cup	42
High Fiber Flax & Granola	1 cup	42
Shredded Oats Vanilla Almond	1 cup	42
Puffins Cinnamon	1 cup	39
Shredded Oats Original	1 cup	37
Puffins Puffs Fruit Medley	1 cup	35
Brown Rice Crisps	1 cup	33
Corn Flakes	1 cup	33
Puffins Honey Rice	1 cup	33
Puffins Multigrain	1 cup	33
Hole 'n Oats Honey Nut	1 cup	32
Puffins Peanut Butter & Chocolate	1 cup	32
Puffins Puffs Crunchy Cocoa	1 cup	32
Shredded Spoonfuls Multigrain	1 cup	32
Shredded Wheat	2 biscuits	31
Puffins Original	1 cup	31
Puffins Peanut Butter	1 cup	31
Hole 'n Oats: Fruit Juice Sweetened	1 cup	29

Bear Naked®	Amount	Carbohydrate (g)
Banana Nut Granola	1 cup	72
Fruit & Nut Ganola	1 cup	72
Nut Cluster Crunch Cereal	1 cup	47
Original Granola, Peak Protein	1 cup	60
Vanila Almond Crucnh Granola	1 cup	88

Cascadian Farm™	Amount	Carbohydrate (g)
Cinnamon Raisin Granola	1 cup	64
Maple Brown Sugar Granola	1 cup	64
Oats & Honey Granola	1 cup	64
Hearty Morning	1 cup	59
Dark Chocolate Almond Granola	1 cup	52
French Vanilla Almond Granola	1 cup	51
Fruit & Nut Granola	1 cup	51
Raisin bran	1 cup	41
Multi Gain Squares	1 cup	33
Purely O's	1 cup	33
Chocolate O's	1 cup	31
Fruit Ful O's	1 cup	31
Honey Nut O's	1 cup	25
Cinnamon Crunch	1 cup	22

CARBOHYDRATES

Erewhon®	Amount	Carbohydrate (g)
Cocoa Crispy Brown Rice	1 cup	44
Corn Flakes	1 cup	40
Raisin Bran	1 cup	40
Brown Rice, Strawberry Crisp	1 cup	37
Rice Twice	1 cup	35
Crispy Brown Rice, Mixed Berries	1 cup	27
Crispy Brown Rice, Gluten Free	1 cup	25
Crispy Brown Rice, No Salt Added	1 cup	25
Crispy Brown Rice, Original	1 cup	25

Ezekiel 4:9	Amount	Carbohydrate (g)
Cinnamon Flax	1 cup	82
Original	1 cup	82
Almond	1 cup	76
Golden Flax	1 cup	74

Cereal, General Mills®	Amount	Carbohydrate (g)
Multi-Bran CHEX	1 cup	52
Raisin Nut Bran	1 cup	52
Wheat Chex	1 cup	52
Honey Nut Clusters	1 cup	48
Oatmeal Crisp, Hearty Raisin	1 cup	46
Basic 4	1 cup	44
Oatmeal Crisp, Crunchy Almond	1 cup	43
Total Raisin Bran	1 cup	42
Honey Nut Chex	1 cup	37
Total Cranberry Crunch	1 cup	36
Golden Gram	1 cup	35
Chocolate Chex	1 cup	34
Cinnamon Chex	1 cup	33
Cinnamon Toast Crunch	1 cup	33
Total Whole Grain	1 cup	31
Cocoa Puffs	1 cup	30
Dora The Explorer	1 cup	30
Cookie Crisp	1 cup	29
Lucky Charms	1 cup	29
Reese's Puffs	1 cup	29
Wheaties	1 cup	29
Trix	1 cup	27
Corn Chex	1 cup	26
Rice Chex	1 cup	23
Berry Berry Kix	1 cup	22
Kix	1 cup	20

CARBOHYDRATES

General Mills® Cheerios®	Amount	Carbohydrate (g)
Yogurt Burst, Strawberry	1 cup	33
Apple Cinnamon	1 cup	32
Banana Nut	1 cup	31
Frosted	1 cup	31
Multi Grain Peanut Butter	1 cup	31
Chocolate	1 cup	30
Fruity	1 cup	30
Berry Burst	1 cup	29
Crunch, Oat Clusters	1 cup	29
Dulce de leche	1 cup	29
Honey Nut	1 cup	29
Cinnamon Burst	1 cup	27
Multi Grain	1 cup	23
Original	1 cup	20

General Mills® Fiber-One®	Amount	Carbohydrate (g)
Original Bran	1 cup	50
Frosted Shredded Wheat	1 cup	49
Raisin Bran Clusters	1 cup	47
Honey Clusters	1 cup	44
Nuty Clusters & Almonds	1 cup	44
Caramel Delight	1 cup	41
80 Calorie Honey Squares	1 cup	33

Glutino®	Amount	Carbohydrate (g)
Apple & Cinnamon Rings	1 cup	52
Honey Nut Cereal	1 cup	52
Frosted Corn & Rice Flakes	1 cup	28
Berry Sensible Beginning	1 cup	27
Corn Rice Flakes	1 cup	27
Corn Rice Flakes with Strawberries	1 cup	27

Health Valley®	Amount	Carbohydrate (g)
Oat Bran Almond Crunch	1 cup	68
Low Fat Date & Almond Flavored Granola	1 cup	56
Low Fat Raisin Cinnamon Granola	1 cup	56
Cranberry Crunch	1 cup	51
Oat Bran Flakes & Raisins	1 cup	43
Oat Bran Flakes	1 cup	39
Fiber 7	1 cup	37
Golden Flax	1 cup	37
Heart Wise	1 cup	37
Multigrain Apple Cinnamon Squares	1 cup	35

CARBOHYDRATES

Continued

Multigrain Maple, Honey, Nut Squares	1 cup	35
Amaranth Flakes	1 cup	34
Corn Crunch-EMS	1 cup	27
Rice Crunch-EMS	1 cup	21

Kashi®	Amount	Carbohydrate (g)
7-Whole Grain Nuggets	1 cup	94
Go Lean Crisp, Toasted Berry Crumble	1 cup	46
Strawberry Fields	1 cup	46
Go Lean Crisp, Cinnamon Crumble	1 cup	45
Heart to Heart, Oat Flakes & Blueberry Clusters	1 cup	44
Island Vanilla	27 biscuits	44
Autum Wheat	29 biscuits	43
Cinnamon Harvest	28 biscuits	43
Good Friends	1 cup	42
Berry Fruitful	29 biscuits	42
Blackberry Hills	1 cup	41
7-Whole Grain Flakes	1 cup	41
Go Lean Crunch	1 cup	38
Go Lean Vanilla Graham	1 cup	36
Go Lean	1 cup	35
Go Lean Crunch, Honey Almond Flax	1 cup	35
Heart to Heart, Honey Toasted Oat	1 cup	34
Heart to Heart, Warm Cinnamon	1 cup	34
Honey Sunshine	1 cup	34
Berry Blossom	1 cup	33
Heart to Heart, Nutty Chia Flax	1 cup	32
Simply Maize	1 cup	30
Indigo morning	1 cup	29
7-Whole Grain Honey Puffs	1 cup	25
7-Whole Grain Puffs	1 cup	15

Kellogg's®	Amount	Carbohydrate (g)
All-Bran Bran Buds	1 cup	72
MUESLIX	1 cup	60
Cracklin' Oat Bran	1 cup	47
All-Bran Original	1 cup	46
Raisin Bran	1 cup	46
Raisin Bran Crunch	1 cup	45
Raisin Bran with Flaxseeds	1 cup	44
Fiberplus Berry Yogurt Crunch	1 cup	43
Smart Start, Strong Heart Antioxidants	1 cup	43
Frosted MINI-Wheats, Big Bite	1 cup	42
Frosted Rice Krispies	1 cup	36
Cocoa Krispies	1 cup	35

CARBOHYDRATES

Continued

Fiberplus Cinnamon Oat Crunch	1 cup	35
Frosted Flakes	1 cup	35
Crunchy Nut Golden Honey Nut Flakes	1 cup	34
Honey Crunch Corn Flakes	1 cup	34
Rice Krispies Treats	1 cup	34
Honey Smacks	1 cup	32
Krave Chocolate	1 cup	32
All-Bran Complete Wheat Flakes	1 cup	31
Crunchy Nut Roasted Nut & Honey O's	1 cup	30
Corn Pops	1 cup	29
Apple Jacks	1 cup	26
Cinnabon	1 cup	25
Crispix	1 cup	25
Froot Loops	1 cup	25
Product 19	1 cup	25
Smorz	1 cup	25
Corn Flakes	1 cup	24
Rice Krispies	1 cup	24

Kellogg's Special-K®	Amount	Carbohydrate (g)
Low Fat Granola	1 cup	78
Multigrain Oats & Honey	1 cup	37
Fruit & Yogurt	1 cup	36
Blueberry	1 cup	34
Chocolately Delight	1 cup	33
Vanilla Almond	1 cup	33
Cinnamon Pecan	1 cup	32
Red Berries	1 cup	27
Original	1 cup	23
Protein Plus	1 cup	18

Mom's Best® Natural	Amount	Carbohydrate (g)
Raisin Bran	1 cup	49
Blue Pom Wheat Fuls	1 cup	45
Sweetened Wheat Fuls	1 cup	45
Toasted Wheat Fuls	1 cup	44
Crispy Coco Rice	1 cup	33
Honey Ful Wheats	1 cup	33
Honey Grahams	1 cup	33
Oats & Honey Blend	1 cup	33
Toasted Cinnamon Squares	1 cup	32
Honey Nut Toasty O's	1 cup	24
Mallow Oats	1 cup	24

CARBOHYDRATES

Nature's Path®	Amount	Carbohydrate (g)
Heritage Crunch	1 cup	59
Flax Plus Raisin Bran Flakes	1 cup	55
Optimum Cranberry Ginger	1 cup	55
Flax Plus Pumpkin Raisin Crunch	1 cup	53
Acai Apple Granola	1 cup	52
Flax Plus Redberry Crunch	1 cup	52
Flax Plus Maple Pecan Crunch	1 cup	51
Optimum Power Blueberry Cinnamon	1 cup	51
Pomegran Cherry Granola	1 cup	51
Pomegran Plus Granola	1 cup	51
AGAVE Plus Granola	1 cup	49
Flax Plus Pumpkin Flax Granola	1 cup	49
Flax Plus Vanilla Almond Granola	1 cup	48
Hemp Plus Granola	1 cup	48
Smart Bran	1 cup	48
Optimum Banana Almond	1 cup	47
Peanut Butter Granola	1 cup	47
Optimum Slim Low Fat Vanilla	1 cup	40
Crunchy Maple Sunrise, Gluten Free	1 cup	38
Crunchy Vanilla Sunrise	1 cup	38
Whole O's	1 cup	38
Honeyed Corn Flakes, Gluten Free	1 cup	35
Heritage Flakes	1 cup	32
Heritage Heirloom Whole Grain	1 cup	32
Mesa Sunrise, Gluten Free	1 cup	32
Multigrain Oat bran	1 cup	32
Flax Plus Multibran Flakes	1 cup	31
OATY BITES Whole Grain	1 cup	31
Organic Millet Rice	1 cup	29

Peace Cereal®	Amount	Carbohydrate (g)
Cherry Almond Clusters & Flakes	1 cup	64
Golden Honey Granola	1 cup	61
Mango Peach Passion Clusters & Flakes	1 cup	46
Maple Pecan	1 cup	42
Vanilla Almond Clusters & Flakes	1 cup	42
Walnut Spice Clusters & Flakes	1 cup	61
Wild Berry Clusters & Flakes	1 cup	61

Post®	Amount	Carbohydrate (g)
Grape-Nuts Cereal	1 cup	93
100% Bran Cereal	1 cup	68
Great Grains, Cranberry Almond Crunch	1 cup	54

CARBOHYDRATES

Continued

Great Grains, Raisin, Date & Pecan	1 cup	53
Great Grains, Crunchy Pecan	1 cup	49
Honey Nut Shredded Wheat	1 cup	49
Raisin Bran	1 cup	46
Great Grains, Banana Nut Crunch	1 cup	44
Shredded Wheat, frosted, spoon-size	1 cup	44
Shredded Wheat, Original spoon-size	1 cup	40
Shredded Wheat n' Bran, spoon-size	1 cup	39
Blueberry Morning	1 cup	36
Shredded Wheat, Sugar and Salt Free	1 cup	36
Cocoa Pebbles	1 cup	34
Fruity Pebbles	1 cup	34
Golden Crisp	1 cup	33
Grape-Nuts Flakes	1 cup	32
OREO O's Cereal	1 cup	29
Honeycomb Cereal	1 cup	19

Post Honey Bunches of Oats®	Amount	Carbohydrate (g)
Just Bunches Honey Roasted	1 cup	65
Just Bunches Cinnamonn	1 cup	64
Vanilla Bunches	1 cup	46
Raisin Medley	1 cup	42
With Almonds	1 cup	35
With Peaches	1 cup	35
With Strawberries	1 cup	35
Honey Roasted	1 cup	33
With Cinnamon	1 cup	33
Pecan Bunches	1 cup	32

Quaker®	Amount	Carbohydrate (g)
Granola, Oats, Honey, Raisins, & Almonds	1 cup	76
Granola, Apple, Cranberry, & Almonds	1 cup	74
Granola, Oats, Honey, & Almonds	1 cup	70
Oatmeal Squares, Brown Sugar	1 cup	44
Oatmeal Squares, Cinnamon	1 cup	44
Oatmeal Squares, Golden Maple	1 cup	44
Oatmeal Squares, Honey Nut	1 cup	44
LIFE Cereal, Crunchtime Strawberry	1 cup	36
Toasted Multigrain Crisp	1 cup	34
LIFE Cereal, Cinnamon	1 cup	33
LIFE Cereal, Maple & Brown Sugar	1 cup	33
LIFE Cereal, Original	1 cup	33
CAP'N Crunch	1 cup	31
Honey Graham OH'S	1 cup	31
CAP'N Crunch with Crunchberries	1 cup	30

CARBOHYDRATES

Continued

Corn Bran Crunch	1 cup	30
Whole Hearts	1 cup	29
CAP'N Crunch's OOPS! All Berries	1 cup	28
CAP'N Crunch's Peanut Butter Crunch	1 cup	28
Puffed Wheat	1 cup	22
Puffed Rice	1 cup	12

Target® Brand Cereal	Amount	Carbohydrate (g)
Raisin Bran	1 cup	46
Frosted Shredded Wheat	1 cup	42
Sugar Frosted Flakes	1 cup	37
Cinnamon Oat Bites	1 cup	34
Honey & Oat Mixers with Almonds	1 cup	34
Honey & Oat Mixers	1 cup	33
Honey & Nut Toasted Oats	1 cup	32
Frosted Bites with Marshmallows	1 cup	30
Toasted Cinnamon Squares	1 cup	30
Corn Flakes	1 cup	28
Crispy Flakes with Red Berrys	1 cup	27
Toasted Oats	1 cup	23
Toasted Rice	1 cup	23

Trader Joe's® Brand Cereal	Amount	Carbohydrate (g)
Super Nutty Toffe Clusters	1 cup	50
Very Berry Clusters	1 cup	42
Organic Raisin Bran Clusters	1 cup	41
Banana Nut Clusters	1 cup	40
Maple Pecan Clusters	1 cup	40
Organic High Fiber O's	1 cup	35
High Fiber Cereal	1 cup	34
Bran Flakes*	1 cup	32
Frosted Flakes*	1 cup	32
Tosted Oatmeal Flakes	1 cup	30
Corn Flakes	1 cup	26
Crispy Rice	1 cup	26
MuitiGrain O's	1 cup	24
Fruity O's	1 cup	23
Puffed Wheat	1 cup	22
Joes O's	1 cup	20

CARBOHYDRATES

Uncle Sam®	Amount	Carbohydrate (g)
Wheat Berry & Flaxseed, Original	1 cup	51
Wheat Berry & Flaxseed, & Strawberry	1 cup	53
Wheat Berry & Flaxseed, Honey Almond	1 cup	49
Skinners Raisin Bran	1 cup	42

Wall Mart® Brand Cereal	Amount	Carbohydrate (g)
Toasted Wheat	1 cup	52
Raisin Bran	1 cup	45
Crunchy Raisin Bran	1 cup	44
Extra Raisin Raisin Bran	1 cup	43
Frosted Shredded Wheats	1 cup	42
Sugar Frosted Flakes	1 cup	37
Cruinchy Honey Oats & Almonds	1 cup	34
Cruinchy Honey Oats	1 cup	33
Honey Nut Spins	1 cup	33
Vanilla Almond Awake	1 cup	33
Cinnamon Crunch	1 cup	32
Berry Crunch	1 cup	30
Bran Flakes	1 cup	30
Apple Blast	1 cup	29
Toasted Corn	1 cup	26
Strawberry Awake	1 cup	25
Toasted Rice	1 cup	23
Toasted Whole-Grain Oats	1 cup	21

Whole Foods® 365 Brand Cereal	Amount	Carbohydrate (g)
Raisin Bran	1 cup	44
High Fiber Morning O's	1 cup	41
Wheat Squares	1 cup	38
Protein & Fiber	1 cup	36
Wheat Waffles	1 cup	33
Honey Flakes & Oat Clusters	1 cup	33
Cocoa Rice Crisps	1 cup	33
Bran Flakes	1 cup	32
Berry Flax Protein & Fiber Crunch	1 cup	32
Whole Wheat Flakes	1 cup	29
Corn Flakes	1 cup	27
Frosted Flakes	1 cup	27
Brown Rice Crisp	1 cup	25
Multi-Grain Morning O's	1 cup	24
Morning O's	1 cup	22
Crunchy Cinnamon Squares	1 cup	22

CARBOHYDRATES

Wild Harvest®	Amount	Carbohydrate (g)
Blueberry Flax Granola	1 cup	60
Cherry Vanilla Granola	1 cup	53
Cranberry Almond	1 cup	40
Crunchy Vanilla Almond Granola	1 cup	62
Golden Honey & Flax Granola	1 cup	60
Mango Crisp	1 cup	47
Maple Pecan Flakes & Clusters	1 cup	42
Wholesome Raisin Bran	1 cup	40
Wild Berry Crisp	1 cup	34

Cereal, Cooked	Amount	Carbohydrate (g)
White corn grits	1 cup	36
Yellow corn grits	1 cup	34
WHEATENA	1 cup	29
Oats, regular, unenriched	1 cup	28
CREAM OF WHEAT, regular	1 cup	26
Farina	1 cup	26
Malt-o-Meal plain	1 serving	23

Cheese	Amount	Carbohydrate (g)
American, pasteurized process, imitation	1 oz	4.59
Swiss	1 oz	1.53
Cream cheese, fat free	1 tbsp	1.38
American, pasteurized process, fortified	1 oz	1.36
Feta	1 oz	1.16
Cream cheese	1 oz	1.15
Parmesan, grated	1 oz	1.15
Pepper Jack, Red & Green Jalapenos	1 oz	1.00
Romano	1 oz	1.00
Muenster, low fat	1 oz	0.99
American, pasteurized process, low fat	1 oz	0.98
Provolone, reduced fat	1 oz	0.98
Colby	1 oz	0.95
Swiss, low fat	1 oz	0.95
Goat cheese, semisoft	1 oz	0.72
Blue cheese	1 oz	0.66
Gouda	1 oz	0.63
Goat cheese, hard	1 oz	0.62
Mozzarel, whole milk	1 oz	0.62
Provolone	1 oz	0.61
Roquefort	1 oz	0.57
Cheddar cheese, low fat	1 oz	0.54
Fotina	1 oz	0.44

CARBOHYDRATES

Cheddar cheese	1 oz	0.36
Muenster	1 oz	0.32
Goat cheese, soft	1 oz	0.25
Monterey, low fat	1 oz	0.20
Monterey	1 oz	0.19
Brie	1 oz	0.13
Gruyere	1 oz	0.10

Chicken	Amount	Carbohydrate (g)
All types	3 oz	0

Cream	Amount	Carbohydrate (g)
Sour Cream, cultured	1 tbsp	1.35
Half & Half	1 tbsp	0.65
Sour Cream, reduced Fat	1 tbsp	0.64
Light Coffe Cream	1 tbsp	0.55
Heavy Whipping	1 tbsp	0.42
Whipped Topping, pressurized	1 tbsp	0.37

Eggs	Amount	Carbohydrate (g)
Egg whites, dried	1 ounce	2.21
Egg substitute, liquid, fat free	1/4 cup	1.20
Egg whole, scrambled	1 large	0.98
Egg yolk	1 large	0.60
Egg whole, hard boiled	1 large	0.56
Egg whole, fried	1 large	0.38
Egg whole, poached	1 large	0.36
Egg whites, dried powder, stabilized	1 tbsp	0.31
Egg whites	1 large	0.24

Fish	Amount	Carbohydrate (g)
All types	3 oz	0

Fruit, Canned	Amount	Carbohydrate (g)
Plums	1 cup	60
Apricots	1 cup	55
Peaches	1 cup	52
Pears	1 cup	51
Pineapple	1 cup	51
Applesauce, sweetened	1 cup	45
Applesauce, unsweetened	1 cup	28
Olives, black	5 large	1.38
Olives, green	5 large	0.52

CARBOHYDRATES

Continued

Fruit, Dried	Amount	Carbohydrate (g)
Pears	1 cup	125
Currants	1 cup	107
Cranberries	1 cup	100
Peaches	1 cup	98
Figs	1 cup	95
Apricots	1 cup	81
Apples	1 cup	57

Fruit, Frozen	Amount	Carbohydrate (g)
Strawberries	1 cup	66
Raspberries	1 cup	65
Peaches	1 cup	60
Blueberries	1 cup	50
Blackberries, unsweetened	1 cup	24

Fruit, Raw	Amount	Carbohydrate (g)
Raisins	1 cup	114
Prunes, uncooked	1 cup	111
Dates	1 cup	110
Stewed prunes	1 cup	70
Plantains	1 cup	47
Pomegrenates	1 cup	33
Grapes, red or green	1 cup	29
Elderberries	1 cup	27
Kiwi	1 cup	26
Tangerine	1 cup	26
Cherries	1 cup	25
Grapefruit, pink & red, sections	1 cup	25
Mango	1 cup	25
Pears	1 cup	24
Pineapple	1 cup	22
Blueberries	1 cup	21
Florida Oranges	1 cup	21
Naval Oranges	1 cup	21
Valencias Oranges	1 cup	21
Avocado, California, pureed	1 cup	20
Plum	1 cup	19
Pummelo, sections	1 cup	18
Apricots	1 cup	18
Avocado, Florida	1 cup	18
Pomelo	1 cup	18
Apples	1 cup	17

CARBOHYDRATES

Continued

Black currants	1 cup	17
Papayas	1 cup	16
Peachs	1 cup	16
Honeydew	1 cup	15
Nectarine	1 cup	15
Raspberries	1 cup	15
Blackberries	1 cup	14
Mulberries	1 cup	14
Cataloupe	1 cup	13
Strawberries	1 cup	13
Cranberries, whole	1 cup	12
Oranges	1 cup	12
Jicama	1 cup	11
Water mellon	1 cup	11
Chayote, 1" pieces	1 cup	6

Fruit, Raw	Amount	Carbohydrate (g)
Pummelo	1 fruit	59
Plantains	1 fruit	57
Pomegranates	1 fruit	53
Mango	1 fruit	50
Cherimoya	1 fruit	42
Raisins	1 small box	34
Persimmons, Japanese	1 fruit	31
Prunes, uncooked	5 fruit	30
Bananas	1 fruit	27
Dates	5 fruit	27
Figs, dried	5 fruit	25
Pears	1 fruit	25
Avocado, Florida	1 fruit	24
Cantaloupe	1/2 fruit	23
Apples	1 fruit	19
Naval Oranges	1 fruit	18
Papayas,	1 small	17
Florida Oranges	1 fruit	16
Nectarine	1 fruit	14
Valencias Oranges	1 fruit	14
Cheeries	10 fruit	13
Grapefruit, pink & red	1/2 fruit	13
Avocado, California	1 fruit	12
Tangerine	1 fruit	11
Kiwi	1 fruit	10
Peaches	1 fruit	9
Chayote	1 fruit	9
Grapes, red or green	10 fruit	9

CARBOHYDRATES

Continued

Persimmons, small native	1 fruit	8
Plums	1 fruit	8
Pineapple, slices	1/2" x 3"	7
Star fruit, Carambola	1 medium	6
Strawberries	5 fruit	5
Apricots	1 fruit	4
Pineapple guava, Feijoa	1 medium	4
Kumquats	1 fruit	3
Olives, Black	5 large	2
Olives, Green	5 large	1

Game Meat, Cooked	Amount	Carbohydrate (g)
All types	3 oz	0

Grains, Cooked	Amount	Carbohydrate (g)
Kamut	1 cup	52
Spelt	1 cup	51
Amaranth	1 cup	46
White rice, enriched	1 cup	46
Brown rice, long grain	1 cup	45
White rice, regular	1 cup	45
Barley, pearled	1 cup	44
Macaroni	1 cup	43
Rice noodles	1 cup	43
Spaghetti	1 cup	43
Millet	1 cup	41
White rice, instant	1 cup	41
Egg noodles	1 cup	40
Quinoa	1 cup	39
Egg & Spinach noodles	1 cup	38
Macaroni, Whole-Wheat	1 cup	37
Spaghetti, Whole-Wheat	1 cup	37
Spaghetti, spinach	1 cup	37
Couscous	1 cup	36
Wild rice	1 cup	35
Buckwheat	1 cup	33
Bulgur	1 cup	33
Oat bran	1 cup	25
Soba noodles	1 cup	24

Juice	Amount	Carbohydrate (g)
Prune	1 cup	45
Grape juice	1 cup	37
Cranberry juice cocktail	1 cup	34

CARBOHYDRATES

Continued

Pomegranate	1 cup	33
Pineapple	1 cup	32
Apple juice	1 cup	28
Orange juice, raw	1 cup	26
Grapefruit juice, raw	1 cup	23
Carrot juice	1 cup	22
Blackberry	1 cup	19
Lemon juice, raw	1 cup	17
Vegetable juice	1 cup	11
Tomato	1 cup	10

Lamb, Cooked	Amount	Carbohydrate (g)
All types	3 oz	0

Milk	Amount	Carbohydrate (g)
Canned, condensed, sweetened	1 cup	166
Canned, evaporated, non fat	1 cup	29
Canned, evaporated	1 cup	25
Human milk	1 cup	17
Soymilk, original, unfortified	1 cup	15
Sheep milk	1 cup	13
Dry, instant, non fat	1/3 cup	12
Buttermilk, low fat	1 cup	12
Low fat milk, 1%	1 cup	12
Non fat, fat free or skim milk	1 cup	12
Whole milk, liquid, 3.25%	1 cup	12
Whole milk, dry powder	1/4 cup	12
Reduced fat, 2%	1 cup	12
Goat milk	1 cup	11
Coconut milk	1 cup	6

Nuts & Seeds	Amount	Carbohydrate (g)
Trail mix, tropical	1 oz	18.6
Trail mix, regular with chocolate chips	1 oz	12.7
Trail mix, regular, salted	1 oz	12.7
Chia seeds	1 oz	11.9
Cashews	1 oz	8.6
Flaxseeds	1 oz	8.2
Mixed nuts, roasted with peanuts, no salt	1 oz	7.2
Pistachio	1 oz	7.2
Sesame seeds	1 oz	6.7
Almonds	1 oz	6.1
Peanut butter, smooth style	1 oz	6.0
Tahini	1 oz	6.0

CARBOHYDRATES

Continued

Peanuts	1 oz	5.9
Sunflower seeds	1 oz	5.7
Hazelnuts	1 oz	4.7
Coconut, raw meat	1 oz	4.3
Pecans	1 oz	3.9
Macadamia	1 oz	3.9
English walnuts	1 oz	3.9
Pine nuts	1 oz	3.7
Brazil nuts	1 oz	3.5
Pumpkin seeds	1 oz	3.0
Black walnuts	1 oz	2.8

Pork, Cooked	Amount	Carbohydrate (g)
All types	3 oz	0

Turkey, Cooked	Amount	Carbohydrate (g)
All types	3 oz	0

Vegetables, Canned	Amount	Carbohydrate (g)
Sweet potato	1 cup	50
Tomato paste	1 cup	49
Corn	1 cup	40
Carrots	1 cup	22
Tomato pure	1 cup	22
Pumpkin	1 cup	20
Green peas	1 cup	19
Stewed tomato	1 cup	16
Tomato sauce	1 cup	13
Beets	1 cup	12
Sauerkraut	1 cup	10
Tomatoes	1 cup	10
Mushrooms	1 cup	8
Spinach	1 cup	7
Green beans	1 cup	6
Asparagus	1 cup	6

Vegetables, Cooked	Amount	Carbohydrate (g)
Sweet potato, mashed	1 cup	58
Taro	1 cup	46
Split peas	1 cup	41
Yams, cubed	1 cup	37
Potatoes, mashed with whole milk	1 cup	35
Corn	1 cup	31
Acorn squash, baked	1 cup	30

CARBOHYDRATES

Continued

Parsnips	1 cup	26
Potatoes, baked, no skin	1 cup	26
Butternut squash	1 cup	22
Hubbard squash	1 cup	22
Onions	1 cup	21
Artichokes	1 cup	20
Shiitake mushrooms	1 cup	20
Winter squash	1 cup	18
Beets	1 cup	17
Carrots	1 cup	13
Pumpkin, mashed	1 cup	12
Rutabagas	1 cup	12
Broccoli	1 cup	11
Brussels sprouts	1 cup	11
Kohlrabi	1 cup	11
Snow peas	1 cup	11
Green beans	1 cup	10
Spaghetti winter squash	1 cup	10
Tomatoes	1 cup	10
Collard greens	1 cup	9
Eggplant	1 cup	9
Beet greens	1 cup	8
Cabbage	1 cup	8
Leeks	1 cup	8
Summer squash	1 cup	8
Turnips, cubes	1 cup	8
White mushrooms	1 cup	8
Asparagus	1 cup	7
Crookneck or Straighneck Squash	1 cup	7
Dandelion greens	1 cup	7
Kale	1 cup	7
Okra	1 cup	7
Spinach	1 cup	7
Swiss chard	1 cup	7
Celery	1 cup	6
Scallop or Pattypan Squash, slices	1 cup	6
Turnip greens	1 cup	6
Cactus pads, nopales	1 cup	5
Cauliflower	1 cup	5
Zucchini	1 cup	5
Broccoli, chinese	1 cup	3
Cabbage, Chinese Bok-Choy	1 cup	3
Mustard greens	1 cup	3
Broccoli, raab	1 cup	3
Cabbage, Napa	1 cup	2

CARBOHYDRATES

Vegetables, Frozen	Amount	Carbohydrate (g)
Rhubarb	1 cup	75
Corn	1 cup	31
Butternut squash	1 cup	24
Green peas	1 cup	22
Brussels sprouts	1 cup	13
Collard greens	1 cup	12
Okra	1 cup	12
Carrots	1 cup	11
Broccoli	1 cup	10
Green beans	1 cup	9
Spinach	1 cup	9
Turnip greens	1 cup	8
Caulifower	1 cup	7
Kale	1 cup	7
Asparagus	1 cup	3

Vegetables, Raw	Amount	Carbohydrate (g)
Butternut squash	1 cup	16.0
Onions	1 cup	15.0
Carrots	1 cup	11.0
Yellow bell peppers	1 cup	9.4
Red bell peppers	1 cup	9.0
Tomatillos	1 cup	7.7
Snow peas	1 cup	7.4
Green bell peppers	1 cup	7.0
Green onions & scallions	1 cup	7.0
Tomatoes	1 cup	7.0
Kale	1 cup	6.7
Broccoli	1 cup	6.0
Mustard spinach	1 cup	5.9
Tomatoes, cherry	1 cup	5.8
Cabbage, Red	1 cup	5.0
Cauliflower	1 cup	5.0
Dandelion greens	1 cup	5.0
Cabbage	1 cup	4.0
Cabbage, Savoy	1 cup	4.0
Celery	1 cup	4.0
Cucumbers	1 cup	4.0
Zucchini	1 cup	3.9
Summer squash	1 cup	3.8
Belgian endive	1 cup	3.6
Cactus pads, nopales	1 cup	2.9
Shiitake mushrooms, dried	1 each	2.7
Cabbage, Napa	1 cup	2.4

CARBOHYDRATES

Continued

White mushrooms	1 cup	2.3
Endive	1 cup	2.0
Radicchio	1 cup	1.8
Romaine lettuce	1 cup	1.8
Green leaf lettuce	1 cup	1.6
Iceburg lettuce	1 cup	1.6
Spirulina	1 tbsp	1.6
Cabbage, Chinese Bok-Choy	1 cup	1.5
Swiss chard	1 cup	1.4
Chicory greens	1 cup	1.4
Butterhead or boston lettuce	1 cup	1.2
Broccoli, raab	1 cup	1.1
Spinach	1 cup	1.1
Arugula	1 cup	0.7
Red leaf lettuce	1 cup	0.6
Watercress	1 cup	0.4

Nutrient Data Collection Form

Food	Amount	Book Numbers	Multiply By	Estimated Nutrient Intake
Nutrient::	RDA:	Estimated:	% of RDA:	Total Estimated:

To download additional forms for free, go to www.TopNutrients4U.com

NOTES

CHOLESTEROL

Cholesterol is a nutrient absolutely essential for life. It is found in nature only in animals, humans, and any products derived from animals. It is an absolute requirement for fetal and child development. In fact, if your blood and tissue levels were zero you would die. Cholesterol is a precursor for the synthesis of steroids in humans. It is required for the synthesis of vitamin D, sex hormones, and bile acids. Without the cholesterol-rich bile synthesized by the liver your body could not absorb any of the fat soluble vitamins (A, D, E, and K). Nor, could it absorb any of the essential fatty acids necessary to sustain life.

The majority of cholesterol in humans is synthesized by the liver, and not from intake of cholesterol rich foods. Cholesterol, however, like all nutrients becomes a problem when the body's total content is out of balance with body requirements which gradually takes place over time.

It is generally accepted that elevated levels of cholesterol is associated with blood clotting and increased risk of atherosclerosis and heart disease. Studies, likewise, show that blood cholesterol concentrations are regulated by varying intake quantities of cholesterol, sugar, and saturated fats.

Cholesterol Intake

Attempts at lowering blood cholesterol levels by reducing intake of cholesterol rich foods has produced variable results. Many consider the changes to be only modest; however, dietary changes alone will accomplish a noticeable reduction of blood cholesterol levels. Text books and studies agree that a decrease of 100 mg of cholesterol intake a day is predicated to lower blood levels by approximately 2 mg to 5 mg/dL (milligrams per deciliter). It is not necessary to completely avoid all foods rich in cholesterol, but it is wise to limit their intake on a rotational basis.

Sugar Intake

Elevated levels of blood cholesterol are usually due to cholesterol synthesized by the liver rather than the dietary intake. In the liver, the step that controls the rate of cholesterol synthesis is under control of the enzyme known as HMG-CoA reductase. It is further known that insulin increases the activity of HMG-CoA reductase, and intake of sugar increases insulin levels. Thus, sugar itself plays a role in the liver's production of cholesterol. Interesting to note, the cholesterol lowering drugs known as statins lower the body's blood amount of cholesterol by inhibiting the activity of the HMG-CoA reductase enzyme.

Saturated Fatty Acid Intake

Observed increases in blood cholesterol due to saturated fats do not appear to be related with the synthesis of cholesterol in the liver.

Instead it appears to disrupt the mechanisms involved in cholesterols uptake by cells and cholesterol's excretion from the body.

If the mechanism responsible for a cells uptake of cholesterol is in some way hindered then un-metabolized amounts of cholesterol will remain circulating in the blood. Normally, cholesterol is converted to bile acids and excreted in the feces. Secretion into bile is the major route the body uses for eliminating excess cholesterol from the body. However, if removal of cholesterol from the body is in some way hindered then the un-metabolized amounts of cholesterol will accumulate in the blood. Saturated fats have been implicated in hindering the uptake of cholesterol by cells and excretion of cholesterol from the body.

In short, saturated fats may cause a larger proportion of cholesterol to linger in circulation for extended periods of time. It is further believed, it is this lingering unused cholesterol that eventually builds up into cholesterol containing arterial plaques.

In animal and human experiments adding cholesterol alone to a diet caused only modest increases in serum cholesterol concentrations. When saturated fats were added along with the intakes of cholesterol, there was nearly a four-fold rise in blood cholesterol levels. There is an incremental increase in blood cholesterol concentrations with the increased intake of saturated fat. In contrast, neither polyunsaturated nor monounsaturated fatty acids raise blood levels of cholesterol.

This helps to explain in part, why diets with a low saturated / polyunsaturated ratio have been shown to reduce serum cholesterol levels and is considered to be beneficial.

Dietary experiments show blood cholesterol is lowered when saturated fat is restricted or replaced with polyunsaturated fatty acids, and reducing the total fat intake without reducing intake of saturated fat does not significantly lower blood cholesterol.

To summarize the above, intake of sugar, cholesterol, and saturated fat all contribute to elevated levels of blood cholesterol.

For the purpose of cholesterol management the intake levels of cholesterol, saturated fats, and sugars should all be modestly reduced while increasing the intake of polyunsaturated fatty acids. This chapter lists the cholesterol amounts in milligrams, mg.

Since the body is capable of synthesizing its own cholesterol, it is not clear if there is a biological requirement for dietary intake of cholesterol. Because of this, the Institute of Medicine decided not to establish a Recommended Daily Allowance, RDA, nor Adequate Intake level for cholesterol. The American Heart Association, on the other hand, strongly advises limiting daily intake to below 300 mg per day.

CHOLESTEROL

Alcohol	Amount	Cholesterol (mg)
White Wine	1 glass	0
Red Wine	1 glass	0
Light Beer	1 bottle	0
Regular Beer	1 bottle	0
Gin, Rum, Vodka, or Whisky	1 shot	0

Beans, Canned	Amount	Cholesterol (mg)
Baked beans, plain	1 cup	0
Black-eyed peas	1 cup	0
Cranberry beans	1 cup	0
Fava beans	1 cup	0
Garbanzo beans	1 cup	0
Great Northern	1 cup	0
Green beans	1 cup	0
Lima beans, large	1 cup	0
Navy beans	1 cup	0
Pinto beans	1 cup	0
Red kidney beans	1 cup	0
Refried beans	1 cup	0
White beans	1 cup	0
Yellow beans	1 cup	0

Beans, Cooked	Amount	Cholesterol (mg)
Adzuki	1 cup	0
Black beans	1 cup	0
Black Turtle beans, mature	1 cup	0
Black-eyed peas	1 cup	0
Cranberry beans	1 cup	0
Edamame	1 cup	0
Fava beans	1 cup	0
Garbanzo beans, chickpeas	1 cup	0
Great Northern	1 cup	0
Green beans	1 cup	0
Hyacinath beans	1 cup	0
Kidney beans	1 cup	0
Lentils	1 cup	0
Lima beans	1 cup	0
Lupini beans	1 cup	0
Mothbeans	1 cup	0
Mung beans, mature seeds	1 cup	0
Natto	1 cup	0
Navy beans	1 cup	0
Pigeon peas	1 cup	0

CHOLESTEROL

Pinto beans	1 cup	0
Soybeans, green	1 cup	0
Soybeans, matured	1 cup	0
Soybeans, matured, dry roasted	1 cup	0
Split peas	1 cup	0
White beans, mature	1 cup	0
White beans, small	1 cup	0
Winged beans	1 cup	0
Yardlong beans, Chinese long beans	1 cup	0
Yellow beans	1 cup	0

Beef, Cooked	Amount	Cholesterol (mg)
Chuck roast, trimmed to 1/8" fat"	3 oz	88
Brisket, lean, trimmed to 0" fat	3 oz	85
Ground beef, 80%	3 oz	77
Ground beef, 75%	3 oz	76
Ground beef, 85%	3 oz	76
London Broil, top round, trim to 0" fat	3 oz	76
Filet Mignon, tenderloin, trimmed to 0" fat	3 oz	73
Ground beef, 90%	3 oz	72
Beef ribs, trimmed to 1/8" fat"	3 oz	71
Top sirloin, lean, trimmed to 1/8" fat"	3 oz	67
Flank steak, lean, trimmed to 0" fat	3 oz	66
Ground beef, 95%	3 oz	65
Ribeye steak, lean, trimmed 0" fat	3 oz	64
Tri Tip Steak, trimmed to 0" fat"	3 oz	58
Porterhouse steak, trimmed to 0" fat	3 oz	57
Skirt Steak, trimmed to 0" fat"	3 oz	51
T-Bone steak, trimmed 0" fat"	3 oz	51

Beef, Cooked	Amount	Cholesterol (mg)
Chuck roast, trimmed to 1/8" fat"	1 lb	468
Brisket, lean, trimmed to 0" fat	1 lb	454
Beef ribs, trimmed to 1/8" fat"	1 lb	381
Flank steak, lean, trimmed to 0" fat	1 lb	354
Tri Tip steak, lean, trimmed to 0" fat"	1 lb	308
Porterhouse steak, trimmed to 0" fat"	1 lb	304
Top Sirloin, trimmed to 1/8" fat"	1 lb	282
Skirt steak, trimmed to 0" fat"	1 lb	272
T-bone steak, trimmed to 0" fat"	1 lb	272
Ribeye steak, boneless, trimmed to 0" fat"	1 steak	159
Filet Mignon, tenderloin, trimmed to 0" fat	1 filet	109
Ribeye filet, lean, trimmed to 0" fat"	1 filet	106
Top Sirloin, choice filet, trimmed to 0" fat"	1 filet	100

CHOLESTEROL

Beef, Ground, cooked	Amount	Cholesterol (mg)
Ground beef, 80%	1/4 lb patty	70
Ground beef, 90%	1/4 lb patty	70
Ground beef, 85%	1/4 lb patty	69
Ground beef, 75%	1/4 lb patty	62
Ground beef, 95%	1/4 lb patty	62

Bread	Amount	Cholesterol (mg)
All types	1 serving	0

Butter	Amount	Cholesterol (mg)
Regular butter, salted	1 tbsp	31
Regular whipped butter, salted	1 tbsp	21

Cereal	Amount	Cholesterol (mg)
All types	1 cup	0

Cheese	Amount	Cholesterol (mg)
Ricotta, whole milk	1 cup	125
Ricotta, part skim milk	1 cup	76
Cottage cheese, creamed, small curd	1 cup	38
Cottage cheese, creamed, large curd	1 cup	36
Cottage cheese, lowfat, 2%	1 cup	23
Cottage cheese, nonfat & uncreamed	1 cup	10
Cottage cheese, lowfat, 1%	1 cup	9

Cheese	Amount	Cholesterol (mg)
Fontina	1 oz	33
Gouda	1 oz	32
Cream cheese	1 oz	31
Gruyere	1 oz	31
Cheddar	1 oz	30
Pepper Jack, Red & Green Jalapenos	1 oz	30
Romano	1 oz	29
American, pasteurized process, fortified	1 oz	28
Brie	1 oz	28
Colby	1 oz	27
Muenster	1 oz	27
Roquefort	1 oz	26
Swiss	1 oz	26
Dubliner	1 oz	25
Feta	1 oz	25
Monterey	1 oz	25

CHOLESTEROL

Continued

Parmesan, grated	1 oz	25
Mozzarella, whole milk	1 oz	22
Velveeta, pasteurized process	1 oz	22
Blue cheese	1 oz	21
Cheez Whiz, pasteurized process	1 oz	21
Provolone	1 oz	20
Monterey, low fat	1 oz	18
Muenster, low fat	1 oz	18
Mozzarella, part skim milk, low moisture	1 oz	15
Provolone, reduced fat	1 oz	15
Ricotta, whole milk	1 oz	14
Goat cheese, soft	1 oz	13
American, pasteurized process, low fat	1 oz	10
Swiss, low fat	1 oz	10
Ricotta, part skim milk	1 oz	9
Cheddar, lowfat	1 oz	6
Cottage cheese, large & small curd	1 oz	5
Mozzarella, nonfat	1 oz	5
Cottage cheese, lowfat 2 %	1 oz	3
Cream cheese, fat free	1 oz	3
American, pasteurized process, imitation	1 oz	2
Cottage cheese, nonfat, uncreamed	1 oz	2
Cottage cheese, lowfat 1 %	1 oz	1

Cheese, Mexican	Amount	Cholesterol (mg)
Queso anejo	1 oz	29
Queso asadero	1 oz	29
Queso chihuahua	1 oz	29
Mexican, blend	1 oz	27
Queso fresco	1 oz	20
Mexican, blend, reduced fat	1 oz	17

Chicken, Cooked	Amount	Cholesterol (mg)
Breast, skin, fried, flour	1/2 breast	87
Thigh, with skin, fried	1 thigh	80
Breast, no skin, roasted	1/2 breast	73
Thigh, meat only, roasted	1 thigh	70
Drumstick, with skin, fried	1 drumstick	44
Drumstick, no skin, roasted	1 drumstick	41
Wing with skin, fried in batter	1 wing	39
Wing with skin, roasted	1 wing	29

CHOLESTEROL

Chicken, Cooked	Amount	Cholesterol (mg)
Thigh meat only, no skin, roasted	3 oz	115
Thigh with skin, roasted	3 oz	115
Drumstick meat only, no skin, roasted	3 oz	110
Drumstick with skin, roasted	3 oz	110
Cornish game hens, meat only	3 oz	90
Thigh with skin, fried in flour	3 oz	82
Breast with skin, fried in flour	3 oz	76
Drumstick with skin, fried in flour	3 oz	76
Breast meat only, no skin, roasted	3 oz	72
Wing meat only, no skin, roasted	3 oz	72
Breast with skin, roasted	3 oz	71
Wing with skin, roasted	3 oz	71
Wing with skin, fried in flour	3 oz	69

Chili, Amy's® Organic	Amount	Cholesterol (mg)
Black Bean Chili	1 can	0
Light in Sodium Medium Chili	1 can	0
Light in Sodium Spicy Chili	1 can	0
Medium Chili	1 can	0
Medium Chili with Vegetables	1 can	0
South Western Black Bean Chili	1 can	0
Spicy Chili	1 can	0

Chili, Cattle Drive®	Amount	Cholesterol (mg)
Cattle drive Golden Chili with beans	1 can	80

Chili, Campbell's® Chunky	Amount	Cholesterol (mg)
Chunky Chili no Beans	1 can	120
Chunky Chili with Beans Roadhouse	1 can	60
Chunky Chili with Beans Firehouse	1 can	60
Chunky Chili with Beans Grilled Steak	1 can	40

Chili, Dennison®	Amount	Cholesterol (mg)
Turkey Chili with Beans	1 can	90
Original Chili Con Carne with Beans	1 can	80
Hot Chili Con Carne with Beans	1 can	80
Chunky Chili Con Carne with Beans	1 can	80
Hot & Chunky Chili with Beans	1 can	80
Vegetarian Chili with Beans	1 can	0

CHOLESTEROL

Chili, Eden Organic	Amount	Cholesterol (mg)
Black Bean & Quinoa Chili	1 can	0
Great Northern Bean & Barley Chili	1 can	0
Kidney Bean & Kamut Chili	1 can	0
Pinto Bean & Spelt Chili	1 can	0

Chili, Healthy Valley	Amount	Cholesterol (mg)
No salt Added Tame Tomato Chili	1 can	0
Santa Fe White Bean Chili	1 can	0
Black Bean Mole Chili	1 can	0
Black Bean Mango Chili	1 can	0
Spicy Tomato Chili	1 can	0
Three Bean Chipotle Chili	1 can	0

Chili, Hormel®	Amount	Cholesterol (mg)
Turkey Chili no Beans	1 can	160
Cook-off White Chicken Chili	1 can	100
Cook-off Chipotle Chicken Chili	1 can	100
Turkey Chili with Beans	1 can	90
Chili no Beans	1 can	80
Less Sodium Chili no Beans	1 can	80
Chili with Beans	1 can	60
Chunky Chili with Beans	1 can	60
Hot Chili with beans	1 can	60
Less Sodium Chili with Beans	1 can	60
Cook-off Roasted Tomato Chili	1 can	50
Vegetarian Chili with Beans 99% Fat Free	1 can	0

Chili, Nalley's®	Amount	Cholesterol (mg)
Thick Chili with beans	1 can	60
Original Chili with beans	1 can	60
Jalapeno Hot Chili with beans	1 can	50
Turkey Chili with beans	1 can	50

Chili, Stagg®	Amount	Cholesterol (mg)
White Chicken Chili with Beans	1 can	140
Steak House Chili no Beans	1 can	130
Ranch House Chicken Chili with Beans	1 can	110
Classi Chili with beans	1 can	90
Laredo Chili with Beans, chili and Jalapno	1 can	90
Country Brand Chili with Beans	1 can	90
Chunkero Chili with Beans	1 can	80
Dynamite Hot Chili with Beans	1 can	80

CHOLESTEROL

Continued

Fiesta Grille Chili with Beans	1 can	80
Country Brand Mild Chil Sweet Bell Peppers	1 can	70
Turkey Ranchero Chili with Beans	1 can	70
Silverado Beef Chili with Beans	1 can	40
Vegetarian Garden Four Bean Chili	1 can	0

Chili, Wolf Brand®	Amount	Cholesterol (mg)
Lean Beef no Beans	1 can	130
Chili no Beans	1 can	110
Chili with Beans	1 can	110
Lean Beef with Beans	1 can	90
Hot Chili no Beans	1 can	80
Turkey Chili no Beans	1 can	70
Homestyle Chili with Beans	1 can	60
Turkey Chili with Beans	1 can	50
Spicy Chili with Beans	1 can	40

Cream	Amount	Cholesterol (mg)
Heavy cream	1 tbsp	21
Light coffe creamer	1 tbsp	10
Half & Half	1 tbsp	6
Sour cream cultured	1 tbsp	6
Sour cream reduced fat	1 tbsp	6
Whipped topping, pressurized	1 tbsp	2

Eggs	Amount	Cholesterol (mg)
Egg whole, hard boiled	1 large	187
Egg whole, poached	1 large	185
Egg whole, fried	1 large	184
Egg yolk	1 large	180
Egg whole, scrambled	1 large	169
Egg whites	1 large	0
Egg substitute, fat free	1 cup	0
Egg whites, dried powder, stabilized	1 tbsp	0
Egg whites, dried	1 ounce	0

Fish, Canned	Amount	Cholesterol (mg)
White (albacore) tuna, in water	3 oz	36
Light tuna, in water	3 oz	31
White (albacore) tuna, in oil	3 oz	26
Light tuna, in oil	3 oz	15

CHOLESTEROL

Fish, Cooked	Amount	Cholesterol (mg)
Walleye pike	3 oz	94
Striped bass	3 oz	88
Keta (chum) salmon	3 oz	81
Atlantic pollock	3 oz	77
Freshwater bass	3 oz	74
Walleye pollock	3 oz	73
Chinook salmon	3 oz	72
Atlantic croaker	3 oz	71
Carp	3 oz	71
Whiting	3 oz	71
Orange roughy	3 oz	68
Swordfish	3 oz	66
Alaskan halibut	3 oz	64
Atlantic mackerel	3 oz	64
Spanish mackerel	3 oz	62
Catfish, wild	3 oz	61
Atlantic salmon, wild	3 oz	60
Catfish, breaded & fried	3 oz	60
Rainbow trout, farmed	3 oz	60
Yellowtail	3 oz	60
Rainbow trout, wild	3 oz	59
King mackerel	3 oz	58
Catfish, farmed	3 oz	56
Haddock	3 oz	56
Atlantic perch	3 oz	54
Atlantic salmon, farmed	3 oz	54
Coho salmon, farmed	3 oz	54
Florida pompano	3 oz	54
Sockeye salmon	3 oz	54
Atlantic & Pacific halibut	3 oz	51
Pacific & Jack mackerel	3 oz	51
Skipjack (aku) tuna	3 oz	51
Greenland halibut	3 oz	50
Flounder & Sole	3 oz	48
Pacific cod	3 oz	48
Tilapia	3 oz	48
Coho salmon, wild	3 oz	47
Pink salmon	3 oz	47
Sea bass	3 oz	45
Bluefin tuna	3 oz	42
Northern pike	3 oz	42
Grouper	3 oz	40
Snapper	3 oz	40

CHOLESTEROL

Continued

Yellowfin tuna	3 oz	40
King salmon, chinook salmon, smoked	3 oz	20
Atlantic herring, pickeled	3 oz	11

Fish, Shellfish, Cooked	Amount	Cholesterol (mg)
Squid, fried	3 oz	221
Shrimp, canned	3 oz	214
Crab cakes	3 oz	128
Northern lobster	3 oz	124
Shrimp, breaded & fried	3 oz	117
Crayfish	3 oz	113
Blue Crab, canned	3 oz	82
Blue crab	3 oz	82
Octopus	3 oz	82
Abalone	3 oz	80
Oysters, breaded & fried	3 oz	60
Queen crab	3 oz	60
Eastern oysters, wild	3 oz	53
Clams, breaded & fried	3 oz	52
Scallops, breaded & fried	3 oz	46
Alaskan king crab	3 oz	45
Clams, canned	3 oz	43
Eastern oysters, farmed	3 oz	32
Alaskan king crab, imitation	3 oz	17

Fruit	Amount	Cholesterol (mg)
All fruit	any size	0

Game Meat, Cooked	Amount	Cholesterol (mg)
Antelope	3 oz	107
Rabbit	3 oz	105
Squirrel	3 oz	103
Deer	3 oz	95
Caribou	3 oz	93
Deer, ground	3 oz	83
Duck	3 oz	76
Bison, ground	3 oz	71
Bufflow, steak, free range	3 oz	70
Elk ground	3 oz	66
Wild boar	3 oz	65
Elk	3 oz	62

CHOLESTEROL

Lamb, Cooked	Amount	Cholesterol (mg)
Foreshank, trimmed to 1/8" fat	3 oz	90
Chops, loin, lean, trimmed to 1/4" fat"	3 oz	85
Ground, broiled	3 oz	82
Leg, whole	3 oz	79
Rib, lean, trimmed to 1/4" fat"	3 oz	77
Cubed, for stew or kabob	3 oz	76

Milk	Amount	Cholesterol (mg)
Canned, condensed, sweetened	1 cup	104
Canned, evaporated	1 cup	73
Sheep milk	1 cup	66
Whole milk, liquid, 3.25%	1 cup	35
Human milk	1 cup	34
Whole milk, dry powder	1/4 cup	31
Goat milk	1 cup	27
Reduced fat, 2%	1 cup	20
Lowfat milk, 1%	1 cup	15
Canned, evaporated, nonfat	1 cup	10
Buttermilk, lowfat	1 cup	10
Nonfat, fat free or skim milk	1 cup	5
Dry, instant, nonfat	1/3 cup	4
Coconut milk	1 cup	0
Soymilk, original & vanilla, unfortified	1 cup	0

Nuts & Seeds	Amount	Cholesterol (mg)
All nuts and seeds	1 oz	0

Oils	Amount	Cholesterol (mg)
Code liver fish oil	1 tbsp	78
Menhaden fish oil	1 tbsp	71
Salmon fish oil	1 tbsp	66
Canola oil	1 tbsp	0
Coconut oil	1 tbsp	0
Cod liver oil	1 tbsp	0
Corn oil	1 tbsp	0
Cottonseed oil	1 tbsp	0
Flaxseed oil	1 tbsp	0
Grapeseed oil	1 tbsp	0
Olive oil	1 tbsp	0
Palm kernal vegetable oil	1 tbsp	0
Peanut oil	1 tbsp	0
Safflower, high linoleic acid, oil	1 tbsp	0
Safflower, high oleic acid, oil	1 tbsp	0

CHOLESTEROL

Continued

Salmon oil	1 tbsp	0
Sesame oil	1 tbsp	0
Soybean lecithin oil	1 tbsp	0
Soybean oil	1 tbsp	0
Soybean, partially hydrogenated oil	1 tbsp	0
Sunflower, high linoleic acid	1 tbsp	0
Sunflower, high oleic acid	1 tbsp	0
Walnut oil	1 tbsp	0

Pork, Cooked	Amount	Cholesterol (mg)
Braunschweiger	3 oz	153
Spareribs	3 oz	103
Bacon	3 oz	94
Backribs	3 oz	71
Sausage	3 oz	71
Pork chops, broiled	3 oz	71
Center loin pork chops	3 oz	71
Pork chops, pan-fried	3 oz	67
Pork chops, lean, pan-fried	3 oz	66
Sirloin pork chops	3 oz	65
Liverwurst spread	1/4 cup	65
Bratwurst	3 oz	63
Tenderloin	3 oz	62
Polish sausage	3 oz	60
Cured ham	3 oz	53
Canadian-style bacon	3 oz	49
Italian sausage	3 oz	48

SALAD DRESSINGS

Annie's® Organic Dressing	Amount	Cholesterol (mg)
Caesar Dressing	2 tbsp	10
Cowgirl Ranch Dressing	2 tbsp	10
Buttermilk Dressing	2 tbsp	5
Creamy Asiago Cheese	2 tbsp	5
Green Goddess Dressing	2 tbsp	5
Thousand Island	2 tbsp	5

Bernstein's® Dressing	Amount	Cholesterol (mg)
Basil Parmesan	2 tbsp	5
Chunky Blue Chees	2 tbsp	5
Creamy Caesar	2 tbsp	5
Light Parmesan Garlic Ranch	2 tbsp	5
Balsamic Italian	2 tbsp	0
Cheese & Garlic Italian	2 tbsp	0

CHOLESTEROL

Continued

Cheese Fantastico	2 tbsp	0
Fat Free Cheese & Garlic Italian	2 tbsp	0
Herb Garden French	2 tbsp	0
Italian & Marinade	2 tbsp	0
Light Fantastic Cheese Fantastico	2 tbsp	0
Light Roasted Garlic Balsamic	2 tbsp	0
Redwine & Garlic Italian	2 tbsp	0
Restaurant Recipe Italian	2 tbsp	0
Sweet Herb Italian	2 tbsp	0

Best Food® Mayonnaise Dressing	Amount	Cholesterol (mg)
Real Mayonnaise	2 tbsp	10
Light Mayonnaise	2 tbsp	10
Mayonnaise with Olive Oil	2 tbsp	10
Mayonesa Con Jugo De Lemon	2 tbsp	10
Low Fat Mayonnaise	2 tbsp	0
Canola Cholesterol Free Mayonnaise	2 tbsp	0

Bob's Big Boy® Dressing	Amount	Cholesterol (mg)
Roquefort	2 tbsp	20
Blue Cheese	2 tbsp	15
Ranch	2 tbsp	15
Thousand Island	2 tbsp	15

Bolthouse Farms® Dressing	Amount	Cholesterol (mg)
Caesar Parmigino Yogurt Dressing	2 tbsp	10
Chunky Bluecheese Yogurt Dressing	2 tbsp	5
Classic Ranch Yogurt Dressing	2 tbsp	5
Honey Mustard Yogurt Dressing	2 tbsp	5
Salsa Ranch Yogurt Dressing	2 tbsp	5
Thousand Island Yogurt Dressing	2 tbsp	5
Asian Ginger & Olive Oil Vinaigrettes	2 tbsp	0
Chunky Blue Cheese & Olive Oil	2 tbsp	0
Classic Balsamic & Olive Oil	2 tbsp	0
Raspberry Merlot & Olive Oil	2 tbsp	0
Zesty French Yogurt	2 tbsp	0

Brianna's® Dressing	Amount	Cholesterol (mg)
Classic Buttermilk Ranch	2 tbsp	10
Asiago Caesar	2 tbsp	5
True Blue Cheese	2 tbsp	5
Blush Wine Vinaigrette	2 tbsp	0
Champagne Caper Vinaigrette	2 tbsp	0
Chipotle Cheddar	2 tbsp	0

CHOLESTEROL

Continued

Dijon Honey Mustard	2 tbsp	0
Ginger Mandarin	2 tbsp	0
Lively Lemon Tarragon	2 tbsp	0
Real French Vinaigrette	2 tbsp	0
Rich Poppy Seed	2 tbsp	0
Rich Santa Fe Blend	2 tbsp	0
The New American	2 tbsp	0
Zesty French	2 tbsp	0

Cardin's® Dressing	Amount	Cholesterol (mg)
Original Caesar	2 tbsp	30
Light Caesar	2 tbsp	30
Aged Parmesan Ranch	2 tbsp	10
Balsamic Vinaigrette	2 tbsp	0
Honey Mustard	2 tbsp	0
Italian	2 tbsp	0
Pear Vinaigrette	2 tbsp	0
Raspberry Pomegranate	2 tbsp	0
Roasted Asian Sesame	2 tbsp	0
Asian Sesame	2 tbsp	0
Fat Free Caesar	2 tbsp	0

Drew's® Dressing	Amount	Cholesterol (mg)
Buttermilk Ranch	2 tbsp	0
Classic Italian	2 tbsp	0
Greek Olive	2 tbsp	0
Honey Dijon	2 tbsp	0
Lemon Goddess	2 tbsp	0
Poppy Seed	2 tbsp	0
Roasted Garlic & Peppercorn	2 tbsp	0
Rosemary Balsamic	2 tbsp	0
Sesame Orange	2 tbsp	0
Shiitake Ginger	2 tbsp	0
Smoked Tomato	2 tbsp	0
Thai Sesame Lime	2 tbsp	0

Girard's® Dressing	Amount	Cholesterol (mg)
Caesar	2 tbsp	10
Light Caesar	2 tbsp	10
Blue Cheese Vinaigrette	2 tbsp	5
Apple Poppy Seed	2 tbsp	0
Champagne	2 tbsp	0
Chinese Chicken Salad	2 tbsp	0
Creamy Balsamic Vinaigrette	2 tbsp	0

CHOLESTEROL

Continued

Greek Feta Vinaigrette	2 tbsp	0
Old Venice Italian	2 tbsp	0
Original French	2 tbsp	0
Peach Mimosa Vinaigrette	2 tbsp	0
Spinach Salad Dressing	2 tbsp	0
White Balsamic Vinaigrette	2 tbsp	0

Hidden Valley® Dressing	Amount	Cholesterol (mg)
Classic Cheese Ranch	2 tbsp	10
Coleslaw	2 tbsp	10
Cracked Peppercorn Ranch	2 tbsp	10
Garden Vegetable Ranch	2 tbsp	10
Old Fashioned Buttermilk Ranch	2 tbsp	10
Original Ranch Dressing	2 tbsp	10
Spicy Ranch	2 tbsp	10
Bacon Ranch	2 tbsp	10
Buttermilk Ranch Light	2 tbsp	5
Original Ranch Light	2 tbsp	5
Original Ranch Fat Free	2 tbsp	0

Hidden Valley® Farm House	Amount	Cholesterol (mg)
Creamy Balsamic with Herb	2 tbsp	10
Creamy Parmesan	2 tbsp	10
Hickory Bacon & Onion	2 tbsp	10
Original Caesar	2 tbsp	10
Roasted Onion Parmesan	2 tbsp	10
Savory Bleu Cheese	2 tbsp	10
Southwest Chipotle	2 tbsp	10
Dijon Mustard Vinaigrette	2 tbsp	0
Garden Tomato & Bacon	2 tbsp	0
Homestyle Italian	2 tbsp	0
Original Italian with Herb	2 tbsp	0
Pomegranate Vinaigrette	2 tbsp	0

Ken's Steak House® Dressing	Amount	Cholesterol (mg)
Russian Dressing	2 tbsp	15
Thousand Island	2 tbsp	15
Creamy Caesar Dressing	2 tbsp	10
Ranch Dressing	2 tbsp	10
Buttermilk Ranch Dressing	2 tbsp	5
Pepper Corn Ranch	2 tbsp	5
3 Cheese Italian	2 tbsp	0
Balsamic & Honey	2 tbsp	0
Balsamic Vinaigrete	2 tbsp	0

CHOLESTEROL

Continued

Caesar Dressing	2 tbsp	0
Chunky Bluecheese	2 tbsp	0
Creamy Italian	2 tbsp	0
Greek & Olive Oil	2 tbsp	0
Honey Mustard	2 tbsp	0
Italian & Aged Romano	2 tbsp	0
Italian Marinade	2 tbsp	0
Italian with Olive Oil	2 tbsp	0
Northern Italian Basil & Romano	2 tbsp	0
Red Wine Vinegar Oil	2 tbsp	0
Sweet Vidalia Onion	2 tbsp	0
Zesty Italian	2 tbsp	0

Ken's® Lite Dressing	Amount	Cholesterol (mg)
Lite Creamy Caesar Dressing	2 tbsp	5
Lite Ranch Dressing	2 tbsp	5
Lite Thousand Island	2 tbsp	5
Lite Asian Sesame Ginger & Soy	2 tbsp	0
Lite Blue Cheese Dressing	2 tbsp	0
Lite Chunky Blue Cheese Dressing	2 tbsp	0
Lite Raspberry & Walnut Vinaigrette	2 tbsp	0
Lite Sweet Vidalia Onion	2 tbsp	0
Lite Zesty Italian	2 tbsp	0

Kraft® Dressing	Amount	Cholesterol (mg)
Classic Caesar Dressing	2 tbsp	15
Buttermilk Ranch	2 tbsp	10
Ranch with Backon	2 tbsp	10
Lite Ranch	2 tbsp	10
Coleslaw Dressing	2 tbsp	5
Ranch	2 tbsp	5
Green Goddnes	2 tbsp	5
Classic Catalina	2 tbsp	0
Creamy French Dressing	2 tbsp	0
Creamy Italian Dressing	2 tbsp	0
Creamy Poppyseed	2 tbsp	0
Cucumber Ranch	2 tbsp	0
Free Thousand Island	2 tbsp	0
Light Thousand Island	2 tbsp	0
Light Zesty Italian Dressing	2 tbsp	0
Peppercorn Ranch	2 tbsp	0
Roka Blue Cheese	2 tbsp	0
Sweet Balsamic Vinaigrette Dressing	2 tbsp	0
Sweet Honey Catalina	2 tbsp	0
Thousand Island	2 tbsp	0

CHOLESTEROL

Zesty Italian Anything Dressing	2 tbsp	0
Zesty Italian Dressing & Marinade	2 tbsp	0
fat Free Ranch	2 tbsp	0
Catalina fat Free	2 tbsp	0

Litehouse® Dressing	Amount	Cholesterol (mg)
Big Bleu Dressing	2 tbsp	15
Ceaser Dressing	2 tbsp	15
Chunky Bleu Cheese	2 tbsp	15
Original Bleu Cheese	2 tbsp	15
Barbecue Ranch	2 tbsp	10
Buttermilk Ranch	2 tbsp	10
Ceaser-Caesar Dressing	2 tbsp	10
Creamy Cilantro	2 tbsp	10
Homestyle Ranch	2 tbsp	10
Honey Mustard	2 tbsp	10
Jalapeno Ranch	2 tbsp	10
Organic Ranch	2 tbsp	10
Original Thousand Island	2 tbsp	10
Ranch Dressing	2 tbsp	10
Chunky Garlic Caesar	2 tbsp	5
Coleslaw Dressing	2 tbsp	5
Coleslaw with Pinapple	2 tbsp	5
Parmesan Caesar	2 tbsp	5
Yogurt Bleu Cheese with Kefir	2 tbsp	5
Yogurt Ranch with Kefir	2 tbsp	5
Harvest Cranberry Greek	2 tbsp	0
Pear Gorzonzola Dressing	2 tbsp	0
Sesame Ginger	2 tbsp	0
Spinach	2 tbsp	0
Sweet French	2 tbsp	0

Litehouse® Lite Dressing	Amount	Cholesterol (mg)
Lite Jalapeno Ranch Dressing	2 tbsp	15
Lite Bleu Cheese Dressing	2 tbsp	10
Lite Ranch Dressing	2 tbsp	10
Lite 1000 Island Dressing	2 tbsp	5
Lite Caesar Dressing	2 tbsp	5
Lite Coleslaw Dressing	2 tbsp	5
Lite Creamy Ranch Dressing	2 tbsp	5
Lite Honey Dijon Vinaigrette	2 tbsp	0

CHOLESTEROL

Litehouse® Vinaigrette Dressing	Amount	Cholesterol (mg)
Bleu Cheese Vinaigrette	2 tbsp	5
Balsamic Vinaigrette	2 tbsp	0
Cherry Vinaigrette	2 tbsp	0
Fuji Apple Vinaigrette	2 tbsp	0
Greek Vinaigrette	2 tbsp	0
Harvest Cranberry Vinaigrette	2 tbsp	0
Huckleberry Vinaigrette	2 tbsp	0
Organic Balsamic Vinaigrette	2 tbsp	0
Pomegranate Blueberry Vinaigrette	2 tbsp	0
Raspberry Walnut Vinaigrette	2 tbsp	0
Red Wine Olive Oil Vinaigrette	2 tbsp	0
White Balsamic Vinaigrette	2 tbsp	0
Zesty Italian Vinaigrette	2 tbsp	0

Marie's® Dressing	Amount	Cholesterol (mg)
Creamy Caesar	2 tbsp	25
Super Blue Cheese	2 tbsp	20
Thousand Island	2 tbsp	15
Yogurt Thousand Island	2 tbsp	15
Caesar	2 tbsp	15
Chunky Blue Cheese	2 tbsp	15
Creamy Ranch	2 tbsp	15
Creamy Chipotle Ranch	2 tbsp	15
Creamy Italian Garlic	2 tbsp	15
Yogurt Blue Cheese	2 tbsp	10
Honey Dijon	2 tbsp	10
Honey Mustard	2 tbsp	10
Coleslaw	2 tbsp	10
Asiago Peppercorn	2 tbsp	10
Poppy Seed	2 tbsp	10
Jalapeno Ranch	2 tbsp	10
Yogurt Coleslaw	2 tbsp	10
Lite Chunky Blue Cheese	2 tbsp	5
Buttermilk Ranch	2 tbsp	5
Yogurt Ranch	2 tbsp	5
Lite Creamy Ranch	2 tbsp	5
Blue Cheese Vinaigrette	2 tbsp	5
Balsamic Vinaigrette	2 tbsp	0
Italian Vinaigrette	2 tbsp	0
Spinach Salad	2 tbsp	0
Sesame Ginger	2 tbsp	0
Greek Vinaigrette	2 tbsp	0
Raspberry Vinaigrette	2 tbsp	0
Red Wine Vinaigrette	2 tbsp	0

CHOLESTEROL

Newman's® Own Dressing	Amount	Cholesterol (mg)
Creamy Ceasar	2 tbsp	20
Ranch Dressing	2 tbsp	10
3 Cheese Balsamic	2 tbsp	0
Balsamic Vinaigrette	2 tbsp	0
Caesar Dressing	2 tbsp	0
Creamy Balsamic	2 tbsp	0
Family Italian	2 tbsp	0
Greek Vinaigrette	2 tbsp	0
Honey French	2 tbsp	0
Olive Oil & Vinegar	2 tbsp	0
Orange Ginger	2 tbsp	0
Parmesan & Roasted Garlic	2 tbsp	0
Poppy Seed	2 tbsp	0

Walden Farm's® Dressing	Amount	Cholesterol (mg)
Asian	2 tbsp	0
Bacon Ranch	2 tbsp	0
Balsamic Vinaigrette	2 tbsp	0
Bleu Cheese	2 tbsp	0
Buttermilk Ranch	2 tbsp	0
Caesar	2 tbsp	0
Chipotle Ranch	2 tbsp	0
Colesaw	2 tbsp	0
Creamy Bacon	2 tbsp	0
Creamy Italian	2 tbsp	0
French	2 tbsp	0
Honey Dijon	2 tbsp	0
Italian	2 tbsp	0
Italian Sun Dried Tomato	2 tbsp	0
Jersey Sweet Onion	2 tbsp	0
Ranch	2 tbsp	0
Raspberry Vinaigrette	2 tbsp	0
Russian	2 tbsp	0
Sesame Ginger	2 tbsp	0
Sweet Onion	2 tbsp	0
Thousand Island	2 tbsp	0
Zesty Italian	2 tbsp	0

Wish Bone® Creamy Dressing	Amount	Cholesterol (mg)
Creamy Caesar	2 tbsp	10
Thousand Island	2 tbsp	10
Chunky Blue Cheese	2 tbsp	5
Light Ranch Dressing	2 tbsp	5

CHOLESTEROL

Continued

Light Ranch Dressing	2 tbsp	5
Ranch Dressing	2 tbsp	5
Creamy Italian Dressing	2 tbsp	0
Delux French	2 tbsp	0
Fat Free Chunky Blue Cheese	2 tbsp	0
Fat Free Ranch Dressing	2 tbsp	0
Fat Free Ranch Dressing	2 tbsp	0
Light Blue Cheese	2 tbsp	0
Light Creamy Caesar	2 tbsp	0
Light Delux French	2 tbsp	0
Light Parmesan Peppercorn Ranch	2 tbsp	0
Light Sweet & Spicy French	2 tbsp	0
Light Thousand Island	2 tbsp	0
Russian	2 tbsp	0
Sweet & Spicy French	2 tbsp	0

Wish Bone® Oil & Vinegar Dressing	Amount	Cholesterol (mg)
Balsamic Italian Vinaigrette	2 tbsp	0
Balsamic Vinaigrette	2 tbsp	0
Bruschetta Italian	2 tbsp	0
Fat Free Italian	2 tbsp	0
Fat Free Red Wine Vinaigrette	2 tbsp	0
Fat Free Red Wine Vinaigrette	2 tbsp	0
Greek Vinaigrette	2 tbsp	0
House Italian	2 tbsp	0
Italian	2 tbsp	0
Light Asian Sesame & Ginger	2 tbsp	0
Light Balsamic & Basil Vinaigrette	2 tbsp	0
Light Honey Dijon	2 tbsp	0
Light Italian dressing	2 tbsp	0
Light Raspberry Walnut	2 tbsp	0
Mediterranean Italian	2 tbsp	0
Olive Oil Vinaigrette	2 tbsp	0
Raspberrt Hazelnut Vinaigrette	2 tbsp	0
Red Wine Vinaigrette	2 tbsp	0
Robusto Italian	2 tbsp	0
Romano Basil Vinaigrette	2 tbsp	0
Superfruit Vinaigrette	2 tbsp	0

Turkey, Cooked	Amount	Cholesterol (mg)
Dark meat	3 oz	109
Ground turkey, 93% lean	3 oz	90
Ground turkey, 85% lean	3 oz	89
Turkey bacon	3 oz	83
Ground turkey	3 oz	79

CHOLESTEROL

Continued

Breast meat	3 oz	71
Light meat	3 oz	68
Ground turkey, fat free	3 oz	55
Turkey sausage, reduced fat	3 oz	49

Veal, Cooked	Amount	Cholesterol (mg)
Leg, top round	3 oz	114
Foreshank	3 oz	105
Breast	3 oz	99
Rib	3 oz	94
Ground	3 oz	88
Loin	3 oz	88
Sirloin	3 oz	87

Vegetables	Amount	Cholesterol (mg)
All vegetables	1 cup	0

Nutrient Data Collection Form

Food	Amount	Book Numbers	Multiply By	Estimated Nutrient Intake
Nutrient::	RDA:	Estimated:	% of RDA:	Total Estimated:

To download additional forms for free, go to www.TopNutrients4U.com

NOTES

COPPER

Copper is a mineral required daily in very small microgram (mcg) quantities. Copper is needed for the production of red blood cells, nerve cells, bone structure, and the connective tissues of hair, nails, skin, arteries, and veins. Copper is used for the production of energy, decreasing inflammation, blood clotting, iron metabolism, and protection against oxidative damage.

Copper toxicity is associated with problems of the liver, thyroid and adrenal glands, and Alzheimer's disease. Toxicity symptoms include chronic fatigue, lack of energy, a tired body with an overactive mind, craving for chocolate, anxiety, migraines, and depression. Toxicity signs include: anemia, nausea, headaches, dizziness, and a metallic taste in the mouth. Toxicity is commonly caused by environmental exposures, vitamin and mineral supplements formulated with the wrong form of copper, hereditary disorders, and zinc deficiencies.

Copper deficiency is associated with arthritis, bone marrow failure, multiple sclerosis, and a lowered immunity. Deficiency signs are loss of skin and hair pigmentation, irregular heartbeat, loss of feelings in lower extremities and finger tips, low body temperature, low white blood cell count and anemia. Causes of deficiency are associated with poor intestinal absorption, gastric bypass surgery, genetic disorders, and dietary intake of zinc.

Some people believe that a copper deficiency state is not a major health concern. However, a number of reported cases prove severe copper deficiency does occur in humans, with patients showing no clinical signs of a copper deficiency.

Early stages of a copper deficiency can easily be treated but have gone unnoticed because of a low clinical suspicion. If untreated, a copper deficiency will eventually end in irreversible neurological damage.

An early condition commonly noticed in a copper deficient patient is a type of anemia that does not respond to iron intake. In this type of anemia, iron absorption is hindered, and iron is redirected and forced to accumulate in tissues. Iron accumulation in joints induced by a copper deficiency has been considered a contributor to rheumatoid arthritis.

COPPER

A common cause associated with a deficiency is the long term dietary imbalance of zinc with copper. Animal and human studies have demonstrated that high intakes of zinc relative to copper induce a copper deficiency state known as hypocupremia. The risk of hypocupremia increases as the zinc / copper (Zn / Cu) ratio increases.

Further, balance studies show the amount of copper required by humans is dependent on the intake of zinc. A research group has shown that 20 mg of dietary zinc requires 1.6 mg of dietary copper for equilibrium. This equates to a Zn / Cu = 12.5.

For a comparison to other ratios, dividing the RDA for zinc by the RDA for copper equates to a Zn / Cu = 12.2 for adults. Thus, based on calculations, the optimal ratio range is 12.2 to 12.5. With these ratios in mind, consider the following experimental dietary studies.

A group of twenty four men were fed a diet with a Zn / Cu = 25. The abnormal outcomes were low plasma copper concentrations, low activity of copper-dependent enzymes, low concentrations of copper-dependent proteins, increased levels of the bad LDL cholesterol, and decreased concentrations of the good HDL cholesterol. The study was stopped after eleven weeks because of cardiac abnormalities. The zinc to copper ratio was believed to be a factor in the induction of the copper deficiency.

In another study, 12 premenopausal women and 12 post-menopausal women were fed similar diets with a Zn / Cu ≈ 18.0 for over eighty days. Although, there was no change in the plasma copper concentrations, there were reductions in copper-dependent enzyme activity and copper-dependent proteins, and a reduction in white blood cells needed for fighting infections.

In summary, zinc induced copper deficiencies has been identified, confirmed and is well grounded in science. Of course it is safe to eat foods with a high zinc / copper ratio but not every day throughout an entire life. Variety is what's important. Because of its low prevalence and nonspecific clinical manifestation, a copper deficiency may go unnoticed due to a lack of suspicion.

COPPER

This chapter list the copper values in micrograms (mcg) followed by the Zn / Cu ratios for the same foods. See reference section for reported cases of copper deficiencies.

Recommend Daily Intakes Levels for Copper

Children	Copper, mcg
1 to 3 year olds	340
4 to 8 year olds	440

Males	
9 to 13 year olds	700
14 to 18 year olds	890
19 to 30 years	900
31 to 50 years	900
51 to 70 years	900
Over 70	900

Females	
9 to 13 year olds	700
14 to 18 year olds	890
19 to 30 years	900
31 to 50 years	900
51 to 70 years	900
Over 70	900
Pregnancy	1000
Lactation	1300

COPPER

Alcohol	Amount	Copper (mcg)
Light Beer	1 bottle	21
Regular Beer	1 bottle	18
Red Wine	1 glass	16
Gin, Rum, Vodka, Whisky	1 shot	9
White Wine	1 glass	6

Beans, Canned	Amount	Copper (mcg)
White beans	1 cup	608
Navy beans	1 cup	545
Lima beans	1 cup	434
Great Northern	1 cup	419
Refried beans	1 cup	395
Pinto beans	1 cup	389
Kidney beans	1 cup	376
Cranberry beans	1 cup	369
Baked beans, plain	1 cup	368
Garbanzo beans	1 cup	367
Blackeyed peas	1 cup	281
Fava beans	1 cup	279
Green beans	1 cup	60
Yellow beans	1 cup	58

Beans, Cooked	Amount	Copper (mcg)
Winged beans	1 cup	1330
Natto	1 cup	1167
Soybeans, matured, dry roasted	1 cup	1003
Soybeans, mature	1 cup	700
Adzuki	1 cup	685
Hyacinath beans	1 cup	662
Garbanzo beans	1 cup	577
Edamame	1 cup	535
White beans, mature	1 cup	514
Black Turtle beans, mature	1 cup	498
Lentils	1 cup	497
Black-eyed peas	1 cup	458
Pigeon peas	1 cup	452
Lima beans	1 cup	442
Fava beans	1 cup	440
Great Northern	1 cup	437
Kidney beans	1 cup	428
Cranberry beans	1 cup	409
Lupini beans	1 cup	383
Navy beans,	1 cup	382

COPPER

Pinto beans	1 cup	374
Black beans	1 cup	359
Split peas	1 cup	355
Mung beans, mature seeds	1 cup	315
Moth beans	1 cup	290
White beans, small	1 cup	267
Soybeans, green	1 cup	211
Yellow beans	1 cup	129
Green beans	1 cup	71
Yardlong beans, Chinese long beans	1 cup	49

Beef, Cooked	Amount	Copper (mcg)
Tri Tip Steak, trimmed to 0" fat	3 oz	138
Ribeye steak, lean, trimmed 0" fat	3 oz	129
T-Bone steak, trimmed 0" fat	3 oz	111
Porterhouse steak, trimmed to 0" fat	3 oz	110
Chuck roast, trimmed to 1/8" fat	3 oz	105
Lond Broil, top round, trim to 0" fat	3 oz	105
Brisket, lean, trimmed to 0" fat	3 oz	98
Ground Beef, 95%, broiled	3 oz	82
Skirt Steak, trimmed to 0" fat	3 oz	79
Ground Beef, 90%	3 oz	77
Top sirloin, lean, trimmed to 1/8" fat	3 oz	74
Ground Beef, 85%, broiled	3 oz	72
Beef ribs, trimmed to 1/8" fat	3 oz	71
Filet Mignon, trimmed to 0" fat	3 oz	70
Flank steak, lean, trimmed to 0" fat	3 oz	69
Ground Beef, 80%	3 oz	68
Ground Beef, 75%	3 oz	64

Beef, Cooked	Amount	Copper (mcg)
Tri Tip steak, lean, trimmed to 0" fat	1 lb cooked	735
T-bone steak, trimmed to 0" fat	1 lb cooked	594
Porterhouse steak, trimmed to 0" fat	1 lb cooked	590
Chuck roast, trimmed to 1/8" fat	1 lb cooked	563
Brisket, lean, trimmed to 0" fat	1 lb cooked	522
Skirt steak, trimmed to 0" fat	1 lb cooked	422
Beef ribs, trimmed to 1/8" fat	1 lb cooked	381
Flank steak, lean, trimmed to 0" fat	1 lb cooked	368
Top Sirloin, trimmed to 1/8" fat	1 lb cooked	368
Ribeye steak, boneless, trimmed to 0" fat	1 steak	322
Flank steak, lean, trimmed to 0" fat	1 steak	310

RDA is 900 mcg for adults

COPPER

Ribeye filet, lean, trimmed to 0" fat	1 filet	181
Top Sirloin, choice filet, trimmed to 0" fat	1 filet	131
Filet Mignon, tenderloin, trimmed to 0" fat	1 steak	108

Beef, Cooked	Amount	Copper (mcg)
Ground beef, 95%	1/4 lb patty	79
Ground beef, 90%	1/4 lb patty	75
Ground beef, 85%	1/4 lb patty	65
Ground beef, 80%	1/4 lb patty	62
Ground beef, 75%	1/4 lb patty	52

Bread	Amount	Copper (mcg)
Bagel, Wheat	4" bagel	171
Indian bread, Naan, whole wheat	1 piece	167
Bagel, oat bran	4" bagel	159
Bagel, cinnamon & raisen	4" bagel	145
Mexican roll, bollilo	1 roll	132
Indian bread, Naan, plain	1 piece	116
Bagel, plain	4" bagel	116
Whole-Wheat	1 slice	106
Hamburger & Hotdog buns, plain	1 bun	95
Bagel, egg	4" bagel	94
Kaiser rolls	1 roll	93
Pumpernickle	1 slice	92
English Muffin, plain	1 muffin	77
Reduced calorie white	1 slice	76
Multigrain, and Whole-Grain	1 slice	73
Egg bread	1 slice	65
White	1 slice	63
Rye bread	1 slice	60
Cracked wheat	1 slice	56
Oatmeal bread	1 slice	56
Raisin bread	1 slice	51
Pita, white	6 inch pita	47
Croissants, butter	1 croissant	46
Tortillas, flour	1 tortilla	45
Tortillas, corn	1 tortilla	40
Wheat	1 slice	40
Dinner Rolls, brown & serve	1 roll	38
Cornbread	1 piece	37
French, italian, sourdough	1 slice	34
Potato bread	1 slice	30

RDA is 900 mcg for adults

COPPER

Butter	Amount	Copper (mcg)
Regular dairy whipped butter, salted	1 tbsp	2
Regular dairy butter, salted	1 tbsp	0

Cereal, General Mills®	Amount	Copper (mcg)
Multi-Bran CHEX	1 cup	241
Wheat Chex	1 cup	226
Raisin Nut Bran	1 cup	190
Oatmeal Crisp, Crunchy Almond	1 cup	120
Whole Grain Total	1 cup	120
Total Raisin Bran	1 cup	116
Total Cranberry Crunch	1 cup	113
Wheaties	1 cup	96
Honey Nut Clusters	1 cup	83
Lucky Charms	1 cup	81
Basic 4	1 cup	80
Oatmeal Crisp, Apple Cinnamon	1 cup	80
Cinnamon Toast Crunch	1 cup	70
Honey Nut Chex	1 cup	60
Golden Grahams	1 cup	58
Rice Chex	1 cup	55
Cocoa Puffs	1 cup	53
Dora The Explorer	1 cup	51
Reese's Puffs	1 cup	45
Cookie Crisp	1 cup	40
Corn Chex	1 cup	38
Kix	1 cup	34
Berry Berry Kix	1 cup	25
Trix	1 cup	15

Cereal, General Mills Cheerios®	Amount	Copper (mcg)
Original	1 cup	108
Oat Cluster Cheerios Crunch	1 cup	102
Honey Nut	1 cup	97
Apple Cinnamon	1 cup	96
Frosted	1 cup	95
Berry Burst, Triple Berry	1 cup	91
Yogurt Burst, Strawberry	1 cup	91
Multi Grain	1 cup	76
Fruity	1 cup	70
Banana Nut	1 cup	64
Chocolate	1 cup	53
Cinnamon Burst	1 cup	x

RDA is 900 mcg for adults

COPPER

Cereal, Kashi®	Amount	Copper (mcg)
7-Whole Grain Flakes	1 cup	x
7-Whole Grain Nuggets	1 cup	x
Berry Blossom	1 cup	x
Berry Fruitful	29 biscuits	x
Blackberry Hills	1 cup	x
Cinnamon Harvest	28 biscuits	x
Go Lean Crisp, Cinnamon Crumble	1 cup	x
Go Lean Crisp, Toasted Berry Crumble	1 cup	x
Go Lean Vanilla Graham	1 cup	x
Granola Cocoa Beach	1 cup	x
Granola Mountain Medley	1 cup	x
Heart to Heart, Nutty Chia Flax	1 cup	x
Heart to Heart, Warm Cinnamon	1 cup	x
Indigo Morning	1 cup	x
Kashi U	1 cup	x
Simply Maize	1 cup	x
Strawberry Fields	1 cup	x
Go Lean Crunch, Honey Almond Flax	1 cup	324
Go Lean	1 cup	312
Heart to Heart, Oat Flakes & Blueberry Clusters	1 cup	224
Autum Wheat	29 biscuits	223
Good Friends	1 cup	205
Go Lean Crunch	1 cup	159
Heart to Heart, Honey Toasted Oat	1 cup	121
7-Whole Grain Honey Puffs	1 cup	112
Island Vanilla	27 biscuits	110
7-Whole Grain Puffs	1 cup	81
Honey Sunshine	1 cup	80

Cereal, Kellogg's®	Amount	Copper (mcg)
All-Bran Original	1 cup	645
All-Bran Bran Buds	1 cup	450
Raisin Bran	1 cup	269
Cracklin' Oat Bran	1 cup	261
All-Bran Complete Wheat Flakes	1 cup	193
MUESLIX	1 cup	164
Raisin Bran Crunch	1 cup	159
Frosted MINI-Wheat's, Big-Bite	1 cup	145
Cocoa Krispies	1 cup	137
Smart Start, Strong Heart, Antioxidants	1 cup	128
Honey Smacks	1 cup	70
Frosted Rice Krispies	1 cup	66
Corn Flakes	1 cup	55
Rice Krispies	1 cup	54

RDA is 900 mcg for adults

COPPER

Continued

Crispix	1 cup	42
Smorz	1 cup	41
Honey Crunch Corn Flakes	1 cup	40
Rice Krispies Treats	1 cup	40
Product 19	1 cup	30
Apple Jacks	1 cup	27
Froot Loops	1 cup	26
Corn Pops	1 cup	25
Frosted Flakes	1 cup	16
CINNABON	1 cup	x
Crunchy Nut, Golden Honey Nut Flakes	1 cup	x
Crunchy Nut, Roasted Nut and Honey O's	1 cup	x
Fiberplus Berry Yogurt Crunch	1 cup	x
Fiberplus Cinnamon Oat Crunch	1 cup	x
Krave Chocolate	1 cup	x

Cereal, Kelloggs Special-K®	Amount	Copper (mcg)
Chocolately Delight	1 cup	157
Blueberry	1 cup	135
Fruit & Yogurt	1 cup	134
Cinnamon Pecan	1 cup	125
Vanilla Almond	1 cup	122
Red Berries	1 cup	53
Original	1 cup	46
Low Fat Granola	1 cup	x
Miltigrain Oats & Honey	1 cup	x
Protein Plus	1 cup	x

Cereal, Post®	Amount	Copper (mcg)
Grape-Nuts Cereal	1 cup	485
Raisin Bran	1 cup	295
Great Grains, Raisin, Date & Pecan	1 cup	293
Great Grains, Crunchy Pecan Cereal	1 cup	277
Bran Flakes	1 cup	240
Great Grains, Banana Nut Crunch	1 cup	236
Honey Nut Shredded Wheat	1 cup	198
Great Grains, Cranberry Almond Crunch	1 cup	192
Shredded Wheat n' Bran, spoon-size	1 cup	173
Shredded Wheat, Original, spoon-size	1 cup	164
Cocoa Pebbles	1 cup	116
Grape-Nuts Flakes	1 cup	116
Alpha-Bits	1 cup	90
Shredded Wheat, Frosted, spoon-size	1 cup	90
Shredded Wheat, Original, big-biscuit	1 cup	90
Blueberry Morning	1 cup	88

RDA is 900 mcg for adults

COPPER

Continued

Golden Crisp	1 cup	72
Fruity Pebbles	1 cup	36
Honeycomb Cereal	1 cup	21

Post® Honey Bunches of Oats®	Amount	Copper (mcg)
Just Bunches Honey Roasted	1 cup	255
With Vanilla Bunches	1 cup	168
With Almonds	1 cup	85
With Strawberries	1 cup	83
With Cinnamon Bunches	1 cup	80
Pecan Bunches	1 cup	77
Honey Roasted	1 cup	72

Cereal, Quaker®	Amount	Copper (mcg)
Oatmeal Squares	1 cup	265
Oatmeal Squares, Cinnamon	1 cup	257
Toasted Multigrain Crisp	1 cup	146
LIFE Cereal, Original	1 cup	116
LIFE Cereal, Cinnamon	1 cup	107
Puffed Wheat	1 cup	68
Puffed Rice	1 cup	45
Corn Bran Crunch	1 cup	42
CAP'N Crunch	1 cup	40
CAP'N Crunch's Peanut Butter Crunch	1 cup	40
CAP'N Crunch & Crunchberries	1 cup	38
Honey Graham OH'S	1 cup	31
CAP'N Crunch's OOPs! All Berries	1 cup	x
Granola, Apple, Cranberry, & Almond	1 cup	x
LIFE Cereal, Maple & Brown Sugar	1 cup	x
Oatmeal Squares, Golden Maple	1 cup	x

Cereal, Cooked in Water	Amount	Copper (mcg)
Oats, regular, unenriched	1 cup	173
WHEATENA	1 cup	126
CREAM OF WHEAT, regular	1 cup	100
Farina	1 cup	98
Malt-o-Meal plain	1 serving	40
Corn grits, white	1 cup	0
Corn grits, yellow	1 cup	0

Cheese	Amount	Copper (mcg)
Ricotta, part skim milk	1 cup	84
Cottage cheese, low fat, 2 %	1 cup	68
Cottage cheese, creamed, small curd	1 cup	65

RDA is 900 mcg for adults

COPPER

Continued

Cottage cheese, low fat, 1 %	1 cup	63
Ricotta, whole milk	1 cup	52
Cottage cheese, non fat, uncreamed	1 cup	44

Cheese	Amount	Copper (mcg)
Goat cheese, soft type	1 oz	208
Goat cheese, hard type	1 oz	178
Goat cheese, semisoft	1 oz	160
Parmesan, grated	1 oz	67
American, pasteurized process, fortified	1 oz	13
Colby	1 oz	12
Swiss	1 oz	12
Blue cheese	1 oz	11
Cream cheese, fat free	1 oz	10
Gouda	1 oz	10
Mozzarella, non fat	1 oz	10
Roquefort	1 oz	10
American, pasteurized process, low fat	1 oz	9
Cheddar	1 oz	9
Feta cheese	1 oz	9
Gruyere	1 oz	9
Monterey	1 oz	9
Monterey, low fat	1 oz	9
Muenster	1 oz	9
Muenster, low fat	1 oz	9
Romano	1 oz	9
Mozzarella, part skim milk, low moisture	1 oz	8
Swiss, low fat	1 oz	8
American, pasteurized process, imitation	1 oz	7
Fontina	1 oz	7
Provolone	1 oz	7
Provolone, reduced fat	1 oz	7
Cheddar, low fat	1 oz	6
Brie	1 oz	5
Cream cheese	1 oz	5
Mozzarella, whole milk	1 oz	3

Cheese, Mexican	Amount	Copper (mcg)
Queso fresco	1 oz	9
Queso seco	1 oz	8
Queso blanco	1 oz	7
Mexican, blend	1 oz	7
Queso asadero	1 oz	7

RDA is 900 mcg for adults

COPPER

Queso chihuahua	1 oz	7
Mexican, blend, reduced fat	1 oz	6
Queso anejo	1 oz	2

Chicken, Cooked	Amount	Copper (mcg)
Breast, with skin, fried with flour	1/2 breast	84
Thigh, with skin, fried	1 thigh	71
Drumstick, with skin, fried	1 drumstick	55
Breast, no skin, roasted	1/2 breast	42
Thigh, no skin, roasted	1 thigh	42
Drumstick, no skin, roasted	1 drumstick	35
Wing with skin, fried in batter	1 wing	31
Wing with skin, roasted	1 wing	19

Chicken, Cooked	Amount	Copper (mcg)
Thigh with skin, fried in flour	3 oz	76
Drumstick with skin, fried in flour	3 oz	68
Drumstick meat only, no skin, roasted	3 oz	57
Drumstick with skin, roasted	3 oz	55
Wing with skin, fried in flour	3 oz	52
Cornish game hens, meat only	3 oz	50
Breast meat only, no skin, roasted	3 oz	48
Wing with skin, roasted	3 oz	48
Thigh meat only, no skin, roasted	3 oz	46
Wing meat only, no skin, roasted	3 oz	46
Thigh with skin, roasted	3 oz	44
Breast with skin, fried in flour	3 oz	42
Breast with skin, roasted	3 oz	42

Cream	Amount	Copper (mcg)
Half & Half	1 tbsp	2
Sour Cream cultured	1 tbsp	2
Sour Cream reduced fat	1 tbsp	2
Heavy Cream	1 tbsp	1
Light Coffe Cream	1 tbsp	1

Eggs	Amount	Copper (mcg)
Egg whole, fried	1 large	36
Egg whole, poached	1 large	36
Egg whole, scrambled	1 large	36
Egg whites, dried	1 ounce	32
Egg substitute, fat free	1/4 cup	13
Egg yolk, raw	1 large	13

RDA is 900 mcg for adults

COPPER

Continued

Egg whites, dried powder, stabilized	1 tbsp	12
Egg whites, raw	1 large	8
Egg whole, hard boiled	1 large	7

Fish, Canned	Amount	Copper (mcg)
White (albacore) tuna, in oil	3 oz	110
Light tuna, in oil	3 oz	60
Light tuna, in water	3 oz	42
White (albacore) tuna, in water	3 oz	33

Fish, Cooked	Amount	Copper (mcg)
Atlantic salmon, wild	3 oz	273
Chinook salmon, smoked	3 oz	196
Walleye pike	3 oz	194
Mullet, striped	3 oz	120
Freshwater bass	3 oz	101
Pacific & Jack mackerel	3 oz	101
Bluefin tuna	3 oz	94
Skipjack (aku) tuna	3 oz	94
Atlantic herring, pickled	3 oz	89
Cat fish, breaded & fried	3 oz	86
Atlantic mackerel	3 oz	80
Coho salmon, farmed	3 oz	76
Florida pompano	3 oz	66
Orange roughy	3 oz	64
Pink salmon	3 oz	64
Tilapia	3 oz	64
Carp	3 oz	62
Sockeye salmon	3 oz	61
Coho salmon, wild	3 oz	60
Keta (chum) salmon	3 oz	60
Atlantic croaker	3 oz	55
Northern pike	3 oz	55
Spanish mackerel	3 oz	55
Atlantic pollock	3 oz	54
Walleye pollock	3 oz	51
Rainbow trout, wild	3 oz	49
Yellowtail	3 oz	49
Rainbow trout, farmed	3 oz	47
King salmon, chinook, smoked	3 oz	45
Atlantic salmon, farmed	3 oz	42
Snapper	3 oz	39
Swordfish	3 oz	39
Grouper	3 oz	38
Yellowfin tuna	3 oz	37

RDA is 900 mcg for adults

COPPER

Continued

Alaskan halibut	3 oz	35
Pacific Rockfish	3 oz	35
Striped bass	3 oz	34
Whiting	3 oz	34
Catfish, farmed	3 oz	33
Catfish, wild caught	3 oz	33
Greenland halibut	3 oz	32
Atlantic cod	3 oz	31
King mackerel	3 oz	28
Surimi	3 oz	27
Atlantic & Pacific halibut	3 oz	24
Atlantic perch	3 oz	22
Haddock	3 oz	22
Flounder & Sole	3 oz	20
Pacific cod	3 oz	20
Sea bass	3 oz	20

Fish, Shellfish, Cooked	Amount	Copper (mcg)
Oysters, breaded & fried	3 oz	3779
Eastern oysters, wild	3 oz	3773
Squid, fried	3 oz	1797
Northern lobster	3 oz	1318
Eastern oysters, farmed	3 oz	1219
Alaskan king crab	3 oz	1005
Blue crab	3 oz	692
Blue crab, canned	3 oz	692
Octopus	3 oz	628
Crayfish	3 oz	582
Queen crab	3 oz	528
Blue crab cakes	3 oz	518
Clams, breaded & fried	3 oz	303
Shrimp, breaded & fried	3 oz	233
Shrimp, canned	3 oz	223
Shrimp	3 oz	219
Abalone	3 oz	194
Clams, canned	3 oz	74
Scallops, breaded & fried	3 oz	66
Alaskan king crab, imitation	3 oz	27

Fruit, Canned	Amount	Copper (mcg)
Pineapple	1 cup	257
Apricots	1 cup	201
Peaches	1 cup	134
Pears	1 cup	130
Plums	1 cup	95

RDA is 900 mcg for adults

COPPER

Applesauce, sweetened	1 cup	82
Applesauce, unsweetened	1 cup	66
Olives, black	5 large	55
Olives, green	5 large	16

Fruit, Dried	Amount	Copper (mcg)
Currants	1 cup	694
Pears	1 cup	668
Peaches	1 cup	582
Apricots	1 cup	446
Figs	1 cup	428
Apples	1 cup	164
Cranberries, sweetened	1 cup	97

Fruit, Frozen	Amount	Copper (mcg)
Raspberries	1 cup	262
Blackberries, unsweetened	1 cup	181
Blueberries	1 cup	90
Peaches	1 cup	60
Strawberries	1 cup	48

Fruit, Raw	Amount	Copper (mcg)
Avocado, Florida	1 cup	715
Prunes, uncooked	1 cup	489
Raisins	1 cup	461
Avocado, California, pureed	1 cup	391
Prunes, stewed	1 cup	305
Dates	1 cup	303
Pomegrenates	1 cup	275
Blackberries	1 cup	238
Kiwi	1 cup	234
Grapes	1 cup	203
Mango	1 cup	183
Pears	1 cup	182
Pineapple	1 cup	182
Apricots	1 cup	129
Nectarine	1 cup	123
Plantains	1 cup	120
Peachs	1 cup	116
Raspberries	1 cup	111
Black currants	1 cup	96
Plum	1 cup	94
Cherries, sweet	1 cup	92
Mulberries	1 cup	84

RDA is 900 mcg for adults

COPPER

Blueberries	1 cup	83
Tangerine	1 cup	82
Oranges	1 cup	81
Strawberries	1 cup	80
Grapefruit, pink & red sections	1 cup	74
Florida Oranges	1 cup	72
Valencias Oranges	1 cup	67
Cataloupe	1 cup	66
Papayas	1 cup	65
Naval Oranges	1 cup	64
Water mellon	1 cup	64
Jicama	1 cup	62
Cranberries	1 cup	61
Honeydew	1 cup	41
Apples	1 cup	34

Fruit, Raw	Amount	Copper (mcg)
Avocado, Florida	1 fruit	945
Pomegranates	1 fruit	446
Mango	1 fruit	373
Pummelo	1 fruit	292
Chayote	1 fruit	250
Avocado, California	1 fruit	231
Persimmons, Japanese	1 fruit	190
Cherimoya	1 fruit	162
Plantains	1 fruit	145
Raisins	1 small box	137
Pears	1 fruit	136
Star fruit, Carambola	1 fruit	125
Prunes, uncooked	5 fruit	118
Nectarine	1 fruit	117
Cantaloupe	1/2 fruit	113
Kiwi	1 fruit	99
Banana	1 fruit	92
Dates	5 fruit	73
Papayas, small	1 fruit	71
Peaches	1 fruit	67
Grapes, red or green	10 fruit	62
Florida Oranges	1 fruit	55
Naval Oranges	1 fruit	55
Olives, Black	5 large	55
Olives, Green	5 large	55
Pineapple, slices	1/2" x 3"	55
Cherries	10 fruit	49
Valencias Oranges	1 fruit	45

RDA is 900 mcg for adults

COPPER

Grapefruit, pink & red	1/2 fruit	39
Plums	1 fruit	38
Apples	1 fruit	37
Tangerine	1 fruit	35
Strawberries	5 fruit	29
Apricots	1 fruit	27
Figs, dried	1 fruit	24
Kumquats	1 fruit	18
Pineapple guava, Feijoa	1 fruit	15
Persimmons, small native	1 fruit	x

Game Meat, Cooked	Amount	Copper (mcg)
Deer	3 oz	255
Caribou	3 oz	224
Duck	3 oz	196
Antelope	3 oz	181
Buffalo, steak, free range	3 oz	161
Rabbit, wild, stewed	3 oz	150
Squirrel	3 oz	126
Bison, ground	3 oz	124
Elk, ground	3 oz	121
Elk, roasted	3 oz	121
Deer, ground	3 oz	85
Wild boar	3 oz	48

Grains, Cooked	Amount	Copper (mcg)
Kamut	1 cup	427
Spelt	1 cup	417
Amaranth	1 cup	367
Quinoa	1 cup	355
Spaghetti, spinach	1 cup	287
Millet	1 cup	280
Buckwheat, groats	1 cup	245
Macaroni, Whole-Wheat	1 cup	234
Spaghetti, Whole-Wheat	1 cup	234
Wild rice	1cup	198
Brown rice	1 cup	195
Oats, regular, unenriched	1 cup	173
Barley, pearled	1 cup	165
Egg noodles	1 cup	157
Oat bran	1 cup	145
Macaroni	1 cup	140
Spaghetti	1 cup	140

RDA is 900 mcg for adults

COPPER

Bulgur	1 cup	136
Egg & Spinach noodles	1 cup	128
White rice, long-grain, paraboiled	1 cup	111
White rice, long-grain, regular	1 cup	109
Rice noodles	1 cup	67
Couscous	1 cup	64
White rice, long-grain, instant	1 cup	61
Soba noodles	1 cup	9

Herbs & Spices	Amount	Copper (mcg)
Mace, ground	1 tsp	42
Pepper, black, whole	1 tsp	39
Pepper, black, ground	1 tsp	31
Basil, dried & ground	1 tsp	29
Celery seeds	1 tsp	27
Chili powder	1 tsp	27
Nutmeg, ground	1 tsp	23
Fennel seed	1 tsp	21
Anise seed	1 tsp	19
Caraway seeds	1 tsp	19
Coriander, seeds	1 tsp	18
Garlic powder	1 tsp	17
Curry powder	1 tsp	16
Paprika, powder	1 tsp	16
Basil, dried leaves	1 tsp	15
Onion powder	1 tsp	14
Tumeric, ground	1 tsp	13
Thyme, dried, ground	1 tsp	12
All spice, ground	1 tsp	11
Capers, canned	1 tsp	11
Coriander, dried	1 tsp	11
Oregano, dried, ground	1 tsp	11
Tarragon, dried, ground	1 tsp	11
Cilantro	1/4 cup	9
Cinnamon powder	1 tsp	9
Ginger, ground	1 tsp	9
Thyme, dried, leaves	1 tsp	9
Cloves, dried, ground	1 tsp	8
Spearmint, dried	1 tsp	8
Marjoram, dried	1 tsp	7
Rosemary, dried	1 tsp	7
Oregano, dried, leaves	1 tsp	6
Dill weed, dried	1 tsp	5
Sage, ground	1 tsp	5
Spearmint, fresh	1 tsp	5

RDA is 900 mcg for adults

COPPER

Parsley, dried	1 tsp	4
Tarragon, dried, leaves	1 tsp	4
Thyme, fresh	1 tsp	4
Basil, fresh, chopped	1 tsp	3
Chervil, dried	1 tsp	3
Dill weed, fresh	1/4 cup	3
Bay leaf, crumbled	1 tsp	2
Chives, raw, chopped	1 tsp	2
Rosemary, fresh	1 tsp	2
Saffron	1 tsp	2

Juice	Amount	Copper (mcg)
Vegetable	1 cup	484
Prune	1 cup	174
Pineapple	1 cup	172
Tomato	1 cup	148
Carrot	1 cup	109
Orange, raw	1 cup	109
Grapefruit juice, raw	1 cup	82
Pomegranate	1 cup	52
Grape	1 cup	46
Lemon juice, raw	1 cup	39
Apple	1 cup	30
Cranberry	1 cup	25

Lamb, Cooked	Amount	Copper (mcg)
Cubed, for stew or kabob	3 oz	128
Rib, lean, trimmed to 1/4" fat	3 oz	118
Chops, loin, lean, trimmed to 1/4" fat	3 oz	110
Ground, broiled	3 oz	109
Foreshank, trimmed to 1/8" fat	3 oz	105
Leg, whole, trimmed to 1/4"	3 oz	98

Milk	Amount	Copper (mcg)
Coconut milk, canned	1 cup	504
Soy milk, original, unfortified	1 cup	311
Human milk	1 cup	128
Sheep milk	1 cup	113
Goat milk	1 cup	112
Buttermilk, whole milk	1 cup	61
Whole milk, 3.25%	1 cup	61
Canned, condensed, sweetened	1 cup	46
Canned, evaporated, nonfat	1 cup	41
Canned, evaporated	1 cup	40
Nonfat, fat free or skim milk	1 cup	32

RDA is 900 mcg for adults

COPPER

Buttermilk, lowfat	1 cup	27
Lowfat, 1%	1 cup	24
Reduced fat, 2%	1 cup	15
Dry, instant, nonfat	1/3 cup	9

Nuts & Seeds	Amount	Copper (mcg)
Sesame seeds	1 oz	1157
Cashews	1 oz	622
Sunflower seeds	1 oz	510
Brazilnuts	1 oz	494
Hazelnuts	1 oz	489
Tahini	1 oz	456
English walnuts	1 oz	450
Black walnuts	1 oz	386
Pumpkin seeds	1 oz	381
Pine nuts	1 oz	375
Pistachio	1 oz	369
Mixed nuts, roasted with peanuts, no salt	1 oz	363
Flaxseeds	1 oz	346
Pecans	1 oz	340
Peanuts	1 oz	324
Almonds	1 oz	282
Trail mix, regular, salted	1 oz	279
Chia seeds	1 oz	262
Trail mix, regular with chocolate chips	1 oz	239
Macadamia	1 oz	214
Trail mix, tropical	1 oz	150
Peanut butter, smooth style	1 oz	134
Coconut, raw meat	1 oz	123

Nuts & Seeds	Amount	Copper (mcg)
Sesame seeds	1/4 cup	1470
Sunflower seeds	1/4 cup	630
Brazilnuts, whole	1/4 cup	580
Flaxseeds	1/4 cup	512
Hazelnuts, chopped	1/4 cup	496
Pine nuts	1/4 cup	447
Mixed nuts, roasted with peanuts, no salt	1/4 cup	438
Pumpkin seeds	1/4 cup	433
Black walnuts, chopped	1/4 cup	425
Peanuts	1/4 cup	418
Pistachio	1/4 cup	400
English walnuts, chopped	1/4 cup	396
Trail mix, regular, salted	1/4 cup	369
Sesame seeds	1 tbsp	367

RDA is 900 mcg for adults

COPPER

Almonds, whole	1/4 cup	356
Trail mix, regular with chocolate chips	1/4 cup	308
Peanut butter, smooth	1/4 cup	305
Pecans, halves	1/4 cup	297
Macadamia	1/4 cup	253
Trail mix, tropical	1/4 cup	185
Peanut butter, smooth	1 tbsp	151
Flaxseeds	1 tbsp	126
Coconut meat, shredded	1/4 cup	87
Cashews	1/4 cup	x
Chia seeds	1/4 cup	x

Pork, Cooked	Amount	Copper (mcg)
Braunschweiger	3 oz	204
Bacon	3 oz	139
Liverwurst spread	1/4 cup	132
Spareribs	3 oz	121
Center loin chops, pan-fried	3 oz	100
Center loin chops, lean, pan-fried	3 oz	100
Chops, lean, pan-fried	3 oz	100
Chops, pan-fried	3 oz	100
Tenderloin	3 oz	94
Backribs	3 oz	91
Bratwurst	3 oz	88
Polish sausage	3 oz	77
Cured ham, lean	3 oz	74
Sausage	3 oz	73
Sirloin chops	3 oz	72
Cured ham	3 oz	71
Italian sausage	3 oz	68
Chops, broiled	3 oz	66
Canadian-style bacon	3 oz	46

Soup (canned)	Amount	Copper (mcg)
Bean with Ham, chunky, ready-to-serve	1 cup	389
Bean with Pork, chunky, add water	1 cup	385
Pea soup, add water	1 cup	293
Chicken Vegetable, chunky, ready to serve	1 cup	240
Clam Chowder, New England	1 cup	240
Chunky Vegetable, ready-to-serve	1 cup	203
Tomato with water	1 cup	200
Minestrone, ready-to-serve	1 cup	196
Tomato with milk	1 cup	195
Cream of Mushroom with water	1 cup	191
Cream of Mushroom with Milk	1 cup	188

RDA is 900 mcg for adults

COPPER

Vegetable beef, add water	1 cup	154
Chicken Noodle, add water	1 cup	146
Beef Noodle, add water	1 cup	139
Cream of Chicken with Milk	1 cup	133
Vegetarian Vegetable, add water	1 cup	132
Clam Chowder, Manhattan	1 cup	128
Chicken with Rice, add water	1 cup	124
Cream of Chicken with water	1 cup	123
Minestrone, add water	1 cup	118

Turkey, Cooked	Amount	Copper (mcg)
Ground turkey, 85% lean	3 oz	218
Ground turkey, 93% lean	3 oz	137
Ground turkey	3 oz	128
Turkey sausage, reduced fat	3 oz	127
Turkey bacon	3 oz	123
Dark meat	3 oz	108
Breast meat	3 oz	60
Light meat	3 oz	54
Ground turkey, fat free	3 oz	52

Veal, Cooked	Amount	Copper (mcg)
Leg, top round	3 oz	119
Sirloin	3 oz	110
Foreshank	3 oz	94
Loin	3 oz	94
Ground	3 oz	88
Rib	3 oz	84
Breast	3 oz	65

Vegetables, Canned	Amount	Copper (mcg)
Tomato paste	1 cup	956
Tomato pure	1 cup	718
Spinach	1 cup	385
Mushrooms	1 cup	367
Sweet potato	1 cup	327
Tomato sauce	1 cup	287
Tomatoes, stewed	1 cup	286
Pumpkin	1 cup	262
Asparagus	1 cup	232
Sauerkraut	1 cup	227
Green peas	1 cup	179
Tomatoes, ripe	1 cup	166
Carrots	1 cup	152

COPPER

Continued

Corn, yellow, sweet	1 cup	101
Beets	1 cup	100
Green beans	1 cup	53

Vegetables, Cooked	Amount	Copper (mcg)
Shitake mushrooms	1 cup	1299
White mushrooms	1 cup	786
Turnip greens	1 cup	364
Beet greens	1 cup	361
Split peas	1 cup	355
Spinach	1 cup	313
Sweet potato, mashed	1 cup	308
Potatoes, mashed with whole milk	1 cup	304
Asparagus	1 cup	297
Swiss chard	1 cup	285
Potatoes, baked flesh	1 cup	262
Pumpkin	1 cup	223
Kohlrabi	1 cup	218
Parsnips	1 cup	215
Artichokes	1 cup	213
Yams, cubed	1 cup	207
Kale	1 cup	203
Summer squash	1 cup	185
Tomatoes	1 cup	180
Acorn squash	1 cup	176
Winter squash	1 cup	168
Scallop or Pattypan Squash, slices	1 cup	149
Onions	1 cup	141
Okra	1 cup	136
Butternut squash	1 cup	133
Brussels sprouts	1 cup	129
Beets	1 cup	126
Snow peas	1 cup	123
Dandelion greens	1 cup	121
Mustard greens	1 cup	118
Crookneck or Straighneck Squash, slices	1 cup	117
Napa cabbage	1 cup	105
Broccoli	1 cup	95
Hubbard Squash	1 cup	92
Zucchini	1 cup	90
Corn	1 cup	73
Prickley pear cactus pads	1 cup	73
Collard greens	1 cup	72
Green beans	1 cup	71
Rutabagas	1 cup	70

RDA is 900 mcg for adults

COPPER

Continued

Leeks	1 cup	64
Raab broccoli	1 cup	64
Eggplant	1 cup	58
Broccolini	1 cup	54
Celery	1 cup	54
Spaghetti Squash	1 cup	54
Bok-Choy	1 cup	32
Carrots	1 cup	27
Cabbage	1 cup	26
Cauliflower	1 cup	22
Turnips, cubes	1 cup	3

Vegetables, Frozen	Amount	Copper (mcg)
Spinach	1 cup	306
Turnip greens	1 cup	246
Asparagus	1 cup	189
Green peas	1 cup	168
Okra	1 cup	140
Carrots	1 cup	120
Collard greens	1 cup	94
Butternut squash	1 cup	86
Green beans	1 cup	80
Corn	1 cup	79
Rhubarb	1 cup	65
Broccoli	1 cup	63
Kale	1 cup	61
Brussels sprouts	1 cup	53
Cauliflower	1 cup	43

Vegetables, Raw	Amount	Copper (mcg)
Spirulina, dried	1 tbsp	427
Crimini mushrooms	1 cup	360
Portabella mushrooms	1 cup	246
White mushrooms	1 cup	223
Oyster mushrooms	1 cup	210
Kale	1 cup	194
Shiitake mushrooms, dried	1 each	186
Yellow bell peppers	1 cup	159
Radicchio	1 cup	136
Mustard spinach	1 cup	112
Tomatoes	1 cup	106
Tomatillos	1 cup	104
Butternut squash	1 cup	101
Green bell peppers	1 cup	98
Dandelion greens	1 cup	94

COPPER

Continued

Tomatoes, cherry	1 cup	88
Chicory greens	1 cup	86
Green onions & scallions	1 cup	83
Snow peas	1 cup	77
Enoki mushrooms	1 cup	70
Swiss chard	1 cup	64
Onions	1 cup	62
Zucchini	1 cup	60
Summer squash	1 cup	58
Carrots	1 cup	50
Endive	1 cup	50
Belgian endive	1 cup	46
Cactus pads, Nopales	1 cup	45
Broccoli	1 cup	43
Cucumbers	1 cup	43
Savoy cabbage	1 cup	43
Celery	1 cup	42
Cauliflower	1 cup	39
Spinach	1 cup	39
Romaine lettuce	1 cup	27
Shiitake mushrooms	1 each	27
Watercress	1 cup	26
Red bell peppers	1 cup	25
Raab broccoli	1 cup	17
Green leaf lettuce	1 cup	16
Iceburg lettuce	1 cup	16
Arugula	1 cup	15
Bok-Choy	1 cup	15
Cabbage	1 cup	13
Red cabbage	1 cup	12
Butterhead & boston lettuce	1 cup	9
Red leaf lettuce	1 cup	8

RDA is 900 mcg for adults

Nutrient Data Collection Form

Food	Amount	Book Numbers	Multiply By	Estimated Nutrient Intake
Nutrient::	RDA:	Estimated:	% of RDA:	Total Estimated:

To download additional forms for free goto www.TopNutrients4U.com

ZINC TO COPPER RATIO

Alcohol	Amount	Zinc / Copper
White Wine	1 glass	30
Red Wine	1 glass	13
Regular Beer	1 bottle	2
Gin, Rum, Vodka, Whisky	1 shot	2
Light Beer	1 bottle	2

Beans, Canned	Amount	Zinc / Copper
Baked beans, plain	1 cup	16
Yellow beans	1 cup	8
Blackeyed peas	1 cup	6
Cranberry beans	1 cup	6
Fava beans	1 cup	6
Green beans	1 cup	5
White beans	1 cup	5
Garbanzo beans	1 cup	5
Kidney beans	1 cup	4
Great Northern	1 cup	4
Refried beans	1 cup	4
Navy beans	1 cup	4
Lima beans	1 cup	4
Pinto beans	1 cup	3

Beans, Cooked	Amount	Zinc / Copper
Hyacinth beans	1 cup	8
Soybeans, green	1 cup	8
Yardlong beans, Chinese long beans	1 cup	8
White beans, small	1 cup	7
Lupini beans	1 cup	6
Adzuki	1 cup	6
Split peas	1 cup	6
Mung beans	1 cup	5
Black beans	1 cup	5
Lentils	1 cup	5
Cranberry beans	1 cup	5
Navy beans,	1 cup	5
Black-eyed peas	1 cup	5
White beans, mature	1 cup	5
Natto	1 cup	5
Pinto beans	1 cup	4
Soybeans, mature, dry roasted	1 cup	4
Kidney beans	1 cup	4
Green beans	1 cup	4
Garbanzo beans	1 cup	4

ZINC TO COPPER RATIO

Continued

Lima beans	1 cup	4
Edamame	1 cup	4
Fava beans	1 cup	4
Mothbeans	1 cup	4
Great Northern	1 cup	4
Yellow beans	1 cup	3
Pigeon peas	1 cup	3
Black Turtle beans, mature	1 cup	3
Soybeans, mature	1 cup	3
Winged beans	1 cup	2

Beef, Cooked	Amount	Zinc / Copper
Ground Beef, 75%	3 oz	82
Ground Beef, 80%	3 oz	78
Skirt Steak, trim to 0" fat	3 oz	78
Ground Beef, 85%, broiled	3 oz	74
Ground Beef, 90%	3 oz	70
Brisket, lean, trim to 0" fat	3 oz	69
Ground Beef, 95%, broiled	3 oz	67
Chuck roast, trim to 1/8" fat	3 oz	67
Beef ribs, trim to 1/8" fat	3 oz	65
Ribeye steak, lean, trim 0" fat	3 oz	63
Flank steak, lean, trim to 0" fat	3 oz	63
Top sirloin, lean, trim to 1/8" fat	3 oz	63
Filet Mignon, trim to 0" fat	3 oz	60
London Broil, top round, trim to 0" fat	3 oz	37
T-Bone steak, trim 0" fat	3 oz	36
Porterhouse steak, trim to 0" fat	3 oz	35

Bread	Amount	Zinc / Copper
Potato bread	1 slice	15
Bagel, plain	4" bagel	15
Pita, white	6 inch pita	11
Cornbread	1 piece	10
Croissants, butter	1 croissant	9
Bagel, egg	4" bagel	9
Tortillas, corn	1 tortilla	9
Reduced calorie wheat	1 slice	8
English Muffin, plain	1 muffin	8
Wheat	1 slice	8
Dinner Rolls, brown & serve	1 roll	7
Bagel, cinnamon & raisen	4" bagel	7
French, italian, sourdough	1 slice	7
Bagel, wheat	4" bagel	6
Multigrain, and Whole-Grain	1 slice	6

ZINC TO COPPER RATIO

Continued

Rye bread	1 slice	6
Bagel, oat bran	4" bagel	6
Kaiser rolls	1 roll	6
Cracked wheat	1 slice	6
Pumpernickle	1 slice	5
Oatmeal bread	1 slice	5
Egg bread	1 slice	5
Reduced calorie rye	1 slice	5
Whole-Wheat	1 slice	5
Reduced calorie white	1 slice	4
Tortillas, flour	1 tortilla	4
Raisin bread	1 slice	4
White	1 slice	3
Hamburger & Hotdog buns, plain	1 bun	3

Cereal, General Mills®	Amount	Zinc / Copper
Trix	1 cup	235
Total Whole Grain	1 cup	167
Frosted Chex	1 cup	139
Total Raisin Bran	1 cup	129
Cookie Crisp	1 cup	125
Kix	1 cup	123
Berry Berry Kix	1 cup	120
Reese's Puffs	1 cup	111
Total Cranberry Crunch	1 cup	106
Wheaties	1 cup	104
Cinnamon Toast Crunch	1 cup	101
Corn Chex	1 cup	99
Dora The Explorer	1 cup	98
Golden Grahams	1 cup	86
Honey Nut Chex	1 cup	83
Cocoa Puffs	1 cup	79
Rice Chex	1 cup	68
Lucky Charms	1 cup	60
Basic 4	1 cup	47
Oatmeal Crisp, Apple Cinnamon	1 cup	47
Honey Nut Clusters	1 cup	45
Cinnamon Toast, 25% Less Sugar	1 cup	37
Wheat Chex	1 cup	31
Raisin Nut Bran	1 cup	22
Multi-Bran CHEX	1 cup	21
Oatmeal Crisp, Crunchy Almond	1 cup	7

ZINC TO COPPER RATIO

Cereal, General Mills Cheerios®	Amount	Zinc / Copper
Chocolate	1 cup	94
Banana Nut	1 cup	78
Fruity	1 cup	71
Berry Burst, Triple Berry	1 cup	55
Yogurt Burst, Strawberry	1 cup	55
Frosted	1 cup	54
Apple Cinnamon	1 cup	52
Honey Nut	1 cup	51
Multi Grain	1 cup	49
Oat Clusters Cherrios Crunch	1 cup	49
Original	1 cup	43

Cereal, General Mill's Fiber One®	Amount	Zinc / Copper
Honey Clusters	1 cup	64
Original Bran Cereal	1 cup	40
Caramel Delight	1 cup	29
Raisin Bran Clusters	1 cup	27
80 Calorie Chocolate Squares	1 cup	x
80 Calorie Honey Squares	1 cup	x
Frosted Shreaded Wheat	1 cup	x
Nutty Clusters & almonds	1 cup	x

Cereal, Kashi®	Amount	Zinc / Copper
Heart to Heart, Honey Toasted Oat	1 cup	15
Organic Promise, Island Vanilla	1 cup	13
Good Friends	1 cup	7
7-Whole Grain Puffs	1 cup	7
7-Whole Grain Honey Puffs	1 cup	7
Good Friends, Cinna- Raisin Crunch	1 cup	5
Organic Promise, Autumn Wheat	1 cup	4
Go Lean Crunch	1 cup	3
Go Lean Crunch, Honey Almond Flax	1 cup	2
Go Lean	1 cup	1

Cereal, Kellogg's®	Amount	Zinc / Copper
Product 19	1 cup	500
Smart Start, Strong Heart, Antioxidants	1 cup	117
All-Bran Complete Wheat Flakes	1 cup	104
Corn Pops	1 cup	60
Froot Loops	1 cup	58
Apple Jacks	1 cup	56
Smorz	1 cup	37
Crispix	1 cup	36

ZINC TO COPPER RATIO

Continued

	Amount	Zinc / Copper
MUESLIX	1 cup	34
Cocoa Krispies	1 cup	15
All-Bran Original	1 cup	12
All-Bran Bran Buds	1 cup	10
Raisin Bran Crunch	1 cup	9
Honey Smacks	1 cup	9
Rice Krispies Treats	1 cup	8
Cracklin' Oat Bran	1 cup	8
Frosted MINI-Wheat's, Big-Bite	1 cup	8
Raisin Bran	1 cup	7
Rice Krispies	1 cup	7
Corn Flakes	1 cup	5
Frosted Rice Krispies	1 cup	5
Frosted Flakes	1 cup	4
Honey Crunch Corn Flakes	1 cup	3
CINNABON	1 cup	x
Crunchy Nut, Golden Honey Nut Flakes	1 cup	x
Crunchy Nut, Roasted Nut and Honey O's	1 cup	x
Fiberplus Berry Yogurt Crunch	1 cup	x
Fiberplus Cinnamon Oat Crunch	1 cup	x
Frosted MINI-Wheat's, Bit-Size	1 cup	x
Krave Chocolate	1 cup	x

Cereal, Kelloggs Special-K®	Amount	Zinc / Copper
Protein Plus	1 cup	10
Red Berries	1 cup	7
Original	1 cup	6
Fruit & Yogurt	1 cup	5
Cinnamon Pecan	1 cup	5
Chocolately Delight	1 cup	4
Vanilla Almond	1 cup	3

Cereal, Post®	Amount	Zinc / Copper
Fruity Pebbles	1 cup	56
Honeycomb Cereal	1 cup	48
Golden Crisp	1 cup	28
Grape-Nuts Flakes	1 cup	26
Cocoa Pebbles	1 cup	17
Alpha-Bits	1 cup	17
Shredded Wheat, Frosted, spoon-size	1 cup	17
Grape-Nuts Cereal	1 cup	13
Great Grains, Cranberry Almond Crunch	1 cup	10
Shredded Wheat, Original, spoon-size	1 cup	9
Shredded Wheat n' Bran, spoon-size	1 cup	9
Bran Flakes	1 cup	8

ZINC TO COPPER RATIO

Continued

Shredded Wheat, Original, big-biscuit	1 cup	8
Blueberry Morning	1 cup	8
Honey Nut Shredded Wheat	1 cup	8
Raisin Bran	1 cup	8
Great Grains, Banana Nut Crunch	1 cup	6
Great Grains, Crunchy Pecan Cereal	1 cup	6
Great Grains, Raisin, Date & Pecan	1 cup	6

Post® Honey Bunches of Oats®	Amount	Zinc / Copper
Honey Roasted	1 cup	28
Just Bunches Honey Roasted	1 cup	9
Pecan Bunches	1 cup	5
With Cinnamon Bunches	1 cup	5
With Strawberries	1 cup	5
With Almonds	1 cup	4
With Vanilla Bunches	1 cup	2

Cereal, Quaker®	Amount	Zinc / Copper
Honey Graham OH'S	1 cup	213
CAP'N Crunch & Crunchberries	1 cup	151
CAP'N Crunch	1 cup	146
CAP'N Crunch's Peanut Butter Crunch	1 cup	138
Corn Bran Crunch	1 cup	131
LIFE Cereal, Cinnamon	1 cup	55
LIFE Cereal, Original	1 cup	41
Toasted Multigrain Crisp	1 cup	22
Oatmeal Squares, Cinnamon	1 cup	16
Oatmeal Squares	1 cup	15
Puffed Wheat	1 cup	7
Puffed Rice	1 cup	5

Cereal, Cooked	Amount	Zinc / Copper
Corn grits, white	1 cup	44
Corn grits, yellow	1 cup	34
Oats, regular, unenriched	1 cup	14
WHEATENA	1 cup	13
Oats, instant, fortified, plain	1 cup	9
Farina	1 cup	6
Malt-o-Meal plain	1 serving	5
CREAM OF WHEAT, regular	1 cup	3

ZINC TO COPPER RATIO

Continued

Cheese	Amount	Zinc / Copper
Ricotta, whole milk	1 cup	55
Ricotta, part skim milk	1 cup	39
Cottage cheese, non fat, uncreamed	1 cup	15
Cottage cheese, low fat, 1%	1 cup	15
Cottage cheese, creamed, small curd	1 cup	14
Cottage cheese, low fat, 2%	1 cup	13

Cheese	Amount	Zinc / Copper
Mozzarella, whole milk	1 oz	277
Fontina	1 oz	141
Swiss, low fat	1 oz	136
Brie	1 oz	134
Provolone	1 oz	131
Provolone, reduced fat	1 oz	129
Gruyere	1 oz	123
Mozzarella, part skim milk, low moisture	1 oz	111
Gouda	1 oz	111
Mozzarella, non fat	1 oz	111
Swiss	1 oz	103
Cheddar	1 oz	98
Monterey	1 oz	94
Monterey, low fat	1 oz	93
Feta cheese	1 oz	91
Muenster	1 oz	89
Muenster, low fat	1 oz	88
Cheddar, low fat	1 oz	87
Romano	1 oz	81
Colby	1 oz	73
Blue cheese	1 oz	68
Roquefort	1 oz	59
American, pasteurized process	1 oz	55
Cream cheese, fat free	1 oz	43
Cream cheese	1 oz	28
Parmesan, grated	1 oz	16
Goat cheese, hard type	1 oz	3
Goat cheese, soft type	1 oz	1
Goat cheese, semisoft	1 oz	1

Cheese, Mexican	Amount	Zinc / Copper
Queso anejo	1 oz	415
Mexican, blend, reduced fat	1 oz	203
Queso chihuahua	1 oz	141
Queso asadero	1 oz	123

ZINC TO COPPER RATIO

Continued

Mexican, blend	1 oz	121
Queso fresco	1 oz	81

Chicken, Cooked	Amount	Zinc / Copper
Wing meat only, no skin, roasted	3 oz	40
Drumstick with skin, fried in flour	3 oz	36
Drumstick meat only, no skin, roasted	3 oz	36
Drumstick with skin, roasted	3 oz	35
Thigh meat only, no skin, roasted	3 oz	33
Thigh with skin, roasted	3 oz	31
Wing with skin, roasted	3 oz	31
Wing with skin, fried in flour	3 oz	29
Thigh with skin, fried in flour	3 oz	28
Cornish game hens, meat only	3 oz	26
Breast with skin, fried in flour	3 oz	22
Breast with skin, roasted	3 oz	21
Breast meat only, no skin, roasted	3 oz	18

Cream	Amount	Zinc / Copper
Half & Half	1 tbsp	40
Light Coffe Cream	1 tbsp	40
Sour Cream reduced fat	1 tbsp	40
Heavy Cream	1 tbsp	30
Sour Cream cultured	1 tbsp	25

Eggs	Amount	Zinc / Copper
Egg whole, hard boiled	1 large	76
Egg substitute, fat free	1/4 cup	45
Egg yolk, raw	1 large	29
Egg whole, fried	1 large	18
Egg whole, poached	1 large	18
Egg whole, scrambled	1 large	18
Egg whites, raw	1 large	1.3
Egg whites, dried	1 ounce	0.9
Egg whites, dried powder, stabilized	1 tbsp	0.8

ZINC TO COPPER RATIO

FISH

Fish, Canned	Amount	Zinc / Copper
Light tuna, in water	3 oz	14
Light tuna, in oil	3 oz	13
White (albacore) tuna, in water	3 oz	12
Atlantic sardines, in oil	3 oz	7
White (albacore) tuna, in oil	3 oz	4

Fish, Cooked	Amount	Zinc / Copper
Carp	3 oz	26
Sea bass	3 oz	22
King mackerel	3 oz	22
Alaskan halibut	3 oz	18
Swordfish	3 oz	17
Flounder & Sole	3 oz	17
Pacific cod	3 oz	17
Atlantic cod	3 oz	16
Catfish, wild caught	3 oz	16
Haddock	3 oz	15
Atlantic & Pacific halibut	3 oz	15
Catfish, farmed	3 oz	15
Atlantic perch	3 oz	14
Greenland halibut	3 oz	13
Northern pike	3 oz	13
Whiting	3 oz	13
Striped bass	3 oz	13
Yellowtail	3 oz	12
Grouper	3 oz	11
King salmon, chinook, smoked	3 oz	11
Pacific Rockfish	3 oz	11
Surimi	3 oz	10
Yellowfin tuna	3 oz	10
Atlantic mackerel	3 oz	10
Rainbow trout, farmed	3 oz	10
Spanish mackerel	3 oz	10
Snapper	3 oz	9
Skipjack (aku) tuna	3 oz	9
Atlantic pollock	3 oz	9
Walleye pollock	3 oz	9
Florida pompano	3 oz	9
Atlantic salmon, farmed	3 oz	9
Rainbow trout, wild	3 oz	9
Keta (chum) salmon	3 oz	9

ZINC TO COPPER RATIO

Continued

Cat fish, breaded & fried	3 oz	8
Atlantic croaker	3 oz	8
Coho salmon, wild	3 oz	8
Pacific & Jack mackerel	3 oz	7
Freshwater bass	3 oz	7
Bluefin tuna	3 oz	7
Sockeye salmon	3 oz	7
Mullet, striped	3 oz	6
Pink salmon	3 oz	6
Tilapia	3 oz	5
Coho salmon, farmed	3 oz	5
Atlantic herring, pickled	3 oz	5
Orange roughy	3 oz	4
Walleye pike	3 oz	3
Atlantic salmon, wild	3 oz	3
Chinook salmon, smoked	3 oz	1

Fish, Shellfish, Cooked	Amount	Zinc / Copper
Eastern oysters, farmed	3 oz	31
Oysters, breaded & fried	3 oz	20
Eastern oysters, wild	3 oz	14
Scallops, breaded & fried	3 oz	14
Alaskan king crab, imitation	3 oz	10
Clams, canned	3 oz	10
Shrimp, canned	3 oz	7
Blue crab cakes	3 oz	7
Alaskan king crab	3 oz	6
Shrimp	3 oz	6
Queen crab	3 oz	6
Shrimp, breaded & fried	3 oz	5
Blue crab	3 oz	5
Blue crab, canned	3 oz	5
Octopus	3 oz	5
Abalone	3 oz	4
Clams, breaded & fried	3 oz	4
Northern lobster	3 oz	3
Crayfish	3 oz	3
Squid, fried	3 oz	1

ZINC TO COPPER RATIO

FRUIT

Fruit, Canned	Amount	Zinc / Copper
Plums	1 cup	1.9
Peaches	1 cup	1.8
Pears	1 cup	1.6
Apricots	1 cup	1.4
Pineapple	1 cup	1.2
Applesauce, unsweetened	1 cup	1.1
Applesauce, sweetened	1 cup	1.0
Olives, black	5 large	0.9
Olives, green	5 large	0.6

Fruit, Dried	Amount	Zinc / Copper
Figs	1 cup	2
Peaches	1 cup	2
Currants	1 cup	1
Cranberries, sweetened	1 cup	1
Apricots	1 cup	1
Pears	1 cup	1
Apples	1 cup	1

Fruit, Frozen	Amount	Zinc / Copper
Strawberries	1 cup	3
Peaches	1 cup	2
Blackberries, unsweetened	1 cup	2
Raspberries	1 cup	2
Blueberries	1 cup	2

Fruit, Raw	Amount	Zinc / Copper
Raspberries	1 cup	5
Cantaloupe	1 cup	4
Avocado, California, pureed	1 cup	4
Honeydew	1 cup	4
Jicama	1 cup	3
Blackberries	1 cup	3
Black currants	1 cup	3
Strawberries	1 cup	3
Blueberries	1 cup	3
Apricots	1 cup	3
Water mellon	1 cup	2
Peachs	1 cup	2
Pomegrenates	1 cup	2

ZINC TO COPPER RATIO

Continued

Grapefruit, pink & red sections	1 cup	2
Florida Oranges	1 cup	2
Naval Oranges	1 cup	2
Nectarine	1 cup	2
Papayas	1 cup	2
Plantains	1 cup	2
Tangerine	1 cup	2
Plum	1 cup	2
Valencias oranges	1 cup	2
Cranberries	1 cup	2
Oranges	1 cup	2
Prunes, uncooked	1 cup	2
Prunes, stewed	1 cup	2
Apples	1 cup	1
Dates	1 cup	1
Avocado, Florida	1 cup	1
Cherries, sweet	1 cup	1
Pineapple	1 cup	1
Kiwi	1 cup	1
Pears	1 cup	1
Mango	1 cup	1
Raisins	1 cup	1
Grapes	1 cup	1

Game Meat, Cooked	Amount	Zinc / Copper
Deer, ground	3 oz	66
Wild boar	3 oz	53
Elk, ground	3 oz	46
Bison, ground	3 oz	35
Buffalo, steak, free range	3 oz	27
Elk, roasted	3 oz	22
Caribou	3 oz	20
Rabbit, wild, stewed	3 oz	13
Squirrel	3 oz	12
Duck	3 oz	11
Deer	3 oz	9
Antelope	3 oz	8

Grains, Cooked	Amount	Zinc / Copper
Soba noodles	1 cup	16
Instant white rice	1 cup	13
Wild rice	1 cup	11
Oat bran	1 cup	8
Egg & Spinach noodles	1 cup	8
Barley, pearled	1 cup	8

ZINC TO COPPER RATIO

Continued

Bulgur	1 cup	8
Kamut	1 cup	7
White rice, regular, long grain	1 cup	7
Egg noodles	1 cup	7
Rice noodles	1 cup	7
Couscous	1 cup	6
Brown rice	1 cup	6
Spelt	1 cup	6
Amaranth	1 cup	6
Quinoa	1 cup	6
Millet	1 cup	6
Macaroni	1 cup	5
Spaghetti	1 cup	5
Buckwheat, groats	1 cup	4
Spaghetti, Whole Wheat	1 cup	1

Herbs & Spices	Amount	Zinc / Copper
Chervil, dried	1 tsp	17
Anise seed	1 tsp	12
Bay leaf, crumbled	1 tsp	10
Dill weed, fresh	5 sprigs	10
Ginger, ground	1 tsp	8
Tumeric, ground	1 tsp	8
Onion powder	1 tsp	8
Thyme, dried	1 tsp	8
Paprika, powder	1 tsp	7
Cloves, dried, ground	1 tsp	6
Dill weed, dried	1 tsp	6
Sage, ground	1 tsp	6
Rosemary, dried	1 tsp	6
Tarragon, dried	1 tsp	5
Garlic powder	1 tsp	5
Celery seeds	1 tsp	5
Chives, raw	1 tsp	5
Cinnamon powder	1 tsp	5
Curry powder	1 tsp	5
Rosemary, fresh	1 tsp	5
Saffron	1 tsp	5
Coriander, seeds	1 tsp	4
Oregano	1 tsp	4
Chili powder	1 tsp	4
Caraway seeds	1 tsp	4
Basil, dried & ground	1 tsp	3

ZINC TO COPPER RATIO

Continued

Parsley, dried	1 tsp	3
Marjoram, dried	1 tsp	3
Coriander, dried	1 tsp	3
Thyme, fresh	1 tsp	3
Cilantro	1/4 cup	2
All spice	1 tsp	2
Capers, canned	1 tsp	1
Pepper, black	1 tsp	1
Basil, fresh, chopped	1 tsp	0.4

Juice	Amount	Zinc / Copper
Pomegranate	1 cup	4
Grape	1 cup	4
Carrot	1 cup	4
Cranberry	1 cup	3
Prune	1 cup	3
Lemon juice, raw	1 cup	3
Tomato	1 cup	2
Apple	1 cup	2
Pineapple	1 cup	2
Grapefruit juice, raw	1 cup	1
Orange, raw	1 cup	1
Vegetable	1 cup	1

Lamb, Cooked	Amount	Zinc / Copper
Foreshank, trim to 1/8" fat	3 oz	62
Cubed, for stew or kabob	3 oz	38
Leg, whole, trim to 1/4"	3 oz	38
Rib, lean, trim to 1/4" fat	3 oz	38
Ground, broiled	3 oz	36
Chops, loin, lean, trim to 1/4" fat	3 oz	27

Milk	Amount	Zinc / Copper
Dry, instant, nonfat	1/3 cup	112
Reduced fat, 2%	1 cup	78
Canned, condensed, sweetened	1 cup	63
Canned, evaporated, nonfat	1 cup	56
Canned, evaporated	1 cup	49
Lowfat, 1%	1 cup	43
Buttermilk, lowfat	1 cup	38
Nonfat, fat free or skim milk	1 cup	32
Buttermilk, whole milk	1 cup	15

ZINC TO COPPER RATIO

Continued

Whole milk, 3.25%	1 cup	15
Sheep milk	1 cup	12
Goat milk	1 cup	7
Human milk	1 cup	3
Coconut milk, canned	1 cup	3
Soy milk, original, unfortified	1 cup	1

Nuts & Seeds	Amount	Zinc / Copper
Peanut butter, smooth style	1 oz	6
Pumpkin seeds	1 oz	6
Chia seeds	1 oz	5
Pine nuts	1 oz	5
Soybeans, mature, dry roasted	1 oz	4
Pecans	1 oz	4
Flaxseeds	1 oz	4
Almonds	1 oz	3
Tahini	1 oz	3
Peanuts	1 oz	3
Sunflower seeds	1 oz	3
Cashews	1 oz	3
Coconut, raw meat	1 oz	3
Black walnuts	1 oz	2
Brazilnuts	1 oz	2
English walnuts	1 oz	2
Sesame seeds	1 oz	2
Macadamia	1 oz	2
Pistachio	1 oz	2
Hazelnuts	1 oz	1

Pork, Cooked	Amount	Zinc / Copper
Spareribs	3 oz	32
Bratwurst	3 oz	31
Canadian-style bacon	3 oz	31
Italian sausage	3 oz	30
Cured ham, lean	3 oz	29
Center loin chops, lean, pan-fried	3 oz	29
Chops, lean, pan-fried	3 oz	29
Backribs	3 oz	29
Cured ham	3 oz	28
Chops, broiled	3 oz	28
Center loin chops, pan-fried	3 oz	27
Chops, pan-fried	3 oz	27
Sirloin chops	3 oz	25
Sausage	3 oz	24
Tenderloin	3 oz	22

ZINC TO COPPER RATIO

Continued

Bacon	3 oz	21
Polish sausage	3 oz	21
Braunschweiger	3 oz	12
Liverwurst spread	1/4 cup	10

Turkey, Cooked	Amount	Zinc / Copper
Ground turkey, fat free	3 oz	36
Dark meat	3 oz	28
Light meat	3 oz	27
Breast meat	3 oz	25
Ground turkey, 93% lean	3 oz	23
Turkey bacon	3 oz	21
Ground turkey	3 oz	21
Turkey sausage, reduced fat	3 oz	15
Ground turkey, 85% lean	3 oz	13

Veal, Cooked	Amount	Zinc / Copper
Foreshank	3 oz	60
Breast	3 oz	55
Rib	3 oz	41
Ground	3 oz	37
Leg, top round	3 oz	28
Loin	3 oz	27
Sirloin	3 oz	26

VEGETABLES

Vegetables, Canned	Amount	Zinc / Copper
Corn	1 cup	10
Green beans	1 cup	7
Green peas	1 cup	6
Asparagus	1 cup	4
Beets	1 cup	4
Mushrooms	1 cup	3
Spinach	1 cup	3
Carrots	1 cup	3
Tomatoes, ripe	1 cup	2
Sauerkraut	1 cup	2
Tomato paste	1 cup	2
Tomato sauce	1 cup	2
Pumpkin	1 cup	2
Tomatos stewed	1 cup	2
Tomato pure	1 cup	1
Sweet potato	1 cup	1

ZINC TO COPPER RATIO

Vegetables, Cooked	Amount	Zinc / Copper
Turnips, cubes	1 cup	63
Corn	1 cup	13
Cabbage	1 cup	12
Carrots	1 cup	11
Cauliflower	1 cup	10
Bok-Choy	1 cup	9
Rutabagas	1 cup	9
Broccoli	1 cup	7
Raab broccoli	1 cup	7
Zucchini	1 cup	7
Broccolini	1 cup	6
Collard greens	1 cup	6
Split peas	1 cup	6
Okra	1 cup	5
Snow peas	1 cup	5
Beets	1 cup	5
Spinach	1 cup	4
Green beans	1 cup	4
Prickley pear cactus pads	1 cup	4
Brussels sprouts	1 cup	4
Celery	1 cup	4
Summer squash	1 cup	4
Asparagus	1 cup	4
Artichokes	1 cup	3
Onions	1 cup	3
Winter squash	1 cup	3
Pumpkin	1 cup	3
Dandelion greens	1 cup	2
Kohlrabi	1 cup	2
Sweet potato, mashed	1 cup	2
Eggplant	1 cup	2
Swiss chard	1 cup	2
Butternut squash	1 cup	2
Beet greens	1 cup	2
Acorn squash	1 cup	2
Potatoes, mashed with whole milk	1 cup	2
Parsnips	1 cup	2
Tomatoes	1 cup	2
White mushrooms	1 cup	2
Kale	1 cup	2
Shitake mushrooms	1 cup	1
Napa cabbage	1 cup	1
Potatoes, flesh	1 cup	1
Yams, cubed	1 cup	1

ZINC TO COPPER RATIO

Continued

Mustard greens	1 cup	1
Leeks	1 cup	1
Turnip greens	1 cup	1

Vegetables, Frozen	Amount	Zinc / Copper
Corn	1 cup	13
Broccoli	1 cup	8
Brussels Sprouts	1 cup	7
Okra	1 cup	6
Green peas	1 cup	6
Cauliflower	1 cup	5
Collard greens	1 cup	5
Carrots	1 cup	4
Green beans	1 cup	4
Asparagus	1 cup	4
Kale	1 cup	4
Butternut squash	1 cup	3
Spinach	1 cup	3
Rhubarb	1 cup	3
Turnip greens	1 cup	3

Vegetables, Raw	Amount	Zinc / Copper
Raab broccoli	1 cup	18
Red bell peppers	1 cup	15
Red cabbage	1 cup	13
Butterhead & boston lettuce	1 cup	12
Cabbage	1 cup	10
Bok-Choy	1 cup	9
Broccoli	1 cup	8
Endive	1 cup	8
Red leaf lettuce	1 cup	8
Shiitake mushrooms	1 each	7
Cauliflower	1 cup	7
Green leaf lettuce	1 cup	6
Arugula	1 cup	6
Zucchini	1 cup	6
Enoki mushrooms	1 cup	6
Summer squash	1 cup	6
Carrots	1 cup	5
Iceburg lettuce	1 cup	5
Prickley pear cactus pads	1 cup	5
Cucumbers	1 cup	5
Romaine lettuce	1 cup	5
Green onions & scallions	1 cup	5
Savoy cabbage	1 cup	4

ZINC TO COPPER RATIO

Continued

Onions	1 cup	4
Spinach	1 cup	4
Celery	1 cup	4
Snow peas	1 cup	3
Oyster mushrooms	1 cup	3
Belgian endive	1 cup	3
Tomatoes	1 cup	3
Tomatoes, cherry	1 cup	3
Tomatillos	1 cup	3
Dandelion greens	1 cup	2
Crimini mushrooms	1 cup	2
Butternut squash	1 cup	2
Swiss chard	1 cup	2
Green bell peppers	1 cup	2
Portabella mushrooms	1 cup	2
Radicchio	1 cup	2
White mushrooms	1 cup	2
Mustard spinach	1 cup	2
Yellow bell peppers	1 cup	2
Watercress	1 cup	2
Shiitake mushrooms, dried	1 each	2
Kale	1 cup	1
Chicory greens	1 cup	1
Spirulina, dried	1 tbsp	0

YOGURT	Amount	Zinc / Copper
Yogurt plain, lowfat	8 ounces	67
Yogurt plain, whole milk	8 ounces	67
Yogurt plain, skim milk	8 ounces	65
Yogurt plain, Greek, nonfat	8 ounces	30

ZINC TO COPPER RATIO

NOTES

ESSENTIAL FATTY ACIDS

There is a widely held misconception that the essential fatty acids known as omega-3 and omega-6 can be found in only a few plants, fish or fish oil. The true essential omega-3 fatty acids, are in fact, found naturally in all foods.

To start with, there are two distinct families of polyunsaturated fatty acids. One begins with an omega-3 fatty acid known as alpha-linolenic acid (ALA) and the other begins with an omega-6 fatty acid known as linoleic acid (LA).

Omega-3 and omega-6 fatty acids are structural components of every living cell membrane in the human body. Although cellular proteins are genetically determined, the essential fatty acid composition of a cell membrane is totally dependent on dietary intake.

Both LA and ALA are obtained from plants, phytoplankton, and anything that feeds on them. They are essential because they cannot be synthesized by the human body but are required for human survival. LA and ALA are the only two fatty acids that are essential and are the precursors for the synthesis of all other omega fatty acids.

LA and ALA have opposing physiological functions but work together to keep the body in balance. However, at one point along their pathways there is a junction at which LA and ALA compete for the same enzyme. It is here, that it is believed, that too much LA in the diet can overtake and use up the enzyme needed by ALA. Because of this, the dietary ratio of LA / ALA has become a heated topic.

It is estimated that Americans consume, on an average, an intake of LA / ALA ratio between 15 and 20. The Institute of Medicine's recommended adequate intake levels equates to an LA / ALA ratio range between 9 and 11. Human breast milk has a LA / ALA ratio of approximately 7. We know from research depending on an individual's health that beneficial ratios for adults have been shown between 5 and 1. Although, many ratios maybe favorable, studies have shown, changing the dietary LA / ALA intake ratio from 8 to 2 resulted in a decrease in serum triglycerides. A ratio of 5 benefited patients with asthma. A ratio of 3 suppressed inflammation in patients with rheumatoid arthritis. And a ratio of 1 reduced C-reactive proteins which are strong markers of inflammation.

ESSENTIAL FATTY ACIDS

Within the body LA is converted into arachidonic acid (AA) which is associated with inflammation if in excess. In contrast, ALA is converted into eicosa-penta-e-noic acid (EPA), and docosa-hexa-e-noic acid (DHA). EPA and DHA have anti-inflammatory properties and a host of positive health effects, if not in excessive quantities.

Several discussions on essential fatty acids have ended with some confusion by leaving an impression that the levels of EPA and DHA synthesized by humans are insufficient to meet human requirements. This is the justification for claiming that everyone should be consuming supplemental fish oils, rich in EPA and DHA.

To believe this, is to believe that humans have evolved with or were created with some type of biochemical flaw that restricts the production of fatty acids required to sustain life. If this were true, we were doomed from the beginning and would already be extinct.

In reality, the human body has no biochemical flaws. The amount of ALA not converted into EPA and DHA has not been wasted, nor does it reflect a biochemical inefficiency, but instead, has been used for bodily functions not requiring any EPA or DHA. The amount synthesized in humans is what the body has determined needs to be allocated for its requirements, and it has worked for thousands of years.

Focusing on chemicals generated within the body from the intake of essential nutrients, in this case, misplaces the importance of the essential nutrient. It is the dietary intake of ALA from food that is, by definition, essential and not EPA nor DHA from fish oils. In short, EPA and DHA are physiological evidence that dietary intake of ALA is essential. Do not confuse dietary essential with physiologically essential.

Further, it is the excessive intake of omega-6 fatty acids from dietary oils that are drowning out the effects of the omega-3 fatty acids normally consumed in a diet. Contrary to what you have been told, heard, or read there is no lack of dietary intake of omega-3 fatty acids in America. Of course, unless you are eating only, a very small variety of foods with exceptionally low concentrations of ALA or eating exclusively non-fat food, since non-fat food by definition will contain no essential omega-3 fatty acids.

Concerning toxicity, doubts have been cast regarding the long-term use of fish oil because of its association with oxidative stress and hair loss. In one study, 25 women fed fish oil capsules for 12 weeks had significantly altered composition of red blood cell membranes and susceptibility to oxidative stress. Although fish oil supplements have some beneficial effects, at the same time, they increase tissue susceptibility to free radical attack and lipid peroxidation.

Excessive or long term use of fish oil supplements can introduce peroxided fatty acids which may contribute to the onset or progression of age-associated diseases.

The components of fish generally recognized for their therapeutic value are in part attributable to their effects on hemostatic function. One dietary experiment investigated the hemostatic effects of fish vs fish oil in mild hyperlipid males. What was found was a daily dose of 4.5 g of EPA and DHA from fish had a greater effect on hemostatis than did 4.5 g of EPA and DHA from fish oil. The noticed effect may be related to compounds in fish that complement the action of the omega-3 fatty acids that cannot be found in supplemental oils.

A body of evidence supports the position that long term or excessive use of supplemental fish oil may counteract the advertised beneficial effects by exceeding threshold levels leading to lipid peroxidation.

Epidemiological studies reported that men who ate at least some fish weekly had a lower heart disease mortality rate than men who ate none. The American Heart Association recommends eating fish at least twice weekly in addition to consuming foods rich in omega-3 fatty acids. Studies show no additional health benefits when fish intake is increased above two servings a week.

Before closing, the issue of mercury poisoning from fish consumption needs to be addressed. The American Medical Association's position is that the benefits of modest fish consumption outweigh the risks. Further, the avoidance of modest fish consumption due to confusion regarding the risk could result in excessive deaths from Coronary Heart Disease and suboptimal neurodevelopment in children.

ESSENTIAL FATTY ACIDS

It is true that mercury does bio-accumulate in the aquatic food chain and, if consumed in excess, can be toxic to humans. The amount of mercury in seafood depends on the predatory nature and lifespan of the species.

The larger carnivorous, high on the food chain, and / or longer lived fish will have higher tissue mercury concentrations than the smaller and shorter lived species. The Environmental Protection Agency has published a chart titled Monthly Fish Consumption Limits for Mercury. The table below shows the amount of fish the EPA believes is safe to consume on a monthly basis depending on the particular specie's mercury concentration in ppm.

Fish Consumption Limits

Fish Concentration, ppm	Fish Meals / Month
> .03 -.06	16
> .06 -.08	12
> .08 -.12	8
> .12 - .24	4
> .24 - .32	3
> .32 - .48	2
> .48 - .97	1
> .97 - 1.9	0.5
> 1.9	None

The above table is based on a human body weight of 70 Kg (154 lbs), with an average fish meal size of 8 ounces with a time averaging period of one month.

As an example, if the mercury levels of the fish you're intending to eat is .4 ppm (parts per million), the EPA then believes you are safe eating two 8 ounce meals per month, or four 4 ounce meals. The above table combined with the table below, showing the Mercury Content of Fish, should give you some guidance in minimizing your mercury exposure.

To summarize the above, a high LA / ALA dietary ratio is associated with inflammation. A lower ratio increases conversion of ALA into anti-inflammatory EPA and DHA. Therefore, it seems sensible to decrease LA intake while increasing ALA intake. The safest way is to eat a variety of foods. Of course it is safe to eat a food or meal with a high LA / ALA ratio, however, a dietary habit of eating only foods taken from the upper end of the range should be reconsidered.

There is no recommended daily allowance, RDA, for omega-3 or omega-6 fatty acids but the Institute of Medicine has set what it considers to be adequate daily intake levels.

Recommend Adequate Intakes Levels

Children	LA, mcg	ALA, mcg
1 to 3 year olds	7000	700
4 to 8 year olds	10000	900
Males		
9 to 13 year olds	12000	1200
14 to 18 year olds	16000	1600
19 to 30 years	17000	1600
31 to 50 years	14000	1600
50 to 70 years	14000	1600
Females		
9 to 13 year olds	10000	1000
14 to 18 year olds	12000	1100
19 to 30 years	12000	1100
31 to 50 years	12000	1100
50 to 70 years	11000	1100
Pregnancy	13000	1400

Mean Averages for Mercury Content in parts per million

Fish	Mercury, ppm
Tilefish, Gulf of Mexico	1.450
Swordfish	0.995
Shark	0.979
King mackerel	0.730
Orange Roughy	0.571
Marlin	0.485
Spanish mackerel, Gulf of Mexico	0.454
Grouper	0.448
Tuna, fresh or frozen	0.391
Bluefish	0.368
Sablefish	0.361
Chilean bass	0.354
Yellow fin tuna	0.354
Albacore or white tuna, canned	0.350
Tuna, canned, Albacore	0.350
Pacific croaker	0.287
Halibut	0.241
Snapper	0.166
Stripped bass	0.152
Perch, freshwater	0.151
Skipjack tuna	0.144
Tilefish, Atlantic	0.144
Perch, Ocean	0.121
Cod	0.117
Carp	0.110
Northern lobster	0.107
Whitefish	0.089
Herring	0.084
Hake	0.079
Light tuna, canned	0.071
Trout, fresh water	0.071
Atlantic croaker	0.065
Crab	0.065
Butterfish	0.058
Sole & Flounder	0.056
Atlantic haddock	0.055
Whiting	0.051
Atlantic mackerel	0.050
Mullet	0.050
American shad	0.045
Crawfish	0.033
Pollock	0.031

ESSENTIAL FATTY ACIDS

Catfish	0.025
Squid	0.023
Salmon, fresh or frozen	0.022
Anchovies	0.017
Sardines	0.013
Tilapia	0.013
Oyster	0.012
Clam	0.009
Shrimp	0.009
Salmon, canned	0.008
Scallops	0.003

Nutrient Data Collection Form

Food	Amount	Book Numbers	Multiply By	Estimated Nutrient Intake
Nutrient::	RDA:	Estimated:	% of RDA:	Total Estimated:

To download additional forms for free, go to www.TopNutrients4U.com

OMEGA-3 ALA

Alcohol	Amount	ALA (mg)
White Wine	1 glass	0
Red Wine	1 glass	0
Light Beer	1 bottle	0
Regular Beer	1 bottle	0
Gin, Rum, Vodka, or Whisky	1 shot	0

Beans, Canned	Amount	ALA (mg)
Refried beans *	1 cup	307
Pinto beans	1 cup	281
Navy beans	1 cup	223
Black-eyed peas	1 cup	209
Great Northern	1 cup	189
Green beans	1 cup	182
Kidney beans *	1 cup	169
White beans	1 cup	149
Cranberry beans	1 cup	143
Baked beans, plain *	1 cup	130
Garbanzo beans	1 cup	79
Lima beans, large	1 cup	55
Yellow beans	1 cup	47
Fava beans	1 cup	18

Beans, Cooked	Amount	ALA (mg)
Adzuki	1 cup	x
Hyacinath beans	1 cup	x
Mothbeans	1 cup	x
Soybeans, dry roasted	1 cup	1342
Natto	1 cup	1284
Soybeans, mature	1 cup	1029
Soybeans, green	1 cup	637
Edamame *	1 cup	555
Navy beans *	1 cup	322
Kidney beans	1 cup	297
Pinto beans	1 cup	234
White beans, small	1 cup	226
Lupini beans	1 cup	222
Black beans	1 cup	181
Winged beans	1 cup	162
Cranberry beans	1 cup	161
Great Northern beans	1 cup	149
Black-eyed peas	1 cup	142
Black Turtle beans, mature	1 cup	126
White beans, mature	1 cup	124

OMEGA-3 ALA

Continued

Green beans	1 cup	111
Yellow beans	1 cup	111
Lima beans	1 cup	98
Lentils	1 cup	73
Garbanzo beans	1 cup	71
Split peas	1 cup	55
Fava beans	1 cup	20
Mung beans, mature seeds	1 cup	18
Yardlong beans, Chinese long beans	1 cup	18
Pigeon peas, mature seeds	1 cup	15

Beef, Cooked	Amount	ALA (mg)
Beef ribs, trim to 1/8" fat	3 oz	264
Chuck roast, trim to 1/8" fat	3 oz	230
Porterhouse steak, trim to 0" fat	3 oz	161
T-Bone steak, trim 0" fat	3 oz	140
Top sirloin, trim to 1/8" fat	3 oz	108
Flank steak, lean, trim to 0" fat	3 oz	62
Filet Mignon, trim to 0" fat	3 oz	60
Skirt Steak, trim to 0" fat	3 oz	54
Ground beef, 85% lean	3 oz	44
Ground beef, 80% lean *	3 oz	42
Tri Tip steak, lean, trim to 0" fat	3 oz	42
Ground beef, 90% lean *	3 oz	40
Ground beef, 75% lean *	3 oz	34
Ground beef, 95% lean *	3 oz	29
Ribeye steak, trim to 0" fat	3 oz	19
London Broil, top round, trim to 0" fat	3 oz	17
Brisket, lean, trim to 0" fat	3 oz	14

Beef, Cooked	Amount	ALA (mg)
Ribeye filet, lean, trim to 0" fat	1 filet	x
Ribeye steak, boneless, trim to 0" fat	1 steak	x
Top Sirloin, choice filet, trim to 0" fat	1 filet	x
Beef ribs, trim to 1/8" fat	1 lb cooked	1407
Chuck roast, trim to 1/8" fat	1 lb cooked	1226
Porterhouse steak, trim to 0" fat	1 lb cooked	857
T-bone steak, trim to 0" fat	1 lb cooked	748
Top Sirloin, trim to 1/8" fat	1 lb cooked	577
Flank steak, lean, trim to 0" fat	1 lb cooked	331
Skirt steak, trim to 0" fat	1 lb cooked	286
Flank steak, lean, trim to 0" fat	1 steak	280
Tri Tip steak, lean, trim to 0" fat	1 lb cooked	227
Brisket, lean, trim to 0" fat	1 lb cooked	77
Filet Mignon, tenderloin, trim to 0" fat *	1 steak	23

OMEGA-3 ALA

Beef, Cooked	Amount	ALA (mg)
Ground beef, 85%	1/4 lb patty	40
Ground beef, 90%	1/4 lb patty	39
Ground beef, 80%	1/4 lb patty	38
Ground beef, 75%	1/4 lb patty	28
Ground beef, 95%	1/4 lb patty	28

Bread	Amount	ALA (mg)
Indian bread, Naan, plain*	1 piece	248
Bagel, Wheat	4" bagel	74
Hamburger & Hotdog buns, plain	1 bun	70
Cornbread, dry mix	1 piece	63
Bagel, plain	4" bagel	57
Dinner Rolls, brown & serve*	1 roll	56
Kaiser rolls	1 roll	55
Multi-Grain, and Whole-Grain	1 slice	53
Mexican roll, bollilo *	1 roll	46
White	1 slice	42
Wheat *	1 slice	38
Indian bread, Naan, whole wheat	1 piece	37
Bagel, cinnamon & raisins	4" bagel	35
Pumpernickel	1 slice	29
English Muffin, plain*	1 muffin	27
Oatmeal bread	1 slice	27
Bagel, egg	4" bagel	23
Bagel, oat bran	4" bagel	23
Italian	1 slice	20
Egg bread	1 slice	19
Rye bread	1 slice	19
Whole-Wheat	1 slice	17
Tortillas, flour	1 tortilla	16
Pita, white	6" pita	14
French, and Sourdough	1 slice	12
Raisin bread	1 slice	10
Tortillas, corn	1 tortilla	9
Cracked wheat	1 slice	8
Potato bread	1 slice	0

Butter	Amount	ALA (mg)
Regular dairy whipped butter, salted	1 tbsp	111
Regular dairy butter, salted *	1 tbsp	45

OMEGA-3 ALA

Cereal, General Mills®	Amount	ALA (mg)
Chocolate Chex	1 cup	x
Dora The Explorer	1 cup	165
Cinnamon Chex	1 cup	140
Cocoa Puffs	1 cup	115
Reese's Puffs	1 cup	99
Cookie Crisp	1 cup	72
Golden Grahams	1 cup	70
Oatmeal Crisp, Crunchy Almond	1 cup	56
Cinnamon Toast Crunch	1 cup	55
Trix	1 cup	51
Oatmeal Crisp, Hearty Raisin	1 cup	45
Raisin Nut Bran	1 cup	43
Berry Berry Kix	1 cup	40
Total Raisin Bran	1 cup	40
Wheat Chex	1 cup	39
Multi-Bran CHEX	1 cup	36
Wheaties	1 cup	27
Basic 4	1 cup	24
Total Cranberry Crunch	1 cup	21
Total Whole Grain	1 cup	20
Honey Nut Chex	1 cup	18
Lucky Charms *	1 cup	16
Honey Nut Clusters	1 cup	14
Corn Chex	1 cup	12
Kix *	1 cup	10
Rice Chex	1 cup	4

Cereal, General Mill's Cheerios®	Amount	ALA (mg)
Cinnamon Burst	1 cup	x
Chocolate	1 cup	93
Apple Cinnamon	1 cup	85
Banana Nut	1 cup	76
Honey Nut	1 cup	36
Berry Burst, Triple Berry	1 cup	34
Yogurt Burst, Strawberry	1 cup	30
Oat Cluster Cherrios Crunch	1 cup	28
Fruity	1 cup	25
Frosted	1 cup	24
Multi Grain	1 cup	20
Original *	1 cup	19

OMEGA-3 ALA

Cereal, General Mill's Fiber One®	Amount	ALA (mg)
Caramel Delight	1 cup	286
Original Bran	1 cup	38
Raisin Bran Clusters	1 cup	25
Honey Clusters	1 cup	22
80 Calorie Chocolate Squares	1 cup	x
80 Calorie Honey Squares	1 cup	x
Frosted Shredded Wheat	1 cup	x
Nutty Clusters & Almonds	1 cup	x

Cereal, Kashi®	Amount	ALA (mg)
Go Lean Crunch, Honey Almond Flax	1 cup	683
Honey Sunshine	1 cup	103
Go Lean Crunch	1 cup	71
Good Friends	1 cup	64
Go Lean	1 cup	55
Heart to Heart, Honey Toasted Oat	1 cup	49
Heart to Heart, Oat Flakes & Blueberry Clusters	1 cup	26
7-Whole Grain Honey Puffs	1 cup	16
Autumn Wheat	1 cup	14
7-Whole Grain Puffs	1 cup	13

Cereal, Kellogg's®	Amount	ALA (mg)
All-Bran Original	1 cup	93
All-Bran Bran Buds	1 cup	79
Smorz	1 cup	49
Mueslix	1 cup	46
Berry Rice Krispies	1 cup	42
Cracklin Oat Bran	1 cup	36
Raisin Bran	1 cup	31
All-Bran Complete Wheat Flakes	1 cup	29
Raisin Bran Crunch	1 cup	29
Smart Start, Strong Heart Antioxidants	1 cup	29
Frosted MINI Wheat's, Big Bite	1 cup	25
Honey Smacks	1 cup	22
Product 19	1 cup	17
Rice Krispies Treats	1 cup	15
Froot Loops	1 cup	11
Frosted Rice Krispies	1 cup	7
Apple Jacks	1 cup	6
Corn Flakes	1 cup	5
Corn Pops	1 cup	4
Honey Crunch Corn Flakes	1 cup	4
Rice Krispies	1 cup	3

Continued

Crispix	1 cup	2
Frosted Flakes	1 cup	2
Cocoa Krispies	1 cup	0

Cereal, Kellogg's Special-K®	Amount	ALA (mg)
Protein Plus	1 cup	241
Cinnamon Pecan	1 cup	46
Original	1 cup	30
Chocolately Delight	1 cup	22
Red Berries	1 cup	18
Vanilla Almond	1 cup	17
Fruit & Yogurt	1 cup	8

Cereal, Post®	Amount	ALA, mg
Great Grains, Banana Nut Crunch	1 cup	409
Great Grains, Crunchy Pecan Cereal	1 cup	115
Grape-Nuts Cereal	1 cup	108
Great Grains, Raisin, Date & Pecan	1 cup	84
Blueberry Morning	1 cup	62
Grape-Nuts Flakes	1 cup	49
Great Grains, Cranberry Almond Crunch	1 cup	46
Honey Nut Shredded Wheat	1 cup	43
Raisin Bran	1 cup	38
Bran Flakes	1 cup	35
Cocoa Pebbles	1 cup	33
Shredded Wheat, Frosted, spoon-size	1 cup	33
Shredded Wheat, Original, spoon-size	1 cup	31
Shredded Wheat n' Bran, spoon size	1 cup	25
Alpha-Bits	1 cup	23
Shredded Wheat, Original, big-biscuit	1 biscuit	20
Golden Crisp	1 cup	14
Honeycomb	1 cup	7
Fruity Pebbles	1 cup	6

Post® Honey Bunches of Oats®	Amount	ALA, mg
With Cinnamon Bunches	1 cup	x
With Strawberries	1 cup	x
Just Bunches, Honey Roasted	1 cup	316
With Vanilla Bunches	1 cup	83
With Almonds	1 cup	54
Honey Roasted *	1 cup	36
Pecan Bunches	1 cup	34

OMEGA-3 ALA

Quaker	Amount	ALA (mg)
Granola, Oats, Wheat & Honey	1 cup	627
Granola, Oats, Wheat, Honey & Raisins	1 cup	530
Low Fat Granola with Raisins	1 cup	113
Toasted Multigrain Crisp	1 cup	39
Oatmeal Squares	1 cup	38
Oatmeal Squares, Cinnamon	1 cup	38
LIFE Cereal, Original	1 cup	26
Toasted Oatmeal Cereal, Honey Nut	1 cup	24
LIFE Cereal, Cinnamon	1 cup	23
Honey Graham OH'S	1 cup	15
Crunchy Bran	1 cup	13
Puffed Rice	1 cup	11
CAP'N Crunch	1 cup	9
CAP'N Crunch & Crunch Berries	1 cup	8
CAP'N Crunch's Peanut Butter Crunch	1 cup	8
Puffed Wheat	1 cup	6

Cereal, Cooked	Amount	ALA (mg)
WHEATENA	1 cup	46
Oats, regular, unenriched *	1 cup	42
CREAM OF WHEAT, regular	1 cup	30
Farina *	1 cup	17
White corn grits	1 cup	0
Yellow corn grits	1 cup	0

Cheese	Amount	ALA (mg)
Ricotta, whole milk	1 cup	276
Ricotta, part skim milk	1 cup	172
Cottage cheese, small curd	1 cup	38
Cottage cheese, low fat, 2 %	1 cup	23
Cottage cheese, low fat, 1 %	1 cup	20
Cottage cheese, non fat & uncreamed	1 cup	0

Cheese	Amount	ALA (mg)
American, pasteurized process, imitation *	1 oz	268
Fontina	1 oz	224
Roquefort	1 oz	200
Gruyere	1 oz	123
Gouda	1 oz	112
Mozzarella, whole milk	1 oz	105
Cheddar	1 oz	103
Swiss	1 oz	100
Brie	1 oz	89

Continued

Romano	1 oz	88
Ricotta, part skim milk	1 oz	87
Colby	1 oz	79
Provolone	1 oz	78
Blue cheese	1 oz	75
Feta	1 oz	75
Monterey	1 oz	74
Muenster, low fat	1 oz	72
Monterey, low fat	1 oz	67
Muenster	1 oz	65
Parmesan, grated	1 oz	54
Provolone, reduced fat	1 oz	50
Cream cheese *	1 oz	49
Mozzarella, part skim, low moisture	1 oz	42
American, pasteurized process, fortified *	1 oz	39
Ricotta	1 oz	32
American, pasteurized process, low fat	1 oz	24
Cheddar, low-fat	1 oz	19
Swiss, low fat	1 oz	18
Cream cheese, fat free *	1 oz	2
Goat cheese, hard type	1 oz	0
Goat cheese, semisoft	1 oz	0
Goat cheese, soft type	1 oz	0
Mozzarella, non fat	1 oz	0

Cheese, Mexican	Amount	ALA (mg)
Queso anejo	1 oz	99
Queso chihuahua	1 oz	98
Mexican, blend	1 oz	93
Queso asadero	1 oz	93
Mexican, blend, reduced fat	1 oz	37
Queso fresco *	1 oz	28

Chicken, Cooked	Amount	ALA (mg)
Wing with skin, fried in batter	1 wing	118
Breast, with skin, fried in flour	1/2 breast	78
Drumstick, with skin, fried in flour	1 drumstick	69
Breast, with skin, roasted	1/2 breast	59
Wing with skin, roasted	1 wing	51
Thigh, meat only, roasted *	1 thigh	30
Breast, no skin, roasted	1/2 breast	26

OMEGA-3 ALA

Chicken, Cooked	Amount	ALA (mg)
Wing with skin, fried in flour	3 oz	178
Wing with skin, roasted	3 oz	128
Drumstick with skin, fried in flour	3 oz	119
Thigh with skin, fried in flour	3 oz	119
Thigh with skin, roasted *	3 oz	100
Breast with skin, fried in flour	3 oz	68
Drumstick with skin, roasted *	3 oz	66
Breast with skin, roasted	3 oz	51
Wing meat only, no skin, roasted	3 oz	51
Thigh meat only, no skin, roasted *	3 oz	49
Drumstick meat only, no skin, roasted *	3 oz	31
Breast meat only, no skin, roasted	3 oz	26
Cornish game hens, meat only	3 oz	26

Cream	Amount	ALA (mg)
Heavy Cream	1 tbsp	81
Light Coffee Cream	1 tbsp	40
Sour Cream, reduced fat, cultured	1 tbsp	26
Half & Half	1 tbsp	25
Sour Cream, cultured	1 tbsp	10
Whipped Cream, pressurized	1 tbsp	10

Eggs	Amount	ALA (mg)
Egg whole, scrambled	1 large	82
Egg whole, fried	1 large	63
Egg whole, poached	1 large	24
Egg whole, hard-boiled	1 large	18
Egg yolk	1 large	18
Egg substitute, fat free	1/4 cup	0
Egg whites	1 large	0
Egg whites, dried	1 ounce	0
Egg whites, dried powder & stabilized	1 tbsp	0

Fish, Canned	Amount	ALA (mg)
Atlantic sardines, in oil	3 oz	424
White (albacore) tuna, in oil	3 oz	173
Light tuna, in oil	3 oz	63
White (albacore) tuna, in water	3 oz	60
Light tuna, in water *	3 oz	2

OMEGA-3 ALA

Fish, Cooked	Amount	ALA (mg)
Atlantic salmon, wild	3 oz	321
Carp	3 oz	294
Rainbow trout, wild	3 oz	159
Cat fish, breaded & fried	3 oz	151
Atlantic croaker	3 oz	133
Freshwater bass	3 oz	121
Spanish mackerel	3 oz	99
Atlantic mackerel	3 oz	96
Atlantic salmon, farmed	3 oz	96
Chinook salmon	3 oz	94
Catfish, wild	3 oz	82
Catfish, farmed	3 oz	74
Sockeye salmon	3 oz	73
Rainbow trout, farmed	3 oz	68
Coho salmon, farmed	3 oz	65
Pacific & Jack mackerel	3 oz	54
Pink salmon	3 oz	48
Coho salmon, wild	3 oz	47
Greenland halibut	3 oz	47
Tilapia*	3 oz	38
Keta, (chum) salmon	3 oz	37
Swordfish	3 oz	29
Northern pike	3 oz	23
Flounder & Sole	3 oz	18
Atlantic perch	3 oz	16
Striped bass	3 oz	16
Walleye pike	3 oz	15
Atlantic & Pacific halibut	3 oz	11
Whiting	3 oz	11
Alaskan halibut*	3 oz	8
Haddock	3 oz	2
Yellowfin tuna	3 oz	2
Atlantic cod	3 oz	1
Pacific cod	3 oz	1
Atlantic hearing, pickled	3 oz	0
Chinook salmon, smoked	3 oz	0
Orange roughy*	3 oz	0
Walleye pollock	3 oz	0

Fish, Shellfish, Cooked	Amount	ALA (mg)
Shrimp, breaded & fried	3 oz	227
Clams, breaded & fried	3 oz	136
Scallops, breaded & fried	3 oz	133
Oysters, breaded & fried	3 oz	133

OMEGA-3 ALA

Continued

Eastern oysters, wild	3 oz	110
Squid, fried	3 oz	85
Abalone	3 oz	81
Blue crab cakes	3 oz	74
Eastern oysters, farmed	3 oz	54
Northern lobster *	3 oz	42
Crayfish	3 oz	24
Clams, canned	3 oz	21
Alaskan king crab	3 oz	12
Shrimp	3 oz	10
Blue crab, canned	3 oz	8
Blue crab *	3 oz	8
Alaskan king crab, imitation *	3 oz	6
Shrimp, canned *	3 oz	3
Queen crab	3 oz	3
Octopus	3 oz	0

Fruit, Canned	Amount	ALA (mg)
Pineapple	1 cup	43
Applesauce, sweetened	1 cup	22
Olives, black	5 large	14
Olives, green	5 large	12
Applesauce, unsweetened	1 cup	7
Peaches	1 cup	3
Apricots	1 cup	0
Plums	1 cup	0
Pears	1 cup	0

Fruit, Dried	Amount	ALA (mg)
Cranberries	1 cup	32
Prunes	1 cup	30
Apples	1 cup	14
Peaches	1 cup	4
Pears	1 cup	4
Apricots	1 cup	0
Currants	1 cup	0
Figs	1 cup	0

Fruit, Frozen	Amount	ALA (mg)
Blueberries	1 cup	174
Blackberries	1 cup	124
Raspberries	1 cup	75
Strawberries	1 cup	74
Peaches	1 cup	5

OMEGA-3 ALA

Fruit, Raw	Amount	ALA (mg)
Avocado, California *	1 cup	255
Avocado, Florida	1 cup	221
Raspberries	1 cup	155
Blackberries	1 cup	135
Elderberries	1 cup	123
Strawberries	1 cup	108
Blueberries	1 cup	86
Kiwi	1 cup	76
Cantaloupe	1 cup	74
Papayas	1 cup	68
Honeydew	1 cup	56
Cherries	1 cup	40
Plantains	1 cup	37
Tangerine	1 cup	35
Prunes, uncooked	1 cup	30
Pineapple	1 cup	28
Jicama	1 cup	18
Grapes, red or green	1 cup	17
Navel oranges	1 cup	15
Raisins	1 cup	12
Apples	1 cup	11
Dates	1 cup	4
Nectarine	1 cup	3
Peaches	1 cup	3
Apricots	1 cup	0
Water mellon	1 cup	0
Plums	1 cup	0
Pears	1 cup	0

Fruit, Raw	Amount	ALA (mg)
Persimmons, small natives	1 fruit	x
Cherimoya*	1 fruit	374
Avocado, Florida	1 fruit	292
Avocado, California *	1 fruit	151
Cantaloupe	1/2 fruit	127
Chayote	1 fruit	73
Plantains	1 fruit	45
Strawberries	5 fruit	39
Banana	1 fruit	32
Kiwi	1 fruit	29
Star fruit, Carambola	1 fruit	25
Cherries	10 cherries	21

OMEGA-3 ALA

Continued

Pineapple guava, Feijoa*	1 fruit	17
Apples	1 fruit	16
Tangerine	1 fruit	16
Oranges, navel	1 fruit	13
Kumquats	1 fruit	9
Pineapple, slices	1/2" x 3" slice	8
Prunes, uncooked	5 prunes	8
Persimmons, Japanese	1 fruit	7
Nectarine	1 fruit	3
Peaches	1 fruit	3
Raisins	1 small box	3
Dates	5 dates	1
Apricots	1 fruit	0
Figs, dried	1 fig	0
Pears	1 fruit	0
Plums	1 plum	0

Game Meat, Cooked	Amount	ALA (mg)
Duck	3 oz	124
Rabbit	3 oz	119
Antelope	3 oz	85
Deer, ground	3 oz	80
Deer	3 oz	76
Bison, ground	3 oz	68
Elk, ground	3 oz	57
Elk	3 oz	51
Caribou	3 oz	26
Squirrel	3 oz	26
Wild boar	3 oz	26
Buffalo, steak, free range *	3 oz	25

Grains, Cooked	Amount	ALA (mg)
Wild rice	1 cup	156
Egg & Spinach noodles	1 cup	77
Millet	1 cup	49
Egg noodles	1 cup	45
Spaghetti, spinach	1 cup	42
Macaroni *	1 cup	34
Spaghetti, enriched *	1 cup	34
Oat bran	1 cup	33
Pearled barley	1 cup	33
Brown rice	1 cup	27
Buckwheat	1 cup	24

Continued

White rice, regular long grain	1 cup	21
Spaghetti, whole wheat	1 cup	14
Bulgur	1 cup	7
Rice noodles	1 cup	7
Couscous	1 cup	5
Soba noodles	1 cup	2

Herbs & Spices	Amount	ALA (mg)
Tarragon, dried leaves	1 tbsp	53
Spearmint, dried	1 tbsp	45
Chili powder *	1 tbsp	42
Cloves, ground *	1 tbsp	40
Rosemary, dried	1 tbsp	36
Oregano, dried, ground	1 tbsp	33
Turmeric, ground	1 tbsp	33
Paprika	1 tbsp	31
Parsley, dried *	1 tbsp	30
Thyme, ground	1 tbsp	30
Curry powder	1 tbsp	27
Saffron	1 tbsp	26
Sage, ground	1 tbsp	25
Bay leaf, crumbled	1 tbsp	19
Thyme, dried, leaves	1 tbsp	19
Capers	1 tbsp	16
Basil, dried & ground *	1 tbsp	13
Celery seeds	1 tbsp	13
Ginger, ground	1 tbsp	12
Thyme, fresh	1 tbsp	12
Caraway seeds	1 tbsp	10
Pepper, black	1 tbsp	10
Basil, fresh, chopped	1 tbsp	8
Rosemary, fresh	1 tbsp	7
All-spice, ground	1 tbsp	4
Cinnamon, ground	1 tbsp	1
Garlic powder *	1 tbsp	1
Onion powder *	1 tbsp	1
Anise seed	1 tbsp	0
Chervil, dried	1 tbsp	0
Chives, raw	1 tbsp	0
Coriander, leaves, cilantro	1/4 cup	0
Dill weed, fresh	1/4 cup	0
Nutmeg	1 tbsp	0

OMEGA-3 ALA

Juice	Amount	ALA (mg)
Cranberry, cocktail	1 cup	58
Pineapple	1 cup	45
Orange juice, raw	1 cup	27
Lemon juice, raw *	1 cup	22
Carrot	1 cup	21
Grapefruit juice, raw	1 cup	18
Apple	1 cup	17
Grape	1 cup	13
Tomato	1 cup	2
Vegetable, cocktail	1 cup	2
Pomegranate	1 cup	0
Prune	1 cup	0

Lamb, Cooked	Amount	ALA (mg)
Chops, loin, lean, trim to 1/4" fat	3 oz	224
Ground	3 oz	221
Leg, whole, trim to 1/4" fat	3 oz	196
Foreshank, trim to 1/8" fat	3 oz	161
Rib, lean, trim to 1/4" fat	3 oz	145
Cubed, for stew or kabob	3 oz	85

Milk	Amount	ALA (mg)
Canned, condensed, sweetened	1 cup	370
Sheep milk	1 cup	311
Whole Milk, dry powder	1/4 cup	261
Canned, evaporated	1 cup	197
Buttermilk, whole milk	1 cup	186
Whole Milk, liquid, 3.25% milk fat	1 cup	183
Soymilk, original, unfortified	1 cup	182
Human milk	1 cup	128
Goat milk	1 cup	98
Buttermilk, low-fat	1 cup	32
Reduced fat, 2% *	1 cup	20
Low-fat, 1% *	1 cup	10
Canned, evaporated, non-fat	1 cup	5
Dry, instant, nonf fat	1/3 cup	3
Non fat, fat-free or skim milk	1 cup	2
Coconut milk, canned	1 cup	0

OMEGA-3 ALA

Nuts & Seeds	Amount	ALA (mg)
Flaxseeds	1 oz	6467
Chia seeds *	1 oz	5005
English walnuts	1 oz	2574
Black walnuts *	1 oz	569
Pecans	1 oz	280
Tahini	1 oz	115
Sesame seeds	1 oz	107
Pistachio	1 oz	73
Macadamia	1 oz	58
Mixed nuts, roasted with peanuts, no salt	1 oz	54
Pumpkin seeds *	1 oz	34
Pine nuts	1 oz	32
Hazelnuts	1 oz	25
Peanut butter, smooth style	1 oz	22
Trail mix, regular with chocolate chips	1 oz	22
Trail mix, regular, salted	1 oz	20
Cashews	1 oz	18
Sunflower seeds	1 oz	17
Trail mix, tropical	1 oz	11
Brazilnuts *	1 oz	5
Almonds *	1 oz	1
Peanuts	1 oz	1
Coconut, raw meat	1 oz	0

Nuts & Seeds	Amount	ALA (mg)
Cashews	1/4 cup	x
Chia seeds	1/4 cup	x
Flaxseeds	1/4 cup	9581
Flaxseeds	1 tbsp	2350
English walnuts, halves	1/4 cup	2270
Black walnuts, chopped	1/4 cup	627
Pecans, halves	1/4 cup	244
Sesame seeds	1/4 cup	135
Pistachio	1/4 cup	80
Macadamia	1/4 cup	69
Mixed nuts, roasted with peanuts, no salt	1/4 cup	65
Peanut butter, smooth	1/4 cup	50
Pumpkin seeds	1/4 cup	39
Pine nuts	1/4 cup	38
Sesame seeds	1 tbsp	34
Trail mix, regular with chocolate chips	1/4 cup	28
Trail mix, regular, salted	1/4 cup	26
Hazelnuts	1/4 cup	25
Sunflower seeds	1/4 cup	21

OMEGA-3 ALA

Continued

Trail mix, tropical	1/4 cup	14
Brazilnuts, whole	1/4 cup	6
Almonds	1/4 cup	1
Peanuts	1/4 cup	1
Coconut meat, shredded	1/4 cup	0

Oils	Amount	ALA (mg)
Flaxseed oil *	1 tbsp	7258
Walnut oil	1 tbsp	1414
Canola oil *	1 tbsp	1279
Soybean oil *	1 tbsp	923
Soybean lecithin oil	1 tbsp	698
Soybean, partially hydrogenated, oil	1 tbsp	354
Menhaden oil	1 tbsp	203
Sardine oil	1 tbsp	180
Corn oil *	1 tbsp	158
Salmon oil	1 tbsp	144
Avocado oil	1 tbsp	134
Cod liver oil	1 tbsp	127
Olive oil	1 tbsp	103
Sesame oil	1 tbsp	41
Cottonseed oil	1 tbsp	27
Sunflower, high oleic acid	1 tbsp	27
Grapeseed oil	1 tbsp	14
Safflower, high oleic acid, oil *	1 tbsp	13
Coconut oil	1 tbsp	0
Peanut oil	1 tbsp	0
Safflower, high linoleic acid, oil	1 tbsp	0
Sunflower, high linoleic acid, oil	1 tbsp	0

Pork, Cooked	Amount	ALA (mg)
Italian sausage	3 oz	399
Braunschweiger	3 oz	291
Polish sausage	3 oz	247
Bacon, pan-fried *	3 oz	170
Cured ham	3 oz	145
Pork sausage	3 oz	118
Sausage *	3 oz	117
Backribs *	3 oz	111
Canadian style bacon	3 oz	102
Spareribs	3 oz	94
Bratwurst	3 oz	84
Liverwurst spread	1/4 cup	72
Chops, pan-fried *	3 oz	62
Cured ham, lean	3 oz	51

Continued

Center loin pork chops*	3 oz	43
Chops, lean, pan-fried *	3 oz	28
Sirloin pork chops *	3 oz	19
Tenderloin *	3 oz	16

Salad dressings, Averages	Amount	ALA (mg)
Mayonnaise, regular *	1 tbsp	736
Caesar, regular	1 tbsp	566
Blue cheese, regular	1 tbsp	479
Ranch, regular	1 tbsp	459
French, regular	1 tbsp	438
Honey Mustard, regular	1 tbsp	404
Thousand Island, regular	1 tbsp	376
Russian	1 tbsp	261
Mayonnaise, light *	1 tbsp	228
Italian, regular *	1 tbsp	211
French, reduced fat	1 tbsp	143
Ranch, reduced fat	1 tbsp	79
Ranch, fat-free *	1 tbsp	19
Thousand Island, fat-free	1 tbsp	14
Blue cheese, light	1 tbsp	10
Italian, fat-free	1 tbsp	4
French, fat-free	1 tbsp	3
Blue cheese, fat-free	1 tbsp	1
Honey Mustard, fat-free	1 tbsp	0.015
Caesar, fat-free	1 tbsp	0.001

Turkey, Cooked	Amount	ALA (mg)
Turkey bacon	3 oz	317
Ground turkey, 85% lean *	3 oz	162
Ground turkey, 93% lean *	3 oz	148
Turkey sausage, reduced fat	3 oz	121
Ground turkey *	3 oz	116
Dark meat *	3 oz	61
Liver *	3 oz	28
Ground turkey, fat free *	3 oz	26
Light meat *	3 oz	17
Breast meat, only	3 oz	0

Veal, Cooked	Amount	ALA (mg)
Loin	3 oz	76
Rib	3 oz	76
Sirloin	3 oz	60
Ground	3 oz	42

Continued

Leg, top round	3 oz	34
Breast	3 oz	28
Foreshank	3 oz	25

Vegetables, Canned	Amount	ALA (mg)
Spinach	1 cup	381
Green beans	1 cup	161
Green peas	1 cup	124
Sauerkraut	1 cup	78
Sweet potato	1 cup	43
Asparagus	1 cup	36
Pumpkin	1 cup	20
Tomato paste	1 cup	18
Carrots	1 cup	16
Corn	1 cup	15
Tomato pure	1 cup	10
Stewed tomato	1 cup	8
Tomato sauce	1 cup	7
Beets	1 cup	7
Tomatoes	1 cup	5
Mushrooms	1 cup	2

Vegetables, Cooked	Amount	ALA (mg)
Brussels sprouts	1 cup	270
Broccolini	1 cup	227
Cauliflower	1 cup	207
Winter squash	1 cup	189
Broccoli	1 cup	186
Collard greens	1 cup	177
Zucchini	1 cup	169
Spinach	1 cup	166
Summer squash	1 cup	148
Kale	1 cup	134
Green beans	1 cup	111
Raab broccoli	1 cup	110
Rutabagas	1 cup	97
Turnip greens	1 cup	92
Acorn squash	1 cup	76
Bok-choy	1 cup	70
Leeks	1 cup	69
Artichokes	1 cup	64
Split peas	1 cup	55
Asparagus	1 cup	52
Turnips,	1 cup	50
Butternut squash	1 cup	49

OMEGA-3 ALA

Continued

Kohlrabi	1 cup	46
Potatoes, mashed with whole milk	1 cup	42
Dandelion greens	1 cup	40
Mustard greens	1 cup	31
Corn	1 cup	27
Snow peas	1 cup	24
Cabbage	1 cup	21
Eggplant	1 cup	15
Potatoes, flesh	1 cup	12
Yams, cubed	1 cup	12
Beet greens	1 cup	9
Beets	1 cup	8
Onions	1 cup	8
Parsnips	1 cup	5
Pumpkin	1 cup	5
Swiss chard	1 cup	5
Tomatoes	1 cup	5
Shitake mushrooms	1 cup	4
Cactus pads, nopales	1 cup	3
Carrots	1 cup	2
Okra	1 cup	2
White mushrooms	1 cup	2
Celery	1 cup	0
Sweet potato, mashed	1 cup	0

Vegetables, Frozen	Amount	ALA (mg)
Spinach	1 cup	705
Collard greens	1 cup	216
Brussels sprouts	1 cup	200
Turnip greens	1 cup	195
Kale	1 cup	162
Cauliflower	1 cup	146
Broccoli	1 cup	77
Green beans	1 cup	65
Carrots	1 cup	64
Butternut squash	1 cup	43
Green peas	1 cup	38
Asparagus	1 cup	18
Yellow corn	1 cup	15
Okra	1 cup	2
Rhubarb	1 cup	0

OMEGA-3 ALA

Vegetables, Raw	Amount	ALA (mg)
Kale	1 cup	121
Zucchini *	1 cup	69
Romaine lettuce	1 cup	63
Summer squash	1 cup	63
Spirulina, dried	1 tbsp	58
Butter head & boston lettuce *	1 cup	46
Raab broccoli	1 cup	45
Spinach	1 cup	41
Bok-choy	1 cup	38
Red bell peppers	1 cup	37
Butternut squash	1 cup	36
Arugula	1 cup	34
Green leaf lettuce	1 cup	32
Red cabbage	1 cup	32
Iceberg lettuce	1 cup	29
Dandelion greens	1 cup	24
Tomatillos	1 cup	21
Enoki mushrooms	1 cup	20
Savoy cabbage	1 cup	20
Broccoli	1 cup	18
Snow peas	1 cup	13
Green bell peppers	1 cup	12
Watercress	1 cup	8
Cauliflower *	1 cup	7
Endive	1 cup	7
Chicory greens	1 cup	6
Onions	1 cup	6
Radicchio	1 cup	6
Belgian endive	1 cup	5
Cucumbers	1 cup	5
Tomatoes	1 cup	5
Green onions & scallions	1 cup	4
Prickley pear cactus pads, nopales	1 cup	4
Tomatoes, cherry	1 cup	4
Swiss chard	1 cup	3
Carrots	1 cup	2
Cabbage	1 cup	0
Celery	1 cup	0
Crimini mushrooms, sliced	1 cup	0
Oyster mushrooms, sliced	1 cup	0
Portabella mushrooms	1 cup	0
Shiitake mushrooms, dried	1 each	0
White mushrooms	1 cup	0

OMEGA-3 ALA

Continued

Yogurt	Amount	ALA (mg)
Yogurt plain, whole milk	8 ounces	61
Yogurt plain, low fat	8 ounces	30
Yogurt plain, skim milk	8 ounces	2
Yogurt, greek, plain, non fat	8 ounces	2

Nutrient Data Collection Form

Food	Amount	Book Numbers	Multiply By	Estimated Nutrient Intake
Nutrient::	RDA:	Estimated:	% of RDA:	Total Estimated:

To download additional forms for free, go to www.TopNutrients4U.com

NOTES

OMEGA-3 DHA

Alcohol	Amount	DHA (mg)
White Wine	1 glass	0
Red Wine	1 glass	0
Light Beer	1 bottle	0
Regular Beer	1 bottle	0
Gin, Rum, Vodka, or Whisky	1 shot	0

Beans, Canned	Amount	DHA (mg)
Great Northern	1 cup	0
Baked beans, plain	1 cup	0
Black-eyed peas	1 cup	0
Cranberry beans	1 cup	0
Fava beans	1 cup	0
Garbanzo beans	1 cup	0
Green beans	1 cup	0
Kidney, red	1 cup	0
Lima beans	1 cup	0
Navy beans	1 cup	0
Pinto beans	1 cup	0
Refried beans	1 cup	0
White beans, mature	1 cup	0
Yellow beans	1 cup	0

Beans, Cooked	Amount	DHA (mg)
Great Northern	1 cup	0
Edamame	1 cup	0
Adzuki	1 cup	0
Black beans	1 cup	0
Black Turtle beans, mature	1 cup	0
Black-eyed peas	1 cup	0
Cranberry beans	1 cup	0
Fava beans	1 cup	0
Garbanzo beans	1 cup	0
Green beans	1 cup	0
Hyacinath beans	1 cup	0
Kidney beans	1 cup	0
Lentils	1 cup	0
Lima beans	1 cup	0
Lupini beans	1 cup	0
Mothbeans	1 cup	0
Mung beans, mature seeds	1 cup	0
Natto	1 cup	0
Navy beans	1 cup	0
Pigeon peas	1 cup	0

OMEGA-3 DHA

Continued

Pinto beans	1 cup	0
Soybeans, green	1 cup	0
Soybeans, mature	1 cup	0
Soybeans, mature, dry roasted	1 cup	0
Split peas	1 cup	0
White beans, mature	1 cup	0
White beans, small	1 cup	0
Winged beans	1 cup	0
Yardlong beans, Chinese long beans	1 cup	0
Yellow beans	1 cup	0

Beef, Cooked	Amount	DHA (mg)
Ribeye steak, trimmed to 0" fat	3 oz	2
Chuck roast, trimmed to 1/8" fat	3 oz	1
Ground beef, 75%	3 oz	1
Ground beef, 80%	3 oz	1
Ground beef, 85%	3 oz	1
Ground beef, 90%,	3 oz	1
Ground beef, 95%	3 oz	1
Top sirloin, trimmed to 1/8" fat	3 oz	1
Filet Mignon, trimmed to 0" fat	3 oz	0
Porterhouse steak, trimmed to 0" fat	3 oz	0
Skirt Steak, trimmed to 0" fat	3 oz	0
T-Bone steak, trimmed 0" Fat	3 oz	0
Beef ribs, trimmed to 1/8" fat	3 oz	x

Bread	Amount	Omega-3 DHA (mg)
All types	1 slice	0

Cheese	Amount	Omega-3 DHA (mg)
All types of cheese	1 oz	0

Chicken, Cooked	Amount	Omega-3 DHA (mg)
Breast, with skin, fried in flour	1/2 breast	29
Breast, with skin, roasted	1/2 breast	29
Drumstick, with skin, fried in flour	1 drumstick	20
Breast, no skin, roasted	1/2 breast	17
Drumstick, no skin, roasted	1 drumstick	12
Thigh, no skin, roasted	1 thigh	2

Chicken, Cooked	Amount	Omega-3 DHA (mg)
Wing meat only, no skin, roasted	3 oz	60
Wing with skin, roasted	3 oz	51

OMEGA-3 DHA

Continued

Thigh with skin, fried in flour	3 oz	42
Wing with skin, fried in flour	3 oz	42
Drumstick with skin, fried in flour	3 oz	34
Breast with skin, fried in flour	3 oz	26
Breast with skin, roasted	3 oz	26
Breast meat only, no skin, roasted	3 oz	17
Drumstick meat only, roasted	3 oz	5
Drumstick with skin, roasted	3 oz	5
Thigh with skin, roasted	3 oz	4
Thigh meat only, no skin, roasted	3 oz	3

Crackers	Amount	Omega-3 DHA (mg)
All types	1-serving	0

Eggs	Amount	Omega-3 DHA (mg)
Egg whole, fried	1 large	29
Egg whole, poached	1 large	29
Egg whole, scrambled	1 large	26
Egg whole, hard boiled	1 large	19
Egg yolk	1 large	19
Egg whites	1 large	0

Fish, Canned	Amount	Omega-3 DHA (mg)
Anchovy, European, in oil	3 oz	1099
Pacific sardines, in tomato sauce	3 oz	734
Pink salmon	3 oz	685
Sockeye salmon	3 oz	564
White (albacore) tuna, in water	3 oz	535
Alaskan stellhead trout	3 oz	459
Atlantic sardines, in oil	3 oz	433
Light tuna, in water	3 oz	167
White (albacore) tuna, in oil	3 oz	151
Atlantic cod	3 oz	130
Light tuna, in oil	3 oz	86

Fish, Cooked	Amount	Omega-3 DHA (mg)
Atlantic salmon, farmed	3 oz	1238
Atlantic salmon, wild	3 oz	1215
Pacific mackerel	3 oz	1016
Bluefin tuna	3 oz	970
Spanish mackerel	3 oz	809
Coho salmon, farmed	3 oz	740
Swordfish	3 oz	656
Striped bass	3 oz	638

OMEGA-3 DHA

Continued

Chinook salmon	3 oz	618
Atlantic mackerel	3 oz	594
Coho salmon, wild	3 oz	559
Rainbow trout, farmed	3 oz	524
Sea bass	3 oz	473
Atlantic herring, pickled	3 oz	464
Alaskan steelhead trout	3 oz	459
Sockeye salmon	3 oz	445
Rainbow trout, wild	3 oz	442
Keta (chum) salmon	3 oz	429
Florida pompano	3 oz	428
Freshwater bass	3 oz	389
Atlantic pollock	3 oz	383
Walleye pollock	3 oz	360
Pink salmon	3 oz	339
Alaskan halibut	3 oz	309
Walleye pike	3 oz	245
Snapper	3 oz	232
Chinook salmon, smoked	3 oz	227
Pacific rockfish	3 oz	202
Skipjack (aku) tuna	3 oz	201
Whiting	3 oz	200
King mackerel	3 oz	193
Catfish, breaded & fried	3 oz	189
Grouper	3 oz	181
Atlantic perch	3 oz	158
Atlantic & Pacific halibut	3 oz	132
Atlantic cod	3 oz	131
Carp	3 oz	124
Catfish, wild	3 oz	116
Flounder & Sole	3 oz	112
Tilapia	3 oz	110
Pacific cod	3 oz	100
Greenland halibut	3 oz	93
Haddock	3 oz	93
Yellowfin tuna	3 oz	89
Northern pike	3 oz	81
Atlantic croaker	3 oz	76
Catfish, farmed	3 oz	59
Orange roughy	3 oz	21
Yellowtail	3 oz	x

OMEGA-3 DHA

Fish, Shellfish, Cooked	Amount	Omega-3 DHA (mg)
Squid, fried	3 oz	323
Shrimp, canned	3 oz	214
Oysters, breaded & fried	3 oz	192
Blue crab cakes	3 oz	184
Eastern oysters, farmed	3 oz	179
Eastern oysters, wild	3 oz	178
Octopus	3 oz	138
Queen crab	3 oz	123
Shrimp	3 oz	120
Shrimp, breaded & fried	3 oz	105
Alaskan king crab	3 oz	100
Clams, canned	3 oz	90
Scallops, breaded & fried	3 oz	88
Northern lobster	3 oz	66
Clams, breaded & fried	3 oz	60
Blue crab	3 oz	57
Blue crab, canned	3 oz	57
Crayfish	3 oz	40
Abalone	3 oz	39
Alaskan king crab, imitation	3 oz	19

Fruit	Amount	Omega-3 DHA (mg)
All fruits	1 cup	0

Grains, Cooked	Amount	Omega-3 DHA (mg)
All grains	1 cup	0

Herbs & Spices	Amount	Omega-3 DHA (mg)
All types	1 tsp	0

Juice	Amount	Omega-3 DHA (mg)
All types	1 cup	0

Milk	Amount	Omega-3 DHA (mg)
All types	1 cup	0

Nuts & Seeds	Amount	Omega-3 DHA (mg)
All types	1 oz	0

OMEGA-3 DHA

Oils	Amount	Omega-3 DHA (mg)
Salmon oil	1 tbsp	2480
Cod liver oil	1 tbsp	1492
Sardine oil	1 tbsp	1449
Menhaden fish oil	1 tbsp	1164
Canola oil	1 tbsp	0
Coconut oil	1 tbsp	0
Corn oil	1 tbsp	0
Flaxseed oil	1 tbsp	0
Grapeseed oil	1 tbsp	0
Olive oil	1 tbsp	0
Palm kernal vegetable oil	1 tbsp	0
Peanut oil	1 tbsp	0
Safflower, high linoleic acid, oil	1 tbsp	0
Safflower, high oleic acid, oil	1 tbsp	0
Sesame oil	1 tbsp	0
Soybean lecithin oil	1 tbsp	0
Soybean oil	1 tbsp	0
Soybean, partially hydrogenated oil	1 tbsp	0
Sunflower, high linoleic acid	1 tbsp	0
Sunflower, high oleic acid	1 tbsp	0
Walnut oil	1 tbsp	0

Pork, Cooked	Amount	Omega-3 DHA (mg)
Back ribs	3 oz	1
Chops, pan-fried	3 oz	1
Spareribs	3 oz	0
Chops, broiled	3 oz	0
Cured Ham, lean	3 oz	0
Sausage	3 oz	0
Canadian bacon	3 oz	0
Bacon, pan-fried	3 oz	0

Turkey, Cooked	Amount	Omega-3 DHA (mg)
Turkey bacon	3 oz	36
Turkey sausage, reduced fat	3 oz	20
Ground turkey, 93% lean	3 oz	9
Breast meat	3 oz	8
Ground turkey	3 oz	8
Ground turkey, 85% lean	3 oz	8
Ground turkey, fat free	3 oz	5
Dark meat *	3 oz	4
Light meat	3 oz	3

OMEGA-3 DHA

Vegetables	Amount	Omega-3 DHA (mg)
All types	1 cup	0

Yogurt	Amount	Omega-3 DHA (mg)
All types	8 oz	0

Nutrient Data Collection Form

Food	Amount	Book Numbers	Multiply By	Estimated Nutrient Intake
Nutrient::	RDA:	Estimated:	% of RDA:	Total Estimated:

To download additional forms for free, go to www.TopNutrients4U.com

OMEGA-3 EPA

Alcohol	Amount	EPA (mg)
White Wine	1 glass	0
Red Wine	1 glass	0
Light Beer	1 bottle	0
Regular Beer	1 bottle	0
Gin, Rum, Vodka, or Whisky	1 shot	0

Beans, Canned	Amount	EPA (mg)
Great Northern	1 cup	0
Baked beans, plain	1 cup	0
Black-eyed peas	1 cup	0
Cranberry beans	1 cup	0
Fava beans	1 cup	0
Garbanzo beans	1 cup	0
Green beans	1 cup	0
Kidney, red	1 cup	0
Lima beans	1 cup	0
Navy beans	1 cup	0
Pinto beans	1 cup	0
Refried beans	1 cup	0
White beans, mature	1 cup	0
Yellow beans	1 cup	0

Beans, Canned	Amount	EPA (mg)
Edamame	1 cup	5
Great Northern	1 cup	0
Adzuki	1 cup	0
Black beans	1 cup	0
Black Turtle beans, mature	1 cup	0
Black-eyed peas	1 cup	0
Cranberry beans	1 cup	0
Fava beans	1 cup	0
Garbanzo beans	1 cup	0
Green beans	1 cup	0
Hyacinath beans	1 cup	0
Kidney beans	1 cup	0
Lentils	1 cup	0
Lima beans	1 cup	0
Lupini beans	1 cup	0
Mothbeans	1 cup	0
Mung beans, mature seeds	1 cup	0
Natto	1 cup	0
Navy beans	1 cup	0
Pigeon peas	1 cup	0

OMEGA-3 EPA

Continued

Pinto beans	1 cup	0
Soybeans, green	1 cup	0
Soybeans, mature	1 cup	0
Soybeans, mature, dry roasted	1 cup	0
Split peas	1 cup	0
White beans, mature	1 cup	0
White beans, small	1 cup	0
Winged beans	1 cup	0
Yardlong beans, Chinese long beans	1 cup	0
Yellow beans	1 cup	0

Beef, Cooked	Amount	EPA (mg)
Chuck roast, trimmed to 1/8" fat	3 oz	3
Ground beef, 75%	3 oz	3
Ground beef, 80%	3 oz	3
Ground beef, 85%	3 oz	3
Ground beef, 90%,	3 oz	3
Ground beef, 95%	3 oz	3
Ribeye steak, trimmed to 0" fat	3 oz	3
Top sirloin, trimmed to 1/8" fat	3 oz	3
Filet Mignon, trimmed to 0" fat	3 oz	0
Porterhouse steak, trimmed to 0" fat	3 oz	0
Skirt Steak, trimmed to 0" fat	3 oz	0
T-Bone steak, trimmed 0" fat	3 oz	0

Bread	Amount	Omega-3 EPA (mg)
All types	slice	0

Cheese	Amount	Omega-3 EPA (mg)
All cheeses	1 oz	0

Chicken, Cooked	Amount	Omega-3 EPA (mg)
Breast, with skin, fried in flour	1/2 breast	10
Breast, with skin, roasted	1/2 breast	10
Breast, no skin, roasted	1/2 breast	9
Drumstick, with skin, fried in flour	1 drumstick	5
Drumstick, no skin, roasted	1 drumstick	2
Thigh, no skin, roasted	1 thigh	3

Chicken, Cooked	Amount	Omega-3 EPA (mg)
Wing meat only, no skin, roasted	3 oz	17
Wing with skin, fried in flour	3 oz	17
Wing with skin, roasted	3 oz	17

OMEGA-3 EPA

Continued

Breast meat only, no skin, roasted	3 oz	8
Breast with skin, fried in flour	3 oz	8
Breast with skin, roasted	3 oz	8
Drumstick with skin, fried in flour	3 oz	8
Thigh with skin, fried in flour	3 oz	8
Thigh with skin, roasted	3 oz	5
Thigh meat only, no skin, roasted	3 oz	4
Drumstick meat only, no skin, roasted	3 oz	3
Drumstick with skin, roasted	3 oz	3

Crackers	Amount	Omega-3 EPA (mg)
All types	serving	0

Eggs	Amount	Omega-3 EPA (mg)
Egg whole, scrambled	1 large	6
Egg whole, hard boiled	1 large	2
Egg yolk	1 large	2
Egg whites	1 large	0
Egg whole, fried	1 large	0
Egg whole, poached	1 large	0

Fish, Canned	Amount	Omega-3 EPA (mg)
Pink salmon	3 oz	718
Anchovy, European, in oil	3 oz	649
Pacific sardines, in tomato sauce	3 oz	452
Sockeye salmon	3 oz	418
Atlantic sardines, in oil	3 oz	402
Alaskan stellhead trout	3 oz	320
White (albacore) tuna, in water	3 oz	198
White (albacore) tuna, in oil	3 oz	56
Light tuna, in water	3 oz	24
Light tuna, in oil	3 oz	23
Atlantic cod	3 oz	3

Fish, Cooked	Amount	Omega-3 EPA (mg)
Chinook salmon	3 oz	858
Atlantic herring, pickled	3 oz	717
Atlantic salmon, farmed	3 oz	586
Greenland halibut	3 oz	573
Pacific mackerel	3 oz	555
Atlantic mackerel	3 oz	428
Rainbow trout, wild	3 oz	398
Atlantic salmon, wild	3 oz	349
Coho salmon, farmed	3 oz	347

Continued

Coho salmon, wild	3 oz	341
Bluefin tuna	3 oz	309
Carp	3 oz	259
Freshwater bass	3 oz	259
Keta (chum) salmon	3 oz	254
Spanish mackerel	3 oz	250
Whiting	3 oz	241
Sockeye salmon	3 oz	228
Rainbow trout, farmed	3 oz	220
Alaskan halibut	3 oz	207
Florida pompano	3 oz	190
Pink salmon	3 oz	185
Striped bass	3 oz	184
Sea bass	3 oz	175
Chinook salmon, smoked	3 oz	156
King mackerel	3 oz	148
Flounder & Sole	3 oz	143
Swordfish	3 oz	108
Catfish, breaded & fried	3 oz	101
Atlantic croaker	3 oz	96
Walleye pike	3 oz	94
Pacific rockfish	3 oz	91
Catfish, wild	3 oz	85
Atlantic pollock	3 oz	77
Skipjack (aku) tuna	3 oz	77
Walleye pollock	3 oz	73
Atlantic & Pacific halibut	3 oz	68
Atlantic perch	3 oz	64
Haddock	3 oz	43
Snapper	3 oz	41
Northern pike	3 oz	36
Pacific cod	3 oz	36
Grouper	3 oz	30
Catfish, farmed	3 oz	17
Yellowfin tuna	3 oz	13
Orange roughy	3 oz	5
Tilapia	3 oz	4
Atlantic cod	3 oz	3

Fish, Shellfish, Cooked	Amount	Omega-3 EPA (mg)
Queen crab	3 oz	282
Alaskan king crab	3 oz	251
Shrimp, canned	3 oz	249
Eastern oysters, wild	3 oz	233
Eastern oysters, farmed	3 oz	195

OMEGA-3 EPA

Continued

Blue crab cakes	3 oz	193
Oysters, breaded & fried	3 oz	178
Squid, fried	3 oz	138
Octopus	3 oz	129
Shrimp	3 oz	115
Crayfish	3 oz	101
Northern lobster	3 oz	99
Shrimp, breaded & fried	3 oz	93
Blue crab	3 oz	86
Blue crab, canned	3 oz	86
Scallops, breaded & fried	3 oz	73
Clams, canned	3 oz	60
Clams, breaded & fried	3 oz	56
Abalone	3 oz	46
Alaskan king crab, imitation	3 oz	0

Fruit	Amount	Omega-3 EPA (mg)
All fruit	1 cup	0

Grains, Cooked	Amount	Omega-3 EPA (mg)
All types	1 cup	0

Herbs & Spices	Amount	Omega-3 EPA (mg)
All types	1 tsp	0

Juice	Amount	Omega-3 EPA (mg)
All types	1 cup	0

Milk	Amount	Omega-3 EPA (mg)
All types	1 cup	0

Nuts and Seeds	Amount	Omega-3 EPA (mg)
All nuts and seeds	1 oz	0

Oils	Amount	Omega-3 EPA (mg)
Menhaden fish oil	1 tbsp	1791
Salmon oil	1 tbsp	1771
Sardine oil	1 tbsp	1379
Cod liver oil	1 tbsp	938
Canola oil	1 tbsp	0
Coconut oil	1 tbsp	0
Corn oil	1 tbsp	0

OMEGA-3 EPA

Continued

Flaxseed oil	1 tbsp	0
Grapeseed oil	1 tbsp	0
Olive oil	1 tbsp	0
Palm kernal vegetable oil	1 tbsp	0
Peanut oil	1 tbsp	0
Safflower, high linoleic acid, oil	1 tbsp	0
Safflower, high oleic acid, oil	1 tbsp	0
Sesame oil	1 tbsp	0
Soybean lecithin oil	1 tbsp	0
Soybean oil	1 tbsp	0
Soybean, partially hydrogenated oil	1 tbsp	0
Sunflower, high linoleic acid	1 tbsp	0
Sunflower, high oleic acid	1 tbsp	0
Walnut oil	1 tbsp	0

Pork, Cooked	Amount	Omega-3 EPA (mg)
Spareribs	3 oz	0
Back ribs	3 oz	0
Chops, pan-fried	3 oz	0
Chops, broiled	3 oz	0
Cured Ham, lean	3 oz	0
Sausage	3 oz	0
Canadian bacon	3 oz	0
Bacon, pan-fried	3 oz	0

Turkey, Cooked	Amount	Omega-3 EPA (mg)
Ground turkey, 85% lean	3 oz	18
Dark meat	3 oz	10
Ground turkey	3 oz	8
Light meat	3 oz	3
Ground turkey, 93% lean	3 oz	3
Ground turkey, fat free	3 oz	3
Breast meat	3 oz	0
Turkey sausage, reduced fat	3 oz	0
Turkey bacon	3 oz	0

Vegetables	Amount	Omega-3 EPA (mg)
All types	1 serving	0

Yogurt	Amount	Omega-3 EPA (mg)
All types	8 oz	0

Nutrient Data Collection Form

Food	Amount	Book Numbers	Multiply By	Estimated Nutrient Intake
Nutrient::	RDA:	Estimated:	% of RDA:	Total Estimated:

To download additional forms for free, go to www.TopNutrients4U.com

OMEGA-6 LA

Alcohol	Amount	LA (mg)
White Table Wine	1 glass	0
Red Table Wine	1 glass	0
Light Beer	1 bottle	0
Regular Beer	1 bottle	0
Gin, Rum, Vodka, or Whisky	1 shot	0

Beans, Canned	Amount	LA (mg)
Garbanzo beans	1 cup	2038
Refried beans *	1 cup	459
Black-eyed peas	1 cup	360
Kidney beans	1 cup	284
Navy beans	1 cup	265
Great Northern	1 cup	233
Fava beans	1 cup	215
Pinto beans	1 cup	206
White beans	1 cup	181
Cranberry beans	1 cup	172
Baked beans, plain	1 cup	140
Lima beans, large	1 cup	125
Green beans	1 cup	112
Yellow beans	1 cup	29

Beans, Cooked	Amount	LA (mg)
Soybeans, dry roasted	1 cup	10011
Natto	1 cup	9583
Soybeans, mature	1 cup	7680
Soybeans, green	1 cup	4783
Edamame *	1 cup	2773
Winged beans	1 cup	2506
Garbanzo beans	1 cup	1825
Lupini beans	1 cup	991
Hyacinath beans	1 cup	475
Pigeon peas	1 cup	329
Lentils	1 cup	271
Split peas	1 cup	269
White beans, small	1 cup	268
Fava beans	1 cup	258
Navy beans	1 cup	248
Black-eyed peas	1 cup	245
Mung beans	1 cup	240
Lima beans	1 cup	222
Black beans	1 cup	217
Cranberry beans	1 cup	191

OMEGA-6 LA

Continued

Kidney beans	1 cup	189
Great Northern beans	1 cup	182
Pinto beans	1 cup	168
Black Turtle beans, mature	1 cup	150
White beans, mature	1 cup	149
Green beans	1 cup	70
Yellow beans	1 cup	70
Adzuki	1 cup	48
Yardlong beans, Chinese	1 cup	25
Mothbeans	1 cup	x

Beef, Cooked	Amount	LA (mg)
Chuck roast, trim to 1/8" fat	3 oz	570
Beef ribs, trim to 1/8" fat	3 oz	561
Porterhouse steak, trim to 0" fat	3 oz	400
Ground beef, 75% lean	3 oz	348
T-Bone steak, trim 0" fat	3 oz	346
Ribeye steak, trim to 0" fat	3 oz	344
Ground beef, 80% lean	3 oz	338
Top sirloin, trim to 1/8" fat	3 oz	313
Ground beef, 85% lean	3 oz	312
Tri Tip, sirloin, steak, lean, trim to 0" fat	3 oz	298
Skirt Steak, trim to 0" fat	3 oz	292
Ground beef, 90% lean	3 oz	267
Filet Mignon, trim to 0" fat	3 oz	258
Ground beef, 95% lean	3 oz	204
Brisket, trim to 0" fat	3 oz	171
Flank steak, trim to 0" fat	3 oz	156
London Broil, top round, trim to 0" fat	3 oz	145

Beef, Cooked	Amount	LA (mg)
Chuck roast, trim to 1/8" fat	1 cooked lb	3042
Beef ribs, trim to 1/8" fat	1 cooked lb	2996
Porterhouse steak, trim to 0" fat	1 cooked lb	2136
T-bone steak, trim to 0" fat	1 cooked lb	1846
Top Sirloin, trim to 1/8" fat	1 cooked lb	1671
Tri Tip steak, lean, trim to 0" fat	1 cooked lb	1588
Skirt steak, trim to 0" fat	1 cooked lb	1560
Brisket, lean, trim to 0" fat	1 cooked lb	913
Ribeye steak, boneless, trim to 0" fat *	1 steak	857
Flank steak, lean, trim to 0" fat	1 cooked lb	831
Flank steak, lean, trim to 0" fat	1 steak	701
Filet Mignon, tenderloin, trim to 0" fat *	1 steak	386
Ribeye filet, lean, trim to 0" fat *	1 filet	217
Top Sirloin, choice filet, trim to 0" fat *	1 filet	145

OMEGA-6 LA

Beef, Cooked	Amount	LA (mg)
Ground beef, 80%	1/4 lb patty	306
Ground beef, 75%	1/4 lb patty	286
Ground beef, 85%	1/4 lb patty	283
Ground beef, 90%	1/4 lb patty	257
Ground beef, 95%	1/4 lb patty	197

Bread	Amount	LA (mg)
Indian bread, Naan, plain *	1 piece	1608
Indian bread, Naan, whole wheat	1 piece	1295
Cornbread, dry mix	1 piece	1135
Kaiser rolls	1 roll	924
Bagel, oat bran	4" bagel	842
Mexican roll, bollilo *	1 roll	833
Dinner Rolls, brown & serve	1 roll	640
Hamburger & Hotdog buns, plain	1 bun	600
Bagel, cinnamon & raisins	4" bagel	562
Bagel, egg	4" bagel	534
Bagel, plain	4" bagel	512
Bagel, Wheat	4" bagel	488
Croissants, butter	1 medium	453
Multi-Grain or Whole-Grain	1 slice	433
Oatmeal bread	1 slice	433
Egg bread	1 slice	399
Tortillas, flour	1 tortilla	395
Pumpernickel	1 slice	366
Wheat	1 slice	362
Tortillas, corn	1 tortilla	360
White	1 slice	354
Pita, white	6" pita	307
Italian	1 slice	258
English Muffin, plain	1 muffin	256
Rye bread	1 slice	239
French, and Sourdough	1 slice	185
Raisin bread	1 slice	167
Cracked Wheat	1 slice	162
Whole-Wheat	1 slice	151
Potato bread	1 slice	0

Butter	Amount	LA (mg)
Regular dairy butter, salted *	1 tbsp	308
Regular dairy whipped butter, salted	1 tbsp	172

OMEGA-6 LA

General Mills®	Amount	LA (mg)
Raisin Nut Bran	1 cup	1261
Reese's Puffs	1 cup	1149
Oatmeal Crisp, Crunchy Almond	1 cup	1043
Multi-Bran CHEX	1 cup	761
Cinnamon Toast Crunch	1 cup	662
Dora The Explorer	1 cup	644
Cocoa Puffs	1 cup	629
Cookie Crisp	1 cup	629
Lucky Charms *	1 cup	535
Wheat Chex	1 cup	494
Honey Nut Chex	1 cup	481
Oatmeal Crisp, Hearty Raisin	1 cup	480
Trix	1 cup	443
Total Raisin Bran	1 cup	384
Total Cranberry Crunch	1 cup	363
Berry Berry Kix	1 cup	356
Golden Grahams	1 cup	335
Wheaties	1 cup	328
Kix *	1 cup	290
Total Whole Grain	1 cup	260
Honey Nut Clusters	1 cup	214
Corn Chex	1 cup	198
Rice Chex	1 cup	83
Basic 4	1 cup	24

General Mill's® Cheerios®	Amount	LA (mg)
Chocolate	1 cup	699
Original *	1 cup	656
Fruity	1 cup	655
Yogurt Burst, Strawberry	1 cup	637
Honey Nut	1 cup	636
Banana Nut	1 cup	634
Oat Cluster Cherrios Crunch	1 cup	620
Apple Cinnamon	1 cup	595
Berry Burst, Triple Berry	1 cup	542
Frosted	1 cup	536
Multi Grain	1 cup	444
Cinnamon Burst	1 cup	x

General Mill's Fiber One	Amount	LA (mg)
Bran Cereal	1 cup	760

OMEGA-6 LA

Kashi	Amount	LA (mg)
Go Lean Crunch, Honey Almond Flax	1 cup	1733
Go Lean Crunch	1 cup	736
Good Friends	1 cup	518
Go Lean	1 cup	517
Heart to Heart, Honey Toasted Oat	1 cup	480
Good Friends, Cinnamon Raisin Cr.	1 cup	308
Organic Promise, Autumn Wheat	1 cup	308
7-Whole Grain Honey Puffs	1 cup	244
7-Whole Grain Puffs	1 cup	197

Kellogg's	Amount	LA (mg)
Mueslix	1 cup	1426
Low Fat Granola with Raisins	1 cup	1315
All-Bran Original	1 cup	1215
Cracklin Oat Bran	1 cup	1191
Smorz	1 cup	1076
All-Bran Bran Buds	1 cup	1045
Frosted MINI-Wheat's, Bite-Size	1 cup	615
Frosted MINI Wheat's, Big-Bite	1 cup	483
Smart Start, Strong Heart Antioxidants	1 cup	455
Raisin Bran	1 cup	396
All-Bran Complete Wheat Flakes	1 cup	395
Raisin Bran Crunch	1 cup	394
Honey Smacks	1 cup	302
Froot Loops	1 cup	286
Honey Crunch Corn Flakes	1 cup	236
Rice Krispies Treats	1 cup	215
Product 19	1 cup	193
Apple Jacks	1 cup	186
Corn Pops	1 cup	156
Cocoa Krispies	1 cup	95
Berry Rice Krispies	1 cup	78
Rice Krispies	1 cup	77
Corn Flakes	1 cup	76
Crispix	1 cup	56
Frosted Flakes	1 cup	37
Frosted Rice Krispies	1 cup	33

Kellogg's Special-K®	Amount	LA (mg)
Protein Plus	1 cup	1846
Cinnamon Pecan	1 cup	744
Vanilla Almond	1 cup	422
Chocolately Delight	1 cup	226

Continued

Original	1 cup	218
Red Berries	1 cup	135
Fruit & Yogurt	1 cup	120

Post®	Amount	LA, mg
Great Grains, Banana Nut Crunch	1 cup	2305
Great Grains, Crunchy Pecan Cereal	1 cup	2034
Great Grains, Raisin, Date & Pecan	1 cup	1456
Grape-Nuts Cereal	1 cup	1285
Great Grains, Cranberry Almond Crunch	1 cup	1041
Honey Nut Shredded Wheat	1 cup	664
Shredded Wheat, Original, spoon-size	1 cup	605
Blueberry Morning	1 cup	598
Shredded Wheat n' Bran, spoon size	1 cup	541
Grape-Nuts Flakes	1 cup	531
Alpha-Bits	1 cup	517
Raisin Bran	1 cup	461
Shredded Wheat, Frosted, spoon-size	1 cup	447
Bran Flakes	1 cup	444
Shredded Wheat, Original, big-biscuit	1 biscuit	295
Golden Crisp	1 cup	202
Honeycomb Cereal	1 cup	185
Cocoa Pebbles	1 cup	33
Fruity Pebbles	1 cup	30

Post® Honey Bunches of Oats®	Amount	LA, mg
Just Bunches, Honey Roasted	1 cup	2491
With Vanilla Bunches	1 cup	869
With Almonds	1 cup	842
Pecan Bunches	1 cup	623
Honey Roasted *	1 cup	480
With Cinnamon Bunches	1 cup	x
With Strawberries	1 cup	x

Cereal, Quaker	Amount	LA (mg)
Granola, Oats, Wheat & Honey	1 cup	2159
Granola, Oats, Wheat, Honey & Raisins	1 cup	1953
Low Fat Granola with Raisins	1 cup	1074
Oatmeal Squares, Cinnamon	1 cup	814
Oatmeal Squares	1 cup	813
CAP'N Crunch's Peanut Butter Crunch	1 cup	775
LIFE Cereal	1 cup	578
LIFE Cereal, Cinnamon	1 cup	525
Toasted Oatmeal Cereal, Honey Nut	1 cup	525

OMEGA-6 LA

Continued

Crunchy Bran	1 cup	430
CAP'N Crunch	1 cup	260
CAP'N Crunch & Crunch Berries	1 cup	253
Honey Graham OH'S	1 cup	27

Cereal, Cooked	Amount	LA (mg)
Oats, regular, unenriched *	1 cup	1264
WHEATENA	1 cup	569
White corn grits	1 cup	424
Yellow corn grits	1 cup	303
CREAM OF WHEAT, regular	1 cup	256
Farina *	1 cup	231
CREAM OF WHEAT, mix'n eat	1 packet	141

Cheese	Amount	LA (mg)
Ricotta, whole milk	1 cup	672
Ricotta, part skim milk	1 cup	467
Cottage cheese, small curd	1 cup	236
Cottage cheese, low fat, 2 %	1 cup	136
Cottage cheese, low fat, 1 %	1 cup	50
Cottage cheese, non fat & uncreamed	1 cup	4

Cheese	Amount	LA (mg)
American, pasteurized process, imitation	1 oz	1842
Gruyere	1 oz	369
Cream cheese	1 oz	293
Parmesan, grated	1 oz	267
Fontina	1 oz	245
Goat cheese, hard type	1 oz	240
American, pasteurized process, fortified *	1 oz	224
Goat cheese, semisoft	1 oz	201
Colby	1 oz	192
Monterey	1 oz	181
Swiss	1 oz	176
Swiss	1 oz	175
Monterey, low fat	1 oz	168
Cheddar	1 oz	163
Blue cheese	1 oz	152
Brie	1 oz	145
Goat cheese, soft type	1 oz	142
Provolone	1 oz	140
Muenster	1 oz	122
Mozzarella, whole milk	1 oz	111
Muenster, low fat	1 oz	111

OMEGA-6 LA

Continued

Mozzarella, part skim, low moisture	1 oz	102
Feta	1 oz	92
Provolone, reduced fat	1 oz	92
Romano	1 oz	81
Ricotta	1 oz	77
Gouda	1 oz	75
Ricotta, part skim milk	1 oz	54
Cheddar, low-fat	1 oz	44
American, pasteurized process, low fat	1 oz	38
Swiss, low fat	1 oz	32
Cream cheese, fat free	1 oz	12
Mozzarella, non fat	1 oz	0

Cheese, Mexican	Amount	LA (mg)
Queso fresco *	1 oz	168
Mexican blend, reduced fat	1 oz	162
Queso anejo	1 oz	156
Queso chihuahua	1 oz	155
Mexican blend	1 oz	149
Queso asadero	1 oz	147

Chicken, Cooked	Amount	LA (mg)
Wing, with skin, fried in batter	1 wing	2225
Breast, with skin, fried in flour	1/2 breast	1656
Drumstick, with skin, fried in flour	1 drumstick	1387
Breast, with skin, roasted	1/2 breast	1382
Wing, with skin, roasted	1 wing	1214
Thigh, meat only, roasted *	1 thigh	723
Breast, no skin, roasted	1/2 breast	507

Chicken, Cooked	Amount	LA (mg)
Wing with skin, fried in flour	3 oz	3689
Wing with skin, roasted	3 oz	3034
Thigh with skin, fried in flour	3 oz	2524
Drumstick with skin, fried in flour	3 oz	2406
Thigh with skin, roasted *	3 oz	2199
Drumstick with skin, roasted *	3 oz	1470
Breast with skin, fried in flour	3 oz	1436
Breast with skin, roasted	3 oz	1411
Thigh meat only, no skin, roasted *	3 oz	1182
Wing meat only, no skin, roasted	3 oz	1096
Drumstick meat only, no skin, roasted *	3 oz	777
Cornish game hens, meat only	3 oz	586
Breast meat only, no skin, roasted	3 oz	502

OMEGA-6 LA

Cream	Amount	LA (mg)
Heavy Cream	1 tbsp	125
Light Coffee Cream	1 tbsp	93
Sour Cream, cultured	1 tbsp	73
Sour Cream, reduced fat, cultured	1 tbsp	41
Half & Half	1 tbsp	39
Whipped Cream, pressurized	1 tbsp	15

Eggs	Amount	LA (mg)
Egg whole, fried	1 large	1279
Egg whole, scrambled	1 large	1261
Egg whole, poached	1 large	775
Egg yolk	1 large	601
Egg whole, hard boiled	1 large	594
Egg substitute, liquid, fat free	1/4 cup	0
Egg whites	1 large	0
Egg whites, dried	1 ounce	0
Egg whites, dried powder, stabilized	1 tbsp	0

FISH

Fish, Canned	Amount	LA (mg)
Light tuna, in oil	3 oz	2281
White (albacore) tuna, in oil	3 oz	2116
White (albacore) tuna, in water	3 oz	47
Light tuna, in water *	3 oz	12

Fish, Cooked	Amount	LA (mg)
Cat fish, breaded & fried	3 oz	2224
Atlantic croaker	3 oz	2020
Catfish, farmed	3 oz	824
Atlantic salmon, farmed	3 oz	566
Carp	3 oz	564
Rainbow trout, farmed	3 oz	500
Chinook salmon, smoked	3 oz	401
Sockeye salmon	3 oz	320
Coho salmon, farmed	3 oz	317
Rainbow trout, wild	3 oz	245
Tilapia	3 oz	242
Atlantic salmon, wild	3 oz	187
Atlantic hearing, pickled	3 oz	179
Greenland halibut	3 oz	134
Florida pompano	3 oz	132

OMEGA-6 LA

Continued

Pacific & Jack mackerel	3 oz	127
Atlantic mackerel	3 oz	125
Catfish, wild	3 oz	121
Chinook salmon	3 oz	116
Freshwater bass	3 oz	95
Spanish mackerel	3 oz	92
Pink salmon	3 oz	82
Swordfish	3 oz	75
Keta, (chum) salmon	3 oz	65
Bluefin tuna	3 oz	58
Orange roughy	3 oz	48
Coho salmon, wild	3 oz	48
Flounder & Sole	3 oz	47
King mackerel	3 oz	43
Atlantic & Pacific halibut	3 oz	35
Northern pike	3 oz	35
Atlantic perch	3 oz	33
Walleye pike	3 oz	28
Sea bass	3 oz	26
Snapper	3 oz	21
Yellowfin tuna	3 oz	20
Pacific cod	3 oz	18
Skipjack (aku) tuna	3 oz	17
Whiting	3 oz	17
Haddock	3 oz	16
Striped bass	3 oz	16
Grouper	3 oz	15
Alaskan halibut	3 oz	15
Atlantic pollock	3 oz	10
Walleye pollock	3 oz	9
Atlantic cod	3 oz	5

Fish, Shellfish, Cooked	Amount	LA (mg)
Shrimp, breaded & fried	3 oz	3834
Clams, breaded & fried	3 oz	2087
Scallops, breaded & fried	3 oz	2077
Oysters, breaded & fried	3 oz	2074
Blue crab cakes	3 oz	1341
Abalone	3 oz	1253
Squid, fried	3 oz	1248
Shrimp	3 oz	162
Crayfish	3 oz	76
Alaskan king crab, imitation *	3 oz	61
Clams, canned	3 oz	60
Eastern oysters, wild	3 oz	54

OMEGA-6 LA

Continued

Eastern oysters, farmed	3 oz	37
Northern lobster *	3 oz	28
Blue crab, canned	3 oz	17
Alaskan king crab	3 oz	17
Octopus	3 oz	15
Blue crab *	3 oz	14
Shrimp, canned *	3 oz	13
Queen crab	3 oz	7

Fruit, Canned	Amount	LA (mg)
Olives, black	5 large	186
Olives, green	5 large	164
Peaches	1 cup	121
Applesauce, sweetened	1 cup	111
Pears	1 cup	80
Pineapple	1 cup	58
Plums	1 cup	57
Applesauce, unsweetened	1 cup	29
Apricots	1 cup	15

Fruit, Dried	Amount	LA (mg)
Cranberries	1 cup	626
Peaches	1 cup	573
Figs	1 cup	514
Pears	1 cup	263
Currants	1 cup	259
Apricots	1 cup	96
Prunes	1 cup	77
Apples	1 cup	66

Fruit, Frozen	Amount	LA (mg)
Blueberries	1 cup	259
Blackberries	1 cup	246
Peaches	1 cup	158
Raspberries	1 cup	148
Strawberries	1 cup	102

Fruit, Raw	Amount	LA (mg)
Avocado, California	1 cup	3850
Avocado, Florida	1 cup	3634
Kiwi	1 cup	443
Raspberries	1 cup	306
Blackberries	1 cup	268
Elderberries	1 cup	235

Continued

Nectarine	1 cup	159
Strawberries	1 cup	149
Blueberries	1 cup	130
Peaches	1 cup	129
Apricots	1 cup	127
Tangerine	1 cup	94
Prunes, uncooked	1 cup	77
Water mellon	1 cup	76
Plums	1 cup	73
Plantains	1 cup	64
Grapes, red or green	1 cup	56
Cantaloupe	1 cup	56
Apples	1 cup	54
Pears	1 cup	47
Honeydew	1 cup	44
Cherries	1 cup	42
Raisins	1 cup	41
Navel oranges	1 cup	38
Jicama	1 cup	38
Pineapple	1 cup	38
Dates	1 cup	24
Papayas	1 cup	16

Fruit, Raw	Amount	LA (mg)
Avocado, Florida	1 fruit	4803
Avocado, California	1 fruit	3850
Cherimoya*	1 fruit	374
Olives, black	5 large	186
Olives, green	5 large	164
Nectarine	1 fruit	143
Star fruit, Carambola	1 fruit	143
Cantaloupe	1/2 fruit	97
Peaches	1 fruit	82
Apples	1 fruit	78
Plantains	1 fruit	77
Chayote	1 fruit	73
Persimmons, Japanese	1 fruit	66
Pineapple guava, Feijoa*	1 fruit	64
Bananas	1 fruit	54
Strawberries	5 fruit	54
Pears	1 fruit	48
Tangerine	1 fruit	42
Grapefruit, pink or red	1/2 fruit	36
Oranges, navel	1 fruit	32
Figs, dried	1 fig	29

OMEGA-6 LA

Continued

Plums	1 plum	29
Apricots	1 fruit	27
Kumquats	1 fruit	24
Cherries	10 cherries	22
Prunes, uncooked	5 prunes	21
Raisins	1 small box	21
Kiwi	1 fruit	17
Pineapple	1/2" x 3" slice	11
Dates	5 dates	6
Persimmons, small natives	1 fruit	x

Game Meat, Cooked	Amount	LA (mg)
Duck	3 oz	1140
Squirrel	3 oz	1139
Bison, ground	3 oz	467
Rabbit	3 oz	459
Wild boar	3 oz	425
Deer	3 oz	340
Antelope	3 oz	280
Caribou	3 oz	264
Deer, ground	3 oz	223
Elk, ground	3 oz	214
Elk	3 oz	196
Buffalo, steak, free range *	3 oz	70

Grains, Cooked	Amount	LA (mg)
Egg noodles	1 cup	835
Millet	1 cup	835
Oat bran	1 cup	710
Brown rice	1 cup	603
Egg & Spinach noodles	1 cup	482
Macaroni	1 cup	413
Spaghetti, enriched	1 cup	413
Spaghetti, spinach	1 cup	318
Pearled barley	1 cup	303
Buckwheat	1 cup	292
Spaghetti, whole wheat	1 cup	284
Wild rice	1 cup	195
Bulgur	1 cup	171
White rice, regular long grain	1 cup	98
Couscous	1 cup	94
Rice noodles	1 cup	33
Soba noodles	1 cup	33

OMEGA-6 LA

Herbs & Spices	Amount	LA (mg)
Chili powder	1 tbsp	598
Paprika	1 tbsp	497
Celery seeds	1 tbsp	229
Anise seed	1 tbsp	211
Caraway seeds	1 tbsp	209
Cloves, ground *	1 tbsp	174
All-spice, ground	1 tbsp	137
Curry powder	1 tbsp	134
Turmeric, ground	1 tbsp	115
Coriander, seeds	1 tbsp	88
Pepper, black	1 tbsp	48
Oregano, dried, ground	1 tbsp	39
Rosemary, dried	1 tbsp	38
Ginger, ground	1 tbsp	37
Chervil, dried	1 tbsp	34
Nutmeg	1 tbsp	24
Bay leaf, crumbled	1 tbsp	22
Thyme, ground	1 tbsp	22
Parsley, dried *	1 tbsp	20
Onion powder	1 tbsp	18
Saffron	1 tbsp	16
Garlic powder	1 tbsp	14
Thyme, dried, leaves	1 tbsp	14
Tarragon, dried leaves	1 tbsp	13
Sage, ground	1 tbsp	11
Capers	1 tbsp	10
Basil, dried & ground	1 tbsp	9
Chives, raw	1 tbsp	8
Rosemary, fresh	1 tbsp	8
Spearmint, dried	1 tbsp	7
Cinnamon, ground	1 tbsp	3
Thyme, fresh	1 tbsp	3
Basil, fresh, chopped	1 tbsp	2
Coriander, leaves, cilantro	1/4 cup	2
Dill weed, fresh	1/4 cup	2

Juice	Amount	LA (mg)
Carrot	1 cup	144
Pomegranate	1 cup	125
Cranberry juice, cocktail	1 cup	89
Vegetable juice, cocktail	1 cup	87
Apple	1 cup	82
Orange juice, raw	1 cup	72
Pineapple	1 cup	60

OMEGA-6 LA

Tomato	1 cup	56
Grape	1 cup	43
Prune	1 cup	18

Lamb, Cooked	Amount	LA (mg)
Ground	3 oz	910
Chops, loin, lean, trim to 1/4" fat	3 oz	806
Leg, whole, trim to 1/4" fat	3 oz	765
Rib, lean, trim to 1/4" fat	3 oz	757
Foreshank, trim to 1/8" fat	3 oz	620
Cubed, for stew or kabob	3 oz	425

Milk	Amount	LA (mg)
Soymilk	1 cup	1419
Human milk	1 cup	920
Canned, condensed, sweet	1 cup	661
Canned, evaporated	1 cup	421
Whole, 3.25% milkfat	1 cup	293
Goat milk	1 cup	266
Coconut milk, canned	1 cup	233
Reduced fat, 2% milkfat *	1 cup	134
Low-fat, 1% milkfat *	1 cup	66
Buttermilk, low-fat	1 cup	49
Canned, evaporated, non fat	1 cup	10
Non fat, fat free or skim	1 cup	5
Dry, instant, non fat	1/3 cup	4

Nuts & Seeds, raw	Amount	LA (mg)
English walnuts	1 oz	10799
Pine nuts	1 oz	9398
Black walnuts	1 oz	9371
Tahini	1 oz	6558
Sunflower seeds	1 oz	6535
Sesame seeds	1 oz	6060
Pumpkin seeds	1 oz	5859
Pecans	1 oz	5848
Brazil nuts	1 oz	5834
Peanuts	1 oz	4410
Almonds *	1 oz	4404
Peanut butter, smooth style	1 oz	3993
Pistachio	1 oz	3823
Hazelnuts	1 oz	2252
Cashews	1 oz	2206
Flaxseeds	1 oz	1674

OMEGA-6 LA

Continued

Chia seeds *	1 oz	1654
Macadamia	1 oz	367
Coconut, raw meat	1 oz	104

Oils	Amount	LA (mg)
Safflower, high linoleic acid, oil	1 tbsp	10149
Grapeseed oil	1 tbsp	9466
Sunflower, high linoleic acid, oil	1 tbsp	8935
Corn oil	1 tbsp	7239
Walnut oil	1 tbsp	7194
Cottonseed oil	1 tbsp	7004
Soybean oil *	1 tbsp	6857
Sesame oil	1 tbsp	5616
Soybean lecithin oil	1 tbsp	5465
Soybean, partially hydrogenated	1 tbsp	4746
Peanut oil	1 tbsp	4320
Canola oil *	1 tbsp	2610
Flaxseed oil *	1 tbsp	1937
Avocado oil	1 tbsp	1754
Safflower, high oleic acid, oil *	1 tbsp	1730
Olive oil	1 tbsp	1318
Canola oil, * partially hydrogenated	1 tbsp	1194
Sunflower, high oleic acid	1 tbsp	505
Menhaden oil	1 tbsp	293
Sardine oil	1 tbsp	274
Coconut oil	1 tbsp	245
Salmon oil	1 tbsp	210
Cod liver oil	1 tbsp	127

Pork, Cooked	Amount	LA (mg)
Pork sausage	3 oz	3727
Bacon, pan-fried *	3 oz	3400
Sausage	3 oz	2798
Backribs *	3 oz	2639
Italian sausage	3 oz	2581
Braunschweiger	3 oz	2424
Polish sausage	3 oz	2373
Spareribs	3 oz	2133
Bratwurst	3 oz	2056
Cured ham, whole	3 oz	1318
Liverwurst spread	1/4 cup	1263
Center loin chops *	3 oz	978
Chops, pan-fried *	3 oz	893
Chops, lean, pan-fried	3 oz	753
Sirloin chops *	3 oz	594

OMEGA-6 LA

Continued

Canadian-style bacon	3 oz	586
Cured ham, lean	3 oz	425
Tenderloin *	3 oz	397

Salad Dressing	Amount	LA (mg)
Mayonnaise, regular	1 tbsp	5374
Caesar, regular	1 tbsp	4259
Ranch, regular *	1 tbsp	3733
Blue cheese, regular	1 tbsp	3648
Honey Mustard, regular	1 tbsp	3018
French, regular	1 tbsp	2927
Thousand Island, regular	1 tbsp	2539
Russian	1 tbsp	1963
Mayonnaise, light *	1 tbsp	1703
Italian, regular *	1 tbsp	1359
French, reduced fat	1 tbsp	473
Blue cheese, light	1 tbsp	126
Ranch, fat-free	1 tbsp	87
Thousand Island, fat-free	1 tbsp	86
Ranch, reduced fat	1 tbsp	79
Honey Mustard, fat-free	1 tbsp	25
Italian, fat-free	1 tbsp	23
Blue cheese, fat-free	1 tbsp	9
French, fat-free	1 tbsp	7
Caesar, fat-free	1 tbsp	1

Turkey, cooked	Amount	LA (mg)
Turkey bacon	3 oz	5150
Ground turkey, 85% lean *	3 oz	3094
Ground turkey, 93% lean *	3 oz	3039
Ground turkey *	3 oz	2132
Turkey sausage, reduced fat	3 oz	1893
Dark meat *	3 oz	1411
Liver *	3 oz	1235
Ground turkey, fat free *	3 oz	508
Light meat *	3 oz	362
Breast meat, only	3 oz	110

Vegetables, Canned	Amount	LA (mg)
Asparagus	1 cup	651
Green peas	1 cup	532
Corn	1 cup	483
Tomato paste	1 cup	398
Sweet potato	1 cup	233

OMEGA-6 LA

Continued

Tomato pure	1 cup	205
Stewed tomato	1 cup	189
Mushrooms	1 cup	173
Tomato sauce	1 cup	169
Tomatoes	1 cup	120
Carrots	1 cup	115
Green beans	1 cup	99
Sauerkraut	1 cup	80
Beets	1 cup	76
Spinach	1 cup	71
Pumpkin	1 cup	17

Veal, Cooked	Amount	LA (mg)
Rib	3 oz	638
Breast	3 oz	530
Loin	3 oz	527
Sirloin	3 oz	442
Ground	3 oz	357
Foreshank	3 oz	353
Leg, top round	3 oz	298

Vegetables, Cooked	Amount	LA (mg)
Corn	1 cup	873
White mushrooms	1 cup	279
Split peas	1 cup	269
Dandelion greens	1 cup	235
Sweet potato, mashed	1 cup	200
Artichokes	1 cup	176
Onions	1 cup	147
Asparagus	1 cup	137
Carrots	1 cup	136
Snow peas	1 cup	136
Collard greens	1 cup	133
Brussels sprouts	1 cup	123
Winter squash	1 cup	113
Celery	1 cup	112
Zucchini	1 cup	104
Kale	1 cup	103
Beets	1 cup	99
Beet greens	1 cup	94
Potatoes, flesh	1 cup	94
Summer squash	1 cup	88
Broccoli	1 cup	80
Eggplant	1 cup	77
Okra	1 cup	72

OMEGA-6 LA

Continued

Green beans	1 cup	70
Yams, cubed	1 cup	68
Broccolini	1 cup	67
Rutabagas	1 cup	65
Parsnips	1 cup	64
Cauliflower	1 cup	62
Bok-Choy	1 cup	53
Leeks	1 cup	47
Acorn squash	1 cup	45
Shitake mushrooms	1 cup	45
Swiss chard	1 cup	44
Turnip greens	1 cup	40
Potatoes, mashed with whole milk	1 cup	39
Kohlrabi	1 cup	36
Mustard greens	1 cup	34
Spinach	1 cup	31
Butternut squash	1 cup	29
Prickley pear pads, Nopales	1 cup	28
Raab broccoli	1 cup	17
Turnips	1 cup	14
Cabbage	1 cup	13
Pumpkin	1 cup	5

Vegetables, Frozen	Amount	LA (mg)
Corn	1 cup	510
Carrots	1 cup	422
Asparagus	1 cup	315
Green peas	1 cup	168
Kale	1 cup	125
Okra	1 cup	116
Collard greens	1 cup	102
Brussels sprouts	1 cup	91
Turnip greens	1 cup	84
Rhubarb	1 cup	60
Green beans	1 cup	49
Cauliflower	1 cup	43
Butternut squash	1 cup	26
Broccoli	1 cup	24
Spinach	1 cup	0

Vegetables, Raw	Amount	LA (mg)
Tomatillos	1 cup	531
Dandelion greens	1 cup	144
Tomatoes	1 cup	144
Carrots	1 cup	126

OMEGA-6 LA

Continued

Tomatoes, cherry	1 cup	119
White mushrooms	1 cup	112
Oyster mushrooms, sliced	1 cup	106
Portabella mushrooms *	1 cup	101
Kale	1 cup	92
Spiulina, dried	1 tbsp	88
Celery	1 cup	80
Green bell peppers	1 cup	80
Snow peas	1 cup	74
Green onions & scallions	1 cup	70
Red bell peppers	1 cup	67
Enoki mushrooms	1 cup	39
Endive	1 cup	38
Prickley pear cactus pads	1 cup	38
Radicchio	1 cup	37
Summer squash	1 cup	37
Zucchini *	1 cup	34
Belgian endive	1 cup	33
Chicory greens	1 cup	32
Bok-choy	1 cup	29
Crimini mushrooms, sliced	1 cup	29
Cucumbers	1 cup	29
Arugula	1 cup	26
Romaine lettuce	1 cup	26
Red cabbage	1 cup	24
Swiss chard	1 cup	23
Butternut squash	1 cup	22
Onions	1 cup	21
Butter head & boston lettuce	1 cup	19
Broccoli	1 cup	15
Savoy cabbage	1 cup	15
Green leaf lettuce	1 cup	13
Cabbage	1 cup	12
Iceberg lettuce	1 cup	12
Spinach	1 cup	8
Raab broccoli	1 cup	7
Cauliflower *	1 cup	6
Shiitake mushrooms, dried	1 each	5
Watercress	1 cup	4

Yogurt	Amount	LA (mg)
Plain, whole milk	8 ounces	148
Plain, low fat	8 ounces	70
Plain, skim milk	8 ounces	9

Nutrient Data Collection Form

Food	Amount	Book Numbers	Multiply By	Estimated Nutrient Intake
Nutrient::	RDA:	Estimated:	% of RDA:	Total Estimated:

To download additional forms for free, go to www.TopNutrients4U.com

259

NOTES

OMEGA-6 TO OMEGA-3 RATIO

Alcohol	Amount	LA / ALA
White Table Wine	1 glass	0
Red Table Wine	1 glass	0
Light Beer	1 bottle	0
Regular Beer	1 bottle	0
Gin, Rum, Vodka, or Whisky	1 shot	0

Beans, Canned	Amount	LA / ALA
Garbanzo beans	1 cup	26.0
Fava beans	1 cup	12.0
Lima beans, large	1 cup	2.30
Black-eyed peas	1 cup	1.70
Red kidney beans	1 cup	1.70
Refried beans *	1 cup	1.50
Cranberry beans	1 cup	1.20
Great Northern	1 cup	1.20
Navy beans	1 cup	1.20
White beans	1 cup	1.20
Baked beans, plain	1 cup	1.10
Pinto beans	1 cup	0.70
Green beans	1 cup	0.60
Yellow beans	1 cup	0.60

Beans, Cooked	Amount	LA / ALA
Garbanzo beans	1 cup	26
Pigeon peas	1 cup	22
Winged beans	1 cup	15
Mung beans	1 cup	13
Fava beans	1 cup	13
Soybeans, green	1 cup	8
Natto	1 cup	7
Soybeans, dry roasted	1 cup	7
Soybeans, mature	1 cup	7
Edamame *	1 cup	5
Split peas	1 cup	5
Lupini beans	1 cup	4
Lentils	1 cup	4
Lima beans	1 cup	2
Black-eyed peas	1 cup	2
Yardlong beans, Chinese long beans	1 cup	1
Great Northern beans	1 cup	1
Black beans	1 cup	1
White beans, mature	1 cup	1
Black Turtle beans, mature	1 cup	1

OMEGA-6 TO OMEGA-3 RATIO

Continued

Cranberry beans	1 cup	1
White beans, small	1 cup	1
Navy beans	1 cup	0.8
Pinto beans	1 cup	0.7
Kidney beans	1 cup	0.6
Green beans	1 cup	0.6
Yellow beans	1 cup	0.6
Adzuki	1 cup	x
Hyacinath beans	1 cup	x
Mothbeans	1 cup	x

Beef, Cooked	Amount	LA / ALA
Brisket, trimmed to 0" fat	3 oz	12
Ground beef, 75% lean	3 oz	10
Ground beef, 80% lean	3 oz	8
Ground beef, 85% lean	3 oz	7
Ground beef, 90% lean	3 oz	7
Ground beef, 95% lean	3 oz	7
Tri-Tip, sirloin, lean, trimmed to 0" fat	3 oz	7
Filet Mignon, trimmed to 0" fat	3 oz	4
Top sirloin, trimmed to 1/8" fat	3 oz	3
Flank steak, trimmed to 0" fat	3 oz	3
Beef ribs, trimmed to 1/8" fat	3 oz	2
Chuck roast, trimmed to 1/8" fat	3 oz	2
Porterhouse steak, trimmed to 0" fat	3 oz	2
Skirt Steak, trimmed to 0" fat	3 oz	2
T-Bone steak, trimmed 0" fat	3 oz	2
Ribeye steak, trimmed to 0" fat	3 oz	x

Bread	Amount	LA / ALA
Tortillas, corn	1 tortilla	40
Tortillas, flour	1 tortilla	25
Bagel, egg	4" bagel	23
Pita, white	6" pita	22
Egg bread	1 slice	21
Cracked wheat	1 slice	20
Cornbread, dry mix	1 piece	18
Kaiser rolls	1 roll	17
Raisin bread	1 slice	17
Bagel, cinnamon & raisins	4" bagel	16
French, and Sourdough	1 slice	15
Italian	1 slice	13
Pumpernickel	1 slice	13
Rye bread	1 slice	13
Dinner Rolls, brown & serve	1 roll	10

OMEGA-6 TO OMEGA-3 RATIO

Continued

Wheat bread *	1 slice	10
Bagel plain	4" bagel	9
English Muffin, plain	1 muffin	9
Hamburger & Hotdog buns, plain	1 bun	9
Whole wheat	1 slice	9
Multigrain or Whole grain	1 slice	8
Oatmeal bread	1 slice	8
White	1 slice	8

Cereal, General Mills®	Amount	LA / ALA
Lucky Charms *	1 cup	33
Kix *	1 cup	29
Honey Nut Chex	1 cup	27
Oatmeal Crisp, Apple Cinnamon	1 cup	24
Basic 4	1 cup	20
Multi-Bran CHEX	1 cup	19
Oatmeal Crisp, Crunchy Almond	1 cup	19
Wheat Chex	1 cup	19
Corn Chex	1 cup	18
KABOOM	1 cup	18
Raisin Nut Bran	1 cup	18
Cocoa Puffs	1 cup	17
Cookie Crisp	1 cup	17
Total Cranberry Crunch	1 cup	17
Honey Nut Clusters	1 cup	15
Total Whole Grain	1 cup	14
Cinnamon Toast Crunch *	1 cup	12
Rice Chex	1 cup	12
Wheaties	1 cup	11
Total Raisin Bran	1 cup	10
Reese's Puffs	1 cup	9
Trix	1 cup	8
Golden Grahams	1 cup	5
Dora The Explorer	1 cup	4
Berry Berry Kix	1 cup	0

General Mill's Cheerios®	Amount	LA / ALA
Cinnamon Burst	1 cup	x
Original	1 cup	34
Fruity	1 cup	26
Frosted	1 cup	22
Multi Grain	1 cup	22
Oat Cluster Cherrios Crunch	1 cup	22
Yogurt Burst, Strawberry	1 cup	21
Honey Nut	1 cup	17

OMEGA-6 TO OMEGA-3 RATIO

Continued

Berry Burst, Triple Berry	1 cup	16
Banana Nut	1 cup	8
Chocolate	1 cup	7.5
Apple Cinnamon	1 cup	7

General Mill's Fiber One®	Amount	LA / ALA
Bran Cereal	1 cup	13

Kashi® Cereal	Amount	LA / ALA
Organic Promise, Autumn Wheat	1 cup	22
7-Whole Grain Honey Puffs	1 cup	15
7-Whole Grain Puffs	1 cup	15
Go Lean Crunch, Honey Almond Flax	1 cup	14
Heart to Heart, Honey Toasted Oat	1 cup	11
Go Lean	1 cup	9
Good Friends	1 cup	8
Good Friends, Cinnamon Raisin Cr.	1 cup	8
Go Lean Crunch	1 cup	3

Kellogg's® Cereal	Amount	LA / ALA
Honey Crunch Corn Flakes	1 cup	59
Corn Pops	1 cup	39
Low Fat Granola with Raisins	1 cup	39
Cracklin Oat Bran	1 cup	33
Apple Jacks	1 cup	31
Mueslix	1 cup	31
Crispix	1 cup	28
Froot Loops	1 cup	26
Rice Krispies	1 cup	26
Smorz	1 cup	22
Frosted Flakes	1 cup	19
Frosted MINI Wheat's, Big-Bite	1 cup	19
Frosted MINI-Wheat's, Bite-Size	1 cup	19
Smart Start, Strong Heart Antioxidants	1 cup	16
Corn Flakes	1 cup	15
Honey Smacks	1 cup	14
Raisin Bran Crunch	1 cup	14
Rice Krispies Treats	1 cup	14
All-Bran Complete Wheat Flakes	1 cup	14
All-Bran Bran Buds	1 cup	13
All-Bran Original	1 cup	13
Raisin Bran	1 cup	13

OMEGA-6 TO OMEGA-3 RATIO

Continued

Product	Amount	LA / ALA
Product 19	1 cup	11
Frosted Rice Krispies	1 cup	5
Berry Rice Krispies	1 cup	2

Kellogg's Special K®	Amount	LA / ALA
Vanilla Almond	1 cup	25
Cinnamon Pecan	1 cup	16
Fruit & Yogurt	1 cup	15
Chocolately Delight	1 cup	10
Protein Plus	1 cup	8
Red Berries	1 cup	8
Original	1 cup	7

Cereal, Post®	Amount	LA / ALA
Honeycomb Cereal	1 cup	26
Great Grains, Cranberry Almond Crunch	1 cup	23
Alpha-Bits	1 cup	23
Shredded Wheat n' Bran, spoon size	1 cup	22
Shredded Wheat, Original, spoon-size	1 cup	20
Great Grains, Crunchy Pecan Cereal	1 cup	18
Great Grains, Raisin, Date & Pecan	1 cup	17
Honey Nut Shredded Wheat	1 cup	15
Shredded Wheat, Original, big-biscuit	1 biscuit	15
Golden Crisp	1 cup	14
Shredded Wheat, Frosted, spoon-size	1 cup	14
Bran Flakes	1 cup	13
Raisin Bran	1 cup	12
Grape-Nuts Cereal	1 cup	12
Grape-Nuts Flakes	1 cup	11
Blueberry Morning	1 cup	10
Great Grains, Banana Nut Crunch	1 cup	6
Fruity Pebbles	1 cup	5
Cocoa Pebbles	1 cup	1

Post® Honey Bunches of Oats®	Amount	LA / ALA
Pecan Bunches	1 cup	18
With Almonds	1 cup	16
Honey Roasted *	1 cup	13
With Vanilla Bunches	1 cup	11
Just Bunches, Honey Roasted	1 cup	8

OMEGA-6 TO OMEGA-3 RATIO

Cereal, Quaker®	Amount	LA / ALA
CAP'N Crunch's Peanut Butter Crunch	1 cup	97
Crunchy Bran	1 cup	33
CAP'N Crunch & Crunch Berries	1 cup	32
CAP'N Crunch	1 cup	29
Oat Cinnamon Life	1 cup	23
Oat LIFE	1 cup	22
Toasted Oatmeal Cereal, Honey Nut	1 cup	22
Cinnamon Oatmeal Squares	1 cup	21
Oatmeal Squares	1 cup	21
Honey Graham OH'S	1 cup	18
Low Fat Granola with Raisins	1 cup	10
Granola, Oats, Wheat, Honey & Raisins	1 cup	4
Granola, Oats, Wheat & Honey	1 cup	3

Cereal, Cooked	Amount	LA / ALA
White corn grits	1 cup	424
Yellow corn grits	1 cup	303
Oats, regular, unenriched	1 cup	30
Farina	1 cup	14
WHEATENA	1 cup	12
Cream of Wheat, regular	1 cup	9

Cheese	Amount	LA / ALA
Cottage cheese, small curd	1 cup	6
Cottage cheese, low fat, 2 %	1 cup	6
Cottage cheese, non fat & uncreamed	1 cup	4
Ricotta, part skim milk	1 cup	3
Cottage cheese, low fat, 1 %	1 cup	3
Ricotta, whole milk	1 cup	2

Cheese	Amount	LA / ALA
Goat cheese, hard type	1 oz	240
Goat cheese, semisoft	1 oz	201
Goat cheese, soft type	1 oz	142
Cream cheese, fat free	1 oz	6
Cream cheese	1 oz	6
Parmesan, grated	1 oz	5
Gruyere	1 oz	3
Monterey, low fat	1 oz	3
Monterey	1 oz	2
Colby	1 oz	2
Mozzarella, part skim, low moisture	1 oz	2
Ricotta	1 oz	2

OMEGA-6 TO OMEGA-3 RATIO

Continued

	Amount	LA / ALA
Cheddar, low-fat	1 oz	2
Blue cheese	1 oz	2
Muenster	1 oz	2
Provolone, reduced fat	1 oz	2
Provolone	1 oz	2
Swiss, low fat	1 oz	2
Swiss	1 oz	2
Brie	1 oz	2
Cheddar	1 oz	2
Muenster, low fat	1 oz	2
Feta	1 oz	1
Fontina	1 oz	1
Mozzarella, whole milk	1 oz	1
Romano	1 oz	1
Roquefort	1 oz	1
Gouda	1 oz	1
Ricotta, part skim milk	1 oz	1
Mozzarella, non fat	1 oz	0

Cheese, Mexican	Amount	LA / ALA
Queso fresco *	1 oz	6
Mexican, blend, reduced fat	1 oz	4
Queso anejo	1 oz	2
Queso chihuahua	1 oz	2
Mexican, blend	1 oz	2
Queso asadero	1 oz	2

Chicken, Cooked	Amount	LA / ALA
Thigh, meat only, roasted *	1 thigh	24
Breast, with skin, roasted	1/2 breast	23
Breast, with skin, fried in flour	1/2 breast	21
Drumstick, with skin, fried in flour	1 drumstick	20
Breast, no skin, roasted	1/2 breast	20

Cream	Amount	LA / ALA
Sour cream, cultured	1 tbsp	7
Light coffee cream	1 tbsp	2
Sour cream, reduced fat, cultured	1 tbsp	2
Half & Half	1 tbsp	2
Heavy cream	1 tbsp	2
Whipped cream, pressurized	1 tbsp	2

OMEGA-6 TO OMEGA-3 RATIO

Eggs	Amount	LA / ALA
Egg whole, hard boiled	1 large	33
Egg yolk	1 large	33
Egg whole, poached	1 large	32
Egg whole, fried	1 large	20
Egg whole, scrambled	1 large	15
Egg whites	1 large	0
Egg whites, dried	1 oz	0

Fish, Canned	Amount	LA / ALA
Light tuna, in oil	3 oz	36
White tuna, in oil	3 oz	12
Atlantic sardines, in oil	3 oz	7
Light tuna, in water	3 oz	4
White tuna, in water	3 oz	0.8

Fish, Cooked	Amount	LA / ALA
Pacific cod	3 oz	18
Atlantic croaker	3 oz	15
Cat fish, breaded & fried	3 oz	15
Catfish, farmed	3 oz	11
Yellowfin tuna	3 oz	10
Haddock	3 oz	8
Rainbow trout, farmed	3 oz	7
Atlantic salmon, farmed	3 oz	6
Atlantic cod	3 oz	5
Coho salmon, farmed	3 oz	5
Sockeye salmon	3 oz	4
Tilapia	3 oz	4
Atlantic & Pacific halibut	3 oz	3
Greenland halibut	3 oz	3
Flounder & Sole	3 oz	3
Swordfish	3 oz	3
Pacific & Jack mackerel	3 oz	2
Atlantic perch	3 oz	2
Carp	3 oz	2
Alaskan halibut	3 oz	2
Walleye pike	3 oz	2
Keta, (chum) salmon	3 oz	2
Pink salmon	3 oz	2
Rainbow trout, wild	3 oz	2
Whiting	3 oz	2
Northern pike	3 oz	2
Catfish, wild	3 oz	1

OMEGA-6 TO OMEGA-3 RATIO

Continued

Atlantic mackerel	3 oz	1
Chinook salmon	3 oz	1
Coho salmon, wild	3 oz	1
Striped bass	3 oz	1
Spanish mackerel	3 oz	0.9
Freshwater bass	3 oz	0.8
Atlantic salmon, wild	3 oz	0.6

Fish, Shellfish, Cooked	Amount	LA / ALA
Blue crab cakes	3 oz	18
Shrimp, breaded & fried	3 oz	17
Shrimp	3 oz	16
Scallops, breaded & fried	3 oz	16
Oysters, breaded & fried	3 oz	16
Abalone	3 oz	15
Clams, breaded & fried	3 oz	15
Squid, fried	3 oz	15
Alaskan king crab, imitation *	3 oz	10
Shrimp, canned *	3 oz	4
Crayfish	3 oz	3
Clams, canned	3 oz	3
Queen crab	3 oz	2
Blue crab, canned	3 oz	2
Blue crab *	3 oz	2
Alaskan king crab	3 oz	1
Eastern oysters, farmed	3 oz	0.7
Northern lobster *	3 oz	0.7
Eastern oysters, wild	3 oz	0.5

Fruit, Canned	Amount	LA / ALA
Pears	1 cup	80
Plums	1 cup	57
Peaches	1 cup	40
Apricots	1 cup	15
Olives, black	5 large	13
Olives, green	5 large	13
Applesauce, sweetened	1 cup	5
Applesauce, unsweetened	1 cup	4
Pineapple	1 cup	1

Fruit, Dried	Amount	LA / ALA
Figs	1 cup	514
Currants	1 cup	259
Apricots	1 cup	96

OMEGA-6 TO OMEGA-3 RATIO

Continued

Pears	1 cup	66
Peaches	1 cup	41
Cranberries	1 cup	20
Apples	1 cup	5
Prunes	1 cup	3

Fruit, Frozen	Amount	LA / ALA
Peaches	1 cup	32
Blackberries, unthawed	1 cup	2
Raspberries	1 cup	2
Blueberries	1 cup	1
Strawberries	1 cup	1

Fruit, Raw	Amount	LA / ALA
Apricots	1 cup	127
Water mellon	1 cup	76
Plums	1 cup	73
Nectarine	1 cup	53
Pears	1 cup	47
Peaches	1 cup	43
Avocado, California	1 cup	25
Avocado, Florida	1 cup	16
Dates	1 cup	6
Kiwi	1 cup	6
Apples	1 cup	5
Raisins	1 cup	3
Grapes, red or green	1 cup	3
Tangerine	1 cup	3
Prunes, uncooked	1 cup	3
Navel oranges	1 cup	3
Jicama	1 cup	2
Blackberries	1 cup	2
Raspberries	1 cup	2
Elderberries	1 cup	2
Plantains	1 cup	2
Blueberries	1 cup	2
Strawberries	1 cup	1
Pineapple	1 cup	1
Cherries	1 cup	1
Honeydew	1 cup	0.8
Cantaloupe	1 cup	0.8
Papayas	1 cup	0.2

OMEGA-6 TO OMEGA-3 RATIO

Fruit, Raw	Amount	LA / ALA
Pears	1 fruit	48
Nectarine	1 fruit	48
Peaches	1 fruit	41
Figs, dried	1 fig	29
Plums	1 plum	29
Apricots	1 fruit	27
Avocado, California	1 fruit	25
Avocado, Florida	1 fruit	16
Raisins	1 small box	7
Dates	5 dates	6
Kiwi	1 fruit	6
Apples	1 fruit	5
Kumquats	1 fruit	3
Prunes, uncooked	5 prunes	3
Tangerine	1 fruit	3
Oranges, navel	1 fruit	2
Plantains	1 fruit	2
Banana	1 fruit	2
Strawberries	5 fruit	1
Pineapple	1/2" x 3" slice	1
Cherries	10 cherries	1

Grains, Cooked	Amount	LA / ALA
Bulgur	1 cup	24
Brown rice	1 cup	22
Oat bran	1 cup	21
Spaghetti, whole wheat	1 cup	20
Couscous	1 cup	19
Egg noodles	1 cup	19
Millet	1 cup	17
Soba noodles	1 cup	16
Buckwheat	1 cup	12
Macaroni	1 cup	12
Spaghetti, enriched	1 cup	12
Pearled barley	1 cup	9
Spaghetti, spinach	1 cup	8
Egg & Spinach noodles	1 cup	6
Rice noodles	1 cup	5
White rice, regular long grain	1 cup	5
Wild rice	1 cup	1

OMEGA-6 TO OMEGA-3 RATIO

Herbs & Spices	Amount	LA / ALA
Anise seed	1 tbsp	211
All-spice, ground	1 tbsp	34
Chervil, dried	1 tbsp	34
Nutmeg	1 tbsp	24
Caraway seeds	1 tbsp	21
Onion powder	1 tbsp	18
Celery seeds	1 tbsp	18
Paprika	1 tbsp	16
Chili powder	1 tbsp	14
Garlic powder	1 tbsp	14
Chives, raw	1 tbsp	8
Curry powder	1 tbsp	5
Pepper, black	1 tbsp	5
Cloves, ground	1 tbsp	4
Turmeric, ground	1 tbsp	3
Ginger, ground	1 tbsp	3
Cinnamon, ground	1 tbsp	3
Coriander, leaves, cilantro	1/4 cup	2
Dill weed, fresh	1/4 cup	2
Oregano, dried, ground	1 tbsp	1
Bay leaf, crumbled	1 tbsp	1
Rosemary, fresh	1 tbsp	1
Rosemary, dried	1 tbsp	1
Thyme, dried, leaves	1 tbsp	0.7
Thyme, ground	1 tbsp	0.7
Basil, dried & ground	1 tbsp	0.7
Parsley, dried *	1 tbsp	0.7
Capers	1 tbsp	0.6
Saffron	1 tbsp	0.6
Sage, ground	1 tbsp	0.4
Basil, fresh, chopped	1 tbsp	0.3
Thyme, fresh	1 tbsp	0.3
Tarragon, dried leaves	1 tbsp	0.2
Spearmint, dried	1 tbsp	0.2

Juice	Amount	LA / ALA
Pomegranate	1 cup	125
Vegetable juice, cocktail	1 cup	44
Tomato juice	1 cup	28
Prune juice	1 cup	18
Carrot juice	1 cup	7
Apple juice	1 cup	5
Grape juice	1 cup	3
Orange juice, raw	1 cup	3

OMEGA-6 TO OMEGA-3 RATIO

Continued

| Cranberry juice, cocktail | 1 cup | 2 |
| Pineapple juice | 1 cup | 1 |

Milk	Amount	LA / ALA
Soymilk	1 cup	7.8
Human milk	1 cup	7.0
Reduced fat, 2% milk fat *	1 cup	6.7
Low-fat, 1% milk fat *	1 cup	6.6
Canned, condensed, sweet	1 cup	3.8
Goat milk	1 cup	2.7
Non fat, fat free or skim	1 cup	2.5
Canned, evaporated, nonfat	1 cup	2.1
Canned, evaporated	1 cup	2.0
Dry, instant, nonf fat	1/3 cup	2.0
Whole, 3.25% milk fat	1 cup	1.6
Buttermilk, low-fat	1 cup	1.5

Nuts & Seeds	Amount	LA / ALA
Peanuts	1 oz	4410
Almonds *	1 oz	4400
Sunflower seeds	1 oz	384
Pine nuts	1 oz	293
Peanut butter, smooth style	1 oz	181
Pumpkin seeds	1 oz	172
Cashews	1 oz	123
Brazil nuts	1 oz	117
Coconut, raw meat	1 oz	104
Hazelnuts	1 oz	90
Tahini	1 oz	57
Sesame seeds	1 oz	57
Pistachio	1 oz	52
Pecans	1 oz	21
Black walnuts	1 oz	16
Macadamia	1 oz	6
English walnuts	1 oz	4
Chia seeds	1 oz	0.3
Flaxseeds	1 oz	0.3

Oils	Amount	LA / ALA
Grapeseed oil	1 tbsp	676
Cottonseed oil	1 tbsp	259
Sesame oil	1 tbsp	137
Safflower, high oleic acid, oil *	1 tbsp	133
Corn oil	1 tbsp	45

OMEGA-6 TO OMEGA-3 RATIO

Continued

Sunflower, high oleic acid	1 tbsp	18
Avocado oil	1 tbsp	13
Olive oil	1 tbsp	13
Soybean, partially hydrogenated, oil	1 tbsp	13
Safflower, high linoleic acid, oil	1 tbsp	10
Sunflower, high linoleic acid, oil	1 tbsp	9
Soybean lecithin oil	1 tbsp	8
Soybean oil *	1 tbsp	7
Walnut oil	1 tbsp	5
Peanut oil	1 tbsp	4
Canola oil *	1 tbsp	2
Salmon oil	1 tbsp	2
Menhaden oil	1 tbsp	1
Cod liver oil	1 tbsp	1
Flaxseed oil *	1 tbsp	0.2

Pork, Cooked	Amount	LA / ALA
Sausage	3 oz	24
Backribs *	3 oz	24
Chops, broiled *	3 oz	23
Spareribs	3 oz	23
Bacon, pan-fried	3 oz	20
Chops, pan-fried	3 oz	14
Cured ham, lean, pan-fried	3 oz	8
Canadian-style bacon	3 oz	6

Salad Dressing	Amount	LA / ALA
Honey Mustard, fat-free	1 tbsp	1667
Caesar, fat-free	1 tbsp	1000
Blue cheese, light	1 tbsp	12.6
Blue cheese, fat-free	1 tbsp	9
Ranch, regular	1 tbsp	8.1
Blue cheese, regular	1 tbsp	7.6
Caesar, regular	1 tbsp	7.5
Russian	1 tbsp	7.5
Honey Mustard, regular	1 tbsp	7.5
Mayonnaise, light *	1 tbsp	7.5
Mayonnaise, regular *	1 tbsp	7.3
Thousand Island, regular	1 tbsp	6.8
French, regular	1 tbsp	6.7
Italian, regular *	1 tbsp	6.4
Thousand Island, fat-free	1 tbsp	6.1
Italian, fat-free	1 tbsp	5.8
Ranch, fat-free *	1 tbsp	4.6

OMEGA-6 TO OMEGA-3 RATIO

Continued

French, reduced fat	1 tbsp	3.3
French, fat-free	1 tbsp	2.3
Ranch, reduced fat	1 tbsp	1

Turkey, Cooked	Amount	LA / ALA
Breast meat, only	3 oz	110
Dark meat *	3 oz	23
Light meat *	3 oz	21
Ground turkey, 93% lean *	3 oz	21
Ground turkey, fat free *	3 oz	20
Ground turkey, 85% lean *	3 oz	19
Ground turkey *	3 oz	18
Turkey bacon	3 oz	16
Turkey sausage, reduced fat	3 oz	16

Vegetables, Canned	Amount	LA / ALA
Mushrooms	1 cup	87
Corn	1 cup	32
Tomato sauce	1 cup	24
Tomatoes	1 cup	24
Stewed tomato	1 cup	24
Tomato paste	1 cup	22
Tomato pure	1 cup	21
Asparagus	1 cup	18
Beets	1 cup	11
Carrots	1 cup	7
Sweet potato	1 cup	5
Green peas	1 cup	4
Sauerkraut	1 cup	1
Pumpkin	1 cup	0.9
Green beans	1 cup	0.6
Spinach	1 cup	0.2

Vegetables, Cooked	Amount	LA / ALA
White mushrooms	1 cup	139
Celery	1 cup	80
Carrots	1 cup	68
Okra	1 cup	36
Yellow sweet corn	1 cup	32
Onions	1 cup	18
Sweet potato	1 potato	15
Parsnips	1 cup	13
Beets	1 cup	12
Shiitake mushrooms	1 cup	11

OMEGA-6 TO OMEGA-3 RATIO

Continued

Beet greens	1 cup	10
Prickley pear pads, Nopales	1 cup	9
Swiss chard	1 cup	9
Dandelion greens	1 cup	6
Snow peas	1 cup	6
Eggplant	1 cup	5
Split peas	1 cup	5
Potatoes	1 potato	3
Artichokes	1 cup	3
Asparagus	1 cup	3
Mustard greens	1 cup	1
Pumpkin	1 cup	1
Kohlrabi	1 cup	0.78
Kale	1 cup	0.76
Bok-choy	1 cup	0.75
Collard greens	1 cup	0.75
Leeks	1 cup	0.68
Rutabagas	1 cup	0.67
Green Beans	1 cup	0.63
Cabbage	1 cup	0.62
Zucchini	1 cup	0.61
Acorn squash	1 cup	0.59
Butternut squash	1 cup	0.59
Summer squash	1 cup	0.59
Winter squash	1 cup	0.59
Brussels sprouts	1 cup	0.45
Broccoli	1 cup	0.43
Turnip greens	1 cup	0.43
Cauliflower	1 cup	0.30
Broccolini	1 cup	0.29
Turnips,	1 cup	0.28
Spinach	1 cup	0.18
Raab broccoli	1 cup	0.15

Vegetables, Frozen	Amount	LA / ALA
Spinach	1 cup	x
Rhubarb	1 cup	60
Okra	1 cup	58
Corn	1 cup	34
Asparagus	1 cup	17.5
Carrots	1 cup	6.59
Green peas	1 cup	4.42
Kale	1 cup	0.77
Green beans	1 cup	0.75
Butternut squash	1 cup	0.60

OMEGA-6 TO OMEGA-3 RATIO

Continued

Collard greens	1 cup	0.47
Brussels sprouts	1 cup	0.45
Turnip greens	1 cup	0.43
Broccoli	1 cup	0.31
Cauliflower	1 cup	0.29

Vegetables, Raw	Amount	LA / ALA
Carrots	1 cup	63
Tomatoes	1 cup	28
Tomatillos	1 cup	25
Green onions & scallions	1 cup	18
Prickley pear cactus pads	1 cup	10
Swiss chard	1 cup	8
Belgian endive	1 cup	7
Green bell peppers	1 cup	7
Radicchio	1 cup	6
Dandelion greens	1 cup	6
Cucumbers	1 cup	6
Snow peas	1 cup	6
Endive	1 cup	5
Chicory greens	1 cup	5
Onions	1 cup	4
Enoki mushrooms	1 cup	2
Red bell peppers	1 cup	2
Spiulina, dried	1 tbsp	2
Celery	1 cup	1
Cauliflower *	1 cup	0.9
Broccoli	1 cup	0.8
Arugula	1 cup	0.8
Bok-choy	1 cup	0.8
Kale	1 cup	0.8
Red cabbage	1 cup	0.8
Savoy cabbage	1 cup	0.8
Butternut squash	1 cup	0.6
Summer squash	1 cup	0.6
Watercress	1 cup	0.5
Zucchini	1 cup	0.5
Butter head & boston lettuce *	1 cup	0.4
Romaine lettuce	1 cup	0.4
Green leaf lettuce	1 cup	0.4
Iceberg lettuce	1 cup	0.4
Spinach	1 cup	0.2
Raab broccoli	1 cup	0.2

OMEGA-6 TO OMEGA-3 RATIO

Yogurt	Amount	LA / ALA
Yogurt, plain, Greek, non fat	6 oz	8.5
Yogurt, plain, skim milk	8 oz	4.5
Yogurt, plain, whole milk	8 oz	2.4
Yogurt, plain, low fat	8 oz	2.3

OMEGA-6 TO OMEGA-3 RATIO

In current public opinion, dietary recommendations would automatically advise lowering intake of total fat. No optimal levels have been established, but upper recommendations are 30% based on caloric intake. These guidelines do not specify a lower safe-limit or how long humans should consume a low-fat diet. Low fat diets have appeal because they are thought to prevent weight gain and reduce the risk of heart disease. However, hard science has not proven this. It is true that groups who subsist on low-fat diets are often thin because of their low calorie intake but hospitals are full of sick people who are thin.

What science has shown is that low-fat diets decrease bile acids required for the absorption of fat soluble vitamins, A, D, E, and K, and that non-fat foods, themselves, are deficient in fat-soluble vitamins and essential fatty acids.

Keep in mind, it is a fundamental principal of chemistry that a fat-soluble compound, by definition, will require some fat to dissolve and chemically react. In fact, all stages of a fat soluble vitamin's absorption and its transport to tissues are linked with absorption and transport of dietary fat.

Consider the following examples of some of the benefits of dietary fat.

(1) Persons consuming vitamin E on a high-fat diet had higher plasma levels of vitamin E than those consuming a low-fat diet. (2) No absorption of carotenoids from salads with fat-free dressings but noticed absorption with full-fat dressings. (3) Increased absorption of carotenoids from salad and salsa by addition of avocado because of avocado's high fat content. In the above study, a salad mix of romaine lettuce, baby spinach, and shredded carrots had a significant increase in absorption of Beta-carotene simply from adding 1/2 of avocado fruit. (4) Green leafy vegetables fed to preschool children with fat had higher concentrations of vitamin A compared to a serving with no fat. (5) Finally, omega-3 fatty acid deficiencies documented in infants and adults as a direct result of being fed only a non-fat diet.

It is true that diets low in saturated fat but high in unsaturated fats have been known to reduce the risk of diseases. However, a strict reduction of total fat may not be necessary and may rob the body of nutrients over a lifetime.

The nutrient content of a low-fat diet is highly dependent on individual food choices. Consider the following dietary example:

Omega-3 fatty acid content in full-fat vs non-fat foods

Full-Fat Foods	Omega-3 ALA, mg
Four large scrambled eggs	328
Two tbsp. olive oil	206
One ounce cheddar cheese	103
One glass whole milk	366
Two tbsp. half & half cream	50
Two tbsp. of butter	90
Eight ounces plain yogurt	61
Two tbsp. blue cheese dressing	956
Total Omega-3 ALA consumed	2160 mg

Non-Fat Foods	Omega-3 ALA, mg
Four large egg whites	0.0
No olive oil	0.0
One ounce low-fat cheddar cheese	19
One glass non-fat milk	4
Two tbsp. non-fat half & half	12
No butter	0.0
Eight ounces non-fat yogurt	2
Two tbsp. fat-free blue cheese	2
Total Omega-3 ALA consumed in mg	39 mg

In this example consuming the non-fat foods reduced the intake of omega-3 fatty acids by 98%.

Research findings do indicate that a fat status in adults can be maintained with low fat during a short period of time. However, trying to maintain an ideal body weight by focusing exclusively on non-fat foods is unlikely to supply enough essential fatty acids or fat soluble vitamins to meet the body's long-term needs.

In summary, dietary fat is a fundamental requirement for the human body to function properly. Let me end by saying that there is nothing wrong with having a fat-free meal or eating fat-free food, I do it now and then myself, but not daily with every meal. This chapter lists the total fat, saturated fats, monounsaturated fats, and polyunsaturated fats in grams (g).

FAT TOTAL

Alcohol	Amount	Total Fat (g)
White Table Wine	1 glass	0
Red Table Wine	1 glass	0
Light Beer	1 bottle	0
Regular Beer	1 bottle	0
Gin, Rum, Vodka, or Whisky	1 shot	0

Beans, Canned	Amount	Total Fat (g)
Garbanzo beans	1 cup	3.75
Refried beans	1 cup	2.78
Pinto beans	1 cup	1.34
Blackeyed peas	1 cup	1.32
Navy beans	1 cup	1.13
Great Northern	1 cup	1.02
Baked beans, plain	1 cup	0.94
Kidney beans	1 cup	0.92
White beans, mature	1 cup	0.76
Cranberry beans	1 cup	0.73
Green beans	1 cup	0.57
Fava beans	1 cup	0.56
Lima beans	1 cup	0.41
Yellow beans	1 cup	0.15

Beans, Cooked	Amount	Total Fat (g)
Soybeans, dry roasted	1 cup	20.11
Natto	1 cup	19.25
Soybeans, mature	1 cup	15.43
Soybeans, green	1 cup	11.52
Winged beans	1 cup	10.04
Edamame	1 cup	8.06
Lupini beans	1 cup	4.85
Garbanzo beans	1 cup	4.25
White beans, small	1 cup	1.15
Hayacinth beans	1 cup	1.13
Navy beans	1 cup	1.13
Pinto beans	1 cup	1.11
Mothbeans	1 cup	0.97
Black beans	1 cup	0.93
Black-eyed peas	1 cup	0.91
Kidney beans	1 cup	0.88
Cranberry beans	1 cup	0.81
Great Northern	1 cup	0.80
Mung beans, mature seeds	1 cup	0.77
Split peas	1 cup	0.76

FAT TOTAL

Continued

Lentils	1 cup	0.75
Lima beans	1 cup	0.71
Fava beans	1 cup	0.68
Black Turtle beans, mature	1 cup	0.65
Pigeon neans	1 cup	0.64
White beans, mature	1 cup	0.63
Green beans	1 cup	0.35
Yellow beans	1 cup	0.35
Adzuki	1 cup	0.23
Yardlong beans, Chinese	1 cup	0.10

Beef, Cooked	Amount	Total Fat (g)
Beef ribs, trimmed to 1/8" fat	3 oz	24
Chuck roast, trimmed to 1/8" fat	3 oz	23
Ground beef, 75%	3 oz	16
Porterhouse steak, trimmed to 0" fat	3 oz	16
Ground Beef, 80%	3 oz	15
T-Bone steak, trimmed to 0" fat	3 oz	14
Ground Beef, 85%	3 oz	13
Ribeye steak, no bone, trimmed 0" fat	3 oz	13
Flat Iron Steak	3 oz	12
Tri Tip steak, lean, trimmed to 0" fat	3 oz	11
Ground Beef, 90%	3 oz	10
Skirt Steak, trimmed to 0" fat	3 oz	10
Filet Mignon, trimmed to 0" fat	3 oz	8
Flank steak, lean, trimmed to 0" fat	3 oz	6
Ground Beef, 95%	3 oz	6
Brisket, lean, trimmed to 0" fat	3 oz	6
Top Sirloin, lean, trimmed to 1/8" fat	3 oz	5
London Broil, top round, trim to 0" fat	3 oz	4

Beef, Cooked	Amount	Total Fat (g)
Beef ribs, trimmed to 1/8" fat	1 lb cooked	128
Chuck roast, trimmed to 1/8" fat	1 lb cooked	124
Porterhouse steak, trimmed to 0" fat	1 lb cooked	87
T-bone steak, trimmed to 0" fat	1 lb cooked	73
Tri Tip steak, lean, trimmed to 0" fat	1 lb cooked	60
Skirt steak, trimmed to 0" fat	1 lb cooked	55
Top Sirloin, trimmed to 1/8" fat	1 lb cooked	44
Flank steak, lean, trimmed to 0" fat	1 lb cooked	34
Ribeye steak, boneless, trimmed to 0" fat	1 steak	33
Brisket, lean, trimmed to 0" fat	1 lb cooked	32
Flank steak, lean, trimmed to 0" fat	1 steak	28

Continued

Filet Mignon, tenderloin, trimmed to 0" fat	1 steak	10
Ribeye filet, lean, trimmed to 0" fat	1 filet	10
Top Sirloin, choice filet, trimmed to 0" fat	1 filet	7

Beef, cooked	Amount	Total Fat (g)
Ground beef, 75%	1/4 lb patty	18
Ground beef, 80%	1/4 lb patty	14
Ground beef, 85%	1/4 lb patty	12
Ground beef, 90%	1/4 lb patty	10
Ground beef, 95%	1/4 lb patty	5

Bread	Amount	Total Fat (g)
Croissants, butter	1 medium	12
Indian bread, Naan, whole wheat	1 piece	7
Cornbread, dry mix	1 piece	6
Mexican roll, bollilo	1 roll	6
Indian bread, Naan, plain	1 piece	5
Tortillas, flour	1 tortilla	2
Kaiser rolls	1 roll	2
Egg bread	1 slice	2
Bagel, egg	4" bagel	2
Hamburger & Hotdog buns, plain	1 bun	2
Dinner Rolls, brown & serve	1 roll	2
Bagel, cinnamon & raisens	4" bagel	2
Bagel, wheat	4" bagel	2
Bagel, plain, enriched	4" bagel	1
Bagel, oat bran	4" bagel	1
Oatmeal bread	1 slice	1
Raisen bread	1 slice	1
Multigrain or Whole grain	1 slice	1
Rye bread	1 slice	1
Potato bread	1 slice	1
Pumpernickle	1 slice	0.99
Cracked Wheat	1 slice	0.98
Wheat	1 slice	0.98
English Muffin, plain, enriched	1 muffin	0.96
Whole-Wheat	1 slice	0.94
White	1 slice	0.82
Tortillas, corn	1 tortilla	0.74
Pita, white	6" pita	0.72
French, Italian, Sourdough	1 slice	0.46

FAT TOTAL

Butter	Amount	Total Fat (g)
Regular dairy butter, salted	1 tbsp	11.52
Regular dairy whipped butter, salted	1 tbsp	7.62

CEREAL

Arrowhead Mills®	Amount	Total Fat (g)
Oat Bran Flakes	1 cup	2.5
Amaranth Flakes	1 cup	2.0
Spelt Flakes	1 cup	1
Sweetened Rice Flakes	1 cup	1
Maple Buckwheat Flakes	1 cup	1
Kamut Flakes	1 cup	1
Sprouted Multigrain Flakes	1 cup	1
Shredded Wheat, Bite Size	1 cup	1
Sweetened Shredded Wheat	1 cup	1

Barbara's®	Amount	Total Fat (g)
High Fiber Flax & Granola	1 cup	3.0
Shredded Oats Cinnamon Crunch	1 cup	3.0
Shredded Oats Vanilla Almond	1 cup	3.0
Shredded Minis Blueberry Burst	1 cup	3.0
Hole 'n Oats Honey Nut	1 cup	2.7
Hole 'n Oats: Fruit & Juice Sweetened	1 cup	2.7
Puffins Peanut Butter	1 cup	2.7
Shredded Oats Original	1 cup	2.0
Shredded Spoonfuls Multigrain	1 cup	2.0
Puffins Cinnamon	1 cup	1.5
High Fiber Original	1 cup	1.5
High Fiber Cranberry	1 cup	1.5
Corn Flakes	1 cup	1.3
Brown Rice Crisps	1 cup	1.3
Puffins Peanut Butter & Chocolate	1 cup	1.3
Puffins Original	1 cup	1.3
Puffins Honey Rice	1 cup	1.3
Puffins Puffs Crunchy Cocoa	1 cup	1.3
Puffins Puffs Fruit Medley	1 cup	1.3
Shredded Wheat	2 biscuits	1.0
Puffins Multigrain	1 cup	0

Cadia®	Amount	Total Fat (g)
Crunch	1 cup	3.0
Organic Honey Kissed Cadi-O's	1 cup	3.0

FAT TOTAL

Continued

Whole Grain Cadi-O's Toasted Oats	1 cup	1.3
Organic All Natural Raisin Bran	1 cup	1.0

Cascadian Farms®	Amount	Total Fat (g)
Oats & Honey Granolia	1 cup	9
Maple & Brown Sugar Granolia	1 cup	8
French Vanilla & Almond Granolia	1 cup	7
Dark Chocolate Almond Granola	1 cup	7
Fruit & Nut Granolia	1 cup	7
Cinnamon & Raisin Granolia	1 cup	5
Hearty Morning	1 cup	4
Cinnamon Crunch	1 cup	3
Chocolate O's	1 cup	1
FruitFul O's	1 cup	1
Honey Nut O's	1 cup	1
Multi Grain Squares	1 cup	1
Purely O's	1 cup	1
Raisin Bran	1 cup	1

Erewhon®	Amount	Total Fat (g)
Cocoa Crispy Brown Rice	1 cup	1.5
Raisin Bran	1 cup	1.0
Crispy Brown Rice, Strawberry Crisp	1 cup	0.6
Crispy Brown Rice, Gluten Free	1 cup	0.5
Crispy Brown Rice, no Salt Added	1 cup	0.5
Crispy Brown Rice, Mixed Berries	1 cup	0.5
Corn Flakes	1 cup	0
Crispy Brown Rice, Original	1 cup	0
Rice Twice	1 cup	0

Ezekiel	Amount	Total Fat (g)
Sprouted Grain Almond, 4:9	1 cup	6
Sprouted Grain Golden Flax, 4:9	1 cup	5
Sprouted Grain Original, 4:9	1 cup	2
Sprouted Grain Cinnamon Flax, 4:9	1 cup	2

General Mills®	Amount	Total Fat (g)
Reese's Puffs	1 cup	4.00
Cinnamon Toast Crunch	1 cup	3.88
Oatmeal Crisp, Crunchy Almond	1 cup	3.68
Raisin Nut Bran	1 cup	3.50
Chocolate Chex	1 cup	3.41
Cinnamon Chex	1 cup	2.64
Basic 4	1 cup	2.20

FAT TOTAL

Continued

Dora The Explorer	1 cup	2.02
Multi-Bran CHEX	1 cup	2.00
Oatmeal Crisp, Apple Cinnamon	1 cup	2.00
Cocoa Puffs	1 cup	1.67
Golden Grahams	1 cup	1.34
Honey Nut Chex	1 cup	1.34
Cookie Crisp	1 cup	1.33
Wheat Chex	1 cup	1.33
Trix	1 cup	1.23
Berry Berry Kix	1 cup	1.20
Lucky Charms	1 cup	1.09
Total Raisin Bran	1 cup	1.00
Honey Nut Clusters	1 cup	0.96
Kix	1 cup	0.83
KABOOM	1 cup	0.80
Total Cranberry Crunch	1 cup	0.80
Whole Grain Total	1 cup	0.67
Wheaties	1 cup	0.54
Corn Chex	1 cup	0.50
Rice Chex	1 cup	0.27

General Mills Cheerios®	Amount	Total Fat (g)
Yogurt Burst, Strawberry	1 cup	2.67
Apple Cinnamon	1 cup	2.00
Cinnamon Burst	1 cup	2.00
Dulce de leche	1 cup	2.00
Multi Grain Peanut Butter	1 cup	2.00
Chocolate	1 cup	1.84
Original	1 cup	1.77
Honey Nut	1 cup	1.61
Banana Nut	1 cup	1.49
Crunch, Oat Clusters	1 cup	1.48
Berry Burst	1 cup	1.44
Frosted	1 cup	1.33
Fruity	1 cup	1.33
Multi grain	1 cup	1.00

General Mills Fiber One®	Amount	Total Fat (g)
Caramel Delight	1 cup	2.90
Original Bran	1 cup	2.00
Honey Clusters	1 cup	1.30
Raisin Bran Clusters	1 cup	1.16
Frosted Shredded Wheat	1 cup	1.02

FAT TOTAL

Glutino® Gluten Free	Amount	Total Fat (g)
Honey Nut Cereal	1 cup	3
Apple & Cinnamon Rings	1 cup	2
Corn Rice Flakes	1 cup	0
Berry Sensible Beginning	1 cup	0
Frosted Corn & Rice Flakes	1 cup	0
Corn Rice Flakes with Strawberries	1 cup	0

Healthy Valley®	Amount	Total Fat (g)
Oat Bran Almond Crunch	1 cup	6
Cranberry Crunch	1 cup	5
Golden Flax	1 cup	4
Low Fat Date & Almond Flavored Granola	1 cup	3
Low Fat Raisin Cinnamon Granola	1 cup	3
Heart Wise	1 cup	3
Amaranth Flakes	1 cup	2
Multigrain Maple, Honey, Nut Squares	1 cup	2
Multigrain Apple Cinnamon Squares	1 cup	2
Oat Bran Flakes	1 cup	2
Oat Bran Flakes & Raisins	1 cup	2
Fiber 7	1 cup	1
Rice Crunch-EMS	1 cup	0
Corn Crunch-EMS	1 cup	0

Kashi®	Amount	Total Fat (g)
Go Lean Crisp, Cinnamon Crumble	1 cup	5.3
Go Lean Crisp, Toasted Berry Crumble	1 cup	4.9
Go Lean Crunch, Honey Almond Flax	1 cup	4.4
7-Whole Grain Nuggets	1 cup	3.3
Go Lean Crunch	1 cup	3.0
Heart to Heart, Warm Cinnamon	1 cup	2.2
Heart to Heart, Honey Toasted Oat	1 cup	2.2
Heart to Heart, Oat Flakes	1 cup	1.9
Good Friends	1 cup	1.7
Honey Sunshine	1 cup	1.6
Berry Blossom	1 cup	1.2
Island Vanilla	1 cup	1.0
Go Lean	1 cup	1.0
7-Whole Grain Flakes	1 cup	1.0
Cinnamon Harvest	1 cup	0.8
Autumn Wheat	1 cup	0.8
7-Whole Grain Honey Puffs	1 cup	0.5
7-Whole Grain Puffs	1 cup	0.5
Strawberry Fields	1 cup	0.1

FAT TOTAL

Kellogg's®	Amount	Total Fat (g)
Cracklin' Oat Bran	1 cup	9.08
Krave Chocolate	1 cup	4.60
Granola with Raisins	1 cup	4.59
MUESLIX	1 cup	4.51
All-Bran Original	1 cup	3.04
Raisin Bran Extra	1 cup	2.50
Cinnabon	1 cup	2.19
Smorz	1 cup	2.07
All-Bran Bran Budds	1 cup	1.94
Rice Krispies Treats	1 cup	1.84
Fiberplus Cinnamon Oat Crunch	1 cup	1.83
Smart Start, Strong Heart Toasted Oat	1 cup	1.82
Crunchy Nut Golden Honey Nut Flakes	1 cup	1.65
Crunchy Nut Roasted Nut & Honey O's	1 cup	1.55
Raisin Bran	1 cup	1.34
Cocoa Krispies	1 cup	1.20
Raisin Bran Crunch	1 cup	1.01
Froot Loops	1 cup	0.99
Frosted MINI-Wheats, Bite Size	1 cup	0.97
Fiberplus Berry Yogurt Crunch	1 cup	0.95
Frosted MINI Wheats, Big Bite	1 cup	0.82
All-Bran Complete Wheat Flakes	1 cup	0.77
Honey Crunch Corn Flakes	1 cup	0.76
Smart Start, Strong Heart Antioxidants	1 cup	0.70
Honey Smacks	1 cup	0.65
Apple Jacks	1 cup	0.60
Product 19	1 cup	0.42
Corn Pops	1 cup	0.40
Berry Rice Krispies	1 cup	0.30
Rice Krispies	1 cup	0.27
Corn Flakes	1 cup	0.17
Frosted Rice Krispies	1 cup	0.16
Simply Cinnamon Corn Flakes	1 cup	0.16
Crispix	1 cup	0.14
Frosted Flakes	1 cup	0.11

Kellogg's Special-K®	Amount	Total Fat (g)
Low Fat Granola	1 cup	6.0
Protein Plus	1 cup	3.7
Chocolately Delight	1 cup	3.0
Cinnamon Pecan	1 cup	2.4
Vanilla Almond	1 cup	1.7
Fruit & Yogurt	1 cup	1.3
Multigrain Oats & Honey	1 cup	0.8

FAT TOTAL

Continued

Blueberry	1 cup	0.6
Original	1 cup	0.5
Red Berries	1 cup	0.4

Mom's Best Naturals®	Amount	Total Fat (g)
Toasted Cinnamon Squares	1 cup	4.6
Honey Grahams	1 cup	4.0
Oats & Honey Blend	1 cup	2.0
Honey Nut Toasty O's	1 cup	1.5
Raisin Bran	1 cup	1.5
Crispy Coco Rice	1 cup	1.3
Mallow Oats	1 cup	1.0
Sweetened Wheat Fuls	1 cup	1.0
Toasted Wheat Fuls	1 cup	1.0
Honey Ful Wheats	1 cup	0

Nature's Path®	Amount	Total Fat (g)
Peanut Butter Granola	1 cup	15
Flax Plus Pumpkin Flax Granola	1 cup	13
Hemp Plus Granola	1 cup	13
AGAVE Plus Granola	1 cup	12
Flax Plus Vanilla Almond Granola	1 cup	12
Pomegran Cherry Granola	1 cup	12
Pomegran Plus Granola	1 cup	12
Acai Apple Granola	1 cup	11
Flax Plus Maple Pecan Crunch	1 cup	9
Optimum Banana Almond	1 cup	8
Flax Plus Pumpkin Raisin Crunch	1 cup	6
Flax Plus Redberry Crunch	1 cup	5
Heritage Crunch	1 cup	4
Optimum Power Blueberry Cinnamon	1 cup	4
Flax Plus Raisin Bran Flakes	1 cup	3
Optimum Cranberry Ginger	1 cup	3
Organic Millet Rice	1 cup	3
Flax Plus Multibran Flakes	1 cup	3
Whole O's	1 cup	2
OATY BITES Whole Grain	1 cup	2
Optimum Slim Low Fat Vanilla	1 cup	2
Smart Bran	1 cup	2
Crunchy Maple Sunrise, Gluten Free	1 cup	1.5
Crunchy Vanilla Sunrise	1 cup	1.5
Heritage Flakes	1 cup	1
Mesa Sunrise, Gluten Free	1 cup	1
Multigrain Oat bran	1 cup	1
Heritage Heirloom Whole Grain	1 cup	0.7

FAT TOTAL

Peace All Natural	Amount	Total Fat (g)
Wild Berry Clusters & Flakes	1 cup	9.0
Walnut Spice Clusters & Flakes	1 cup	9.0
Cherry Almond Clusters & Flakes	1 cup	9.0
Golden Honey Granola	1 cup	9.0
Vanilla Almond Clusters & Flakes	1 cup	6.0
Maple Pecan	1 cup	6.0
Mango Peach Passion Clusters & Flakes	1 cup	2.5

Post®	Amount	Total Fat (g)
Great Grains, Cruncy Pecan	1 cup	7.28
Great Grains, Banana Nut Crunch	1 cup	5.72
Great Grains, Raisin, Date & Pecan	1 cup	5.21
Great Grains, Cranberry Almond Crunch	1 cup	3.78
Grape-Nuts Cereal	1 cup	2.44
Blueberry Morning	1 cup	2.33
Honey Nut Shredded Wheat	1 cup	1.71
Cocoa Pebbles	1 cup	1.59
Friuty Pebbles	1 cup	1.44
Grape-Nuts Flakes	1 cup	1.43
Alpha-Bits	1 cup	1.38
Shredded Wheat, Original, spoon-size	1 cup	1.03
Raisin Bran	1 cup	1.00
Shredded Wheat n' Bran, spoon-size	1 cup	0.99
Shredded Wheat, frosted, spoon-size	1 cup	0.99
Bran Flakes	1 cup	0.88
Honeycomb Cereal	1 cup	0.64
Golden Crisp	1 cup	0.61
Shredded Wheat, Original, big-biscuit	1 biscuit	0.55

Post® Honey Bunches of Oats®	Amount	Total Fat (g)
Just Bunches, Honey Roasted	1 cup	9.70
With Almonds	1 cup	3.11
With Vanilla Bunches	1 cup	2.86
Honey Roasted	1 cup	2.18
Pecan Bunches	1 cup	2.17
With Strawberries	1 cup	2.03
With Cinnamon Bunches	1 cup	2.00

Quaker®	Amount	Total Fat (g)
Granola, Apple Cranberry Almond	1 cup	10.0
CAP'N Crunch's Peanut Butter Crunch	1 cup	3.3
Oatmeal Squares, Golden Maple	1 cup	3.0
Oatmeal Squares	1 cup	2.7

FAT TOTAL

Continued

Honey Gram OH'S	1 cup	2.7
Oatmeal Squares, Cinnamon	1 cup	2.5
Toasted Multigrain Crisp	1 cup	2.4
LIFE Cereal, Cinnamon	1 cup	2.0
LIFE Cereal, Maple & Brown Sugar	1 cup	2.0
LIFE Cereal, Original	1 cup	2.0
CAP'N Crunch	1 cup	1.8
CAP'N Crunch & Crunch Berries	1 cup	1.7
Corn Bran Crunch	1 cup	1.5
CAP'N Crunch's OOPs! All Berries	1 cup	1.3
Puffed Rice	1 cup	0
Puffed Wheat	1 cup	0

Cereal, Uncle Sam®	Amount	Total Fat (g)
Flaxseed, Honey Almond	1 cup	8
Flaxseed, Original	1 cup	7
Flaxseed, & Strawberry	1 cup	7
Skinners Raisin Bran	1 cup	1

Cereal, Wild Harvest®	Amount	Total Fat (g)
Blueberry Flax Granola	1 cup	12
Cherry Vanilla Granola	1 cup	9
Crunchy Vanilla Almond Granola	1 cup	9
Golden Honey & Flax Granola	1 cup	9

Cereal, Cooked	Amount	Total Fat (g)
Oats, regular, unenriched	1 cup	3.6
WHEATENA, cooked	1 cup	1.2
White corn grits	1 cup	1.1
Yellow corn grits	1 cup	0.9
Farina	1 cup	0.8
CREAM OF WHEAT, regular, 10 minute cooking	1 cup	0.5
Malt-o-Meal plain	1 serving	0.4
CREAM OF WHEAT, mix'n eat	1 packet	0.3

Cheese	Amount	Total Fat (g)
Goat cheese, hard type	1 oz	10.09
Cheddar	1 oz	9.36
Gruyere	1 oz	9.17
Colby	1 oz	9.10
Dubliner	1 oz	9.00
Pepper Jack & Red & Green Jalapenos	1 oz	9.00
Fontina	1 oz	8.83
American, pasteurized process, fortified	1 oz	8.71

FAT TOTAL

Roquefort	1 oz	8.69
Monterey	1 oz	8.58
Muenster	1 oz	8.52
Goat cheese, semisoft	1 oz	8.46
Blue cheese	1 oz	8.15
Parmesan, grated	1 oz	8.11
Swiss	1 oz	7.88
Brie	1 oz	7.85
Gouda	1 oz	7.78
Romano	1 oz	7.64
Cream cheese	1 oz	7.60
Provolone	1 oz	7.55
Mozzarella, whole milk	1 oz	6.34
Monterey, low fat	1 oz	6.05
Feta	1 oz	6.03
Goat cheese, soft type	1 oz	5.98
Mozzarella, part skim milk, low moisture	1 oz	5.68
American, pasteurized process, imitation	1 oz	5.53
Muenster, low fat	1 oz	4.93
Provolone, reduced fat	1 oz	4.93
Cheddar, low fat	1 oz	1.98
American, pasteurized process, low fat	1 oz	1.96
Swiss, low fat	1 oz	1.43
Cream cheese, fat free	1 oz	0.28
Mozzarella, non fat	1 oz	0

Chicken, Cooked	Amount	Total Fat (g)
Thigh, with skin, fried	1 thigh	14.22
Wing with skin, fried in batter	1 wing	10.69
Breast, skin, fried, flour	1/2 breast	8.69
Drumstick, with skin, fried	1 drumstick	6.72
Wing with skin, roasted	1 wing	6.62
Thigh, no skin, roasted	1 thigh	5.66
Breast, no skin, roasted	1/2 breast	3.07
Drumstick, no skin, roasted	1 drumstick	2.49

Chicken, Cooked	Amount	Total Fat (g)
Wing with skin, fried in flour	3 oz	18.84
Wing with skin, roasted	3 oz	16.54
Thigh with skin, fried in flour	3 oz	12.73
Thigh with skin, roasted	3 oz	12.59
Drumstick with skin, fried in flour	3 oz	11.68
Drumstick with skin, roasted	3 oz	8.47
Breast with skin, fried in flour	3 oz	7.54
Thigh meat only, no skin, roasted	3 oz	7.03

FAT TOTAL

Continued

Wing meat only, no skin, roasted	3 oz	6.91
Breast with skin, roasted	3 oz	6.61
Drumstick meat only, no skin, roasted	3 oz	4.67
Cornish game hems, meat only	3 oz	3.29
Breast meat only, no skin, roasted	3 oz	3.03

CHILI

Chili, Amy's®	Amount	Total Fat (g)
Light in Sodium Medium Chili	1 can	18
Light in Sodium Spicy Chili	1 can	18
Medium Chili	1 can	18
Spicy Chili	1 can	18
Medium Chili with Vegetables	1 can	12
Southwestern Black Bean Chili	1 can	8
Black Bean Chili	1 can	6

Chili, Campbell's® Chunky	Amount	Total Fat (g)
Chili no Beans	1 can	12
Chili with Beans Roadhouse	1 can	12
Chili with Beans Firehouse	1 can	12
Chili with Beans Grilled Steak	1 can	6

Chili, Cattle Drive®	Amount	Total Fat (g)
Cattle Drive Golden Chili wirh Beans	1 can	12

Chili, Dennison's®	Amount	Total Fat (g)
Original Chili Con Carne with Beans	1 can	28
Hot Chili Con Carne with Beans	1 can	28
Chunky Chili Con Carne with Beans	1 can	20
Hot & Chunky Chili with Beans	1 can	20
Turkey Chili with Beans	1 can	6
Vegetarian Chili with Beans	1 can	3

Chili, Eden's®	Amount	Total Fat (g)
Kidney Bean & Kamut Chili	1 can	4
Black Bean & Quinoa Chili	1 can	3
Pinto Bean & Spelt Chili	1 can	3
Great Northern Bean & Barley Chili	1 can	2

FAT TOTAL

Chili, Healthy Valley®	Amount	Total Fat (g)
Santa Fe White Bean Chili	1 can	6
Black Bean Mole Chili	1 can	6
Black Bean Mango Chili	1 can	6
Spicy Tomato Chili	1 can	6
Three Bean Chipotle Chili	1 can	6
Vegetarian no salt added Tame Tomato Chili	1 can	5

Chili, Hardy Jack's®	Amount	Total Fat (g)
Chili no beans	1 can	50
Chili with beans	1 can	32

Chili, Hormel®	Amount	Total Fat (g)
Chili No Beans	1 can	18
Less Sodium Chili no Beans	1 can	18
Cook- off White Chicken Chili	1 can	16
Chili with Beans	1 can	14
Chunky Chili with Beans	1 can	14
Hot Chili with beans	1 can	14
Less Sodium Chili with Beans	1 can	14
Cook-off Chipotle Chicken Chili	1 can	14
Cook-off Roasted Tomato Chili	1 can	14
Turkey Chili with Beans	1 can	6
Turkey Chili no Beans	1 can	6
Vegetarian Chili & Beans 99% Fat Free	1 can	2

Chili, Nalley's®	Amount	Total Fat (g)
Jalapeno Hot Chili with beans	1 can	16
Thick Chili with beans	1 can	16
Original Chili with beans	1 can	14
Turkey Chili with beans	1 can	7

Chili, Stagg®	Amount	Total Fat (g)
Steak House Chili no Beans	1 can	44
Classi Chili with beans	1 can	34
Dynamite Hot Chili with Beans	1 can	34
Country Brand Chili, Sweet Bell Peppers	1 can	34
Chunkero Chili with Beans	1 can	32
Country Brand Chili with Beans	1 can	32
Laredo Chili & Beans, Chili and Jalapno	1 can	30
White Chicken Chili with Beans	1 can	24
Fiesta Grille Chili with Beans	1 can	20
Ranch House Chicken Chili with Beans	1 can	16

FAT TOTAL

Continued

Silverado Beef Chili with Beans	1 can	14
Turkey Ranchero Chili with Beans	1 can	6
Vegetarian Garden Four Bean Chili	1 can	2

Chili, Wolf Brand	Amount	Total Fat (g)
Chili no Beans	1 can	56
Hot Chili no Beans	1 can	56
Chili with Beans	1 can	38
Spicy Chili with Beans	1 can	30
Homestyle Chili with Beans	1 can	28
Lean Beaf no Beans	1 can	12
Lean Beaf with Beans	1 can	10
Turkey Chili no Beans	1 can	5
Turkey Chili with Beans	1 can	5

Cream	Amount	Total Fat (g)
Heavy Cream	1 tbsp	5.55
Light Coffe Cream	1 tbsp	2.90
Sour Cream, cultured	1 tbsp	2.37
Sour Cream, reduced fat	1 tbsp	1.80
Half & Half	1 tbsp	1.73
Whipped Topping, pressurized	1 tbsp	0.67

Eggs	Amount	Total Fat (g)
Egg whole, fried	1 large	6.83
Egg whole, scrambled	1 large	6.70
Egg whole, hard-boiled	1 large	5.31
Egg whole, poached	1 large	4.74
Egg yolk	1 large	4.41
Egg substitute, liquid, fat free	1/4 cup	0
Egg white	1 large	0
Egg whites, dried	1 ounce	0
Egg whites, dried powder, stabilized	1 tbsp	0

FISH

Fish, Canned	Amount	Total Fat (g)
Atlantic Sardines, in oil	3 oz	9.74
Light tuna, in oil	3 oz	6.98
White (albacore) tuna, in oil	3 oz	6.87
White (albacore) tuna, in water	3 oz	2.52
Light tuna, in water	3 oz	0.82

FAT TOTAL

Fish, Cooked	Amount	Total Fat (g)
Atlantic herring, pickled	3 oz	15.31
Atlantic mackerel	3 oz	15.14
Halibut, Greenland	3 oz	15.08
Shark	3 oz	11.75
King salmon, chinook, dry heated	3 oz	11.37
Catfish, breaded & fried	3 oz	11.33
Atlantic croaker	3 oz	10.77
Atlantic salmon, farmed	3 oz	10.50
Florida pompano	3 oz	10.32
Pacific & Jack mackerel	3 oz	8.60
Coho salmon, farmed	3 oz	7.00
Atlantic salmon, wild	3 oz	6.91
Swordfish	3 oz	6.74
Rainbow trout, farmed	3 oz	6.27
Catfish, farmed	3 oz	6.11
Carp	3 oz	6.09
Sockeye salmon	3 oz	5.69
Spanish mackerel	3 oz	5.37
Bluefin tuna	3 oz	5.34
Rainbow trout, wild	3 oz	4.95
Pink salmon	3 oz	4.49
Keta (chun) salmon	3 oz	4.11
Freshwater bass	3 oz	4.02
King salmon, chinook, smoked	3 oz	3.67
Coho salmon, wild	3 oz	3.66
Striped bass	3 oz	2.54
Catfish, wild	3 oz	2.42
Halibut, Alaskan	3 oz	2.32
Tilapia	3 oz	2.25
King mackerel	3 oz	2.18
Sea bass	3 oz	2.18
Flounder & Sole	3 oz	2.01
Atlantic perch	3 oz	1.59
Snapper	3 oz	1.46
Whiting	3 oz	1.44
Halibut, Atlantic & Pacific	3 oz	1.37
Walleye pike	3 oz	1.33
Grouper	3 oz	1.10
Skipjack (aku) tuna	3 oz	1.10
Atlantic pollock	3 oz	1.07
Walleye pollock	3 oz	1.00
Orange roughy	3 oz	0.76
Northern pike	3 oz	0.75
Atlantic cod	3 oz	0.73

FAT TOTAL

Continued

Yellowfin tuna	3 oz	0.50
Haddock	3 oz	0.47
Pacific cod	3 oz	0.42

Fish, Shellfish, Cooked	Amount	Total Fat (g)
Oysters, breaded & fried	3 oz	10.69
Shrimp, breaded & fried	3 oz	10.44
Clams, breaded & fried	3 oz	9.48
Scallops, breaded & fried	3 oz	9.30
Blue crab cakes	3 oz	6.39
Squid, fried	3 oz	6.36
Abalone	3 oz	5.76
Eastern oysters, wild	3 oz	2.25
Eastern oysters, farmed	3 oz	1.80
Octopus	3 oz	1.77
Shrimp,	3 oz	1.44
Clams, canned	3 oz	1.35
Alaskan king crab	3 oz	1.31
Queen crab	3 oz	1.28
Shrimp, canned	3 oz	1.16
Crayfish	3 oz	1.02
Northern lobster	3 oz	0.73
Scallops, bay & sea, steamed	3 oz	0.71
Blue crab, canned	3 oz	0.63
Blue crab	3 oz	0.63
Alaskan king crab, imitation	3 oz	0.39

Game Meat, Cooked	Amount	Total Fat (g)
Bison, ground	3 oz	12.86
Duck	3 oz	9.52
Elk, ground	3 oz	7.43
Deer, ground	3 oz	6.99
Squirrel	3 oz	3.99
Caribou	3 oz	3.76
Wild boar	3 oz	3.72
Rabbit	3 oz	2.98
Deer	3 oz	2.71
Antelope	3 oz	2.27
Elk	3 oz	1.62
Buffalo, steak, free range	3 oz	1.53

FAT TOTAL

Juice	Amount	Total Fat (g)
Pomegranate	1 cup	0.72
Lemon juice, raw	1 cup	0.59
Orange, raw	1 cup	0.50
Carrot	1 cup	0.35
Grape, unsweetened	1 cup	0.33
Apple	1 cup	0.32
Grapefruit juice, raw	1 cup	0.32
Pineapple, unsweetened	1 cup	0.30
Cranberry	1 cup	0.25
Vegetable	1 cup	0.22
Tomato	1 cup	0.12
Prune	1 cup	0.08

Lamb, Cooked	Amount	Total Fat (g)
Chops, loin, lean, trimmed to 1/4" fat	3 oz	19.62
Ground	3 oz	16.70
Leg, whole, trimmed to 1/4" fat	3 oz	14.01
Foreshank, trimmed to 1/8" fat	3 oz	11.44
Rib, lean, trimmed to 1/4" fat	3 oz	11.01
Cubed, for stew or kabob	3 oz	6.23

Milk	Amount	Total Fat (g)
Coconut milk, canned	1 cup	48.21
Canned, condensed, sweetened	1 cup	26.62
Canned, evaporated	1 cup	19.05
Sheep milk	1 cup	17.15
Human milk	1 cup	10.77
Goat milk	1 cup	10.10
Buttermilk, whole milk	1 cup	8.11
Whole milk, 3.25%	1 cup	7.93
Meyenberg, goat milk, whole milk	1 cup	7.20
Reduced fat, 2%	1 cup	4.83
Soy- milk	1 cup	4.25
Meyenberg low fat goat milk	1 cup	2.40
Low fat, 1% milk	1 cup	2.37
Buttermilk, cultured, low fat	1 cup	2.16
Canned, evaporated, non fat	1 cup	0.51
Non fat, fat free or skim liquid milk	1 cup	0.20
Dry, instant, non fat	1/3 cup	0.17

FAT TOTAL

Nuts & Seeds	Amount	Total Fat (g)
Macadamia	1 oz	21.48
Pecans	1 oz	20.40
Pine nuts	1 oz	19.38
Brazilnuts	1 oz	18.83
English walnuts	1 oz	18.49
Peanuts	1 oz	17.97
Hazelnuts	1 oz	17.22
Black walnuts	1 oz	16.73
Tahini	1 oz	15.24
Sunflower seed	1 oz	14.59
Mixed nuts, roasted with peanuts, no salt	1 oz	14.59
Peanut butter, smooth	1 oz	14.29
Sesame seeds	1 oz	14.08
Almonds	1 oz	14.01
Pumpkin seeds	1 oz	13.91
Pistachio	1 oz	12.87
Cashews	1 oz	12.43
Flax seeds	1 oz	11.95
Coconut, raw meat	1 oz	9.49
Trail mix, regular with chocolate chips	1 oz	9.04
Chia seeds	1 oz	8.71
Trail mix, regular, salted	1 oz	8.33
Trail mix, tropical	1 oz	4.85

Oils	Amount	Total Fat (g)
Canola oil	1 tbsp	14.0
Sunflower, high oleic acid	1 tbsp	14.0
Cod liver oil	1 tbsp	13.6
Corn oil	1 tbsp	13.6
Cottonseed oil	1 tbsp	13.6
Coconut oil	1 tbsp	13.6
Flaxseed oil	1 tbsp	13.6
Grapeseed oil	1 tbsp	13.6
Safflower oil	1 tbsp	13.6
Salmon oil	1 tbsp	13.6
Sesame oil	1 tbsp	13.6
Soybean oil	1 tbsp	13.6
Sunflower, high linoleic acid, oil	1 tbsp	13.6
Walnut oil	1 tbsp	13.6
Olive oil	1 tbsp	13.5
Peanut oil	1 tbsp	13.5

FAT TOTAL

Pork, Cooked	Amount	Total Fat (g)
Bacon	3 oz	35.5
Spareribs	3 oz	25.8
Liverwurst spread	1/4 cup	25.5
Bratwurst	3 oz	24.8
Polish sausage	3 oz	24.4
Braunschweiger	3 oz	24.2
Sausage	3 oz	24.1
Italian sausage	3 oz	23.2
Backribs	3 oz	18.3
Cured ham	3 oz	14.3
Chops, pan-fried	3 oz	11.3
Center loin pork chops	3 oz	9.4
Chops, broiled	3 oz	9.4
Canadian-style bacon	3 oz	7.2
Chops, lean, pan-fried	3 oz	6.5
Sirloin pork chops	3 oz	4.7
Cured ham, lean	3 oz	4.7
Tenderloin	3 oz	3.4

SALAD DRESSING

Annies's Organic Dressing	Amount	Total Fat (g)
Redwine & Olive Oil	2 tbsp	15
Shiitake Sesame	2 tbsp	13
Oil & Vinegar	2 tbsp	13
Goddnes	2 tbsp	12
Asian Sesame	2 tbsp	12
Caesar Dressing	2 tbsp	11
Cowgirl Ranch Dressing	2 tbsp	11
French Dressing	2 tbsp	11
Green Goddness Dressing	2 tbsp	11
Roasted Garlic Vinaigrette	2 tbsp	11
Balsamic Vinaigrette	2 tbsp	10
Papaya Poppy Seed	2 tbsp	8
Sesame Ginger Vinaigrette	2 tbsp	8
Thousand Island	2 tbsp	8
Creamy Asiago Cheese	2 tbsp	8
Green Garlic	2 tbsp	8
Pomegranate Vinaigrette	2 tbsp	7
Buttermilk Dressing	2 tbsp	6

FAT TOTAL

Bernstein's Dressing	Amount	Total Fat (g)
Chunky Blue Chees	2 tbsp	13
Herb Garden French	2 tbsp	12
Balsamic Italian	2 tbsp	11
Redwine & Garlic Italian	2 tbsp	11
Restaurant Recipe Italian	2 tbsp	11
Sweet Herb Italian	2 tbsp	11
Basil Parmesan	2 tbsp	10
Cheese Fantastico	2 tbsp	10
Creamy Caesar	2 tbsp	10
Italian & Marinade	2 tbsp	9
Cheese & Garlic Italian	2 tbsp	8

Best Food® Mayonnaise Dressing	Amount	Total Fat (g)
Real Mayonnaise	2 tbsp	20
Mayonesa Con Jugo De Limon	2 tbsp	20
Mayonnaise with Olive Oil	2 tbsp	8
Canola Cholesterol Free Mayonnaise	2 tbsp	8
Light Mayonnaise	2 tbsp	7

Bob's Big Boy® Dressing	Amount	Total Fat (g)
Ranch	2 tbsp	16
Blue Cheese	2 tbsp	15
Roquefort	2 tbsp	15
Thousand Island	2 tbsp	14

Bolthouse® Farm's Desssing	Amount	Total Fat (g)
Chunky Blue Cheese & Olive Oil	2 tbsp	3.0
Classic Ranch Yogurt Dressing	2 tbsp	3.0
Salsa Ranch Yogurt Dressing	2 tbsp	3.0
Asian Ginger & Olive Oil Vinaigrettes	2 tbsp	2.5
Caesar Parmigino Yogurt Dressing	2 tbsp	2.5
Chunky Bluecheese Yogurt Dressing	2 tbsp	2.5
Thousand Island Yogurt Dressing	2 tbsp	2.0
Honey Mustard Yogurt Dressing	2 tbsp	1.5
Zesty French Yogurt	2 tbsp	1.5
Classic Balsamic & Olive Oil	2 tbsp	0
Raspberry Merlot & Olive Oil	2 tbsp	0

FAT TOTAL

Brianna's® Dressing	Amount	Total Fat (g)
The New American	2 tbsp	17
Classic Buttermilk Ranch	2 tbsp	17
Zesty French	2 tbsp	15
Asiago Caesar	2 tbsp	15
Champagne Caper Vinaigrette	2 tbsp	15
Dijon Honey Mustard	2 tbsp	14
Ginger Mandarin	2 tbsp	14
Rich Poppy Seed	2 tbsp	14
Real French Vinaigrette	2 tbsp	14
True Blue Cheese	2 tbsp	11
Chipotle Cheddar	2 tbsp	11
Blush Wine Vinaigrette	2 tbsp	7
Lively Lemon Tarragon	2 tbsp	0
Rich Santa Fe Blend	2 tbsp	0

Cardini's Dressing	Amount	Total Fat (g)
Original Caesar	2 tbsp	17
Aged Parmesan Ranch	2 tbsp	16
Honey Mustard	2 tbsp	13
Roasted Asian Sesame	2 tbsp	10
Pear Vinaigrette	2 tbsp	9
Balsamic Vinaigrette	2 tbsp	8
Italian Dressing	2 tbsp	8
Raspberry Pomegranate	2 tbsp	8

Drew's® Dressing	Amount	Total Fat (g)
Rosemary Balsamic	2 tbsp	18
Thai Sesame Lime	2 tbsp	18
Shiitake Ginger	2 tbsp	16
Poppy Seed	2 tbsp	16
Classic Italian	2 tbsp	15
Roasted Garlic & Peppercorn	2 tbsp	15
Sesame Orange	2 tbsp	15
Organic Peppercorn Ranch	2 tbsp	15
Lemon Goddess	2 tbsp	14
Buttermilk Ranch	2 tbsp	14
Honey Dijon	2 tbsp	14
Organic Classic Ceasar	2 tbsp	14
Organic Asian Ginger	2 tbsp	14
Organic Harvest Ranch	2 tbsp	14
Greek Olive	2 tbsp	12
Smoked Tomato	2 tbsp	10
Organic Aged Balsamic	2 tbsp	10

FAT TOTAL

Girard's® Dressing	Amount	Total Fat (g)
Champagne Dressing	2 tbsp	15
Caesar Dressing	2 tbsp	13
Original French Dressing	2 tbsp	13
Old Venice Italian	2 tbsp	13
Romano Cheese Italian	2 tbsp	13
Greek Feta Vinaigrette	2 tbsp	11
Chinese Chicken Salad	2 tbsp	10
Blue Cheee Vinaigrette	2 tbsp	9
Apple Poppy Seed	2 tbsp	9
Creamy Balsamic Vinaigrette	2 tbsp	9
White Balsamic	2 tbsp	9
Peach Mimosa Vinaigrette	2 tbsp	8
Light Caesar Dressing	2 tbsp	7
Light Champagne Dressing	2 tbsp	5
Spinach Salad Dressing	2 tbsp	2

Hidden Valley® Dressing	Amount	Total Fat (g)
Spicy Ranch	2 tbsp	16
Coleslaw Dressing	2 tbsp	15
Classic Cheese Ranch	2 tbsp	14
Old Fashioned Buttermilk Ranch	2 tbsp	14
Original Ranch Dressing	2 tbsp	14
Bacon Ranch	2 tbsp	14
Cracked Peppercorn Ranch	2 tbsp	12
Garden Vegetable Ranch	2 tbsp	12
Original Ranch Light	2 tbsp	7
Buttermilk Ranch Light	2 tbsp	5
Original Ranch Fat Free	2 tbsp	0

Hidden Valley® Farm House Dressing	Amount	Total Fat (g)
Creamy Parmesan	2 tbsp	14
Hickory Bacon & Onion	2 tbsp	12
Roasted Onion Parmesan	2 tbsp	12
Savory Bleu Cheese	2 tbsp	12
Garden Tomato & Bacon	2 tbsp	11
Original Caesar	2 tbsp	11
Creamy Balsamic with Herb	2 tbsp	10
Homestyle Italian	2 tbsp	10
Southwest Chipotle	2 tbsp	10
Dijon Mustard Vinaigrette	2 tbsp	9
Original Italian with Herb	2 tbsp	7
Pomegranate Vinaigrette	2 tbsp	6

FAT TOTAL

Ken's® Steak House Dressings	Amount	Total Fat (g)
Buttermilk Ranch Dressing	2 tbsp	20
Pepper Corn Ranch	2 tbsp	20
Caesar Dressing	2 tbsp	18
Creamy Caesar Dressing	2 tbsp	18
Italian Marinade	2 tbsp	17
Chunky Blue Cheese	2 tbsp	16
Ranch Dressing	2 tbsp	15
Russian Dressing	2 tbsp	14
Creamy Italian	2 tbsp	13
Thousand Island	2 tbsp	13
Italian & Aged Romano	2 tbsp	12
Red Wine Vinegar Oil	2 tbsp	12
3 Cheese Italian	2 tbsp	11
Greek & Olive Oil	2 tbsp	11
Honey Mustard	2 tbsp	11
Balsamic Vinaigrete	2 tbsp	10
Italian with Olive Oil	2 tbsp	8
Zesty Italian	2 tbsp	8
Balsamic & Honey	2 tbsp	7
Sweet Vidalia Onion	2 tbsp	4.5

Ken's® Lite Dressings	Amount	Total Fat (g)
Lite Creamy Caesar Dressing	2 tbsp	8
Lite Ranch Dressing	2 tbsp	7
Lite Bluecheese Dressing	2 tbsp	7
Lite Raspberry & Walnut Vinaigrette	2 tbsp	6
Lite Thousand Island	2 tbsp	5
Lite Zesty Italian	2 tbsp	4.5
Lite Asian Sesame Ginger & Soy	2 tbsp	4

Kraft's® Dressing	Amount	Total Fat (g)
Ranch with Backon	2 tbsp	15
Creamy French Dressing	2 tbsp	13
Green Goddnes	2 tbsp	13
Roka Blue Cheese	2 tbsp	13
Classic Caesar Dressing	2 tbsp	12
Peppercorn Ranch	2 tbsp	12
Buttermilk Ranch	2 tbsp	12
Cucumber Ranch	2 tbsp	12
Thousand Island	2 tbsp	12
Ranch	2 tbsp	11
Creamy Italian	2 tbsp	10
Creamy Poppyseed	2 tbsp	9

FAT TOTAL

Continued

Coleslaw Dressing	2 tbsp	8
Sweet Honey Catalina	2 tbsp	8
Classic Catalina	2 tbsp	6
Zesty Italian Dressing & Marinade	2 tbsp	6
Zesty Italian Anything Dressing	2 tbsp	6
Sweet Balsamic Vinaigrette Dressing	2 tbsp	5
Lite Ranch	2 tbsp	4.5
Light Thousand Island	2 tbsp	2
Light Zesty Italian	2 tbsp	1.5
Free Thousand Island	2 tbsp	0
Fat Free Ranch	2 tbsp	0
Catalina Fat Free	2 tbsp	0

Litehouse® Dressing	Amount	Total Fat (g)
Big Bleu Dressing	2 tbsp	17
Chunky Bleu Cheese	2 tbsp	16
Chunky Garlic Caesar	2 tbsp	16
Original Bleu Cheese	2 tbsp	16
Ceaser-Caesar Dressing	2 tbsp	15
Ceaser Dressing	2 tbsp	13
Organic Ranch	2 tbsp	13
Buttermilk Ranch	2 tbsp	12
Homestyle Ranch	2 tbsp	12
Honey Mustard	2 tbsp	12
Jalapeno Ranch	2 tbsp	12
Original Thousand Island	2 tbsp	12
Ranch Dressing	2 tbsp	12
Barbecue Ranch	2 tbsp	10
Coleslaw with Pinapple	2 tbsp	10
Creamy Cilantro	2 tbsp	10
Parmesan Caesar	2 tbsp	10
Coleslaw Dressing	2 tbsp	9
Sweet French	2 tbsp	8
Yogurt Bleu Cheese with Kefir	2 tbsp	7
Yogurt Ranch with Kefir	2 tbsp	5
Pear Gorzonzola Dressing	2 tbsp	2.5
Spinach	2 tbsp	0.5
Harvest Cranberry Greek	2 tbsp	0
Sesame Ginger	2 tbsp	0

Litehouse® Lite Dressing	Amount	Total Fat (g)
Bleu Cheese	2 tbsp	8
1000 Island	2 tbsp	7
Caesar Dressing	2 tbsp	7
Creamy Ranch Dressing	2 tbsp	6

FAT TOTAL

Continued

Jalapeno Ranch Dressing	2 tbsp	6
Ranch Dressing	2 tbsp	6
Honey Dijon Vinaigrette	2 tbsp	5
Coleslaw Dressing	2 tbsp	3

Litehouse® Vinaigrette Dressing	Amount	Total Fat (g)
Balsamic Vinaigrette	2 tbsp	10
Raspberry Walnut Vinaigrette	2 tbsp	9
Red Wine Olive Oil Vinaigrette	2 tbsp	9
White Balsamic Vinaigrette	2 tbsp	9
Bleu Cheese Vinaigrette	2 tbsp	7
Fuji Apple Vinaigrette	2 tbsp	7
Organic Balsamic Vinaigrette	2 tbsp	7
Zesty Italian Vinaigrette	2 tbsp	5
Greek Vinaigrette	2 tbsp	5
Cherry Vinaigrette	2 tbsp	3
Harvest Cranberry Vinaigrette	2 tbsp	0
Huckleberry Vinaigrette	2 tbsp	0
Pomegranate Blueberry Vinaigrette	2 tbsp	0

Marie's Dressing	Amount	Total Fat (g)
Caesar	2 tbsp	19
Creamy Ranch	2 tbsp	19
Creamy Chipotle Ranch	2 tbsp	19
Creamy Italian Garlic	2 tbsp	19
Chunky Blue Cheese	2 tbsp	17
Asiago Peppercorn	2 tbsp	17
Super Blue Cheese	2 tbsp	17
Jalapeno Ranch	2 tbsp	17
Buttermilk Ranch	2 tbsp	16
Thousand Island	2 tbsp	15
Creamy Caesar	2 tbsp	13
Honey Mustard	2 tbsp	13
Coleslaw	2 tbsp	13
Poppy Seed	2 tbsp	13
Honey Dijon	2 tbsp	12
Greek Vinaigrette	2 tbsp	12
Blue Cheese Vinaigrette	2 tbsp	11
Italian Vinaigrette	2 tbsp	8
Sesame Ginger	2 tbsp	8
Yogurt Blue Cheese	2 tbsp	7
Lite Chunky Blue Cheese	2 tbsp	7
Yogurt Ranch Dressing	2 tbsp	7
Yogurt Thousand Island	2 tbsp	6
Lite Creamy Ranch	2 tbsp	6

FAT TOTAL

Continued

Yogurt Coleslaw Dressing	2 tbsp	6
Balsamic Vinaigrette	2 tbsp	4.5
Red Wine Vinaigrette	2 tbsp	4
Raspberry Vinaigrette	2 tbsp	3
Spinach Salad Dressing	2 tbsp	1.5

Newman's® Own Dressing	Amount	Total Fat (g)
Creamy Ceasar	2 tbsp	18
Ranch Dressing	2 tbsp	16
Caesar Dressing	2 tbsp	16
Olive Oil & Vinegar	2 tbsp	16
Family Italian	2 tbsp	13
Poppy Seed	2 tbsp	13
Honey French	2 tbsp	11
Parmesan & Garlic	2 tbsp	11
3 Cheese Balsamic	2 tbsp	11
Creamy Balsamic	2 tbsp	10
Greek Vinaigrette	2 tbsp	10
Balsamic Vinaigrette	2 tbsp	9
Orange Ginger	2 tbsp	4.5

Walden Farm's Dressing	Amount	Total Fat (g)
Asian	2 tbsp	0
Bacon Ranch	2 tbsp	0
Balsamic Vinaigrette	2 tbsp	0
Bleu Cheese	2 tbsp	0
Buttermilk Ranch	2 tbsp	0
Caesar	2 tbsp	0
Chipotle Ranch	2 tbsp	0
Colesaw	2 tbsp	0
Creamy Bacon	2 tbsp	0
Creamy Italian	2 tbsp	0
French	2 tbsp	0
Honey Dijon	2 tbsp	0
Italian	2 tbsp	0
Italian Sun Dried Tomato	2 tbsp	0
Jersey Sweet Onion	2 tbsp	0
Ranch	2 tbsp	0
Raspberry Vinaigrette	2 tbsp	0
Russian	2 tbsp	0
Sesame Ginger	2 tbsp	0
Sweet Onion	2 tbsp	0
Thousand Island	2 tbsp	0
Zesty Italian	2 tbsp	0

FAT TOTAL

Wish Bone® Creamy Dressing	Amount	Total Fat (g)
Creamy Caesar	2 tbsp	18
Chunky Blue Cheese	2 tbsp	15
Ranch Dressing	2 tbsp	13
Sweet & Spicy French	2 tbsp	12
Thousand Island	2 tbsp	12
Delux French	2 tbsp	11
Creamy Italian Dressing	2 tbsp	10
Russian	2 tbsp	6
Light Blue Cheese	2 tbsp	6
Light Creamy Caesar	2 tbsp	6
Light Ranch Dressing	2 tbsp	5
Light Thousand Island	2 tbsp	5
Light Delux French	2 tbsp	5
Light Parmesan Peppercorn Ranch	2 tbsp	5
Light Sweet & Spicy French	2 tbsp	3.5
Fat Free Ranch Dressing	2 tbsp	0
Fat Free Chunky Blue Cheese	2 tbsp	0

Wish Bone® Oil & Vinegar Dressing	Amount	Total Fat (g)
House Italian	2 tbsp	10
Italian	2 tbsp	7
Robusto Italian	2 tbsp	7
Balsamic Italian Vinaigrette	2 tbsp	6
Romano Basil Vinaigrette	2 tbsp	5
Balsamic Vinaigrette	2 tbsp	5
Red Wine Vinaigrette	2 tbsp	5
Raspberrt Hazelnut Vinaigrette	2 tbsp	5
Olive Oil Vinaigrette	2 tbsp	5
Bruschetta Italian	2 tbsp	5
Greek Vinaigrette	2 tbsp	5
Superfruit Vinaigrette	2 tbsp	5
Mediterranean Italian	2 tbsp	5
Light Balsamic & Basil Vinaigrette	2 tbsp	5
Light Raspberry Walnut	2 tbsp	5
Light Honey Dijon	2 tbsp	5
Light Asian Sesame & Ginger	2 tbsp	5
Light Italian dressing	2 tbsp	3
Fat Free Red Wine Vinaigrette	2 tbsp	0
Fat Free Italian Dressing	2 tbsp	0
Fat Free Red Wine Vinaigrette	2 tbsp	0

FAT TOTAL

Turkey, Cooked	Amount	Total Fat (g)
Turkey bacon	3 oz	24
Ground turkey, 85% lean	3 oz	14
Turkey sausage, reduced fat	3 oz	13
Ground turkey, 93% lean	3 oz	10
Ground turkey	3 oz	9
Dark meat	3 oz	5
Ground turkey, fat free	3 oz	2
Light meat	3 oz	2
Breast meat	3 oz	1

Veal, Cooked	Amount	Total Fat (g)
Rib	3 oz	12
Loin	3 oz	10
Sirloin	3 oz	9
Breast	3 oz	8
Ground	3 oz	6
Leg, top round	3 oz	5
Foreshank	3 oz	5

Nutrient Data Collection Form

Food	Amount	Book Numbers	Multiply By	Estimated Nutrient Intake
Nutrient::	RDA:	Estimated:	% of RDA:	Total Estimated:

To download additional forms for free, go to www.TopNutrients4U.com

FAT SATURATED

Alcohol	Amount	Saturated Fat (g)
White Wine	1 glass	0
Red Wine	1 glass	0
Beer, light, all types	1 bottle	0
Beer, regular, all types	1 bottle	0
Gin, Rum, Vodka, Whisky	1 Shot	0

Beans, Canned	Amount	Saturated Fat (g)
Refried beans	1 cup	0.93
Garbanzo beans	1 cup	0.49
Black-eyed peas	1 cup	0.35
Great Northern	1 cup	0.31
Navy beans	1 cup	0.29
Pinto beans	1 cup	0.28
White beans, mature	1 cup	0.20
Cranberry beans	1 cup	0.19
Kidney beans	1 cup	0.19
Baked beans, plain	1 cup	0.18
Green beans	1 cup	0.13
Fava beans	1 cup	0.10
Lima beans	1 cup	0.09
Yellow beans	1 cup	0.03

Beans, Cooked	Amount	Saturated Fat (g)
Soybeans, dry roasted	1 cup	2.91
Natto	1 cup	2.78
Soybeans, mature	1 cup	2.23
Winged beans	1 cup	1.42
Soybeans, green	1 cup	1.33
Edamame	1 cup	0.96
Lupini beans	1 cup	0.57
Garbanzo beans	1 cup	0.44
White beans, small	1 cup	0.30
Great Northern	1 cup	0.25
Black beans	1 cup	0.24
Black-eyed peas	1 cup	0.24
Mung beans, mature seeds	1 cup	0.23
Pinto beans	1 cup	0.23
Mothbeans	1 cup	0.22
Cranberry beans	1 cup	0.21
Hyacinth beans	1 cup	0.19
Navy beans	1 cup	0.18
Lima beans	1 cup	0.17
Black Turtle beans, mature	1 cup	0.17

FAT SATURATED

Continued

White beans, mature	1 cup	0.16
Pigeon peas	1 cup	0.14
Kidney beans	1 cup	0.13
Fava beans	1 cup	0.11
Split peas	1 cup	0.11
Lentils	1 cup	0.11
Adzuki	1 cup	0.08
Green beans	1 cup	0.08
Yellow beans	1 cup	0.08
Yardlong beans, Chinese long beans	1 cup	0.03

Beef, Cooked	Amount	Saturated Fat (g)
Beef ribs, trim to 1/8" fat	3 oz	9.6
Chuck roast, trim to 1/8" fat	3 oz	9.2
Porterhouse steak, lean, trim to 0" fat	3 oz	6.2
Ground beef, 75%	3 oz	6.2
Ground beef, 80%	3 oz	5.7
T-Bone steak, trim 0" fat	3 oz	5.2
Ground beef, 85%	3 oz	5.0
Tri Tip Steak, trim to 0" fat	3 oz	4.9
Top sirloin, lean, trim to 1/8" fat	3 oz	4.8
Ribeye steak, trim 0" fat	3 oz	4.7
Skirt Steak, trim to 0" fat	3 oz	4.0
Ground beef, 90%	3 oz	3.9
Filet Mignon, trim to 0" fat	3 oz	3.7
Flank steak, lean, trim to 0" fat	3 oz	2.6
Ground beef, 95%	3 oz	2.5
Brisket, lean, trim to 0" fat	3 oz	2.3
London Broil, top round, trim to 0" fat	3 oz	1.5

Beef, Cooked	Amount	Saturated Fat (g)
Beef ribs, trim to 1/8" fat	1 lb	51.4
Chuck roast, trim to 1/8" fat	1 lb	49.3
Porterhouse steak, trim to 0" fat	1 lb	33.0
T-bone steak, trim to 0" fat	1 lb	27.6
Top Sirloin, trim to 1/8" fat	1 lb	25.4
Tri Tip steak, lean, trim to 0" fat	1 lb	22.1
Skirt steak, trim to 0" fat	1 lb	21.2
Brisket, lean, trim to 0" fat	1 lb	12.0
Flank steak, lean, trim to 0" fat	1 steak	11.8
Ribeye steak, boneless, trim to 0" fat	1 steak	11.6
Filet Mignon, tenderloin, trim to 0" fat	1 steak	4.1
Ribeye filet, lean, trim to 0" fat	1 filet	3.3
Top Sirloin, choice filet, trim to 0" fat	1 filet	2.5

FAT SATURATED

Beef, Ground, Cooked	Amount	Saturated Fat (g)
Ground beef, 75%	1/4 lb patty	5.1
Ground beef, 80%	1/4 lb patty	5.2
Ground beef, 85%	1/4 lb patty	4.5
Ground beef, 90%	1/4 lb patty	3.8
Ground beef, 95%	1/4 lb patty	2.4

Bread	Amount	Saturated Fat (g)
Croissants, butter	1 medium	6.65
Indian bread, Naan, whole wheat	1 piece	3.08
Mexican roll, bollilo	1 roll	1.37
Indian bread, Naan, plain	1 piece	1.25
Egg bread	1 slice	0.64
Tortillas, flour	1 tortilla	0.60
Hamburger & Hotdog buns, plain	1 bun	0.47
English Muffin, plain, enriched	1 muffin	0.42
Dinner rolls, brown & serve	1 roll	0.39
Bagel, egg	4" bagel	0.38
Bagel, plain, enriched	4" bagel	0.35
Kaiser rolls	1 roll	0.35
Raisen bread	1 slice	0.28
Bagel, cinnamon & raisens	4" bagel	0.24
Cracked Wheat	1 slice	0.23
Multigrain or Whole grain	1 slice	0.23
Whole-Wheat	1 slice	0.21
Bagel, oat bran	4" bagel	0.20
Wheat	1 slice	0.20
Rye bread	1 slice	0.20
Oatmeal bread	1 slice	0.19
White bread	1 slice	0.18
Italian bread	1 slice	0.17
Pumpernickle	1 slice	0.14
French, or Sourdough	1 slice	0.12
Tortillas, corn	1 tortilla	0.12
Pita, white	6" pita	0.05
Bagel, wheat	4" bagel	0
Potatao bread	1 slice	0

Butter	Amount	Saturated Fat (g)
Regular dairy butter, salted	1 tbsp	7.29
Regular dairy whipped butter, salted	1 tbsp	4.75

FAT SATURATED

General Mills®	Amount	Saturated Fat (g)
Reese's Puffs	1 cup	0.65
Oatmeal Crisp, Crunchy Almond	1 cup	0.61
Cinnamon Toast Crunch	1 cup	0.59
Raisin Nut Bran	1 cup	0.56
Chocolate Chex	1 cup	0.51
Oatmeal Crisp, Apple Cinnampn	1 cup	0.50
Multi-Bran CHEX	1 cup	0.45
Basic 4	1 cup	0.44
Cocoa Puffs	1 cup	0.42
Dora The Explorer	1 cup	0.36
Cinnamon Chex	1 cup	0.24
Honey Nut Chex	1 cup	0.23
Trix	1 cup	0.21
Wheat Chex	1 cup	0.21
Cookie Crisp	1 cup	0.21
Lucky Charms	1 cup	0.18
Wheaties	1 cup	0.18
Whole Grain Total	1 cup	0.16
Total Raisin Bran	1 cup	0.16
Berry Berry Kix	1 cup	0.15
Kix	1 cup	0.14
Golden Grahams	1 cup	0.13
Honey Nut Clusters	1 cup	0.13
Corn Chex	1 cup	0.12
Rice Chex	1 cup	0.06

General Mills® Cheerios®	Amount	Saturated Fat (g)
Yogurt Burst, Strawberry	1 cup	0.67
Original	1 cup	0.42
Apple Cinnamon	1 cup	0.40
Frosted	1 cup	0.37
Honey Nut Cheerios	1 cup	0.37
Berry Burst, Triple Berry	1 cup	0.36
Chocolate	1 cup	0.36
Dulce De Leche Cheerios	1 cup	0.36
Oat Cluster Cheerios Crunch	1 cup	0.36
Honey Nut Cheerios, Medley Crunch	1 cup	0.36
Crunch Oat Clusters	1 cup	0.32
Banana Nut	1 cup	0.26
Fruity Cheerios	1 cup	0.25
Multi grain	1 cup	0.23
Cinnamon Burst	1 cup	0.22

FAT SATURATED

General Mills Fiber One®	Amount	Saturated Fat (g)
Caramel Delight	1 cup	0.5
Honey Clusters	1 cup	0
Original	1 cup	0
Raisin Bran Clusters	1 cup	0

Kashi®	Amount	Saturated Fat (g)
Blackberry Hills	1 cup	x
Heart to Heart, Nutty Chia Flax	1 cup	x
7-Whole Grain Nuggets	1 cup	0.70
Go Lean Crisp, Toasted Berry Crumble	1 cup	0.54
Go Lean Crunch, Honey Almond Flax	1 cup	0.53
Heart to Heart, Honey Toasted Oat	1 cup	0.40
Heart to Heart, Warm Cinnamon	1 cup	0.40
Heart to Heart, Oat Flakes & Blueberry Clusters	1 cup	0.33
Go Lean Crunch	1 cup	0.32
Good Friends	1 cup	0.27
Honey Sunshine	1 cup	0.24
Island Vanilla	27 biscuits	0.22
Indigo Morning	1 cup	0.22
Simply Maize	1 cup	0.22
Go Lean	1 cup	0.21
Autum Wheat	29 biscuits	0.16
Berry Blossom	1 cup	0.16
7-Whole Grain Flakes	1 cup	0.15
Berry Fruitful	29 biscuits	0.11
Cinnamon Harvest	28 biscuits	0.11
Go Lean Crisp, Cinnamon Crumble	1 cup	0.11
7-Whole Grain Honey Puffs	1 cup	0.11
7-Whole Grain Puffs	1 cup	0.09
Strawberry Fields	1 cup	0.06

Kellogg's®	Amount	Saturated Fat (g)
Cracklin' Oat bran	1 cup	3.99
Granola with Raisins	1 cup	1.26
Raisin Bran Extra	1 cup	1.13
Cocoa Krispies	1 cup	0.82
MUESLIX	1 cup	0.66
Smorz	1 cup	0.54
Froot Loops	1 cup	0.52
All-Bran Original	1 cup	0.40
Fiberplus Berry Yogurt Crunch	1 cup	0.37
All-Bran Bran Buds	1 cup	0.36
Rice Krispies Treats	1 cup	0.36

FAT SATURATED

Continued

Fiberplus Cinnamon Oat Crunch	1 cup	0.34
Smart Start, Strong Heart, Toasted Oat	1 cup	0.34
CINNABON	1 cup	0.33
All-Bran Strawberry Medley	1 cup	0.28
Crunchy Nut Golden Honey Nut Flakes	1 cup	0.25
Crunchy Nut Roasted Nut & Honey O's	1 cup	0.22
Raisin Bran	1 cup	0.22
Raisin Bran Crunch	1 cup	0.21
Frosted MINI-Wheats Bite size	1 cup	0.20
Frosted MINI-Wheats Big Bite	1 cup	0.18
Smart Start, Strong Heart, Antioxidants	1 cup	0.14
Corn Pops	1 cup	0.13
Honey Crunch Corn Flakes	1 cup	0.12
All-Bran Complete Wheat Flakes	1 cup	0.12
Apple Jacks	1 cup	0.11
Honey Smacks	1 cup	0.11
Berry Rice Krispies	1 cup	0.09
Product 19	1 cup	0.09
Rice Krispies	1 cup	0.06
Corn Flakes	1 cup	0.05
Frosted Rice Krispies	1 cup	0.04
Simply Cinnamon Corn Flakes	1 cup	0.03
Crispix	1 cup	0.03
Frosted Flakes	1 cup	0.03

Kellogg's Special-K®	Amount	Saturated Fat (g)
Chocolately Delight	1 cup	2.60
Low Fat Granolia	1 cup	1.14
Protein Plus	1 cup	0.77
Fruit & Yogurt	1 cup	0.60
Cinnamon Pecan	1 cup	0.28
Multigrain Oats & Honey	1 cup	0.17
Blueberry	1 cup	0.16
Vanilla Almond	1 cup	0.16
Original	1 cup	0.12
Red Berries	1 cup	0.06

Natures Path®	Amount	Saturated Fat (g)
Optimum Slim Low Fat Vanilla	1 cup	x
Pomegran Plus Granola	1 cup	3.3
Acai Apple Granola	1 cup	2.7
Pumpkin Flax Plus Granola	1 cup	2.1
Hemp Plus Granola	1 cup	2.0
Peanut Butter Granola	1 cup	2.0
Flax Plus Vanilla Almond Granola	1 cup	2.0

· FAT SATURATED

Continued

Flax Plus Maple Pecan Crunch	1 cup	1.3
Flax Plus Pumpkin Raisin Crunch	1 cup	0.7
Flax Plus Redberry Crunch	1 cup	0.7
Heritage Crunch	1 cup	0.7
Sunrise Crunchy Maple	1 cup	0
Sunrise Crunchy Vanilla	1 cup	0
Flax Plus Multibran Flakes	1 cup	0
Flax Plus Raisin Bran Flakes	1 cup	0
Optimum Cranberry Ginger	1 cup	0
Optimum Blueberry Cinnamon	1 cup	0

Post®	Amount	Saturated Fat (g)
Cocoa Pebbles	1 cup	1.39
Fruity Pebbles	1 cup	1.30
Great Grains, Banana Nut Crunch	1 cup	0.77
Great Grains, Crunchy Pecan Cereal	1 cup	0.69
Great Grains, Raisin, Date & Pecan	1 cup	0.59
Great Grains, Cranberry Almond Crunch	1 cup	0.51
Grape-Nuts Cereal	1 cup	0.46
Alpha-Bits	1 cup	0.33
Honeycomb Cereal	1 cup	0.28
Blueberry Morning	1 cup	0.26
Honey Nut Shredded Wheat	1 cup	0.24
Shredded Wheat, Original, spoon-size	1 cup	0.20
Grape-Nuts Flakes	1 cup	0.19
Shredded Wheat n' Bran, spoon-size	1 cup	0.19
Raisin Bran	1 cup	0.19
Bran Flakes	1 cup	0.16
Shredded Wheat, Frosted, spoon-size	1 cup	0.16
Shredded Wheat, Original, big-biscuit	1 biscuit	0.11
Golden Crisp	1 cup	0.07

Post® Honey Bunches of Oats®	Amount	Saturated Fat (g)
Just Bunches, Honey Roasted	1 cup	1.02
With Almonds	1 cup	0.34
With Vanilla Bunches	1 cup	0.34
Honey Roasted	1 cup	0.28
With Strawberries	1 cup	0.25
With Cinnamon Bunches	1 cup	0.24
Pecan Bunches	1 cup	0.23

FAT SATURATED

Quaker®	Amount	Saturated Fat (g)
Honey Graham OH'S	1 cup	2.01
CAP'N Crunch's Peanut Butter Crunch	1 cup	1.46
CAP'N Crunch	1 cup	1.21
Granola Apple Cranberry Almond	1 cup	1.13
CAP'N Crunch & Crunch Berries	1 cup	1.07
CAP'N Crunch's OOPs! All Berries	1 cup	0.73
Corn Bran Crunch	1 cup	0.73
Oatmeal Squares, Cinnamon	1 cup	0.49
Oatmeal Squares	1 cup	0.49
Oatmeal Squares, Golden Maple	1 cup	0.49
Toasted Multigrain Crisp	1 cup	0.42
LIFE Cereal, Original	1 cup	0.35
LIFE Cereal, Cinnamon	1 cup	0.33
LIFE Cereal, Maple & Brown Sugar	1 cup	0.33
Puffed Wheat	1 cup	0.06
Puffed Rice	1 cup	0.06

Cereal, Cooked	Amount	Saturated Fat (g)
Oats, regular, unenriched	1 cup	0.73
WHEATENA	1 cup	0.18
White corn grits	1 cup	0.16
Farina	1 cup	0.16
Yellow corn grits	1 cup	0.15
Malt-o-Meal plain	1 serving	0.09
CREAM OF WHEAT, regular, 10 minute	1 cup	0.08

Cheese	Amount	Saturated Fat (g)
Ricotta, whole milk	1 cup	20.41
Ricotta, part skim milk	1 cup	12.12
Cottage cheese, creamed, small curd	1 cup	3.87
Cottage cheese, lowfat, 2 %	1 cup	2.21
Cottage cheese, lowfat, 1 %	1 cup	1.46
Cottage cheese, nonfat, uncreamed	1 cup	0.25

Cheese	Amount	Saturated Fat (g)
Goat cheese, hard type	1 oz	6.98
Dubliner	1 oz	6.00
Cheddar	1 oz	5.98
Goat cheese, semisoft type	1 oz	5.85
Colby	1 oz	5.71
Cream cheese	1 oz	5.47

FAT SATURATED

Roquefort	1 oz	5.46
Fontina	1 oz	5.44
Muenster	1 oz	5.42
Monterey	1 oz	5.41
Gruyere	1 oz	5.36
Blue cheese	1 oz	5.29
American, pasteurized process, fortified	1 oz	5.12
Swiss	1 oz	5.04
Pepper Jack with Red & Green Jalapenos	1 oz	5.00
Gouda	1 oz	4.99
Brie	1 oz	4.94
Parmesan, grated	1 oz	4.91
Romano	1 oz	4.85
Provolone	1 oz	4.84
Feta	1 oz	4.24
Goat cheese, soft type	1 oz	4.13
Monterey, low fat	1 oz	3.93
Mozzarella, whole milk	1 oz	3.73
Provolone, reduced fat	1 oz	3.16
Muenster, low fat	1 oz	3.10
Mozzarella, part skim milk, low moisture	1 oz	3.08
American, pasteurized process, imitation	1 oz	2.27
American, pasteurized process, low fat	1 oz	1.24
Cheddar, lowfat	1 oz	1.23
Swiss, low fat	1 oz	0.93
Cream cheese, fat free	1 oz	0.18
Mozzarella, nonfat	1 oz	0

Cheese, Mexican	Amount	Saturated Fat (g)
Queso anejo	1 oz	5.40
Queso chihuahua	1 oz	5.34
Queso asadero	1 oz	5.09
Mexican, blend	1 oz	4.83
Queso fresco	1 oz	3.67
Mexican, blend, reduced fat	1 oz	3.28

Chicken, Cooked	Amount	Saturated Fat (g)
Breast, with skin, fried in batter	1/2 breast	4.93
Thigh, with skin, fried in batter	1 thigh	3.79
Drumstick, with skin, fried in batter	1 drumstick	2.98
Wing with skin, fried in batter	1 wing	2.86
Breast, with skin, fried with flour	1/2 breast	2.40
Breast, with skin, roasted	1/2 breast	2.15

FAT SATURATED

Wing with skin, roasted	1 wing	1.85
Drumstick, with skin, fried in flour	1 drumstick	1.79
Thigh, no skin, roasted	1 thigh	1.58
Drumstick, no skin, roasted	1 drumstick	1.36
Breast, no skin, roasted	1/2 breast	0.87

Chicken, Cooked	Amount	Saturated Fat (g)
Wing with skin, fried in flour	3 oz	5.15
Wing with skin, roasted	3 oz	4.63
Thigh with skin, fried in flour	3 oz	3.48
Thigh with skin, roasted	3 oz	3.47
Drumstick with skin, fried in flour	3 oz	3.11
Drumstick with skin, roasted	3 oz	2.25
Breast with skin, fried in flour	3 oz	2.08
Thigh meat only, no skin, roasted	3 oz	1.94
Wing meat only, no skin, roasted	3 oz	1.92
Breast with skin, roasted	3 oz	1.86
Drumstick meat only, no skin, roasted	3 oz	1.19
Breast meat only, no skin, roasted	3 oz	0.86
Cornish game hens, meat only	3 oz	0.84

CHILI

Chili, Amy's®	Amount	Saturated Fat (g)
Light in Sodium Medium Chili	1 can	2
Light in Sodium Spicy Chili	1 can	2
Medium Chili	1 can	2
Spicy Chili	1 can	2
Medium Chili with Vegetables	1 can	1
Southwestern Black Bean Chili	1 can	1
Black Bean Chili	1 can	0

Chili, Campbell's® Chunky	Amount	Saturated Fat (g)
Chunky Chili with Beans Roadhouse	1 can	6
Chunky Chili with Beans Firehouse	1 can	6
Chunky Chili no Beans	1 can	5
Chunky Chili with Beans Grilled Steak	1 can	2

Chili, Cattle Drive®	Amount	Saturated Fat (g)
Cattle Drive Golden Chili with beans	1 can	12

FAT SATURATED

Chili, Dennison's®	Amount	Saturated Fat (g)
Original Chili Con Carne with Beans	1 can	12
Hot Chili Con Carne with Beans	1 can	12
Chunky Chili Con Carne With Beans	1 can	9
Hot & Chunky Chili with Beans	1 can	9
Turkey Chili with Beans	1 can	3
Vegetarian Chili With Beans	1 can	0

Chili, Eden® Organic	Amount	Saturated Fat (g)
Kidney Bean & Kamut Chili	1 can	0
Black Bean & Quinoa Chili	1 can	0
Pinto Bean & Spelt Chili	1 can	0
Great Northern Bean & Barley Chili	1 can	0

Chili, Hardy Jack's®	Amount	Saturated Fat (g)
Chili no Beans	1 can	22
Chili with Beans	1 can	14

Chili, Healthy Valley®	Amount	Saturated Fat (g)
Santa Fe White Bean Chili	1 can	0
Black Bean Mole Chili	1 can	0
Black Bean Mango Chili	1 can	0
Spicy Tomato Chili	1 can	0
Three Bean Chipotle Chili	1 can	0
No salt Added Tame Tomato Chili	1 can	0

Chili, Hormel®	Amount	Saturated Fat (g)
Chili no Beans	1 can	8
Less Sodium Chili no Beans	1 can	8
Cook- off White Chicken Chili	1 can	8
Chili with Beans	1 can	6
Chunky Chili with Beans	1 can	6
Hot Chili with beans	1 can	6
Less Sodium Chili with Beans	1 can	6
Cook-off Roasted Tomato Chili	1 can	6
Cook-off Chipotle Chicken Chili	1 can	4
Turkey Chili with Beans	1 can	2
Turkey Chili no Beans	1 can	2
Vegetarian Chili with Beans, 99% Fat Free	1 can	0

FAT SATURATED

Chili, Nalley's®	Amount	Saturated Fat (g)
Thick Chili with beans	1 can	6
Original Chili with beans	1 can	6
Jalapeno Hot Chili with beans	1 can	5
Turkey Chili with beans	1 can	2

Chili, Stagg®	Amount	Saturated Fat (g)
Steak House Chili no Beans	1 can	20
Classi Chili with beans	1 can	16
Country Brand Chili with Beans	1 can	14
Country Brand Mild Chili Sweet Bell Peppers	1 can	14
Dynamite Hot Chili with Beans	1 can	14
Laredo Chili with Beans, chili & Jalapno	1 can	14
Chunkero Chili with Beans	1 can	12
White Chicken Chili with Beans	1 can	10
Fiesta Grille Chili with Beans	1 can	8
Silverado Beef Chili with Beans	1 can	6
Ranch House Chicken Chili with Beans	1 can	4
Turkey Ranchero Chili with Beans	1 can	2
Vegetarian Garden Four Bean Chili	1 can	0

Chili, Wolf Brand	Amount	Saturated Fat (g)
Chili no Beans	1 can	22
Hot Chili no Beans	1 can	22
Chili with Beans	1 can	10
Homestyle Chili with Beans	1 can	10
Spicy Chili with Beans	1 can	9
Lean Beaf no Beans	1 can	4
Lean Beaf with Beans	1 can	3
Turkey Chili with Beans	1 can	1
Turkey Chili no Beans	1 can	1

Cream	Amount	Saturated Fat (g)
Heavy Cream	1 tbsp	5.6
Light Coffe Cream	1 tbsp	2.9
Sour Cream, cultured	1 tbsp	2.4
Sour Cream, reduced fat	1 tbsp	1.8
Half & Half	1 tbsp	1.1
Whipped Topping, pressurized	1 tbsp	0.4

Eggs	Amount	Saturated Fat (g)
Egg whole, scrambled	1 large	2.03
Egg whole, fried	1 large	1.99

FAT SATURATED

Continued

Egg whole, hard boiled	1 large	1.63
Egg yolk	1 large	1.59
Egg whole, poached	1 large	1.56
Egg substitute, liquid, fat free	1/4 cup	0
Egg whites	1 large	0
Egg whites, dried	1 ounce	0
Egg whites, dried powder, stabilized	1 tbsp	0

Fish, Canned	Amount	Saturated Fat (g)
Light tuna, in oil	3 oz	1.30
Atlantic Sardines, in oil	3 oz	1.30
White (albacore) tuna, in oil	3 oz	1.09
White (albacore) tuna, in water	3 oz	0.67
Light tuna, in water	3 oz	0.18

Fish, Cooked	Amount	Saturated Fat (g)
Yellowtail	3 oz	x
Florida pompano	3 oz	3.82
Atlantic mackerel	3 oz	3.55
Atlantic croaker	3 oz	2.96
Catfish, breaded & fried	3 oz	2.80
King salmon, chinook, dry heated	3 oz	2.73
Shark	3 oz	2.72
Greenland halibut	3 oz	2.64
Pacific & Jack mackerel	3 oz	2.45
Atlantic salmon, farmed	3 oz	2.13
Atlantic herring, pickled	3 oz	2.03
Coho salmon, farmed	3 oz	1.65
Swordfish	3 oz	1.62
Spanish mackerel	3 oz	1.53
Rainbow trout, farmed	3 oz	1.40
Rainbow trout, wild	3 oz	1.38
Bluefin tuna, fresh	3 oz	1.37
Catfish, farmed	3 oz	1.35
Carp	3 oz	1.18
Atlantic salmon, wild	3 oz	1.07
Keta (chum) salmon	3 oz	0.92
Coho salmon, wild	3 oz	0.90
Freshwater bass	3 oz	0.85
Pink salmon	3 oz	0.83
Tilapia	3 oz	0.80
King salmon, chinook, smoked	3 oz	0.79
Sockeye salmon	3 oz	0.77
Catfish, wild	3 oz	0.63
Sea bass	3 oz	0.56

FAT SATURATED

Continued

Striped bass	3 oz	0.55
Flounder & Sole	3 oz	0.46
Alaskan halibut	3 oz	0.42
King mackerel	3 oz	0.40
Skipjack (aku) tuna	3 oz	0.36
Whiting	3 oz	0.34
Snapper	3 oz	0.31
Atlantic & Pacific halibut	3 oz	0.30
Atlantic perch	3 oz	0.28
Walleye pike	3 oz	0.27
Grouper	3 oz	0.25
Yellowfin tuna	3 oz	0.17
Atlantic pollock	3 oz	0.15
Atlantic cod	3 oz	0.14
Walleye pollock	3 oz	0.14
Northern pike	3 oz	0.13
Haddock	3 oz	0.09
Pacific cod	3 oz	0.09
Orange roughy	3 oz	0.03

Fish, Shellfish, Cooked	Amount	Saturated Fat (g)
Oysters, breaded & fried	3 oz	2.72
Clams, breaded & fried	3 oz	2.28
Scallops, breaded & fried	3 oz	2.27
Shrimp, breaded & fried	3 oz	1.77
Squid, fried	3 oz	1.60
Abalone	3 oz	1.40
Blue crab cakes	3 oz	1.26
Eastern oysters, wild	3 oz	0.63
Eastern oysters, farmed	3 oz	0.58
Shrimp	3 oz	0.44
Octopus	3 oz	0.39
Clams, canned	3 oz	0.26
Northern lobster	3 oz	0.18
Blue crab	3 oz	0.17
Shrimp, canned	3 oz	0.16
Queen crab	3 oz	0.16
Crayfish	3 oz	0.15
Alaskan king crab, imitation	3 oz	0.15
Alaskan king crab	3 oz	0.11

FAT SATURATED

Game Meat, Cooked	Amount	Saturated Fat (g)
Bison, ground	3 oz	5.49
Elk, ground	3 oz	3.40
Deer, ground	3 oz	3.39
Duck	3 oz	3.36
Caribou	3 oz	1.45
Wild boar	3 oz	1.11
Deer	3 oz	1.06
Rabbit	3 oz	0.89
Antelope	3 oz	0.82
Squirrel	3 oz	0.72
Elk	3 oz	0.60
Buffalo, steak, free range	3 oz	0.51

Ice Cream	Amount	Saturated Fat (g)
Haagen-Dazs Vanilla	1 cup	20
Haagen-Dazs Chocolate	1 cup	20
Haagen-Dazs Strawberry	1 cup	18
Haagen-Dazs Rocky Road	1 cup	16
Blue Bunny Vanilla	1 cup	10
Blue Bunny Butter Pecan	1 cup	9
Breyers Chocolate	1 cup	9
Nestle Drumstick	1 drumstick	9
Party Pail Vanilla Ice Cream	1 cup	9
Blue Bunny Homemade Chocolate	1 cup	9
Breyers Vanilla	1 cup	8
Dreyers Rocky Road	1 cup	8
Dreyers Chocolate	1 cup	8
Blue Bunny Rocky Road	1 cup	7
Breyers Rocky Road	1 cup	7
Dreyers Strawberry	1 cup	6
Breyers Natural Strawberry	1 cup	6
Breyers Butter Pecan	1 cup	4
Dreyers Sherbet, Orange	1 cup	2
Dreyers Slow Churned Rocky Road	1 cup	2
Albertson's Sherbet, pineapple	1 cup	1
Kroger Delux Mango Sherbet, Fat Free	1 cup	0

FAT SATURATED

Lamb, Cooked	Amount	Saturated Fat (g)
Chops, loin, lean, trim to 1/4" fat	3 oz	8.36
Ground	3 oz	6.90
Leg, whole	3 oz	5.86
Foreshank, trim to 1/8" fat	3 oz	4.79
Rib, lean, trim to 1/4" fat	3 oz	3.95
Cubed, for stew or kabob	3 oz	2.23

Milk	Amount	Saturated Fat (g)
Coconut milk, canned	1 cup	42.75
Canned milk, condensed, sweetened	1 cup	16.79
Canned milk , evaporated	1 cup	11.57
Sheep milk	1 cup	11.28
Goat milk	1 cup	6.51
Human milk	1 cup	4.94
Buttermilk, whole milk	1 cup	4.65
Whole milk, liquid, 3.25%	1 cup	4.55
Reduced fat, 2%	1 cup	3.07
Lowfat, 1%	1 cup	1.55
Buttermilk, lowfat	1 cup	1.34
Soy milk, original, unfortified	1 cup	0.50
Canned milk, evaporated, nonfat	1 cup	0.31
Nonfat, fat free or skim milk	1 cup	0.14
Dry, instant, non fat	1 cup	0.11

Nuts & Seeds	Amount	Saturated Fat (g)
Coconut, raw meat	1 oz	8.42
Brazilnuts	1 oz	4.29
Macadamia	1 oz	3.42
Peanut butter, smooth style	1 oz	2.98
Pumpkin seeds	1 oz	2.46
Trail mix, tropical	1 oz	2.40
Cashews	1 oz	2.21
Tahini	1 oz	2.13
Sesame seeds	1 oz	1.97
Mixed nuts, roasted with peanuts & salt	1 oz	1.96
Mixed nuts, roasted with peanuts, no salt	1 oz	1.96
Peanuts	1 oz	1.94
Pecans	1 oz	1.75
English walnuts	1 oz	1.74
Trail mix, regular with chocolate chips	1 oz	1.73
Pistachio	1 oz	1.58
Trail mix, regular with salt	1 oz	1.57
Trail mix, regular, salted	1 oz	1.57

FAT SATURATED

Continued

Pine nuts	1 oz	1.39
Hazelnuts	1 oz	1.27
Sunflower seeds	1 oz	1.26
Almonds	1 oz	1.06
Flaxseeds	1 oz	1.04
Black walnuts	1 oz	0.96
Chia seeds	1 oz	0.94

Nuts & Seeds	Amount	Saturated Fat (g)
Peanut butter, smooth	1/4 cup	6.78
Coconut meat, shredded	1/4 cup	5.94
Brazilnuts, whole	1/4 cup	5.03
Macadamia, whole	1/4 cup	4.04
Trail mix, tropical	1/4 cup	2.97
Pumpkin seeds	1/4 cup	2.79
Sesame seeds	1/4 cup	2.51
Peanuts	1/4 cup	2.49
Mixed nuts, roasted with peanuts, no salt	1/4 cup	2.36
Trail mix, regular with chocolate chips	1/4 cup	2.22
Trail mix, regular, salted	1/4 cup	2.08
Pistachio	1/4 cup	1.71
Pine nuts	1/4 cup	1.65
Sunflower seeds	1/4 cup	1.56
Flaxseeds	1/4 cup	1.54
English walnuts	1/4 cup	1.53
Pecans, halves	1/4 cup	1.53
Almonds	1/4 cup	1.33
Hazelnuts, chopped	1/4 cup	1.28
Black walnuts, chopped	1/4 cup	1.05
Sesame seeds	1 tbsp	0.63
Flaxseeds	1 tbsp	0.38
Cashews	1/4 cup	x
Chia seeds	1/4 cup	x

Oils	Amount	Saturated Fat (g)
Coconut oil	1 tbsp	11.76
Palm kernal vegetable oil	1 tbsp	11.08
Menhaden fish oil	1 tbsp	4.14
Sardine oil	1 tbsp	4.06
Cottonseed oil	1 tbsp	3.52
Code liver fish oil	1 tbsp	3.08
Salmon fish oil	1 tbsp	2.70
Peanut oil	1 tbsp	2.28
Soybean oil	1 tbsp	2.13
Soybean lecithin oil	1 tbsp	2.04

FAT SATURATED

Continued

Soybean, partially hydrogenated	1 tbsp	2.03
Sesame oil	1 tbsp	1.93
Olive oil	1 tbsp	1.86
Corn oil	1 tbsp	1.76
Acocado oil	1 tbsp	1.62
Sunflower, high linoleic acid	1 tbsp	1.40
Sunflower, high oleic acid	1 tbsp	1.38
Canola oil, partially hydrogenated	1 tbsp	1.38
Grapeseed oil	1 tbsp	1.31
Walnut oil	1 tbsp	1.24
Flaxseed oil	1 tbsp	1.22
Canola oil	1 tbsp	1.03
Safflower, high oleic acid, oil	1 tbsp	1.03
Safflower, high linoleic acid, oil	1 tbsp	0.84

Pork, Cooked	Amount	Saturated Fat (g)
Bacon	3 oz	11.68
Spareribs	3 oz	9.45
Polish sausage	3 oz	8.79
Bratwurst	3 oz	8.50
Italian sausage	3 oz	8.21
Braunschweiger	3 oz	7.91
Sausage	3 oz	7.78
Backribs	3 oz	6.63
Liverwurst spread	1/4 cup	5.46
Cured ham	3 oz	5.08
Pork chops, pan fried	3 oz	4.14
Center loin pork chops	3 oz	2.99
Pork chops, brioled	3 oz	2.99
Bacon	3 slices	2.61
Sausage	2 links	2.38
Pork chops, lean, pan fried	3 oz	2.21
Pork chops, lean, brioled	3 oz	1.83
Cured ham, lean	3 oz	1.56
Sirloin pork chops	3 oz	1.52
Canadian-style bacon	2 slices	1.34
Tenderloin	3 oz	1.15

FAT SATURATED

SALAD DRESSING

Annie's Organic Dressings	Amount	Saturated Fat (g)
Redwine & Olive Oil	2 tbsp	2
Green Goddness Dressing	2 tbsp	1.5
Asian Sesame	2 tbsp	1
Balsamic Vinaigrette	2 tbsp	1
Buttermilk Dressing	2 tbsp	1
Caesar Dressing	2 tbsp	1
Cowgirl Ranch Dressing	2 tbsp	1
Creamy Asiago Cheese	2 tbsp	1
French Dressing	2 tbsp	1
Goddnes	2 tbsp	1
Oil & Vinegar	2 tbsp	1
Papaya Poppy Seed	2 tbsp	1
Roasted Garlic Vinaigrette	2 tbsp	1
Sesame Ginger Vinaigrette	2 tbsp	1
Shiitake Sesame	2 tbsp	1
Thousand Island	2 tbsp	1
Green Garlic	2 tbsp	0.5
Pomegranate Vinaigrette	2 tbsp	0.5

Bernstein's Dressing	Amount	Saturated Fat (g)
Creamy Caesar	2 tbsp	2.0
Restaurant Recipe Italian	2 tbsp	2.0
Balsamic Italian	2 tbsp	1.5
Cheese & Garlic Italian	2 tbsp	1.5
Chunky Blue Chees	2 tbsp	1.5
Italian & Marinade	2 tbsp	1.5
Basil Parmesan	2 tbsp	1.0
Cheese Fantastico	2 tbsp	1.0
Herb Garden French	2 tbsp	1.0
Redwine & Garlic Italian	2 tbsp	1.0
Light Fantastic Cheese Fantastico	2 tbsp	0.5
Light Parmesan Garlic Ranch	2 tbsp	0.5
Sweet Herb Italian	2 tbsp	0.5
Fat Free Cheese & Garlic Italian	2 tbsp	0
Light Roasted Garlic Balsamic	2 tbsp	0

FAT SATURATED

Best Food® Mayonnaise Dressing	Amount	Saturated Fat (g)
Real Mayonnaise	2 tbsp	3
Mayonesa Con Jugo De Lemon	2 tbsp	3
Light Mayonnaise	2 tbsp	1
Mayonnaise with Olive Oil	2 tbsp	1
Canola Cholesterol Free Mayonnaise	2 tbsp	0

Bob's Big Boy® Dressing	Amount	Saturated Fat (g)
Blue Cheese	2 tbsp	3
Roquefort	2 tbsp	3
Ranch	2 tbsp	2
Thousand Island	2 tbsp	1

Bolthouse Farms Desssing	Amount	Saturated Fat (g)
Caesar Parmigino Yogurt Dressing	2 tbsp	1.0
Chunky Bluecheese Yogurt Dressing	2 tbsp	1.0
Chunky Blue Cheese & Olive Oil	2 tbsp	0.5
Classic Ranch Yogurt Dressing	2 tbsp	0.5
Honey Mustard Yogurt Dressing	2 tbsp	0.5
Salsa Ranch Yogurt Dressing	2 tbsp	0.5
Asian Ginger & Olive Oil Vinaigrettes	2 tbsp	0
Classic Balsamic & Olive Oil	2 tbsp	0
Raspberry Merlot & Olive Oil	2 tbsp	0
Thousand Island Yogurt Dressing	2 tbsp	0
Zesty French Yogurt	2 tbsp	0

Brianna's Dressing	Amount	Saturated Fat (g)
Asiago Caesar	2 tbsp	2.0
Classic Buttermilk Ranch	2 tbsp	1.5
True Blue Cheese	2 tbsp	1.5
Chipotle Cheddar	2 tbsp	1.0
Dijon Honey Mustard	2 tbsp	1.0
Ginger Mandarin	2 tbsp	1.0
Real French Vinaigrette	2 tbsp	1.0
Rich Poppy Seed	2 tbsp	1.0
The New American	2 tbsp	1.0
Zesty French	2 tbsp	1.0
Blush Wine Vinaigrette	2 tbsp	0.5
Champagne Caper Vinaigrette	2 tbsp	0.5
Lively Lemon Tarragon	2 tbsp	0
Rich Santa Fe Blend	2 tbsp	0

FAT SATURATED

Cardin's Dressing	Amount	Saturated Fat (g)
Aged Parmesan Ranch	2 tbsp	2.5
Original Caesar	2 tbsp	2.5
Asian Sesame	2 tbsp	1.5
Balsamic Vinaigrette	2 tbsp	1.5
Honey Mustard	2 tbsp	1.5
Pear Vinaigrette	2 tbsp	1.5
Raspberry Pomegranate	2 tbsp	1.5
Roasted Asian Sesame	2 tbsp	1.5
Italian	2 tbsp	1.0
Light Caesar	2 tbsp	1.0
Fat Free Caesar	2 tbsp	0

Drew's® Dressing	Amount	Saturated Fat (g)
Greek Olive	2 tbsp	2.0
Honey Dijon	2 tbsp	2.0
Lemon Goddess	2 tbsp	2.0
Poppy Seed	2 tbsp	2.0
Rosemary Balsamic	2 tbsp	2.0
Shiitake Ginger	2 tbsp	2.0
Smoked Tomato	2 tbsp	2.0
Thai Sesame Lime	2 tbsp	2.0
Buttermilk Ranch	2 tbsp	1.0
Classic Italian	2 tbsp	1.0
Roasted Garlic & Peppercorn	2 tbsp	1.0
Sesame Orange	2 tbsp	1.0

Girard's® Dressing	Amount	Saturated Fat (g)
Blue Cheese Vinaigrette	2 tbsp	2.0
Caesar	2 tbsp	2.0
Champagne	2 tbsp	2.0
Old Venice Italian	2 tbsp	2.0
Original French	2 tbsp	2.0
Apple Poppy Seed	2 tbsp	1.5
Chinese Chicken Salad	2 tbsp	1.5
Creamy Balsamic Vinaigrette	2 tbsp	1.5
Greek Feta Vinaigrette	2 tbsp	1.5
Light Caesar	2 tbsp	1.5
White Balsamic Vinaigrette	2 tbsp	1.5
Spinach Salad Dressing	2 tbsp	0

FAT SATURATED

Hidden Valley® Creamy Dressing	Amount	Saturated Fat (g)
Bacon Ranch	2 tbsp	2.5
Classic Cheese Ranch	2 tbsp	2.5
Coleslaw	2 tbsp	2.5
Original Ranch Dressing	2 tbsp	2.5
Cracked Peppercorn Ranch	2 tbsp	2.0
Garden Vegetable Ranch	2 tbsp	2.0
Old Fashioned Buttermilk Ranch	2 tbsp	2.0
Spicy Ranch	2 tbsp	2.0
Buttermilk Ranch Light	2 tbsp	1.0
Original Ranch Light	2 tbsp	1.0
Original Ranch Fat Free	2 tbsp	0

Hidden Valley® Farm House Dressing	Amount	Saturated Fat (g)
Creamy Parmesan	2 tbsp	2.0
Hickory Bacon & Onion	2 tbsp	2.0
Roasted Onion Parmesan	2 tbsp	2.0
Savory Bleu Cheese	2 tbsp	2.0
Creamy Balsamic with Herb	2 tbsp	1.5
Garden Tomato & Bacon	2 tbsp	1.5
Original Caesar	2 tbsp	1.5
Southwest Chipotle	2 tbsp	1.5
Dijon Mustard Vinaigrette	2 tbsp	0.5
Homestyle Italian	2 tbsp	0.5
Original Italian with Herb	2 tbsp	0
Pomegranate Vinaigrette	2 tbsp	0

Ken's Steak House Dressing	Amount	Saturated Fat (g)
Buttermilk Ranch Dressing	2 tbsp	3.0
Creamy Caesar Dressing	2 tbsp	3.0
Pepper Corn Ranch	2 tbsp	3.0
Caesar Dressing	2 tbsp	2.5
Chunky Blue Cheese	2 tbsp	2.5
Italian Marinade	2 tbsp	2.5
Ranch Dressing	2 tbsp	2.5
3 Cheese Italian	2 tbsp	2.0
Creamy Italian	2 tbsp	2.0
Italian & Aged Romano	2 tbsp	2.0
Red Wine Vinegar Oil	2 tbsp	2.0
Russian Dressing	2 tbsp	2.0
Thousand Island	2 tbsp	2.0
Balsamic Vinaigrete	2 tbsp	1.5
Greek & Olive Oil	2 tbsp	1.5
Honey Mustard	2 tbsp	1.5

FAT SATURATED

Continued

Balsamic & Honey	2 tbsp	1.0
Italian with Olive Oil	2 tbsp	1.0
Northern Italian Basil & Romano	2 tbsp	1.0
Zesty Italian	2 tbsp	1.0
Sweet Vidalia Onion	2 tbsp	0.5

Ken's Lite Dressings	Amount	Saturated Fat (g)
Ken's Lite Creamy Caesar Dressing	2 tbsp	1.5
Ken's Lite Blue Cheese Dressing	2 tbsp	1.0
Ken's Lite Caesar	2 tbsp	1.0
Lite Chunky Blue Cheese Dressing	2 tbsp	1.0
Lite Ranch Dressing	2 tbsp	1.0
Lite Raspberry & Walnut Vinaigrette	2 tbsp	1.0
Lite Sweet Vidalia Onion	2 tbsp	1.0
Lite Asian Sesame Ginger & Soy	2 tbsp	0.5
Lite Thousand Island	2 tbsp	0.5
Lite Zesty Italian	2 tbsp	0.5

Kraft® Dressings	Amount	Saturated Fat (g)
Classic Caesar Dressing	2 tbsp	2.5
Green Goddnes	2 tbsp	2.5
Ranch with Backon	2 tbsp	2.5
Buttermilk Ranch	2 tbsp	2.0
Creamy French Dressing	2 tbsp	2.0
Cucumber Ranch	2 tbsp	2.0
Peppercorn Ranch	2 tbsp	2.0
Roka Blue Cheese	2 tbsp	2.0
Thousand Island	2 tbsp	2.0
Coleslaw Dressing	2 tbsp	1.5
Creamy Italian Dressing	2 tbsp	1.5
Creamy Poppyseed	2 tbsp	1.5
Ranch	2 tbsp	1.5
Classic Catalina	2 tbsp	1.0
Sweet Honey Catalina	2 tbsp	1.0
Sweet Balsamic Vinaigrette Dressing	2 tbsp	0.5
Zesty Italian Anything Dressing	2 tbsp	0.5
Zesty Italian Dressing & Marinade	2 tbsp	0.5
Lite Ranch	2 tbsp	0.5
Free Thousand Island	2 tbsp	0
Light Thousand Island	2 tbsp	0
Light Zesty Italian Dressing	2 tbsp	0
Fat Free Ranch	2 tbsp	0
Catalina Fat Free	2 tbsp	0

FAT SATURATED

Litehouse Salad Dressings	Amount	Saturated Fat (g)
Big Bleu Dressing	2 tbsp	2
Organic Ranch	2 tbsp	2
Ceaser-Caesar Dressing	2 tbsp	1.5
Chunky Bleu Cheese	2 tbsp	1.5
Original Bleu Cheese	2 tbsp	1.5
Barbecue Ranch	2 tbsp	1
Buttermilk Ranch	2 tbsp	1
Ceaser Dressing	2 tbsp	1
Chunky Garlic Caesar	2 tbsp	1
Creamy Cilantro	2 tbsp	1
Homestyle Ranch	2 tbsp	1
Honey Mustard	2 tbsp	1
Jalapeno Ranch	2 tbsp	1
Original Thousand Island	2 tbsp	1
Parmesan Caesar	2 tbsp	1
Ranch Dressing	2 tbsp	1
Yogurt Bleu Cheese with Kefir	2 tbsp	1.0
Coleslaw Dressing	2 tbsp	0.5
Coleslaw with Pineapple	2 tbsp	0.5
Spinach	2 tbsp	0.5
Sweet French	2 tbsp	0.5
Yogurt Ranch with Kefir	2 tbsp	0.5
Harvest Cranberry Greek	2 tbsp	0.0
Pear Gorzonzola Dressing	2 tbsp	0
Sesame Ginger	2 tbsp	0

Litehouse Lite Dressings	Amount	Saturated Fat (g)
Bleu Cheese Dressing	2 tbsp	1
Jalapeno Ranch Dressing	2 tbsp	1
Caesar Dressing	2 tbsp	1
Ranch Dressing	2 tbsp	1
1000 Island Dressing	2 tbsp	0
Coleslaw Dressing	2 tbsp	0
Creamy Ranch Dressing	2 tbsp	0

Litehouse Vinaigrette Dressing	Amount	Saturated Fat (g)
Bleu Cheese Vinaigrette	2 tbsp	1
Organic Balsamic Vinaigrette	2 tbsp	1
Balsamic Vinaigrette	2 tbsp	1
Raspberry Walnut Vinaigrette	2 tbsp	1
White Balsamic Vinaigrette	2 tbsp	1
Cherry Vinaigrette	2 tbsp	0
Fuji Apple Vinaigrette	2 tbsp	0

FAT SATURATED

Continued

Greek Vinaigrette	2 tbsp	0
Harvest Cranberry Vinaigrette	2 tbsp	0
Huckleberry Vinaigrette	2 tbsp	0
Pomegranate Blueberry Vinaigrette	2 tbsp	0
Zesty Italian Vinaigrette	2 tbsp	0

Marie's Dressings	Amount	Saturated Fat (g)
Caesar	2 tbsp	3.5
Chunky Blue Cheese	2 tbsp	3.5
Super Blue Cheese	2 tbsp	3.5
Asiago Peppercorn	2 tbsp	3.0
Creamy Chipotle Ranch	2 tbsp	3.0
Creamy Italian Garlic	2 tbsp	3.0
Creamy Ranch	2 tbsp	3.0
Jalapeno Ranch	2 tbsp	3.0
Blue Cheese Vinaigrette	2 tbsp	2.5
Buttermilk Ranch	2 tbsp	2.5
Creamy Caesar	2 tbsp	2.5
Thousand Island	2 tbsp	2.5
Coleslaw	2 tbsp	2.0
Greek Vinaigrette	2 tbsp	2.0
Honey Dijon	2 tbsp	2.0
Honey Mustard	2 tbsp	2.0
Poppy Seed	2 tbsp	2.0
Italian Vinaigrette	2 tbsp	1.5
Lite Chunky Blue Cheese	2 tbsp	1.5
Sesame Ginger	2 tbsp	1.5
Yogurt Blue Cheese	2 tbsp	1.5
Lite Creamy Ranch	2 tbsp	1
Yogurt Coleslaw	2 tbsp	1
Yogurt Ranch	2 tbsp	1
Yogurt Thousand Island	2 tbsp	1
Balsamic Vinaigrette	2 tbsp	0.5
Red Wine Vinaigrette	2 tbsp	0.5
Raspberry Vinaigrette	2 tbsp	0
Spinach Salad with Bacon	2 tbsp	0

Newman's® Own Dressings	Amount	Saturated Fat (g)
Creamy Ceasar Dressing	2 tbsp	3.0
Caesar Dressing	2 tbsp	2.5
Olive Oil & Vinegar	2 tbsp	2.5
Ranch Dressing	2 tbsp	2.5
Family Italian	2 tbsp	2.0
Parmesan & Roasted Garlic	2 tbsp	2.0
Poppy Seed	2 tbsp	2.0

FAT SATURATED

Continued

3 Cheese Balsamic	2 tbsp	1.5
Creamy Balsamic	2 tbsp	1.5
Greek Vinaigrette	2 tbsp	1.5
Honey French	2 tbsp	1.5
Balsamic Vinaigrette	2 tbsp	1.0
Orange Ginger	2 tbsp	0.5

Newman's® Lite Dressing	Amount	Saturated Fat (g)
Caesar	2 tbsp	1
Italian Dressing	2 tbsp	1
Balsamic Dressing	2 tbsp	0.5
Cranberry Walnut	2 tbsp	0.5
Honey Mustard	2 tbsp	0.5
Raspberry Walnut Dressing	2 tbsp	0.5
Roasted Garlic Balsamic	2 tbsp	0.5

Walden Farm's Dressings	Amount	Saturated Fat (g)
Asian	2 tbsp	0
Bacon Ranch	2 tbsp	0
Balsamic Vinaigrette	2 tbsp	0
Bleu Cheese Dressing	2 tbsp	0
Buttermilk Ranch Dressing	2 tbsp	0
Caesar Dressing	2 tbsp	0
Chipotle Ranch Dressing	2 tbsp	0
Colesaw	2 tbsp	0
Creamy Bacon	2 tbsp	0
Creamy Italian	2 tbsp	0
French Dressing	2 tbsp	0
Honey Dijon Dressing	2 tbsp	0
Italian	2 tbsp	0
Italian Sun Dried Tomato	2 tbsp	0
Jersey Sweet Onion	2 tbsp	0
Ranch	2 tbsp	0
Raspberry Vinaigrette	2 tbsp	0
Russian	2 tbsp	0
Sesame Ginger Dressing	2 tbsp	0
Sweet Onion	2 tbsp	0
Thousand Island Dressing	2 tbsp	0
Zesty Italian	2 tbsp	0

Wish Bone® Creamy Dressings	Amount	Saturated Fat (g)
Creamy Caesar	2 tbsp	3.0
Chunky Blue Cheese	2 tbsp	2.5
Ranch Dressing	2 tbsp	2

FAT SATURATED

Continued

	Amount	Saturated Fat (g)
Sweet & Spicy French	2 tbsp	2
Thousand Island	2 tbsp	2
Creamy Italian Dressing	2 tbsp	2
Delux French	2 tbsp	2
Light Blue Cheese	2 tbsp	1
Light Creamy Caesar	2 tbsp	1
Light Parmesan Peppercorn Ranch	2 tbsp	1
Light Ranch Dressing	2 tbsp	1
Light Ranch Dressing	2 tbsp	1
Light Thousand Island	2 tbsp	1
Russian	2 tbsp	1
Light Delux French	2 tbsp	0.5
Light Sweet & Spicy French	2 tbsp	0.5
Fat Free Chunky Blue Cheese	2 tbsp	0
Fat Free Ranch Dressing	2 tbsp	0
Fat Free Ranch Dressing	2 tbsp	0

Wish Bone® Oil & Vinegar Dressings	Amount	Saturated Fat (g)
House Italian	2 tbsp	1.5
Balsamic Italian Vinaigrette	2 tbsp	1
Bruschetta Italian	2 tbsp	1
Greek Vinaigrette	2 tbsp	1
Italian	2 tbsp	1
Light Asian Sesame & Ginger	2 tbsp	1
Light Honey Dijon	2 tbsp	1
Light Raspberry Walnut	2 tbsp	1
Mediterranean Italian	2 tbsp	1
Raspberrt Hazelnut Vinaigrette	2 tbsp	1
Robusto Italian	2 tbsp	1
Romano Basil Vinaigrette	2 tbsp	1
Superfruit Vinaigrette	2 tbsp	1
Balsamic Vinaigrette	2 tbsp	0.5
Light Balsamic & Basil Vinaigrette	2 tbsp	0.5
Olive Oil Vinaigrette	2 tbsp	0.5
Red Wine Vinaigrette	2 tbsp	0.5
Fat Free Italian	2 tbsp	0
Fat Free Italian Dressing	2 tbsp	0
Fat Free Red Wine Vinaigrette	2 tbsp	0
Fat Free Red Wine Vinaigrette	2 tbsp	0
Light Italian dressing	2 tbsp	0

FAT SATURATED

SOUP

Amy's Organic Soups	Amount	Saturated Fat (g)
Amy's Lentil Soup	1 can	5.0
Amy's Light Lentil Soup	1 can	5.0
Fire Roasted Southwest Vegetable Soup	1 can	4.0
Lentil Vegetable Soup	1 can	4.0
Light Lentil Vegetable Soup	1 can	4.0
Chunky Tomato Bisque Soup	1 can	3.5
Butternut Squash Soup	1 can	3.0
Cream of Tomato Soup	1 can	3.0
Light Cream of Tomato Soup	1 can	2.5
Light Butternut Squash Soup	1 can	2.0
Black Bean Vegetable Soup	1 can	1.5
Light Minestrone Soup	1 can	1.5
Vegetable Barley Soup	1 can	1.0
Chunky Vegetable Soup	1 can	0
Light Split Pea Soup	1 can	0
Minestrone Soup	1 can	0
Split Pea Soup	1 can	0

Andersen's Soup	Amount	Saturated Fat (g)
Creamy Lentil Soup	1 can	2
Creamy Tomato Soup	1 can	0
Creamy Split Pea with Bacon Soup	1 can	0
Creamy Split Pea Soup	1 can	0

Campbell's® Chunky Soup	Amount	Saturated Fat (g)
Potato Ham Chowder	1 can	8
Baked Potato with Cheddar & Bacon Bits	1 can	6
Chicken Broccoli, Cheese & Potato	1 can	6
Chicken Corn Chowder Soup	1 can	6
Creamy Chicken & Dumplings	1 can	4
New England Clam Chowder	1 can	3
Grilled Chicken Sausage Gumbo	1 can	3
Beef with Country Vegetables	1 can	2
Classic Chicken Noodle Soup	1 can	2
Grilled Sirloin Steak & Vegetables	1 can	2
Old Fashioned Vegetable Beef	1 can	2
Sirloin Burger & Country Vegetable	1 can	2
Roasted Beef & Mushrooms & Vegetables	1 can	2

FAT SATURATED

Continued

Split Pea & Ham	1 can	2
Heart Italian Style Wedding	1 can	2
Beef with White Wild Rice	1 can	1
Hearty Beef Barley	1 can	1
Hearty Beef Noodle	1 can	1
Steak "N" Potato Soup	1 can	1
Savory Vegetable	1 can	1
Grilled Chicken with Vegetables & Pasta	1 can	1
Fajita Chicken with Rice & Beans	1 can	1
Savory Chicken & White Wild Rice	1 can	1
Savory Pot Roast	1 can	1
Hearty Bean & Ham	1 can	1
Hearty Chicken with Vegetables	1 can	1

Campbell's® Chunky Healthy Request	Amount	Saturated Fat (g)
Chicken Corn Chowder Soup	1 can	2
Classic Chicken Noodle Soup	1 can	2
Grilled Chicken & Sausage Gumbo Soup	1 can	2
Hearty Italian Style Wedding	1 can	2
Italian Style Wedding	1 can	2
Old Fashioned Vegetable Beef	1 can	2
Sirloin Burger & Country Vegetable	1 can	2
Split Pea & Ham	1 can	2
Beef with Country Vegetables	1 can	1
Roasted Chicken & Country Vegetables	1 can	1
Savory Vegetable	1 can	1
New England Clam Chowder	1 can	0

Campbell's® Home Style Soup	Amount	Saturated Fat (g)
Creamy Gouda Bisque with Chicken	1 can	6
Italian Style Wedding, Micro Wavable	1 can	5
Butternut Squash Bisque	1 can	4
Creole-Style Chicken with Red Beans & Rice	1 can	3
Creamy Chicken & Herb Dumplings	1 can	2
Chicken Noodle, Micro Wavable	1 can	1
Chicken with Whole Grain Pasta	1 can	1
Harvest Tomato with Basil	1 can	1
Light Italian Style Wedding	1 can	1
Chicken with White & Wild Rice	1 can	0
Light Chicken Noodle	1 can	0
Spicy Vegetable Chili	1 can	0

FAT SATURATED

Campbell's® Kettle Style Soup	Amount	Saturated Fat (g)
Tomato with Sweet Basil	1 can	16
Portobello Mushroom & Maderia Bisque	1 can	12
Burgurdy Beef Stew	1 can	3
Southwest Style Chicken Chili	1 can	1
Tuscan Style Chicken & White Beans	1 can	2

Campbell's® Microwavable Soup	Amount	Saturated Fat (g)
Chunky New England Clam Chowder	1 can	4
Chunky Grilled Chicken & Sausage Gumbo	1 can	4
Creamy Tomato	1 can	2
Chunky Classic Chicken Noodle	1 can	2
Chunky Beef & Country Vegetables	1 can	2
Chunky Sirloin Burger & Country Vegetables	1 can	2
Original Chicken Noodle	1 can	1
Homestyle Chicken Noodle	1 can	1

Campbell's® 100 % Natural	Amount	Saturated Fat (g)
Creamy Gouda Bisque with Chicken	1 cup	6.0
Creamy Potato & Roasted Garlic	1 cup	6.0
New England Clam Chowder	1 cup	4.0
Potato Broccoli & Cheese	1 cup	4.0
Butternut Squash Bisque	1 cup	3.0
Creole-Style Chicken & Red Beans & Rice	1 cup	3.0
Italian Style Wedding	1 cup	2.0
Chicken & Egg Noodle	1 cup	2.0
Mexican-Style Chicken Tortilla	1 cup	2.0
Nesty Tomato Bisque	1 cup	2.0
Savory Chicken & Long Grain Rice	1 cup	2.0
Chicken Tuscany	1 cup	1.0
Carmelized French Onion	1 cup	1.0
Southwestern White Chicken Chili	1 cup	1.0
98 % Light New England Clam Chowder	1 cup	1.0
Harvest Tomato with Basil	1 cup	0
Southwestern Style Vegetables	1 cup	0

Campbell's® Soup at Hand Soup	Amount	Saturated Fat (g)
Cream of Broccoli Soup	1 canister	2
Creamy Tomato Parmesan Bisque	1 canister	2
New England Clam Chowder	1 canister	2
Creamy Chicken Soup	1 canister	1.5
CreamyTomato Soup	1 canister	1.5
Chicken with Mini Noodles Soup	1 canister	1.0
Chicken & Stars Soup	1 canister	0.5

FAT SATURATED

Continued

	Amount	Saturated Fat (g)
Vegetable Beef, 70 Calories	1 canister	0.5
Chicken & Mini Noodles, 25% Less Sodium	1 canister	0.5
Classic Tomato Soup	1 canister	0
Vegetable with Mini Round Noodles	1 canister	0
Classic Tomato, 25% Less Sodium Soup	1 canister	0

Campbell's® V8 Soup	Amount	Saturated Fat (g)
V8 Garden Broccoli	1 can	2
V8 Potato Leek	1 can	1
V8 Sweet Red Pepper	1 can	1
V8 Garden Vegetable	1 can	1
V8 South West Corn	1 can	1
V8 Golden ButterNut Squash	1 can	0
V8 Tomato Herb	1 can	0

Muir Glen's Organic Soup	Amount	Saturated Fat (g)
Creamy Tomato Bisque	1 cup	6
Beef & Vegetable	1 cup	3
Chicken Tortilla	1 cup	3
Beef Barley	1 cup	2
Chicken & Wild Rice	1 cup	2
Chicken Noodle	1 cup	2
Classic Minestrone	1 cup	2
Reduced Sodium Chicken Noodle	1 cup	2
Tomato Basil Soup	1 cup	2
Garden Vegetable	1 cup	1
Homestyle Split Pea	1 cup	1
Reduced Sodium Garden Vegetable	1 cup	1
Savory Lentil Soup	1 cup	1
South West Black Bean Soup	1 cup	1

Wolfgang Puck's Organic Soup	Amount	Saturated Fat (g)
Creamy Butternut Squash	1 cup	11
Chicken & Dumplings	1 cup	7
Classic Tomato with Basil	1 cup	6
Chicken & Egg Noodles	1 cup	5
Thick Hearty Vegetable	1 cup	5
Chicken with White & Wild Rice	1 cup	4
Hearty Garden Vegetable	1 cup	4
Tortilla	1 cup	4
Classic Minestrone	1 cup	3
Black Bean	1 cup	1
Vegetable Barley	1 cup	1
Thick Hearty Lentil & Vegetable	1 cup	1

FAT SATURATED

Healthy Choice MicroWavable Soup	Amount	Saturated Fat (g)
Mediterranean Style Chicken with Orzo	1 can	x
Chicken Tortilla	1 can	3
Thai Style Chicken Brown Rice	1 can	2
Butternut Squash	1 can	2
Chicken with Rice	1 can	1
Beef Pot Roast	1 can	0
Chicken Noodles	1 can	0
Hearty Vegetable Barley	1 can	0
Cheese Tortellini	1 can	0
Tomato Basil	1 can	0
Country Vegetable	1 can	0

Turkey, Cooked	Amount	Saturated Fat (g)
Turkey bacon	3 oz	7.05
Ground turkey, 85% lean	3 oz	3.51
Ground turkey, 93% lean	3 oz	2.51
Turkey sausage, reduced fat	3 oz	2.44
Ground turkey	3 oz	2.27
Dark meat	3 oz	1.54
Liver	3 oz	1.22
Ground turkey, fat free	3 oz	0.57
Light meat	3 oz	0.50
Breast meat	3 oz	0.20

Tofu	Amount	Saturated Fat (g)
House Foods Organic Extra Firm	3 oz	1.00
Vitasoy USA, Nasoya Extra Firm	3 oz	0.60
Vitasoy USA, Azumaya Extra Firm	3 oz	0.51
House Foods Organic Cubed	3 oz	0.50
House Foods Organic Firm	3 oz	0.50
House Foods Organic Grilled	3 oz	0.50
House Foods Organic Medium Firm	3 oz	0.50
House Foods Organic Super Firm	3 oz	0.50
House Foods Premium Cubed	3 oz	0.50
House Foods Premium Extra Firm	3 oz	0.50
House Foods Premium Firm	3 oz	0.50
House Foods Premium Super Firm	3 oz	0.50
Vitasoy USA, Nasoya Firm	3 oz	0.43
Vitasoy USA, Azumaya Firm	3 oz	0.42
Mori-Nu, Silken, firm	3 oz	0.34
Mori-Nu, Silken, soft	3 oz	0.30
Vitasoy USA, Azumaya Silken	3 oz	0.26
Vitasoy USA, Nasoya Plus Firm	3 oz	0.26

FAT SATURATED

Continued

Vitasoy USA, Nasoya Silken	3 oz	0.26
Mori-Nu, Silken, extra firm	3 oz	0.25
Vitasoy USA, Nasoya Lite Firm	3 oz	0.17
Vitasoy USA, Nasoya Lite Silken	3 oz	0.17
Mori-Nu, Silken, lite firm	3 oz	0.11
Mori-Nu, Silken, lite extra firm	3 oz	0.10
House Foods Organic Soft (Silken)	3 oz	0
House Foods Premium Grilled	3 oz	0
House Foods Premium Medium Firm	3 oz	0
House Foods Premium Soft (silken)	3 oz	0

Veal, Cooked	Amount	Saturated Fat (g)
Rib	3 oz	4.60
Loin	3 oz	4.47
Sirloin	3 oz	3.83
Breast	3 oz	3.16
Ground	3 oz	2.58
Leg, top round	3 oz	2.15
Foreshank	3 oz	1.77

Nutrient Data Collection Form

Food	Amount	Book Numbers	Multiply By	Estimated Nutrient Intake
Nutrient::	RDA:	Estimated:	% of RDA:	Total Estimated:

NOTES

FAT MONOUNSATURATED

Alcohol	Amount	Monounsaturated (g)
White Wine	1 glass	0
Red Wine	1 glass	0
Beer, light	1 bottle	0
Beer, regular all types	1 bottle	0
Gin, Rum, Vodka, Whisky	1 Shot	0

Beans, Canned	Amount	Monounsaturated (g)
Garbanzo beans	1 cup	1.07
Refried beans	1 cup	0.91
Pinto beans	1 cup	0.27
Baked beans, plain	1 cup	0.24
Fava beans	1 cup	0.11
Kidney beans	1 cup	0.11
Blackeyed peas	1 cup	0.11
Navy beans	1 cup	0.10
White beans, mature	1 cup	0.07
Cranberry beans	1 cup	0.06
Great Northern beans	1 cup	0.05
Lima beans	1 cup	0.04
Green beans	1 cup	0.02
Yellow beans	1 cup	0.01

Beans, Cooked	Amount	Monounsaturated (g)
Soybeans, dry roasted	1 cup	4.44
Natto	1 cup	4.25
Winged beans	1 cup	3.70
Soybeans, mature	1 cup	3.41
Soybeans, green	1 cup	2.18
Edamame	1 cup	1.99
Lupini beans	1 cup	1.96
Garbanzo	1 cup	0.96
Navy beans	1 cup	0.26
Pinto beans	1 cup	0.23
Split peas	1 cup	0.16
Fava beans	1 cup	0.13
Lentils	1 cup	0.13
Blackeyed peas	1 cup	0.11
Mung beans, mature seeds	1 cup	0.11
White beans, small	1 cup	0.10
Black beans	1 cup	0.08
Mothbeans	1 cup	0.08
Cranberry beans	1 cup	0.07
Kidney beans	1 cup	0.07

FAT MONOUNSATURATED

Continued

Lima beans	1 cup	0.06
Black Turtle beans, mature	1 cup	0.06
White beans, mature	1 cup	0.06
Hyacinath beans	1 cup	0.05
Great Northern	1 cup	0.04
Adzuki	1 cup	0.02
Yellow beans	1 cup	0.02
Green beans	1 cup	0.02
Yardlong beans, Chinese long beans	1 cup	0.01
Pigeon peas	1 cup	0.01

Beef, Cooked	Amount	Monounsaturated (g)
Beef ribs, trimmed to 1/8" fat	3 oz	10.27
Chuck roast, trimmed to 1/8" fat	3 oz	10.01
Porterhouse steak, trimmed to 0" fat	3 oz	7.35
Ground beef, 75%	3 oz	7.31
Ground beef, 80%	3 oz	6.70
T-Bone steak, trimmed 0" fat	3 oz	6.12
Tri Tip Steak, trimmed to 0" fat	3 oz	5.89
Ribeye steak, lean, trimmed 0" fat	3 oz	5.74
Ground beef, 85%	3 oz	5.66
Skirt Steak, trimmed to 0" fat	3 oz	5.15
Ground beef, 90%	3 oz	4.20
Filet Mignon, trimmed to 0" fat	3 oz	3.87
Brisket, lean, trimmed to 0" fat	3 oz	2.53
Flank steak, lean, trimmed to 0" fat	3 oz	2.48
Ground beef, 95%, broiled	3 oz	2.31
Top sirloin, lean, trimmed to 1/8" fat	3 oz	1.98
London Broil, top round, trim to 0" fat	3 oz	1.65

Beef, Cooked	Amount	Monounsaturated (g)
Beef ribs, trimmed to 1/8" fat	1 lb of cooked	54.84
Chuck roast, trimmed to 1/8" fat	1 lb of cooked	53.48
Porterhouse steak, trimmed to 0" fat	1 lb of cooked	39.24
T-bone steak, trimmed to 0" fat	1 lb of cooked	32.68
Tri Tip steak, lean, trimmed to 0" fat	1 lb of cooked	31.43
Skirt steak, trimmed to 0" fat	1 lb of cooked	27.47
Top Sirloin, trimmed to 1/8" fat	1 lb of cooked	26.92
Ribeye steak, boneless, trimmed to 0" fat	1 steak	14.27
Brisket, lean, trimmed to 0" fat	1 lb of cooked	13.52
Flank steak, lean, trimmed to 0" fat	1 lb of cooked	13.24
Flank steak, lean, trimmed to 0" fat	1 steak	11.17
Filet Mignon, tenderloin, trimmed to 0" fat	1 steak	4.66
Ribeye filet, lean, trimmed to 0" fat	1 filet	4.14
Top Sirloin, choice filet, trimmed to 0" fat	1 filet	3.37

FAT MONOUNSATURATED

Beef, Cooked	Amount	Monounsaturated (g)
Ground beef, 75%	1/4 lb patty	6.02
Ground beef, 80%	1/4 lb patty	6.07
Ground beef, 85%	1/4 lb patty	5.13
Ground beef, 90%	1/4 lb patty	4.05
Ground beef, 95%	1/4 lb patty	2.23

Bread	Amount	Monounsaturated (g)
Croissants, butter	1 medium	3.15
Cornbread, dry mix, prepared	1 piece	3.08
Mexican roll, bollilo	1 roll	2.61
Buscuits, buttermilk, refrigerated dough	2.5 " biscuit	2.42
Indian bread, Naan, whole wheat	1 piece	2.06
Indian bread, Naan, plain	1 piece	1.62
Tortillas, flour	1 tortilla	1.25
Egg bread	1 slice	0.92
Kaiser rolls	1 roll	0.65
Raisen bread	1 slice	0.60
Dinner Rolls, brown & serve	1 roll	0.53
Hamburger & Hotdog buns, plain	1 bun	0.48
Cracked wheat	1 slice	0.48
Bagel plain, enriched	4" bagel	0.46
Whole-Wheat	1 slice	0.45
Oatmeal bread	1 slice	0.43
Rye bread	1 slice	0.42
Bagel, egg	4" bagel	0.37
Pumpernickel	1 slice	0.30
Bagel, wheat	4" bagel	0.28
Bagel, oat bran	4" bagel	0.26
English Muffin, plain, enriched	1 muffin	0.22
Wheat	1 slice	0.21
Multigrain or Whole grain	1 slice	0.20
Tortillas, corn	1 tortilla	0.18
White	1 slice	0.17
Bagel, cinnamon & raisens	4" bagel	0.16
French or Sourdough	1 slice	0.09
Pita, white	6" pita	0.03
Potato bread	1 slice	0

Butter	Amount	Monounsaturated (g)
Regular dairy butter, salted	1 tbsp	2.99
Regular dairy whipped butter, salted	1 tbsp	2.20

FAT MONOUNSATURATED

Cereal, General Mills®	Amount	Monounsaturated (g)
Cinnamon Toast Crunch	1 cup	2.72
Chocolate Chex	1 cup	2.13
Reese's Puffs	1 cup	1.82
Cinnamon Chex	1 cup	1.72
Oatmeal Crisp, Crunchy Almond	1 cup	1.65
Raisin Nut Bran	1 cup	1.57
Oatmeal Crisp, Hearty Raisin	1 cup	0.74
Dora The Explorer	1 cup	0.68
Golden Grahams	1 cup	0.66
Basic 4	1 cup	0.66
Cocoa Puffs	1 cup	0.61
Trix	1 cup	0.58
Lucky Charms	1 cup	0.57
Multi-Bran CHEX	1 cup	0.50
Cookie Crisp	1 cup	0.49
Honey Nut Chex	1 cup	0.48
Berry Berry Kix	1 cup	0.42
Kix	1 cup	0.24
Wheat Chex	1 cup	0.19
Corn Chex	1 cup	0.19
Total Raisin Bran	1 cup	0.16
Total Cranberry Crunch	1 cup	0.15
Wheaties	1 cup	0.14
Total Whole Grain	1 cup	0.12
Honey Nut Clusters	1 cup	0.11
Rice Chex	1 cup	0.08

General Mills Cheerios®	Amount	Monounsaturated (g)
Apple Cinnamon	1 cup	1.04
Honey Nut	1 cup	0.68
Berry Burst	1 cup	0.67
Original	1 cup	0.54
Yogurt Burst Strawberry	1 cup	0.50
Chocolate	1 cup	0.43
Fruity	1 cup	0.39
Frosted	1 cup	0.37
Multi grain	1 cup	0.29
Crunch, Oat Clusters	1 cup	0.27
Banana Nut	1 cup	0.26

FAT MONOUNSATURATED

General Mills Fiber One®	Amount	Monounsaturated (g)
Caramel Delight	1 cup	1.05
Honey Clusters	1 cup	0.31
Original	1 cup	0.26
Raisin Bran Clusters	1 cup	0.22

Kashi®	Amount	Monounsaturated (g)
Go Lean Crisp, Cinnamon Crumble	1 cup	2.31
Go Lean Crunch, Honey Almond Flax	1 cup	2.17
Go Lean Crunch	1 cup	1.71
7-Whole Grain Nuggets	1 cup	0.70
Heart to Heart, Honey Toasted Oat	1 cup	0.48
Heart to Heart, Warm Cinnamon	1 cup	0.48
Honey Sunshine	1 cup	0.44
Berry blossom	1 cup	0.36
Good Friends	1 cup	0.32
Go Lean	1 cup	0.21
7-Whole Grain Flakes	1 cup	0.20
7-Whole Grain Honey Puffs	1 cup	0.17
Island Vanilla	1 cup	0.17
7-Whole Grain Puffs	1 cup	0.11
Berry Fruitful	1 cup	0.11
Cinnamon Harvest	1 cup	0.11
Autumn Wheat	29 biscuits	0.11
Strawberry Fields	1 cup	0.00

Kellogg's®	Amount	Monounsaturated (g)
Cracklin' Oat Bran	1 cup	3.07
MUESLIX	1 cup	2.30
Low Fat Granola with Raisins	1 cup	1.71
Crunchy Nut Golden Honey Nut Flakes	1 cup	1.16
Crunchy Nut Roasted Nut & Honey O's	1 cup	0.97
Cinnabon	1 cup	0.90
Fiberplus Cinnamon Oat Crunch	1 cup	0.64
Rice Krispies Treats	1 cup	0.64
Smart Start, Strong Heart, Toasted Oat	1 cup	0.53
All-Bran Bran Buds	1 cup	0.45
Raisin Bran Extra	1 cup	0.44
All-Bran Original	1 cup	0.42
Honey Crunch Corn Flakes	1 cup	0.40
Raisin Bran Crunch	1 cup	0.37
Smorz	1 cup	0.30
All-Bran Strawberry Medley	1 cup	0.22
Honey Smacks	1 cup	0.22

FAT MONOUNSATURATED

Continued

	Amount	Monounsaturated (g)
All-Bran Complete Wheat Flakes	1 cup	0.19
Raisin Bran	1 cup	0.17
Cocoa Krispies	1 cup	0.17
Froot Loops	1 cup	0.15
Apple Jacks	1 cup	0.14
Frosted MINI-Wheat's, Bite-Size	1 cup	0.13
Frosted MINI-Wheat's, Big-Bite	1 cup	0.12
Frosted MINI-Wheat's, Little-Bite	1 cup	0.12
Product 19	1 cup	0.12
Berry Rice Krispies	1 cup	0.09
Smart Start, Strong Heart, Antioxidants	1 cup	0.09
Rice Krispies	1 cup	0.08
Corn Pops	1 cup	0.06
Fiberplus Berry Yogurt Crunch	1 cup	0.05
Frosted Rice Krispies	1 cup	0.04
Corn Flakes, Simply Cinnamon	1 cup	0.03
Crispix	1 cup	0.03
Corn Flakes	1 cup	0.03
Frosted Flakes	1 cup	0.02

Kellogg's Special-K®	Amount	Monounsaturated (g)
Low Fat Granolia	1 cup	1.77
Cinnamon Pecan	1 cup	1.13
Protein Plus	1 cup	0.89
Vanilla Almond	1 cup	0.88
Original	1 cup	0.54
Multigrain Oats & Honey	1 cup	0.22
Red Berries	1 cup	0.09
Chocolately Delight	1 cup	0.08
Fruit & Yogurt	1 cup	0.04
Blueberry	1 cup	0.04

Post®	Amount	Monounsaturated (g)
Great Grains, Crunchy Pecan	1 cup	4.02
Great Grains, Raisin, Date & Pecan	1 cup	2.79
Great Grains, Banana Nut Crunch	1 cup	2.01
Great Grains, Cranberry Almond Crunch	1 cup	1.92
Blueberry Morning	1 cup	1.28
Honey Nut Shredded Wheat	1 cup	0.71
Grape-Nuts Flakes	1 cup	0.58
Grape-Nuts Cereal	1 cup	0.35
Alpha-Bits	1 cup	0.30
Raisin Bran	1 cup	0.22
Golden Crisp	1 cup	0.22
Shredded Wheat, Original, spoon-size	1 cup	0.15

FAT MONOUNSATURATED

Continued

Shredded Wheat n' Bran, spoon-size	1 cup	0.14
Shredded Wheat, Frosted, spoon-size	1 cup	0.14
Honeycomb	1 cup	0.13
Bran Flakes	1 cup	0.12
Shredded Wheat, Original, big-biscuit	1 biscuit	0.09
Cocoa Pebbles	1 cup	0.08
Fruity Pebbles	1 cup	0.04

Post® Honey Bunches of Oats®	Amount	Monounsaturated (g)
Just Bunches, Honey Roasted	1 cup	5.36
With Almonds	1 cup	1.71
With Vanilla Bunches	1 cup	1.40
Pecan Bunches	1 cup	1.16
Honey Roasted	1 cup	1.13
With Strawberries	1 cup	1.03
With Cinnamon Bunches	1 cup	1.00

Quaker®	Amount	Monounsaturated (g)
Granola Apple Cranberry Almond	1 cup	6.53
CAP'N Crunch's Peanut Butter Crunch	1 cup	0.96
Oatmeal Squares, Cinnamon	1 cup	0.90
Oatmeal Squares	1 cup	0.89
Oatmeal Squares, Golden Maple	1 cup	0.89
Toasted Multigrain Crisp	1 cup	0.72
LIFE Cereal, Original	1 cup	0.62
LIFE Cereal, Cinnamon	1 cup	0.58
LIFE Cereal, Maple & Brown Sugar	1 cup	0.58
Crunchy Bran	1 cup	0.28
Honey Graham OH'S	1 cup	0.25
CAP'N Crunch	1 cup	0.23
CAP'N Crunch with Crunch Berries	1 cup	0.22
CAP'N Crunch's OOPs! All Berries	1 cup	0.19
Puffed Wheat	1 cup	0.05
Puffed Rice	1 cup	0.03

Cereal, Cooked	Amount	Monounsaturated (g)
Oats, regular, unenriched, cooked	1 cup	1.02
WHEATENA, cooked	1 cup	0.17
White corn grits	1 cup	0.16
Yellow corn grits	1 cup	0.15
Farina	1 cup	0.09
Cream of Wheat, regular, 10 minute	1 cup	0.07
Malt-o-Meal plain	1 serving	0.05

FAT MONOUNSATURATED

Cheese	Amount	Monounsaturated (g)
Ricotta, whole milk	1 cup	8.92
Ricotta, part skim milk	1 cup	5.69
Cottage cheese, creamed, small curd	1 cup	1.75
Cottage cheese, lowfat, 2 %	1 cup	1.00
Cottage cheese, lowfat, 1 %	1 cup	0.66
Cottage cheese, nonfat, uncreamed	1 cup	0.12

Cheese	Amount	Monounsaturated (g)
Cheez Whiz, pasteurized process	1 oz	x
Gruyere	1 oz	2.85
Cheddar	1 oz	2.65
Colby	1 oz	2.63
Monterey	1 oz	2.48
Muenster	1 oz	2.47
Fontina	1 oz	2.46
Cream cheese	1 oz	2.44
Roquefort	1 oz	2.40
Parmesan, grated	1 oz	2.37
American, pasteurized process, fortified	1 oz	2.34
Goat cheese, hard type	1 oz	2.30
Brie	1 oz	2.27
Romano	1 oz	2.22
Blue cheese	1 oz	2.21
Gouda	1 oz	2.20
Provolone	1 oz	2.10
Swiss	1 oz	2.06
Goat cheese, semisoft type	1 oz	1.93
Mozzarella, whole milk	1 oz	1.86
Monterey, low fat	1 oz	1.58
Muenster, low fat	1 oz	1.43
Mozzarella, part skim milk, low moisture	1 oz	1.38
Provolone, reduced fat	1 oz	1.37
Goat cheese, soft type	1 oz	1.36
Feta	1 oz	1.31
American, pasteurized process, imitation	1 oz	0.88
American, pasteurized process, low fat	1 oz	0.56
Swiss, low fat	1 oz	0.38
Cheddar, lowfat	1 oz	0.25
Cream cheese, fat free	1 oz	0.07
Mozzarella, nonfat	1 oz	0

FAT MONOUNSATURATED

Cheese, Mexican	Amount	Monounsaturated (g)
Queso anejo	1 oz	2.42
Queso chihuahua	1 oz	2.39
Queso asadero	1 oz	2.28
Mexican, blend	1 oz	2.20
Queso fresco	1 oz	1.69
Mexican, blend, reduced fat	1 oz	1.42

Chicken, Cooked	Amount	Monounsaturated (g)
Breast, with skin, fried in batter	1/2 breast	7.64
Thigh, with skin, fried in batter	1 thigh	5.76
Drumstick, with skin, fried in batter	1 drumstick	4.63
Wing, with skin, fried in batter	1 wing	4.39
Breast, with skin, fried in flour	1/2 breast	3.43
Drumstick, with skin, fried in flour	1 drumstick	2.66
Wing with skin, roasted	1 wing	2.60
Thigh, no skin, roasted	1 thigh	2.16
Breast, no skin, meat only, roasted	1/2 breast	1.07
Drumstick, no skin, meat only, roasted	1 drumstick	0.82

Chicken, Cooked	Amount	Monounsaturated (g)
Wing with skin, fried in flour	3 oz	7.56
Wing with skin, roasted	3 oz	6.49
Thigh with skin, roasted	3 oz	5.32
Thigh with skin, fried in flour	3 oz	4.99
Drumstick with skin, fried in flour	3 oz	4.61
Drumstick with skin, roasted	3 oz	3.43
Breast with skin, fried in flour	3 oz	2.98
Thigh meat only, no skin, roasted	3 oz	2.86
Breast with skin, roasted	3 oz	2.58
Wing meat only, no skin, roasted	3 oz	2.22
Drumstick meat only, no skin, roasted	3 oz	1.74
Liver	3 oz	1.20
Breast meat only, no skin, roasted	3 oz	1.05
Cornish game hen, meat only	3 oz	1.05

Cream	Amount	Monounsaturated (g)
Heavy Cream	1 tbsp	1.60
Light Coffe Cream	1 tbsp	0.84
Sour Cream, cultured	1 tbsp	0.61
Sour Cream, reduced fat	1 tbsp	0.52
Half & Half	1 tbsp	0.50
Whipped Topping, pressurized	1 tbsp	0.19

FAT MONOUNSATURATED

Eggs	Amount	Monounsaturated (g)
Egg whole, fried	1 large	2.84
Egg whole, scrambled	1 large	2.71
Egg whole, hard boiled	1 large	2.04
Egg yolk	1 large	1.95
Egg whole, poached	1 large	1.82
Egg substitute, fat free	1/4 cup	0
Egg whites, dried	1 ounce	0
Egg whites, dried powder, stabilzed	1 tbsp	0
Egg whites	1 large	0

Fish, Canned	Amount	Monounsaturated (g)
White (albacore) tuna, in oil	3 oz	2.77
Light tuna, in oil	3 oz	2.51
White (albacore) tuna, in water	3 oz	0.67
Light tuna, in water	3 oz	0.09

Fish, Cooked	Amount	Monounsaturated (g)
Yellowtail	3 oz	x
Atlantic herring, pickled	3 oz	10.16
Greenland halibut	3 oz	9.13
Atlantic mackerel	3 oz	5.96
Shark	3 oz	5.05
King salmon, chinook , dry heat	3 oz	4.88
Catfish, breaded & fried	3 oz	4.77
Atlantic croaker	3 oz	4.52
Atlantic salmon, farmed	3 oz	3.77
Coho salmon, farmed	3 oz	3.08
Swordfish	3 oz	3.01
Pacific & Jack mackerel	3 oz	2.87
Florida pompano	3 oz	2.82
Catfish, farmed	3 oz	2.65
Carp	3 oz	2.54
Atlantic salmon, wild caught	3 oz	2.29
Rainbow trout, farmed	3 oz	2.01
Spanish mackerel	3 oz	1.82
Bluefin tuna	3 oz	1.75
King salmon, chinook , smoked	3 oz	1.72
Keta (chum) salmon	3 oz	1.68
Freshwater bass	3 oz	1.56
Rainbow trout, wild	3 oz	1.48
Pink salmon	3 oz	1.37
Coho salmon, wild	3 oz	1.34
Sockeye salmon	3 oz	1.22

FAT MONOUNSATURATED

Catfish, wild	3 oz	0.93
King mackerel	3 oz	0.83
Tilapia	3 oz	0.81
Striped bass	3 oz	0.72
Alaskan halibut	3 oz	0.72
Flounder & Sole	3 oz	0.56
Atlantic perch	3 oz	0.49
Atlantic & Pacific halibut	3 oz	0.49
Sea bass	3 oz	0.46
Whiting	3 oz	0.38
Orange roughy	3 oz	0.37
Walleye pike	3 oz	0.32
Snapper	3 oz	0.27
Grouper	3 oz	0.23
Skipjack (aku) tuna	3 oz	0.21
Northern pike	3 oz	0.17
Atlantic pollock	3 oz	0.12
Yellowfin tuna	3 oz	0.12
Walleye pollock	3 oz	0.11
Atlantic cod	3 oz	0.11
Pacific cod	3 oz	0.08
Haddock	3 oz	0.06

Fish, Shellfish, Cooked	Amount	Monounsaturated (g)
Oysters, breaded & fried	3 oz	4.00
Clams, breaded & fried	3 oz	3.86
Scallops, breaded & fried	3 oz	3.82
Shrimp, breaded & fried	3 oz	3.24
Blue crab cakes	3 oz	2.39
Squid, fried	3 oz	2.34
Abalone	3 oz	2.33
Eastern oysters, wild	3 oz	0.33
Shrimp	3 oz	0.31
Queen crab	3 oz	0.28
Octopus	3 oz	0.28
Northern lobster	3 oz	0.22
Crayfish	3 oz	0.21
Eastern oysters, farmed	3 oz	0.20
Clams, canned	3 oz	0.17
Alaskan king crab	3 oz	0.16
Blue crab	3 oz	0.11
Blue crab, canned	3 oz	0.11
Alaskan king crab, imitation	3 oz	0.10
Shrimp, canned	3 oz	0.09

FAT MONOUNSATURATED

Fruit, Canned	Amount	Monounsaturated (g)
Olives, black	5 large	1.74
Olives, green	5 large	1.53
Plums	1 cup	0.17
Peaches	1 cup	0.09
Apricoits	1 cup	0.09
Pears	1 cup	0.07
Pineapple	1 cup	0.03
Applesauce, sweetened	1 cup	0.02
Applesauce, unsweetened	1 cup	0.01

Fruit, Dried	Amount	Monounsaturated (g)
Peaches	1 cup	0.45
Cranberries	1 cup	0.24
Pears	1 cup	0.24
Figs	1 cup	0.24
Apricots	1 cup	0.10
Currants	1 cup	0.07
Apples	1 cup	0.01

Fruit, Frozen	Amount	Monounsaturated (g)
Peaches	1 cup	0.12
Blackberries, unsweetened	1 cup	0.06
Strawberries	1 cup	0.05
Blueberries	1 cup	0.04
Raspberries	1 cup	0.04

Fruit, Raw	Amount	Monounsaturated (g)
Avocado California	1 cup	22.54
Avocado, Florida	1 cup	12.68
Stewed prunes	1 cup	0.20
Pomegrenates	1 cup	0.16
Valencias Oranges	1 cup	0.10
Prunes, uncooked	1 cup	0.09
Raspberries	1 cup	0.08
Raisins	1 cup	0.07
Florida Oranges	1 cup	0.07
Sweet cherries	1 cup	0.07
Strawberries	1 cup	0.07
Blackberries	1 cup	0.07
Blueberries	1 cup	0.07
Black currants	1 cup	0.07

FAT MONOUNSATURATED

Continued

Mulberries	1 cup	0.06
Water Mellon	1 cup	0.06
Dates	1 cup	0.05
Naval Oranges	1 cup	0.05
Grapefruit, pink & red, sections	1 cup	0.05
Pineapple	1 cup	0.02
Grapes	1 cup	0.01
Cataloupe	1 cup	0.01
Honeydew	1 cup	0.01

Fruit, Raw	Amount	Monounsaturated (g)
Avocado, Florida	1 fruit	16.76
Avocado, California	1 fruit	13.33
Olives, canned	5 large	1.74
Mango	1 fruit	0.29
Pomegranates	1 fruit	0.26
Papya	1 fruit	0.22
Nectarine	1 fruit	0.12
Plums	1 fruit	0.09
California valencias oranges	1 fruit	0.07
Peachs	1 fruit	0.07
Apricots	1 fruit	0.06
Asian Pears	1 fruit	0.06
Plantains	1 fruit	0.06
Florida oranges	1 fruit	0.06
Tangerine	1 fruit	0.05
Pears	1 fruit	0.04
Naval oranges	1 fruit	0.04
Banana	1 fruit	0.04
Kiwi, green	1 fruit	0.04
Oranges	1 fruit	0.03
Grapefruit, pink & red	1/2 fruit	0.03
Apples	1 fruit	0.01
Cantaloupe	1/2 fruit	0.01

Game Meat, Cooked	Amount	Monounsaturated (g)
Bison, ground	3 oz	5.02
Duck	3 oz	3.28
Elk, ground	3 oz	2.34
Deer, ground	3 oz	1.65
Wild boar	3 oz	1.45
Caribou	3 oz	1.13
Squirrel	3 oz	1.13

FAT MONOUNSATURATED

Continued

Rabbit, wild	3 oz	0.81
Deer	3 oz	0.75
Antelope	3 oz	0.54
Buffalo, steak, free range	3 oz	0.52
Elk	3 oz	0.41

Lamb, Cooked	Amount	Monounsaturated (g)
Chops, loin, lean, trimmed to 1/4" fat	3 oz	8.25
Ground	3oz	7.07
Leg, whole, trimmed to 1/4" fat	3 oz	5.92
Foreshank, trimmed to 1/8" fat	3 oz	4.83
Rib, lean, trimmed to 1/4" fat	3 oz	4.43
Cubed, for stew or kabob	3 oz	2.51

Milk	Amount	Monounsaturated (g)
Canned, condensed, sweetened	1 cup	7.43
Canned, evaporated	1 cup	5.88
Sheep milk	1 cup	4.22
Human milk	1 cup	4.08
Goat milk	1 cup	2.71
Coconut milk, canned	1 cup	2.05
Buttermilk, whole milk	1 cup	2.03
Whole milk, 3.25%	1 cup	1.98
Reduced fat, 2%	1 cup	1.37
Soy milk, original, unfortified	1 cup	0.97
Low fat, 1%	1 cup	0.68
Buttermilk, lowfat	1 cup	0.62
Canned, evaporated, non fat	1 cup	0.16
Non fat, fat free or skim liquid milk	1 cup	0.05
Dry, instant, non fat	1/3 cup	0.04

Nuts & Seeds	Amount	Monounsaturated (g)
Macadamia	1 oz	16.69
Hazelnuts	1 oz	12.94
Pecans	1 oz	11.57
Mixed nuts, roasted with peanuts, no salt	1 oz	8.90
Almonds	1 oz	8.76
Brazilnuts	1 oz	6.96
Peanuts	1 oz	6.93
Peanut butter, smooth style	1 oz	6.87
Pistachio	1 oz	6.75
Cashews	1 oz	6.75
Tahini, sesame butter	1 oz	5.76
Pine nuts	1 oz	5.32

FAT MONOUNSATURATED

Continued

Sesame seeds	1 oz	5.32
Sunflower seeds	1 oz	5.25
Trail mix, regular with chocolate chips	1 oz	4.76
Pumpkin seeds	1 oz	4.61
Black walnuts	1 oz	4.25
Trail mix, regular, salted	1 oz	3.55
English walnuts	1 oz	2.53
Flaxseeds	1 oz	2.13
Trail mix, tropical	1 oz	0.71
Chia seeds	1 oz	0.66
Coconut, raw meat	1 oz	0.40

Nuts & Seeds	Amount	Monounsaturated (g)
Cashews	1/4 cup	x
Chia seeds	1/4 cup	x
Macadamia	1/4 cup	19.72
Peanut butter, smooth style	1/4 cup	15.62
Hazelnuts	1/4 cup	13.13
Almonds	1/4 cup	11.04
Mixed nuts, roasted with peanuts, no salt	1/4 cup	10.75
Pecans, halves	1/4 cup	10.10
Peanuts	1/4 cup	8.92
Brazilnuts	1/4 cup	8.16
Pistachio	1/4 cup	7.35
Sesame seeds	1/4 cup	6.75
Sunflower seeds	1/4 cup	6.49
Pine nuts	1/4 cup	6.33
Pumpkin seeds	1/4 cup	5.24
Trail mix, regular with chocolate chips	1/4 cup	4.76
Trail mix, regular, salted	1/4 cup	4.70
Black walnuts, chopped	1/4 cup	4.69
Flaxseeds	1/4 cup	3.16
English walnuts	1/4 cup	2.22
Sesame seeds	1 tbsp	1.69
Trail mix, tropical	1/4 cup	0.87
Flaxseeds	1 tbsp	0.78
Coconut meat, shredded	1/4 cup	0.29

Oil	Amount	Monounsaturated (g)
Sunflower oil, high oleic acid	1 tbsp	11.72
Safflower oil, high oleic acid	1 tbsp	10.23
Avocado	1 tbsp	9.88
Olive oil	1 tbsp	9.85
Canola oil, partially hydrogenated	1 tbsp	9.67
Canola oil	1 tbsp	8.86

FAT MONOUNSATURATED

Continued

Cod liver oil	1 tbsp	6.35
Peanut oil	1 tbsp	6.24
Soybean, partially hydrogenated	1 tbsp	5.85
Sesame oil	1 tbsp	5.40
Sardine oil	1 tbsp	4.60
Salmon fish oil	1 tbsp	3.95
Corn oil	1 tbsp	3.75
Menhaden fish oil	1 tbsp	3.63
Walnut oil	1 tbsp	3.10
Soybean oil	1 tbsp	3.10
Sunflower, high Linoleic acid, oil	1 tbsp	2.65
Flaxseed oil	1 tbsp	2.51
Cottonseed oil	1 tbsp	2.42
Grapeseed oil	1 tbsp	2.19
Safflower oil, high linoleic acid	1 tbsp	1.95
Palm kernal oil	1 tbsp	1.55
Soybean lecithin oil	1 tbsp	1.49
Coconut oil	1 tbsp	0.79

Pork, Cooked	Amount	Monounsaturated (g)
Bacon, pan-fried	3 oz	15.74
Bratwurst	3 oz	12.49
Polish sausage	3 oz	11.50
Spareribs	3 oz	11.46
Italian sausage	3 oz	10.86
Braunschweiger	3 oz	10.82
Sausage	3 oz	10.52
Backribs	3 oz	7.90
Liverwurst spread	1/4 cup	6.76
Cured ham	3 oz	6.70
Pork chops, pan-fried	3 oz	4.66
Pork chops, broiled	3 oz	3.59
Center loin pork chops	3 oz	3.59
Canadian-style bacon	3 oz	3.43
Pork chops, lean, pan-fried	3 oz	2.57
Cured ham, lean	3 oz	2.15
Sirloin pork chops	3 oz	1.79
Tenderloin	3 oz	1.29

FAT MONOUNSATURATED

Turkey, Cooked	Amount	Monounsaturated (g)
Turkey bacon	3 oz	9.26
Ground turkey, 85% lean	3 oz	4.64
Turkey sausage, reduced fat	3 oz	3.30
Ground turkey, 93% lean	3 oz	3.29
Ground turkey	3 oz	2.94
Dark meat	3 oz	1.75
Turkey liver	3 oz	0.88
Ground turkey, fat free	3 oz	0.60
Light meat	3 oz	0.53
Breast meat	3 oz	0.11

Veal, Cooked	Amount	Monounsaturated (g)
Rib	3 oz	4.62
Loin	3 oz	4.06
Breast	3 oz	3.83
Sirloin	3 oz	3.47
Ground	3 oz	2.41
Leg, top round	3 oz	2.01
Foreshank	3 oz	1.99

Nutrient Data Collection Form

Food	Amount	Book Numbers	Multiply By	Estimated Nutrient Intake
Nutrient::	RDA:	Estimated:	% of RDA:	Total Estimated:

To download additional forms for free, go to www.TopNutrients4U.com

FAT POLYUNSATURATED

Alcohol	Amount	Polyunsaturated (g)
White Wine	1 glass	0
Red Wine	1 glass	0
Beer, light	1 bottle	0
Beer, regular all types	1 bottle	0
Gin, Rum, Vodka, Whisky	1 Shot	0

Beans, Canned	Amount	Polyunsaturated (g)
Garbanzo beans, mature	1 cup	2.11
Refried beans	1 cup	0.79
Black-eyed peas	1 cup	0.57
Kidney beans, mature	1 cup	0.55
Navy beans	1 cup	0.49
Pinto beans	1 cup	0.49
Great Northern beans	1 cup	0.42
White beans, mature	1 cup	0.33
Cranberry beans	1 cup	0.31
Baked beans, plain	1 cup	0.31
Green beans	1 cup	0.30
Fava beans	1 cup	0.23
Lima beans	1 cup	0.18
Yellow beans	1 cup	0.08

Beans, Cooked	Amount	Polyunsaturated (g)
Soybeans, dry roasted	1 cup	11.35
Natto	1 cup	10.87
Soybeans, mature	1 cup	8.71
Soybeans, green	1 cup	5.42
Edamame	1 cup	3.34
Winged beans	1 cup	2.67
Garbanzo beans	1 cup	1.90
Lupini beans	1 cup	1.21
Navy beans	1 cup	0.89
White beans, small	1 cup	0.49
Kidney beans	1 cup	0.49
Hyacinath beans	1 cup	0.48
Mothbeans	1 cup	0.45
Pinto beans	1 cup	0.40
Black beans	1 cup	0.40
Black-eyed peas	1 cup	0.39
Cranberry beans	1 cup	0.35
Lentils	1 cup	0.35
Pigeon peas	1 cup	0.34
Great Northern beans	1 cup	0.33

FAT POLYUNSATURATED

Continued

Split peas	1 cup	0.32
Lima beans, mature	1 cup	0.32
Fava beans	1 cup	0.28
Black Turtle beans, mature	1 cup	0.28
White beans, mature	1 cup	0.27
Mung beans, mature seeds	1 cup	0.26
Green beans	1 cup	0.18
Yellow beans	1 cup	0.18
Adzuki	1 cup	0.05
Yardlong beans, Chinese long beans	1 cup	0.04

Beef, Cooked	Amount	Polyunsaturated (g)
Beef ribs, trim to 1/8" fat	3 oz	0.85
Chuck roast, trim to 1/8" fat	3 oz	0.82
Porterhouse steak, trim to 0" fat	3 oz	0.59
T-Bone steak, trim 0" fat	3 oz	0.52
Ribeye steak, boneless, lean, trim 0" fat	3 oz	0.49
Ground beef, 75%	3 oz	0.45
Ground beef, 80%	3 oz	0.44
Ground beef, 85%	3 oz	0.41
Tri Tip Steak, trim to 0 " fat	3 oz	0.39
Skirt Steak, trim to 0" fat	3 oz	0.37
Ground beef, 90%, (ground sirloin)	3 oz	0.36
Filet Mignon, trim to 0" fat	3 oz	0.35
Ground beef, 95%	3 oz	0.28
Flank steak, lean, trim to 0" fat	3 oz	0.25
Brisket, lean, trim to 0" fat	3 oz	0.21
Top sirloin, lean, trim to 1/8" fat	3 oz	0.19
London Broil, top round, trim to 0" fat	3 oz	0.19

Beef, Cooked	Amount	Polyunsaturated (g)
Beef ribs, trim to 1/8" fat	1 lb	4.54
Chuck roast, trim to 1/8" fat	1 lb	4.40
Porterhouse steak, trim to 0" fat	1 lb	3.13
T-bone steak, trim to 0" fat	1 lb	2.80
Tri Tip steak, lean, trim to 0" fat	1 lb	2.09
Skirt steak, trim to 0" fat	1 lb	1.98
Top Sirloin, trim to 1/8" fat	1 lb	1.67
Flank steak, lean, trim to 0" fat	1 lb	1.33
Ribeye steak, boneless, trim to 0" fat	1 steak	1.23
Flank steak, lean, trim to 0" fat	1 steak	1.12
Filet Mignon, tenderloin, trim to 0" fat	1 steak	0.72
Brisket, lean, trim to 0" fat	1 steak	0.66
Ribeye filet, lean, trim to 0" fat	1 filet	0.33
Top Sirloin, choice filet, trim to 0" fat	1 filet	0.21

FAT POLYUNSATURATED

Beef, Ground, Cooked	Amount	Polyunsaturated (g)
Ground beef, 80%	1/4 lb patty	0.40
Ground beef, 85%	1/4 lb patty	0.37
Ground beef, 75%	1/4 lb patty	0.37
Ground beef, 90%	1/4 lb patty	0.35
Ground beef, 95%	1/4 lb patty	0.27

Bread	Amount	Polyunsaturated (g)
Indian bread, Naan, plain	1 piece	1.89
Indian bread, Naan, whole wheat	1 piece	1.33
Mexican roll, bollilo	1 roll	1.00
Kaiser rolls	1 roll	0.98
Bagel, wheat	4" bagel	0.92
Hamburger & hotdog buns, plain	1 bun	0.85
Cornbread, dry mix, prepared	1 piece	0.73
Dinner rolls, brown & serve	1 roll	0.70
Croissants, butter	1 medium	0.62
Bagel, cinnamon & raisens	4" bagel	0.60
Bagel, egg	4" bagel	0.57
Bagel, plain, enriched	4" bagel	0.57
Tortillas, flour	1 tortilla	0.51
Bagel, oat bran	4" bagel	0.50
Multigrain or whole grain	1 slice	0.49
Oatmeal bread	1 slice	0.46
Egg bread	1 slice	0.44
Pumpernickel	1 slice	0.40
Tortillas, corn	1 tortilla	0.40
Wheat bread	1 slice	0.36
White bread	1 slice	0.34
English muffin, plain, enriched	1 muffin	0.28
Rye bread	1 slice	0.26
Reduced calorie wheat	1 slice	0.22
French or Sourdough	1 slice	0.20
Raisen bread	1 slice	0.18
Cracked wheat	1 slice	0.17
Whole-Wheat	1 slice	0.17
Pita, white	6" pita	0.15
Potato bread	1 slice	0

Butter	Amount	Polyunsaturated (g)
Regular dairy butter, salted	1 tbsp	0.43
Regular dairy whipped butter, salted	1 tbsp	0.28

FAT POLYUNSATURATED

Cheese	Amount	Polyunsaturated (g)
American, pasteurized process, imitation	1 oz	2.14
Gruyere	1 oz	0.49
Fontina	1 oz	0.47
Cream cheese	1 oz	0.41
Roquefort	1 oz	0.37
American, pasteurized process, fortified	1 oz	0.37
Parmesan, grated	1 oz	0.33
Swiss	1 oz	0.28
Colby	1 oz	0.27
Cheddar	1 oz	0.27
Monterey	1 oz	0.26
Goat cheese, hard type	1 oz	0.24
Monterey, low fat	1 oz	0.24
Brie	1 oz	0.23
Blue cheese	1 oz	0.23
Provolone	1 oz	0.22
Mozzarella, whole milk	1 oz	0.22
Goat cheese, semisoft type	1 oz	0.20
Muenster	1 oz	0.19
Gouda	1 oz	0.19
Muenster, low fat	1 oz	0.18
Feta	1 oz	0.17
Romano	1 oz	0.17
Mozzarella, part skim milk, low moisture	1 oz	0.14
Provolone, reduced fat	1 oz	0.14
Goat cheese, soft type	1 oz	0.14
Cheddar, lowfat	1 oz	0.06
American, pasteurized process, low fat	1 oz	0.06
Swiss, low fat	1 oz	0.05
Cream cheese, fat free	1 oz	0.02
Mozzarella, nonfat	1 oz	0

Cheese, Mexican	Amount	Polyunsaturated (g)
Queso fresco	1 oz	0.31
Queso anejo	1 oz	0.26
Queso chihuahua	1 oz	0.25
Mexican, blend	1 oz	0.25
Queso asadero	1 oz	0.24
Mexican, blend, reduced fat	1 oz	0.21

FAT POLYUNSATURATED

Chicken, Cooked	Amount	Polyunsaturated (g)
Breast, with skin, fried in batter	1/2 breast	4.31
Thigh, with skin, fried in batter	1 thigh	3.35
Drumstick, with skin, fried in batter	1 drumstick	2.73
Wing, with skin, fried in batter	1 wing	2.48
Thigh, with skin, fried in flour	1 thigh	2.11
Breast, with skin, fried in flour	1/2 breast	1.92
Breast, with skin, roasted	1/2 breast	1.63
Drumstick, with skin, fried in flour	1 drumstick	1.58
Wing, with skin, roasted	1 wing	1.41
Thigh, no skin, meat only, roasted	1 thigh	1.29
Breast, no skin, roasted	1/2 breast	0.66
Drumstick, no skin, meat only, roasted	1 drumstick	0.60

Chicken, Cooked	Amount	Polyunsaturated (g)
Wing with skin, fried in flour	3 oz	4.21
Wing with skin, roasted	3 oz	3.52
Thigh with skin, fried in flour	3 oz	2.90
Drumstick with skin, fried in flour	3 oz	2.75
Thigh with skin, roasted	3 oz	2.50
Drumstick with skin, roasted	3 oz	1.72
Breast with skin, fried in flour	3 oz	1.67
Wing meat only, no skin, roasted	3 oz	1.51
Breast with skin, roasted	3 oz	1.41
Thigh meat only, no skin, roasted	3 oz	1.39
Drumstick meat only, no skin, roasted	3 oz	0.96
Cornish game hens, meat only	3 oz	0.80
Breast meat only, no skin, roasted	3 oz	0.65

Cream	Amount	Polyunsaturated (g)
Heavy Cream	1 tbsp	0.21
Light Coffe Cream	1 tbsp	0.11
Sour Cream, cultured	1 tbsp	0.10
Sour Cream, reduced fat	1 tbsp	0.07
Half & Half	1 tbsp	0.06
Whipped Topping, pressurized	1 tbsp	0.03

Eggs	Amount	Polyunsaturated (g)
Egg whole, fried	1 large	1.50
Egg whole, scrambled	1 large	1.48
Egg whole, poached	1 large	0.95
Egg whole, hard boiled	1 large	0.71
Egg yolk	1 large	0.70

FAT POLYUNSATURATED

Continued

Egg substitute, liquid, fat free	1/4 cup	0
Egg whites	1 large	0
Egg whites, dried	1 ounce	0
Egg whites, dried powder, stabilized	1 tbsp	0

Fish, Canned	Amount	Polyunsaturated (g)
Atlantic Sardines, in oil	3 oz	4.38
White (albacore) tuna, in oil	3 oz	2.53
Light tuna, in oil	3 oz	2.45
White (albacore) tuna, in water	3 oz	0.94
Light tuna, in water	3 oz	0.24

Fish, Cooked	Amount	Polyunsaturated (g)
Atlantic salmon, farmed	3 oz	3.76
Atlantic mackerel	3 oz	3.66
Catfish, breaded & fried	3 oz	2.83
Atlantic salmon, wild	3 oz	2.77
Atlantic croaker	3 oz	2.48
Chinook salmon	3 oz	2.26
Pacific & Jack mackerel	3 oz	2.12
Coho salmon, farmed	3 oz	1.67
Bluefin tuna	3 oz	1.57
Carp	3 oz	1.56
Rainbow trout, wild	3 oz	1.56
Spanish mackerel	3 oz	1.53
Rainbow trout, farmed	3 oz	1.53
Greenland halibut	3 oz	1.49
Atlantic herring	3 oz	1.43
Sockeye salmon	3 oz	1.27
Florida pompano	3 oz	1.24
Swordfish	3 oz	1.16
Freshwater bass	3 oz	1.16
Catfish, farmed	3 oz	1.15
Coho salmon, wild	3 oz	1.08
Keta (chum) salmon	3 oz	0.98
Sea bass	3 oz	0.85
Striped bass	3 oz	0.85
Chinook salmon, smoked, (lox),	3 oz	0.85
Pink salmon	3 oz	0.83
Alaskan halibut	3 oz	0.62
Catfish, wild	3 oz	0.54
Atlantic pollock	3 oz	0.53
Tilapia	3 oz	0.51
King mackerel	3 oz	0.50
Snapper	3 oz	0.50

FAT POLYUNSATURATED

Continued

Whiting	3 oz	0.50
Walleye pollock	3 oz	0.50
Walleye pike	3 oz	0.49
Sole & Flounder	3 oz	0.39
Grouper	3 oz	0.34
Skipjack (aku) tuna	3 oz	0.34
Atlantic perch	3 oz	0.31
Atlantic & Pacific halibut	3 oz	0.30
Atlantic cod	3 oz	0.25
Northern pike	3 oz	0.22
Haddock	3 oz	0.17
Pacific cod	3 oz	0.17
Orange roughy	3 oz	0.16
Yellowfin tuna	3 oz	0.15

Fish, Shellfish, Cooked	Amount	Polyunsaturated (g)
Shrimp, breaded & fried	3 oz	4.32
Oysters, breaded & fried	3 oz	2.82
Clams, breaded & fried	3 oz	2.44
Scallops, breaded & fried	3 oz	2.43
Blue crab cakes	3 oz	1.93
Squid, fried	3 oz	1.82
Abalone	3 oz	1.43
Eastern oysters, wild	3 oz	0.70
Eastern oysters, farmed	3 oz	0.61
Shrimp canned	3 oz	0.58
Shrimp	3 oz	0.50
Queen crab	3 oz	0.46
Alaskan king crab	3 oz	0.46
Octopus	3 oz	0.41
Crayfish	3 oz	0.31
Northern lobster	3 oz	0.29
Clams	3 oz	0.27
Blue crab	3 oz	0.22
Alaskan king crab, imitation	3 oz	0.09

Game Meat, Cooked	Amount	Polyunsaturated (g)
Duck	3 oz	1.26
Squirrel	3 oz	1.24
Bison, ground	3 oz	0.60
Rabbit	3 oz	0.58
Wild boar	3 oz	0.54
Caribou	3 oz	0.53
Deer	3 oz	0.53
Antelope	3 oz	0.49

FAT POLYUNSATURATED

Continued

Deer, ground	3 oz	0.38
Elk, ground	3 oz	0.35
Elk	3 oz	0.34
Buffalo, steak, free range	3 oz	0.15

Lamb, Cooked	Amount	Polyunsaturated (g)
Chops, loin, lean, trim to 1/4" fat	3 oz	1.43
Ground	3 oz	1.19
Leg, whole, trim to 1/4" fat	3 oz	1.00
Rib, lean, trim to 1/4" fat	3 oz	1.00
Foreshank, trim to 1/8" fat	3 oz	0.82
Cubed, for stew or kabob	3 oz	0.57

Milk	Amount	Polyunsaturated (g)
Soy milk, original, unfortified	1 cup	2.34
Human milk	1 cup	1.22
Canned, condensed, sweetened	1 cup	1.03
Sheep milk	1 cup	0.76
Canned, evaporated	1 cup	0.62
Coconut milk, canned	1 cup	0.53
Buttermilk, whole milk	1 cup	0.49
Whole milk, 3.25%	1 cup	0.48
Goat milk	1 cup	0.36
Reduced fat, 2%	1 cup	0.18
Lowfat milk, 1%	1 cup	0.09
Buttermilk, lowfat	1 cup	0.08
Canned, evaporated, non fat	1 cup	0
Nonfat, fat free or skim liquid milk	1 cup	0
Dry, instant, non fat	1/3 cup	0

Nuts & Seeds	Amount	Polyunsaturated (g)
English walnuts	1 oz	13.38
Black walnuts	1 oz	9.94
Pine nuts	1 oz	9.66
Flaxseeds	1 oz	8.15
Chia seeds	1 oz	6.71
Tahini	1 oz	6.68
Sunflower seed	1 oz	6.56
Sesame seeds	1 oz	6.17
Pecans	1 oz	6.13
Pumpkin seed	1 oz	5.95
Brazilnuts	1 oz	5.83
Peanuts	1 oz	4.41
Peanut butter, smooth style	1 oz	4.02

FAT POLYUNSATURATED

Continued

Pistachio nuts	1 oz	3.90
Almonds	1 oz	3.42
Trail mix, regular with chocolate chips	1 oz	3.08
Mixed nuts, roasted with peanuts, no salt	1 oz	3.04
Trail mix, regular, salted	1 oz	2.74
Hazelnuts	1 oz	2.25
Cashews	1 oz	2.22
Trail mix, tropical	1 oz	1.46
Macadamia	1 oz	0.43
Coconut, raw meat	1 oz	0.10

Nuts & Seeds	Amount	Polyunsaturated (g)
Flaxseeds	1/4 cup	12.07
English walnuts, chopped	1/4 cup	11.79
Pine nuts	1/4 cup	11.50
Black walnuts, chopped	1/4 cup	10.96
Peanut butter, smooth	1/4 cup	9.13
Sunflower seeds	1/4 cup	8.10
Sesame seeds	1/4 cup	7.84
Brazilnuts, whole	1/4 cup	6.84
Pumpkin seeds	1/4 cup	6.77
Peanuts	1/4 cup	5.68
Pecans, halves	1/4 cup	5.35
Almonds, whole	1/4 cup	4.32
Pistachio	1/4 cup	4.23
Trail mix, regular with chocolate chips	1/4 cup	3.97
Mixed nuts, roasted with peanuts, no salt	1/4 cup	3.69
Trail mix, regular, salted	1/4 cup	3.62
Flaxseeds	1 tbsp	2.96
Hazelnuts, chopped	1/4 cup	2.23
Sesame seeds	1 tbsp	1.96
Trail mix, tropical	1/4 cup	1.81
Macadamia	1/4 cup	0.50
Coconut meat, shredded	1/4 cup	0.07
Cashews	1/4 cup	x
Chia seeds	1/4 cup	x

Oil	Amount	Polyunsaturated (g)
Safflower oil, high linoleic	1 tbsp	10.15
Grapeseed oil	1 tbsp	9.51
Flaxseed oil	1 tbsp	9.23
Sunflower oil, 65% linoleic	1 tbsp	8.94
Walnut oil	1 tbsp	8.61
Soybean oil	1 tbsp	7.85
Corn oil	1 tbsp	7.44

FAT POLYUNSATURATED

Continued .

Cottonseed oil	1 tbsp	7.06
Sesame oil	1 tbsp	5.67
Salmon oil	1 tbsp	5.48
Soybean, partially hydrogenated	1 tbsp	5.11
Sardine oil	1 tbsp	4.33
Peanut oil	1 tbsp	4.32
Canola oil, rapeseed	1 tbsp	3.94
Cod liver oil	1 tbsp	3.07
Canola oil, partially hydrogenated	1 tbsp	1.91
Avocado	1 tbsp	1.89
Safflower oil, high oleic	1 tbsp	1.74
Olive oil	1 tbsp	1.42
Sunflower oil, 70% or more, high oleic	1 tbsp	0.53
Coconut oil	1 tbsp	0.25

Pork, Cooked	Amount	Polyunsaturated (g)
Bacon, pan-fried	3 oz	3.87
Sausage	3 oz	3.17
Backribs	3 oz	3.00
Italian sausage	3 oz	2.98
Braunschweiger	3 oz	2.71
Polish sausage	3 oz	2.62
Spareribs	3 oz	2.32
Bratwurst	3 oz	2.24
Pork chops, pan-fried	3 oz	1.81
Cured ham	3 oz	1.54
Liverwurst spread	1/4 cup	1.34
Center loin pork chops	3 oz	1.16
Pork chops, broiled	3 oz	1.16
Sausage	1 patty	1.01
Sausage	2 links	0.97
Pork chops, lean, pan-fried	3 oz	0.90
Bacon, pan-fried	3 slices	0.86
Sirloin pork chops	3 oz	0.70
Canadian-style bacon	3 oz	0.69
Cured ham, lean	3 oz	0.54
Tenderloin	3 oz	0.48
Canadian-style bacon	2 slices	0.38

Turkey, Cooked	Amount	Polyunsaturated (g)
Turkey bacon	3 oz	5.79
Ground turkey, 85% lean	3 oz	3.54
Ground turkey, 93% lean	3 oz	3.01
Ground turkey	3 oz	2.48
Turkey sausage, reduced fat	3 oz	2.16

FAT POLYUNSATURATED

Continued

	Amount	Polyunsaturated (g)
Dark meat	3 oz	1.41
Ground turkey, fat free	3 oz	0.65
Light meat	3 oz	0.45
Breast meat	3 oz	0.17

Veal, Cooked	Amount	Polyunsaturated (g)
Rib	3 oz	0.81
Loin	3 oz	0.69
Breast	3 oz	0.67
Sirloin	3 oz	0.58
Ground	3 oz	0.47
Foreshank	3 oz	0.46
Leg, top round	3 oz	0.40

Nutrient Data Collection Form

Food	Amount	Book Numbers	Multiply By	Estimated Nutrient Intake
Nutrient::	RDA:	Estimated:	% of RDA:	Total Estimated:

To download additional forms for free, go to www.TopNutrients4U.com

FIBER

Fiber is a macronutrient needed daily in gram quantities.

The fiber content of foods is linked with normalizing bowel movement, controlling blood sugar, and lowering blood cholesterol. On the other hand, diets lacking fiber have been linked to diverticulitis. However, too much fiber may cause constipation, gas, bloating, and interfere with absorption of some nutrients.

Fiber like every other nutrient cannot be too high or too low but must be held within a level that one would normally expect to find from consuming a variety of foods.

It is estimated that Americans consume about 15 grams/ day of dietary fiber, which professionals consider to be too low. The Institute of Medicine recommends 14 grams / day per 1,000 calories or 25 grams / day for women and 38 grams / day for men.

This chapter deals with fiber known as dietary fiber. Dietary fiber consists of two types known as soluble and insoluble. Soluble form is fermented in the human body, binds to bile acids and plays numerous functions. The insoluble form absorbs water throughout the digestive system and softens the stool. This chapter lists fiber in gram quantities.

FIBER

Recommend Daily Intakes Levels for Fiber

Children	Fiber, grams
1 to 3 year olds	19
4 to 8 year olds	25

Males	
9 to 13 year olds	31
14 to 18 year olds	38
19 to 30 years	38
31 to 50 years	38
51 to 70 years	30
Over 70	30

Females	
9 to 13 year olds	26
14 to 18 year olds	26
19 to 30 years	5
31 to 50 years	25
51 to 70 years	21
Over 70	21
Pregnancy	28
Lactation	29

FIBER

Alcohol	Amount	Fiber (g)
Gin, Rum, Vodka, Whisky	1 shot	0
Light Beer	1 bottle	0
Red Wine	1 glass	0
Regular Beer	1 bottle	0
White Wine	1 glass	0

Beans, Canned	Amount	Fiber (g)
Cranberry beans	1 cup	16
Kidney beans	1 cup	14
Navy beans	1 cup	13
Great Northern beans	1 cup	13
White beans	1 cup	13
Refried beans	1 cup	12
Lima beans	1 cup	12
Pinto beans	1 cup	11
Garbanzo beans	1 cup	11
Baked beans, plain	1 cup	10
Fava beans	1 cup	10
Black-eyed peas	1 cup	8
Green beans	1 cup	4

Beans, Cooked	Amount	Fiber (g)
Navy beans	1 cup	19.1
White beans, small	1 cup	18.6
Cranberry beans	1 cup	17.7
Adzuki	1 cup	16.8
Split peas	1 cup	16.3
Lentils	1 cup	15.6
Pinto beans	1 cup	15.4
Black beans	1 cup	15.0
Black Turtle beans, mature	1 cup	15.0
Mung beans, mature seeds	1 cup	15.0
Lima beans	1 cup	13.2
Kidney beans	1 cup	13.1
Garbanzo beans	1 cup	12.5
Great Northern	1 cup	12.4
Pigeon peas	1 cup	11.3
White beans, mature	1 cup	11.3
Black-eyed peas	1 cup	11.1
Soybeans, mature	1 cup	10.3
Natto	1 cup	9.5
Fava beans	1 cup	9.2
Edamame	1 cup	8.1

FIBER

Soybeans, green	1 cup	7.6
Soybeans, dryroasted	1 cup	7.5
Lupini beans	1 cup	4.6
Yellow beans	1 cup	4.1
Green beans	1 cup	4.0
Hyacinath beans	1 cup	x
Mothbeans	1 cup	x
Winged beans	1 cup	x
Yardlong beans, Chinese long beans	1 cup	x

Beef, Cooked	Amount	Fiber (g)
Beef ribs, trimmed to 1/8" fat	3 oz	0
Chuck roast, trimmed to 1/8" fat	3 oz	0
Filet Mignon, trimmed to 0" fat	3 oz	0
Ground beef, 75%	3 oz	0
Ground beef, 80%	3 oz	0
Ground beef, 85%	3 oz	0
Ground beef, 90%,	3 oz	0
Ground beef, 95%	3 oz	0
Porterhouse steak, trimmed to 0" fat	3 oz	0
Ribeye steak, trimmed to 0" fat	3 oz	0
Skirt Steak, trimmed to 0" fat	3 oz	0
T-Bone steak, trimmed 0" fat	3 oz	0
Top sirloin, trimmed to 1/8" fat	3 oz	0

Bread	Amount	Fiber (g)
Indian bread, Naan, whole wheat	1 piece	5
Bagel, wheat	4" bagel	4
Bagel, oat bran	4" bagel	4
Pumpernickel	1 slice	2
Bagel, cinnamon & raisins	4" bagel	2
Bagel, egg	4" bagel	2
Bagel, plain	4" bagel	2
English muffin, plain	1 muffin	2
Indian bread, Naan, plain	1 piece	2
Mexican roll, bollilo	1 roll	2
Potato bread	1 slice	2
Potato bread	1 slice	2
Multi-Grain, and Whole-Grain	1 slice	2
Rye bread	1 slice	2
Whole-Wheat	1 slice	2
Croissants, butter	1 medium	2
Cornbread	1 piece	1
Cracked wheat	1 slice	1
Kaiser rolls	1 roll	1

FIBER

Continued

Pita, white	6 inch pita	1
Oatmeal bread	1 slice	1
White	1 slice	1
Tortillas, corn	1 tortilla	1
Tortillas, flour	1 tortilla	1
Egg bread	1 slice	1
Hamburger & Hotdog buns, plain	1 bun	1
Wheat	1 slice	1
Dinner Rolls, brown & serve	1 roll	1
French, Italian, sourdough	1 slice	1

CEREAL

Arrowhead Mills	Amount	Fiber (g)
Shredded Wheat, Bite Size	1 cup	6
Sweetened Shredded Wheat	1 cup	5
Oat Bran Flakes	1 cup	4
Spelt Flakes	1 cup	3
Amaranth Flakes	1 cup	3
Sprouted Multigrain Flakes	1 cup	3
Kamut Flakes	1 cup	2
Sweetened Rice Flakes	1 cup	1
Maple Buckwheat Flakes	1 cup	1

Barbara's	Amount	Fiber (g)
High Fiber Original	1 cup	14
High Fiber Flax & Granola	1 cup	10
High Fiber Cranberry	1 cup	10
Puffins Cinnamon	1 cup	9
Puffins Original	1 cup	7
Shredded Spoonfuls Multigrain	1 cup	5
Shredded Wheat	2 biscuits	5
Shredded Oats Original	1 cup	4
Shredded Oats Cinnamon Crunch	1 cup	4
Shredded Oats Vanilla Almond	1 cup	4
Shredded Minis Blueberry Burst	1 cup	4
Puffins Peanut Butter & Chocolate	1 cup	4
Puffins Multigrain	1 cup	4
Puffins Honey Rice	1 cup	4
Puffins Puffs Crunchy Cocoa	1 cup	4
Hole 'n Oats Honey Nut	1 cup	3
Puffins Peanut Butter	1 cup	3
Corn Flakes	1 cup	1
Hole 'n Oats: Fruit Juice, Sweetened	1 cup	1

FIBER

Continued

Brown Rice Crisps	1 cup	1
Puffins Puffs Fruit Medley	1 cup	1

Cereal, Bear Naked®	Amount	Fiber (g)
Original Granola	1 cup	12
Banana Nut Granola	1 cup	8
Fruit & Nut Ganola	1 cup	8
Vanila Almond Crucnh Granola	1 cup	8
Nut Cluster Crunch Cereal	1 cup	3

Cereal, Cascadian Farm	Amount	Fiber (g)
Hearty Morning	1 cup	12
Raisin bran	1 cup	6
Dark Chocolate Almond Granola	1 cup	5
Cinnamon Raisin Granola	1 cup	5
Maple Brown Sugar Granola	1 cup	5
Oats & Honey Granola	1 cup	5
Chocolate O's	1 cup	4
Fruit Ful O's	1 cup	4
French Vanilla Almond Granola	1 cup	4
Fruit & Nut Granola	1 cup	4
Cinnamon Crunch	1 cup	3
Honey Nut O's	1 cup	3
Purel O's	1 cup	3
Multi Gain Squares	1 cup	3

Cereal, Erewhon	Amount	Fiber (g)
Raisin Bran	1 cup	6
Corn Flakes	1 cup	1
Cocoa Crispy Brown Rice	1 cup	1
Crispy Brown Rice, mixed Berries	1 cup	1
Crispy Brown Rice, Strawberry Crisp	1 cup	1
Crispy Brown Rice, Original	1 cup	0
Rice Twice	1 cup	0
Crispy Brown Rice, Gluten Free	1 cup	0
Crispy Brown Rice, No Salt Added	1 cup	0

Cereal, Ezekiel	Amount	Fiber (g)
Sprouted Grain Golden Flax, 4:9	1 cup	12
Sprouted Grain Almond, 4:9	1 cup	12
Sprouted Grain Original, 4:9	1 cup	10
Sprouted Grain Cinnamon Flax, 4:9	1 cup	10

FIBER

Cereal, General Mills®	Amount	Fiber (g)
Multi-Bran CHEX	1 cup	8
Raisin-Nut Bran	1 cup	7
Wheat Chex	1 cup	7
Total Raisin Bran	1 cup	5
Oatmeal Crisp, Crunchy Almond	1 cup	5
Honey Nut Clusters	1 cup	4
Total Whole Grain	1 cup	4
Dora The Explorer	1 cup	4
Basic 4	1 cup	4
Wheaties	1 cup	4
Total Cranberry Crunch	1 cup	3
Cocoa Puffs	1 cup	3
Kix	1 cup	2
Corn Chex	1 cup	2
Berry Berry Kix	1 cup	2
Cinnamon Toast Crunch	1 cup	2
Lucky Charms	1 cup	1
Chocolate Chex	1 cup	1
Cinnamon Chex	1 cup	1
Cookie Crisp	1 cup	1
Golden Grams	1 cup	1
Honey Nut Chex	1 cup	1
Reese's Puffs	1 cup	1
Trix	1 cup	1
Rice Chex	1 cup	1

General Mills Cheerios®	Amount	Fiber (g)
Multi Grain	1 cup	3
Original	1 cup	3
Apple Cinnamon	1 cup	3
Berry Burst	1 cup	3
Frosted	1 cup	3
Fruity	1 cup	3
Honey Nut	1 cup	3
Yogurt Burst, Strawberry	1 cup	3
Crunch, Oat Clusters	1 cup	3
Banana Nut	1 cup	2
Chocolate	1 cup	2

FIBER

General Mills Fiber One®	Amount	Fiber (g)
Original	1 cup	28
Honey Clusters	1 cup	14
Raisin Bran Clusters	1 cup	12
Caramel Delight	1 cup	10
Frosted Shredded Wheat	1 cup	9

Cereal, Glutino®	Amount	Fiber (g)
Honey Nut Cereal	1 cup	2
Apple & Cinnamon Rings	1 cup	2
Corn Rice Flakes	1 cup	1
Berry Sensible Beginning	1 cup	1
Frosted Corn & Rice Flakes	1 cup	1
Corn Rice Flakes with Strawberries	1 cup	1

Cereal, Health Valley	Amount	Fiber (g)
Oat Bran Almond Crunch	1 cup	10
Low Fat Date & Almond Flavored Granola	1 cup	8
Low Fat Raisin Cinnamon Granola	1 cup	8
Fiber 7	1 cup	7
Golden Flax	1 cup	6
Multigrain Maple, Honey, Nut Squares	1 cup	6
Multigrain Apple Cinnamon Squares	1 cup	6
Heart Wise	1 cup	5
Oat Bran Flakes	1 cup	4
Amaranth Flakes	1 cup	4
Oat Bran Flakes & Raisins	1 cup	4
Cranberry Crunch	1 cup	4
Rice Crunch-EMS	1 cup	2
Corn Crunch-EMS	1 cup	2

Cereal, Kashi®	Amount	Fiber (g)
7-Whole Grain Nuggets	1 cup	14
Go Lean Crisp, Cinnamon Crumble	1 cup	12
Good Friends	1 cup	12
Go Lean	1 cup	10
Go Lean Crisp, Toasted Berry Crumble	1 cup	10
Go Lean Vanilla Graham	1 cup	9
Go Lean Crunch	1 cup	8
Go Lean Crunch, Honey Almond Flax	1 cup	8
Heart to Heart, Nutty Chia Flax	1 cup	8
Berry Blossom	1 cup	8

FIBER

Honey Sunshine	1 cup	7
Autum Wheat	29 biscuits	6
Berry Fruitful	29 biscuits	6
Island Vanilla	27 biscuits	6
7-Whole Grain Flakes	1 cup	6
Cinnamon Harvest	28 biscuits	5
Heart to Heart, Honey Toasted Oat	1 cup	5
Heart to Heart, Warm Cinnamon	1 cup	5
Heart to Heart, Oat Flakes & Blueberry Clusters	1 cup	4
Blackberry Hills	1 cup	3
Indigo Morning	1 cup	3
Simply Maize	1 cup	3
Strawberry Fields	1 cup	3
7-Whole Grain Honey Puffs	1 cup	2
7-Whole Grain Puffs	1 cup	1

Cereal, Kellogg's®	Amount	Fiber (g)
All-Bran Buds	1 cup	39
All-Bran Original	1 cup	20
Fiberplus Cinnamon Oat Crunch	1 cup	12
Fiberplus Berry Yogurt Crunch	1 cup	10
All-Bran Strawberry Medley	1 cup	10
Cracklin' Oat bran	1 cup	8
All-Bran Complete Wheat Flakes	1 cup	7
Raisin Bran	1 cup	7
Low Fat Granola with Raisins	1 cup	7
Frosted MINI-Wheat's Bite Size	1 cup	6
Raisin Bran Extra	1 cup	6
MUESLIX	1 cup	6
Frosted MINI-Wheat's, Big Bite	1 cup	5
Raisin Bran with Flaxseeds	1 cup	5
Smart Start, Strong Heart Toasted Oat	1 cup	4
Krave Chocolate	1 cup	4
Raisin Bran Crunch	1 cup	4
Froot Loops	1 cup	3
Apple Jacks	1 cup	3
Corn Pops	1 cup	3
Smart Start, Strong Heart Antioxidants	1 cup	3
Crunchy Nut Roasted Nut & Honey O's	1 cup	3
Honey Crunch Corn Flakes	1 cup	1
Honey Smacks	1 cup	1
Cinnabon	1 cup	1
Product 19	1 cup	1
Cocoa Krispies	1 cup	0.8
Crispix	1 cup	0.8

FIBER

Continued

Smorz	1 cup	0.8
Corn Flakes	1 cup	0.7
Frosted Flakes	1 cup	0.7
Crunchy Nut Golden Honey Nut Flakes	1 cup	0.6
Simply Cinnamon Corn Flakes	1 cup	0.4
Frosted Rice Krispies	1 cup	0.2
Rice Krispies	1 cup	0.2
Berry Rice Krispies	1 cup	0.1
Rice Krispies Treats	1 cup	0.1

Kellogg's Special-K®	Amount	Fiber (g)
Low Fat Granola	1 cup	10
Protein Plus	1 cup	7
Blueberry	1 cup	4
Multigrain Oats & Honey	1 cup	4
Cinnamon Pecan	1 cup	3
Chocolately Delight	1 cup	3
Fruit & Yogurt	1 cup	3
Vanilla Almond	1 cup	3
Original	1 cup	3
Red Berries	1 cup	3

Cereal, Mom's Best Natural	Amount	Fiber (g)
Toasted Wheat Fuls	1 cup	7
Raisin Bran	1 cup	6
Sweetened Wheat Fuls	1 cup	6
Honey Nut Toasty O's	1 cup	2
Honey Grahams	1 cup	1
Mallow Oats	1 cup	1
Oats & Honey Blend	1 cup	1
Toasted Cinnamon Squares	1 cup	1
Crispy Coco Rice	1 cup	0
Honey Ful Wheats	1 cup	0

Cereal, Natures Path	Amount	Fiber (g)
Smart Bran	1 cup	26
Optimum Power Blueberry Cinnamon	1 cup	12
Flax Plus Raisin Bran Flakes	1 cup	11
Optimum Cranberry Ginger	1 cup	11
Flax Plus Pumpkin Raisin Crunch	1 cup	9
Heritage Crunch	1 cup	8
Heritage Heirloom Whole Grain Bites	1 cup	7
Flax Plus Multibran Flakes	1 cup	7
Flax Plus Maple Pecan Crunch	1 cup	7

FIBER

Continued

Flax Plus Redberry Crunch	1 cup	7
Heritage Flakes	1 cup	7
Multigrain Oat bran	1 cup	7
Hemp Plus Granola	1 cup	7
Flax Plus Pumpkin Flax Granola	1 cup	7
Flax Plus Vanilla Almond Granola	1 cup	7
Optimum Banana Almond	1 cup	7
Optimum Slim Low Fat Vanilla	1 cup	6
Peanut Butter Granola	1 cup	5
Pomegran Plus Granola	1 cup	5
Acai Apple Granola	1 cup	5
Pomegran Cherry Granola	1 cup	5
AGAVE Plus Granola	1 cup	5
Crunchy Maple Sunrise, Gluten Free	1 cup	5
Crunchy Vanilla Sunrise	1 cup	5
Whole O's	1 cup	5
Mesa Sunrise, Gluten Free	1 cup	4
Organic Millet Rice	1 cup	4
Honeyed Corn Flakes, Gluten Free	1 cup	3
OATY BITES Whole Grain	1 cup	3

Cereal, Peace All Natural	Amount	Fiber (g)
Walnut Spice Clusters & Flakes	1 cup	8
Wild Berry Clusters & Flakes	1 cup	6
Golden Honey Granola	1 cup	6
Cherry Almond Clusters & Flakes	1 cup	5
Vanilla Almond Clusters & Flakes	1 cup	3
Maple Pecan	1 cup	3
Mango Peach Passion Clusters & Flakes	1 cup	2

Cereal, Post®	Amount	Fiber (g)
Grape-Nuts Cereal	1 cup	13.8
Raisin Bran	1 cup	7.8
Bran Flakes	1 cup	7.0
Great Grains, Banana Nut Crunch	1 cup	7.0
Great Grains, Cranberry Almond Crunch	1 cup	7.0
Shredded Wheat n' Bran	1 cup	6.9
Great Grains, Raisin, Date & Pecan	1 cup	6.8
Great Grains, Cruncy Pecan Cereal	1 cup	6.7
Honey Nut Shredded Wheat	1 cup	6.3
Shredded Wheat, Original, spoon-size	1 cup	6.1
Shredded Wheat, Frosted, spoon-size	1 cup	5.0
Grape-Nuts Flakes	1 cup	3.9
Shredded Wheat, Original, big biscuit	1 biscuit	3.0

FIBER

Continued

Alpha-Bits	1 cup	2.0
Blueberry Morning	1 cup	1.8
Golden Crisp	1 cup	1.8
Honeycomb Cereal	1 cup	0.7
Cocoa Pebbles	1 cup	0.6
Fruity Pebbles	1 cup	0.3

Post® Honey Bunches Of Oats®	Amount	Fiber (g)
Just Bunches, Honey Roasted	1 cup	5
With Vanilla Bunches	1 cup	4
Honey Roasted	1 cup	2
Pecan Bunches	1 cup	2
With Almonds	1 cup	2
With Cinnamon Bunches	1 cup	2
With Strawberries	1 cup	2

Cereal, Quaker®	Amount	Fiber (g)
Granola, Oats, Honey, Raisins, & Almonds	1 cup	10
Granola, Apple, Cranberry, & Almonds	1 cup	10
Granola, Oats, Honey, & Almonds	1 cup	10
LIFE Cereal, Crunchtime Strawberry	1 cup	8
Corn Bran Crunch	1 cup	6
Oatmeal Squares, Brown Sugar	1 cup	5
Oatmeal Squares, Golden Maple	1 cup	5
Oatmeal Squares, Honey Nut	1 cup	5
Toasted Multigrain Crisp	1 cup	5
Oatmeal Squares, Cinnamon	1 cup	5
Whole Hearts	1 cup	4
LIFE Cereal, Cinnamon	1 cup	3
LIFE Cereal, Maple & Brown Sugar	1 cup	3
LIFE Cereal, Original	1 cup	3
Honey Graham OH'S	1 cup	2
Puffed Wheat	1 cup	1.4
CAP'N Crunch's OOPS! All Berries	1 cup	1
CAP'N Crunch's Peanut Butter Crunch	1 cup	1
CAP'N Crunch	1 cup	1
CAP'N Crunch with Crunchberries	1 cup	1
Puffed Rice	1 cup	0.3

Cereal, Uncle Sam	Amount	Fiber (g)
Flaxseed, Original	1 cup	13
Flaxseed, & Strawberry	1 cup	11
Flaxseed, Honey Almond	1 cup	8
Skinners Raisin Bran	1 cup	6

FIBER

Cereal, Wild Harvest	Amount	Fiber (g)
Wholesome Raisin Bran	1 cup	7
Blueberry Flax Granola	1 cup	6
Golden Honey & Flax Granola	1 cup	6
Crunchy Vanilla Almond Granola	1 cup	5
Cherry Vanilla Granola	1 cup	4
Cranberry Almond	1 cup	2
Mango Crisp	1 cup	2
Maple Pecan Flakes & Clusters	1 cup	2
Wild Berry Crisp	1 cup	1

Cereal, Cooked	Amount	Fiber (g)
Oats, regular, unenriched	1 cup	4
Farina	1 cup	2
White corn grits	1 cup	2
Yellow corn grits	1 cup	2
CREAM OF WHEAT, regular	1 cup	1
Malt-o-Meal plain	1 serving	1

Cheese	Amount	Fiber (g)
All types	1 oz	0

Chicken, Cooked	Amount	Fiber (g)
All types	1 oz	0

CHILI

Chili, Amy's	Amount	Fiber (g)
Black Bean Chili	1 can	26
Southwestern Black Bean Chili	1 can	20
Medium Chili with Vegetables	1 can	18
Light in Sodium Medium Chili	1 can	14
Light in Sodium Spicy Chili	1 can	14
Medium Chili	1 can	14
Spicy Chili	1 can	14

Chili, Campbell's® Chunky	Amount	Fiber (g)
Chunky Chili with Beans Roadhouse	1 can	14
Chunky Chili with Beans Firehouse	1 can	14
Chunky Chili with Beans Grilled Steak	1 can	14
Chunky Chili no Beans	1 can	10

FIBER

Chili, Cattle Drive®	Amount	Fiber (g)
Cattlee Drive Golden Chili with beans	1 can	10

Chili, Dennison's®	Amount	Fiber (g)
Original Chili Con Carne with Beans	1 can	22
Hot Chili Con Carne with Beans	1 can	22
Chunky Chili Con Carne with Beans	1 can	18
Hot & Chunky Chili with Beans	1 can	18
Vegetarian Chili with Beans	1 can	18
Turkey Chili with Beans	1 can	14

Chili, Eden	Amount	Fiber (g)
Kidney Bean & Kamut Chili	1 can	22
Great Northern Bean & Barley Chili	1 can	16
Pinto Bean & Spelt Chili	1 can	16
Black Bean & Quinoa Chili	1 can	12

Chili, Hardy Jack's	Amount	Fiber (g)
Chili with beans	1 can	14
Chili no beans	1 can	6

Chili, Healthy Valley	Amount	Fiber (g)
Santa Fe White Bean Chili	1 can	18
No salt Added Tame Tomato Chili	1 can	16
Spicy Tomato Chili	1 can	16
Three Bean Chipotle Chili	1 can	16
Black Bean Mole Chili	1 can	14
Black Bean Mango Chili	1 can	14

Chili, Hormel®	Amount	Fiber (g)
Vegetarian Chili, Beans 99% Fat Free	1 can	20
Chili With Beans	1 can	14
Chunky Chili with Beans	1 can	14
Hot Chili with beans	1 can	14
Less Sodium Chili with Beans	1 can	14
Cook-off Chipotle Chicken Chili	1 can	14
Cook-off Roasted Tomato Chili	1 can	14
Turkey Chili with Beans	1 can	12
Cook- off White Chicken Chili	1 can	8
Chili no Beans	1 can	6
Turkey Chili no Beans	1 can	6
Less Sodium Chili no Beans	1 can	6

FIBER

Chili, Stagg®	Amount	Fiber (g)
Vegetarian Garden Four Bean Chili	1 can	16
Dynamite Hot Chili with Beans	1 can	16
Ranch House Chicken Chili & Beans	1 can	14
Laredo Chili, Beans, Chili & Jalapeno	1 can	12
Silverado Beef Chili with Beans	1 can	12
Turkey Ranchero Chili with Beans	1 can	12
Chunkero Chili with Beans	1 can	12
Fiesta Grille Chili with Beans	1 can	12
Country Brand Chili & Sweet Peppers	1 can	12
Classic Chili with beans	1 can	10
Country Brand Chili with Beans	1 can	10
White Chicken Chili with Beans	1 can	8
Steak House Chili no Beans	1 can	4

Chili, Wolf Brand	Amount	Fiber (g)
Chili with Beans	1 can	20
Spicy Chili with Beans	1 can	20
Turkey Chili with Beans	1 can	20
Lean Beaf with Beans	1 can	18
Homestyle Chili with Beans	1 can	16
Chili no Beans	1 can	10
Hot Chili no Beans	1 can	10
Lean Beaf no Beans	1 can	10
Turkey Chili no Beans	1 can	8

FISH	Amount	Fiber (g)
All fish	3 oz	0

FRUIT

Fruit, Canned	Amount	Fiber (g)
Pears	1 cup	4
Apricots	1 cup	4
Peaches	1 cup	3
Applesauce, sweetened	1 cup	3
Applesauce, unsweetened	1 cup	3
Plums,	1 cup	2
Pineapple	1 cup	2
Olives, black	5 large	0.7
Olives, green	5 large	0.4

Fruit, Dried	Amount	Fiber (g)

FIBER

Continued

Figs	1 cup	15
Pears	1 cup	14
Peaches	1 cup	13
Currants	1 cup	10
Apricots	1 cup	10
Apples	1 cup	8
Cranberries	1 cup	7

Fruit, Frozen	Amount	Fiber (g)
Raspberries	1 cup	11
Blackberries, unsweetened	1 cup	8
Blueberries	1 cup	5
Strawberries	1 cup	5
Peaches	1 cup	5

Fruit, Raw	Amount	Fiber (g)
Pineapple	1 cup	22
Avocado, California	1 cup	16
Avocado, Florida	1 cup	13
Prunes, dried, uncooked	1 cup	12
Dates	1 cup	12
Elderberries	1 cup	10
Stewed prunes	1 cup	8
Blackberries	1 cup	8
Pomegrenates	1 cup	7
Raspberries	1 cup	6
Jicama	1 cup	6
Kiwi	1 cup	5
Raisins	1 cup	5
Pears	1 cup	5
Cranberries	1 cup	5
Valencias oranges	1 cup	5
Florida oranges	1 cup	4
Oranges	1 cup	4
Grapefruit, pink & red, sections	1 cup	4
Naval oranges	1 cup	4
Blueberries	1 cup	4
Plantains	1 cup	3
Apricots	1 cup	3
Strawberries	1 cup	3
Tangerine	1 cup	3
Cherries	1 cup	3
Apples	1 cup	3
Mango	1 cup	3
Papaya	1 cup	3

FIBER

Continued

Nectarine	1 cup	2
Peach's	1 cup	2
Plums	1 cup	2
Cantaloupe	1 cup	1
Grapes	1 cup	1
Honeydew	1 cup	1
Water mellon	1 cup	0.6

Fruit, Raw	Amount	Fiber (g)
Avocado, Florida	1 fruit	17
Pomegranates	1 fruit	11
Avocado, California	1 fruit	9
Pears	1 fruit	5
Plantains	1 fruit	4
Florida Oranges	1 fruit	3
Prunes, dried, uncooked	5 prunes	3
Apples	1 fruit	3
Bananas	1 fruit	3
Naval Oranges	1 fruit	3
Oranges	1 fruit	3
Pineapple guava, Feijoa	1 fruit	3
Star fruit, Carambola	1 fruit	3
Valencias Oranges	1 fruit	3
Dates	5 dates	3
Cantaloupe	1/2 fruit	3
Nectarine	1 fruit	2
Kiwi	1 fruit	2
Grapefruit, pink & red	1/2 fruit	2
Peaches	1 fruit	2
Cheeries	10 fruit	2
Raisins	1 small box	2
Kumquats	1 fruit	1
Strawberries	5 fruit	1
Tangerine	1 fruit	1
Plums	1 fruit	0.9
Figs, dried	1 fruit	0.8
Apricots	1 fruit	0.7
Olives, black	5 large	0.7
Pineapple	1/2" x 3" slice	0.7
Olives, green	5 large	0.4

FIBER

Grains, Cooked	Amount	Fiber (g)
Bulgur	1 cup	8
Spelt	1 cup	8
Kamut	1 cup	7
Whole-Wheat spaghetti	1 cup	6
Pearled barley	1 cup	6
Oat bran	1 cup	6
Amaranth	1 cup	5
Quinoa	1 cup	5
Buckwheat	1 cup	5
Macaroni, Whole-Wheat	1 cup	4
Egg & Spinach noodles	1 cup	4
Brown rice	1 cup	4
Wild rice	1 cup	3
Macaroni	1 cup	3
Spaghetti	1 cup	3
Millet	1 cup	2
Couscous	1 cup	2
Egg noodles	1 cup	2
Chow mein noodles	1 cup	2
Rice noodles	1 cup	2
White rice, long-grain, enriched	1 cup	1
White rice, long-grain, instant	1 cup	1
White rice, long-grain, regular	1 cup	0.6

Juice	Amount	Fiber (g)
Prune	1 cup	3
Carrot	1 cup	2
Vegetable	1 cup	2
Tomato	1 cup	1
Lemon juice, raw	1 cup	0.7
Apple	1 cup	0.5
Grape	1 cup	0.5
Orange juice, raw	1 cup	0.5
Pineapple	1 cup	0.5
Grapefruit juice, raw	1 cup	0.2
Pomegranate	1 cup	0.2
Cranberry	1 cup	0

Milk	Amount	Fiber (g)
All types	1 cup	0

FIBER

Nuts & Seeds	Amount	Fiber (g)
Chia seeds	1 oz	10
Flaxseeds	1 oz	8
Almonds	1 oz	4
Sesame seeds	1 oz	3
Peanuts	1 oz	3
Mixed nuts, roasted with peanuts, no salt	1 oz	3
Pistachio	1 oz	3
Hazelnuts	1 oz	3
Pecans	1 oz	3
Coconut, raw meat	1 oz	3
Tahini	1 oz	3
Macadamia	1 oz	2
Sunflower seeds	1 oz	2
Brazil nuts	1 oz	2
Black walnuts	1 oz	2
English walnuts	1 oz	2
Peanut butter, smooth style	1 oz	2
Pumpkin seed	1 oz	2
Trail mix, regular with chocolate chips	1 oz	1
Pine nuts	1 oz	1
Cashews	1 oz	1
Trail mix, regular, salted	1 oz	x
Trail mix, tropical	1 oz	x

VEGETABLES

Vegetables, Canned	Amount	Fiber (g)
Tomato paste	1 cup	10.7
Green peas	1 cup	8.3
Pumpkin	1 cup	7.1
Sauerkraut	1 cup	6.8
Spinach	1 cup	5.1
Tomato pure	1 cup	4.8
Sweet Potato	1 cup	4.6
Yellow corn	1 cup	4.2
Asparagus	1 cup	3.9
Mushrooms	1 cup	3.7
Tomato sauce	1 cup	3.7
Beets	1 cup	3.1
Green beans	1 cup	3.1
Stewed tomato	1 cup	2.6
Tomatoes	1 cup	2.4
Carrots	1 cup	2.2

FIBER

Vegetables, Cooked	Amount	Fiber (g)
Cabbage, Napa	1 cup	x
Split Peas	1 cup	16.3
Artichokes	1 cup	14.4
Hubbard Squash	1 cup	10.0
Acorn squash	1 cup	9.0
Sweet potato, mashed	1 cup	8.2
Butternut squash	1 cup	6.6
Winter squash	1 cup	5.7
Parsnips	1 cup	5.6
Collard greens	1 cup	5.3
Yams, cubed	1 cup	5.3
Broccoli	1 cup	5.1
Turnip greens	1 cup	5.0
Carrots	1 cup	4.7
Spinach	1 cup	4.3
Beet greens	1 cup	4.2
Brussels sprouts	1 cup	4.1
Green beans	1 cup	4.0
Okra	1 cup	4.0
Sweet potato	1 cup	3.9
Swiss chard	1 cup	3.7
Asparagus	1 cup	3.6
Yellow corn	1 cup	3.6
Beets	1 cup	3.4
Scallop or Pattypan Squash, slices	1 cup	3.4
White mushrooms	1 cup	3.4
Potatoes, mashed with whole milk	1 cup	3.2
Rutabagas	1 cup	3.1
Turnips	1 cup	3.1
Dandelion greens	1 cup	3.0
Shiitake mushrooms	1 cup	3.0
Cabbage	1 cup	2.9
Cauliflower	1 cup	2.9
Onions	1 cup	2.9
Mustard greens	1 cup	2.8
Pumpkin	1 cup	2.7
Kale	1 cup	2.6
Eggplant,	1 cup	2.5
Snow peas	1 cup	2.5
Summer squash	1 cup	2.5
Celery	1 cup	2.4
Spaghetti Squash	1 cup	2.2
Crookneck or Straighneck Squash, slices	1 cup	2.0
Kohlrabi	1 cup	1.8

FIBER

Potatoes, flesh, baked	1 cup	1.8
Zucchini	1 cup	1.8
Cabbage, Chinese Bok-Choy	1 cup	1.7
Tomatoes	1 cup	1.7
Leeks	1 cup	1.0

Vegetables, Frozen	Amount	Fiber (g)
Green peas	1 cup	8.8
Spinach	1 cup	7.0
Brussels sprouts	1 cup	6.4
Turnip greens	1 cup	5.6
Broccoli	1 cup	5.5
Carrots	1 cup	4.8
Collard greens	1 cup	4.8
Rhubarb	1 cup	4.8
Green beans	1 cup	4.1
Corn	1 cup	3.9
Okra	1 cup	3.9
Asparagus	1 cup	2.9
Kale	1 cup	2.8

Vegetables, Raw	Amount	Fiber (g)
Mustard spinach	1 cup	4.2
Carrots	1 cup	3.1
Red bell peppers	1 cup	3.1
Cactus pad, Nopales	1 cup	3.0
Belgian endive	1 cup	2.8
Onions	1 cup	2.7
Green onions & scallions	1 cup	2.6
Green bell peppers	1 cup	2.5
Snow peas	1 cup	2.5
Broccoli	1 cup	2.3
Cabbage, Savoy	1 cup	2.2
Tomatoes	1 cup	2.2
Cauliflower	1 cup	2.0
Oyster mushrooms	1 cup	2.0
Celery	1 cup	1.9
Dandelion greens	1 cup	1.9
Cabbage	1 cup	1.8
Enoki mushrooms	1 cup	1.8
Tomatoes, cherry	1 cup	1.8
Endive	1 cup	1.6

FIBER

Cabbage, Red	1 cup	1.5
Kale	1 cup	1.3
Yellow bell peppers	1 cup	1.3
Romaine lettuce	1 cup	1.2
Summer squash	1 cup	1.2
Broccoli, raab	1 cup	1.1
Portabella mushrooms	1 cup	1.1
Zucchini	1 cup	1.1
Cabbage, Chinese Bok-Choy	1 cup	0.7
Green leaf lettuce	1 cup	0.7
Iceberg lettuce	1 cup	0.7
Spinach	1 cup	0.7
White mushrooms	1 cup	0.7
Butterhead or boston lettuce	1 cup	0.6
Swiss Chard	1 cup	0.6
Cucumber	1 cup	0.5
Shiitake mushrooms	1 each	0.5
Crimini mushrooms	1 cup	0.4
Radicchio	1 cup	0.4
Arugula	1 cup	0.3
Red leaf lettuce	1 cup	0.3
Watercress	1 cup	0.2

Nutrient Data Collection Form

Food	Amount	Book Numbers	Multiply By	Estimated Nutrient Intake
Nutrient::	RDA:	Estimated:	% of RDA:	Total Estimated:

To download additional forms for free, go to www.TopNutrients4U.com

IRON

Iron is a mineral needed daily in milligram (mg) quantities. It is necessary for transporting oxygen to all living cells, regulating of cell growth, and reproducing. When iron deficiency limits the supply of oxygen to cells it results in fatigue, decreased physical performance, and a decreased immunity which, if not corrected, leads to anemia. The type of anemia may be mild, moderate, or severe depending on the cause and how long a person was deficient. The iron deficiency type of anemia is closely associated with a low dietary intake and excessive blood losses.

A diet consisting of a variety of foods normally contains a sufficient amount of iron, but women, menstruating or pregnant, and children are at a high risk of deficiency. Adult men and post-menopausal women are at high risk of consuming too much iron.

Unlike other nutritional minerals, excess iron is not easily excreted and stays in the body longer. Symptoms of excess iron includes low blood pressure, irregular heart rhythm, a change in skin color, absences of periods, hair loss, depression, and a rise in blood sugar. Vegetarians who exclude all animal foods may need to increase their dietary iron intake because of the lower intestinal absorption of iron from plant food.

Recommended daily allowance (RDA) for iron is in milligram, mg, quantities.

Recommend Daily Intakes Levels for Iron

Children	Iron, mg
1 to 3 year olds	7
4 to 8 year olds	10

Males	
9 to 13 year olds	8
14 to 18 year olds	11
19 to 30 years	8
31 to 50 years	8
51 to 70 years	8
Over 70	8

Females	
9 to 13 year olds	8
14 to 18 year olds	15
19 to 30 years	18
31 to 50 years	18
51 to 70 years	8
Over 70	8
Pregnancy	27
Lactation	9

IRON

Alcohol	Amount	Iron (mg)
Red Wine	1 glass	0.68
White Wine	1 glass	0.40
Light Beer	1 bottle	0.11
Regular Beer	1 bottle	0.07
Gin, Rum, Vodka, Whisky	1 shot	0.02

Beans, Canned	Amount	Iron (mg)
White beans, mature	1 cup	7.83
Navy	1 cup	4.85
Lima beans	1 cup	4.36
Great Northern	1 cup	4.11
Cranberry beans	1 cup	4.03
Refried beans	1 cup	3.57
Pinto	1 cup	3.53
Kidney beans, red	1 cup	3.25
Baked beans, plain	1 cup	3.02
Garbanzo beans	1 cup	2.95
Fava	1 cup	2.56
Blackeyed peas	1 cup	2.33
Yellow beans	1 cup	1.38
Green beans	1 cup	1.35

Beans, Cooked	Amount	Iron (mg)
Natto	1 cup	15.05
Hyacinath beans	1 cup	8.89
Soybeans, mature	1 cup	8.84
Winged beans	1 cup	7.45
White beans, mature	1 cup	6.62
Lentils	1 cup	6.59
Mothbeans	1 cup	5.56
Black Turtle beans, mature	1 cup	5.27
Kidney beans	1 cup	5.20
White beans, small	1 cup	5.08
Garbanzo beans	1 cup	4.74
Adzuki	1 cup	4.60
Soybeans, green	1 cup	4.50
Lima beans	1 cup	4.49
Navy beans	1 cup	4.30
Black-eyed peas	1 cup	4.29
Great Northern	1 cup	3.77
Cranberry beans	1 cup	3.70
Soybeans, mature, dry roasted	1 cup	3.67
Black beans	1 cup	3.61

IRON

Continued

Pinto beans	1 cup	3.57
Edamame	1 cup	3.52
Mung beans, mature seeds	1 cup	2.83
Fava beans	1 cup	2.55
Split peas	1 cup	2.53
Lupini beans	1 cup	1.99
Pigeon peas	1 cup	1.86
Yellow beans	1 cup	1.60
Yardlong beans, Chinese long beans	1 cup	1.02
Green beans	1 cup	0.81

Beef, Cooked	Amount	Iron (mg)
Tri Tip Steak, trimmed to 0" fat	3 oz	3.18
T-Bone steak, trimmed 0" fat	3 oz	2.85
London Broil, top round, trim to 0" fat	3 oz	2.82
Chuck roast, trimmed to 1/8" fat	3 oz	2.62
Ribeye steak, lean, trimmed 0" fat	3 oz	2.58
Porterhouse steak, trimmed to 0" fat	3 oz	2.50
Ground beef, 95%,	3 oz	2.41
Brisket, lean, trimmed to 0" fat	3 oz	2.40
Skirt Steak, trimmed to 0" fat	3 oz	2.35
Ground beef, 90%	3 oz	2.30
Ground beef, 85%	3 oz	2.21
Ground beef, 80%,	3 oz	2.11
Beef ribs, trimmed to 1/8" fat	3 oz	2.01
Ground beef, 75%,	3 oz	2.01
Top sirloin, lean, trimmed to 1/8" fat	3 oz	1.59
Filet Mignon, tenderloin, trimmed to 0" fat	3 oz	1.50
Flank steak, lean, trimmed to 0" fat	3 oz	1.48

Beef, Cooked	Amount	Iron (mg)
Tri Tip steak, lean, trimmed to 0" fat	1 lb	16.96
T-bone steak, trimmed to 0" fat	1 lb	15.20
Chuck roast, trimmed to 1/8" fat	1 lb	13.98
Porterhouse steak, trimmed to 0" fat	1 lb	13.34
Brisket, lean, trimmed to 0" fat	1 lb	12.80
Skirt steak, trimmed to 0" fat	1 lb	12.56
Beef ribs, trimmed to 1/8" fat	1 lb	10.76
Flank steak, lean, trimmed to 0" fat	1 lb	7.90
Top Sirloin, trimmed to 1/8" fat	1 lb	7.85
Flank steak, lean, trimmed to 0" fat	1 steak	6.66
Ribeye steak, boneless, trim to 0" fat	1 steak	6.42
Ribeye filet, lean, trimmed to 0" fat	1 filet	4.59
Filet Mignon, tenderloin, trimmed to 0" fat	1 steak	3.79
Top Sirloin, choice filet, trimmed to 0" fat	1 filet	3.58

RDA for adults in 8 mg for males and 18 mg for females

IRON

Beef, Ground, Cooked	Amount	Iron (mg)
Ground beef, 95%	1/4 lb patty	2.32
Ground beef, 90%	1/4 lb patty	2.22
Ground beef, 85%	1/4 lb patty	2.00
Ground beef, 80%	1/4 lb patty	1.91
Ground beef, 75%	1/4 lb patty	1.66

Bread	Amount	Iron (mg)
Bagel plain	4" bagel	5.38
Mexican roll, bollilo	1 roll	3.82
Bagel, egg, enriched	4" bagel	3.54
Bagel, cinnamon & raisens	4 " bagel	3.36
Bagel, oat bran	4" bagel	3.23
Indian bread, Naan, plain	1 piece	2.92
Bagel, wheat	4" bagel	2.70
English Muffin, plain	1 muffin	2.28
Kaiser rolls	1 roll	1.87
Indian bread, Naan, whole wheat	1 piece	1.83
Pita, white	6" pita	1.57
Hamburger & Hotdog buns, plain	1 bun	1.43
Egg bread	1 slice	1.22
Croissants, butter	1 medium	1.16
Cornbread	1 piece	1.14
Tortillas, flour	1 tortilla	1.07
Dinner Rolls, brown & serve	1 roll	1.04
Pumpernickle	1 slice	0.92
French, italian, sourdough	1 slice	0.91
Rye bread	1 slice	0.91
Wheat	1 slice	0.87
Raisen bread	1 slice	0.75
Oatmeal bread	1 slice	0.73
Potato bread	1 slice	0.72
Potato bread	1 slice	0.72
Whole-Wheat	1 slice	0.68
Multigrain bread	1 slice	0.65
Tortillas, corn	1 tortilla	0.32
Cracked wheat	1 slice	0.07

Butter	Amount	Iron (mg)
Regular whipped butter, salted	1 tbsp	0.02
Regular butter, salted	1 tbsp	0.00

RDA for adults in 8 mg for males and 18 mg for females

IRON

Cereal, General Mills®	Amount	Iron (mg)
Total Whole Grain	1 cup	24.00
Multi-Bran CHEX	1 cup	21.62
Wheat Chex	1 cup	19.18
Total Raisin Bran	1 cup	18.02
Total Cranberry Crunch	1 cup	14.40
Wheaties	1 cup	11.99
Chocolate Chex	1 cup	11.52
Cinnamon Chex	1 cup	10.80
Dora The Explorer	1 cup	10.80
Corn Chex	1 cup	8.99
Oatmeal Crisp, Hearty Raisin	1 cup	8.99
Rice Chex	1 cup	8.99
Oatmeal Crisp, Crunchy Almond	1 cup	8.25
Lucky Charms	1 cup	8.02
Kix	1 cup	7.68
Berry Berry Kix	1 cup	7.39
Cocoa Puffs	1 cup	6.01
Raisin Nut Bran	1 cup	6.01
Cookie Crisp	1 cup	6.00
Honey Nut Chex	1 cup	6.00
Golden Grams	1 cup	5.99
Reese's Puffs	1 cup	5.99
Cinnamon Toast Crunch	1 cup	5.33
Basic 4	1 cup	4.51
Trix	1 cup	4.51
Honey Nut Clusters	1 cup	4.50

Cereal, General Mills Cheerios®	Amount	Iron (mg)
Multi Grain	1 cup	18
Original	1 cup	9
Banana Nut	1 cup	6
Chocolate	1 cup	6
Crunch, Oat Clusters	1 cup	6
Apple Cinnamon	1 cup	6
Berry Burst	1 cup	6
Frosted	1 cup	6
Fruity	1 cup	6
Honey Nut	1 cup	6
Yogurt Burst, Strawberry	1 cup	6

RDA for adults in 8 mg for males and 18 mg for females

IRON

Cereal, General Mills Fiber One®	Amount	Iron (mg)
Frosted Shredded Wheat	1 cup	17.88
Original Bran	1 cup	9.00
Honey Clusters	1 cup	4.52
Raisin Bran Clusters	1 cup	4.51
Caramel Delight	1 cup	4.50

Cereal, Kashi®	Amount	Iron (mg)
7-Whole Grain Nuggets	1 cup	27.84
Heart to Heart, Warm Cinnamon	1 cup	3.83
Go Lean	1 cup	2.60
Heart to Heart, Honey Toasted Oat	1 cup	2.42
Go Lean Crisp, Cinnamon Crumble	1 cup	2.38
Good Friends	1 cup	2.17
Heart to Heart, Oat Flakes & Blueberry Clusters	1 cup	2.04
Go Lean Crisp, Toasted Berry Crumble	1 cup	1.75
Go Lean Crunch	1 cup	1.70
Autumn Wheat	1 cup	1.67
Berry Fruitful	29 biscuits	1.65
Cinnamon Harvest	28 biscuits	1.54
Island Vanilla	27 biscuits	1.54
Go Lean Crunch, Honey Almond Flax	1 cup	1.48
7-Whole Grain Flakes	1 cup	1.45
Berry Blossom	1 cup	1.36
Honey Sunshine	1 cup	1.28
Strawberry Fields	1 cup	0.99
Indigo Morning	1 cup	0.94
Simply Maize	1 cup	0.94
7-Whole Grain Honey Puffs	1 cup	0.75
7-Whole Grain Puffs	1 cup	0.57
Blackberry Hills	1 cup	x
Go Lean Vanilla Graham	1 cup	x
Heart to Heart, Nutty Chia Flax	1 cup	x

Cereal, Kellogg's®	Amount	Iron (mg)
All-Bran Complete Wheat Flakes	1 cup	23.97
Product 19	1 cup	18.09
Smart Start, Strong Heart, Antioxidants	1 cup	18.00
Frosted MINI-Wheats Bite Size	1 cup	16.96
Frosted MINI wheats, Big Bite	1 cup	16.32
All-Bran Bran Buds	1 cup	13.51
All-Bran Original	1 cup	10.91
Fiberplus Cinnamon Oat Crunch	1 cup	10.79
Crispix	1 cup	9.74

RDA for adults in 8 mg for males and 18 mg for females

IRON

Rice Krispies	1 cup	9.63
Cocoa Krispies	1 cup	9.18
Frosted Flakes	1 cup	9.13
Simply Cinnamon Corn Flakes	1 cup	8.99
Corn Flakes	1 cup	8.12
Frosted Rice Krispies	1 cup	7.56
Raisin Bran	1 cup	7.53
MUESLIX	1 cup	6.73
Crunchy Nut Roasted Nut & Honey O's	1 cup	6.01
Crunchy Nut Golden Honey Nut Flakes	1 cup	5.99
Berry Rice Krispies	1 cup	5.40
Apple Jacks	1 cup	4.83
Raisin Bran Extra	1 cup	4.80
CINNABON	1 cup	4.71
Froot Loops	1 cup	4.65
All-Bran Strawberry Medley	1 cup	4.51
Raisin Bran Crunch	1 cup	4.50
Smorz	1 cup	4.50
Low Fat Granola with Raisins	1 cup	3.78
Smart Start, Strong Heart, Toasted Oat	1 cup	3.60
Honey Crunch Corn Flakes	1 cup	2.48
Rice Krispies Treats	1 cup	2.48
Cracklin' Oat Bran	1 cup	2.42
Corn Pops	1 cup	1.79
Fiberplus Berry Yogurt Crunch	1 cup	1.43
Honey Smacks	1 cup	0.47

Cereal, Kellogg's Special-K®	Amount	Iron (mg)
Multigrain Oats & Honey	1 cup	12.15
Vanilla Almond	1 cup	11.12
Chocolately Delight	1 cup	10.83
Protein Plus	1 cup	10.83
Blueberry	1 cup	10.80
Cinnamon Pecan	1 cup	10.80
Fruit & Yogurt	1 cup	10.79
Original	1 cup	8.68
Red Berries	1 cup	8.09

Cereal, Post®	Amount	Iron (mg)
Grape-Nuts Cereal	1 cup	44.15
Honey Nut Shredded Wheat	1 cup	16.52
Great Grains, Banana Nut Crunch	1 cup	16.22
Great Grains, Raisin, Date & Pecan	1 cup	12.03
Great Grains, Crunchy Pecan	1 cup	11.99
Bran Flakes	1 cup	10.80

RDA for adults in 8 mg for males and 18 mg for females

IRON

Continued

Raisin Bran	1 cup	10.80
Grape-Nuts Flakes	1 cup	10.79
Alpha-Bits	1 cup	9.00
Great Grains, Cranberry Almond Crunch	1 cup	2.43
Fruity Pebbles	1 cup	2.41
Golden Crisp	1 cup	2.41
Cocoa Pebbles	1 cup	2.40
Shredded Wheat n' Bran, spoon size	1 cup	1.84
Shredded Wheat, Frosted, spoon-size	1 cup	1.80
Honeycomb	1 cup	1.79
Blueberry Morning	1 cup	1.45
Shredded Wheat, Original, spoon-size	1 cup	1.22
Shredded Wheat, Oiginal, big-biscuit	1 biscuit	0.74

Post® Honey Bunches Of Oats®	Amount	Iron (mg)
With Vanilla Bunches	1 cup	16.2
With Almonds	1 cup	14.4
Honey Roasted	1 cup	13.9
Just Bunches, Honey Roasted	1 cup	12.1
With Cinnamon Bunches	1 cup	10.8
With Strawberries	1 cup	10.8
Pecan Bunches	1 cup	5.9

Cereal, Quaker®	Amount	Iron (mg)
Oatmeal Squares, Golden Maple	1 cup	18.34
Oatmeal Squares, Cinnamon	1 cup	16.53
Oatmeal Squares	1 cup	16.41
Toasted Multigrain Crisp	1 cup	13.66
LIFE Cereal, Original	1 cup	12.32
LIFE Cereal, Maple & Brown Sugar	1 cup	12.24
Corn Bran Crunch	1 cup	11.15
LIFE Cereal, Cinnamon	1 cup	9.91
Honey Graham OH'S	1 cup	7.92
CAP'N Crunch	1 cup	6.99
CAP'N Crunch's OOPs! All Berries	1 cup	6.90
CAP'N Crunch & Crunchberries	1 cup	6.89
CAP'N Crunch's Peanut Butter Crunch	1 cup	6.61
Granola, Apple, Cranberry, & Almond	1 cup	2.42
Puffed Wheat	1 cup	0.66
Puffed Rice	1 cup	0.53

IRON

Cereal, Cooked	Amount	Iron (mg)
Malt-o-Meal, plain	1 serving	17.23
Farina	1 cup	12.74
Cream of Wheat, regular	1 cup	9.39
Oats, regular, unenriched	1 cup	2.11
White corn grits	1 cup	1.38
Yellow corn grits	1 cup	1.38
WHEATENA	1 cup	1.36

Cheese	Amount	Iron (mg)
Ricotta, part skim milk	1 cup	1.08
Ricotta, whole milk	1 cup	0.93
Cottage cheese, lowfat, 2 %	1 cup	0.34
Cottage cheese, lowfat, 1 %	1 cup	0.32
Cottage cheese, nonfat, uncreamed	1 cup	0.22
Cottage cheese, creamed, small curd	1 cup	0.16

Cheese	Amount	Iron (mg)
Goat cheese, soft	1 oz	0.54
Goat cheese, hard	1 oz	0.53
Goat cheese, semisoft	1 oz	0.46
Mozzarella, nonfat	1 oz	0.35
Parmesan, grated	1 oz	0.26
Colby	1 oz	0.22
Romano	1 oz	0.22
Monterey	1 oz	0.20
Monterey, low fat	1 oz	0.20
American, pasteurized process, imitation	1 oz	0.19
Cheddar cheese	1 oz	0.19
American, pasteurized process, fortified	1 oz	0.18
Feta cheese	1 oz	0.18
Roqufort	1 oz	0.16
Provolone	1 oz	0.15
Provolone, reduced fat	1 oz	0.15
Brie	1 oz	0.14
American, pasteurized process, low fat	1 oz	0.12
Cheddar cheese, lowfat	1 oz	0.12
Mozzarella, whole milk	1 oz	0.12
Muenster	1 oz	0.12
Cream cheese	1 oz	0.11
Muenster, low fat	1 oz	0.11
Blue cheese	1 oz	0.09
Fontina	1 oz	0.07
Gouda	1 oz	0.07

RDA for adults in 8 mg for males and 18 mg for females

IRON

Mozzarella, part skim milk, low moisture	1 oz	0.07
Swiss	1 oz	0.06
Cream cheese, fat free	1 oz	0.05
Gruyere	1 oz	0.05
Swiss, low fat	1 oz	0.05

Cheese, Mexican	Amount	Iron (mg)
Mexican, blend	1 oz	0.17
Queso seco	1 oz	0.17
Queso asadero	1 oz	0.14
Queso anejo	1 oz	0.13
Queso chihuahua	1 oz	0.13
Queso fresco	1 oz	0.06
Queso blanco	1 oz	0.05
Mexican, blend, reduced fat	1 oz	0.04

Chicken, Cooked	Amount	Iron (mg)
Thigh, with skin, fried	1 thigh	1.25
Breast, with skin, fried, flour	1/2 breast	1.17
Breast, no skin, roasted	1/2 breast	0.89
Thigh, no skin, roasted	1 thigh	0.68
Drumstick, with skin, fried	1 drumstick	0.66
Wing with skin, fried in batter	1 wing	0.63
Drumstick, no skin, roasted	1 drumstick	0.57
Wing with skin, roasted	1 wing	0.43

Chicken, Cooked	Amount	Iron (mg)
Thigh with skin, fried in flour	3 oz	1.27
Drumstick with skin, fried in flour	3 oz	1.14
Wing with skin, roasted	3 oz	1.08
Wing with skin, fried in flour	3 oz	1.06
Breast meat only, no skin, roasted	3 oz	1.01
Wing meat only, no skin, roasted	3 oz	0.99
Thigh meat only, no skin, roasted	3 oz	0.92
Breast with skin, roasted	3 oz	0.91
Thigh with skin, roasted	3 oz	0.89
Breast with skin, fried in flour	3 oz	0.88
Drumstick meat only, no skin, roasted	3 oz	0.83
Drumstick with skin, roasted	3 oz	0.82
Cornish game hens, meat only	3 oz	0.65

IRON

Cream	Amount	Iron (mg)
Sour Cream, cultured	1 tbsp	0.02
Half & Half	1 tbsp	0.01
Light Coffe Cream	1 tbsp	0.01
Sour Cream, reduced fat	1 tbsp	0.01
Heavy Cream	1 tbsp	0
Whipped Topping, pressurized	1 tbsp	0

Eggs	Amount	Iron (mg)
Egg substitute, liquid, fat free	1/4 cup	1.19
Egg whole, poached	1 large	0.88
Egg whole, fried	1 large	0.87
Egg whole, scrambled	1 large	0.80
Egg whole, hard boiled	1 large	0.60
Egg yolk	1 large	0.45
Egg whites, dried	1 ounce	0.04
Egg whites	1 large	0.03
Egg whites, dried powder, stabilized	1 tbsp	0.02

Fish, Canned	Amount	Iron (mg)
Atlantic Sardines, in oil	3 oz	2.48
Light tuna, in water	3 oz	1.39
Light tuna, in oil	3 oz	1.18
White (albacore) tuna, in water	3 oz	0.82
White (albacore) tuna, in oil	3 oz	0.55

Fish, Cooked	Amount	Iron (mg)
King mackerel	3 oz	1.94
Freshwater bass	3 oz	1.62
Walleye pike	3 oz	1.42
Skipjack (aku) tuna	3 oz	1.36
Carp	3 oz	1.35
Pacific mackerel	3 oz	1.27
Catfish, breaded & fried	3 oz	1.22
Atlantic mackerel	3 oz	1.13
Bluefin tuna	3 oz	1.11
Atlantic herring, pickeled	3 oz	1.04
Grouper	3 oz	0.97
Orange roughy	3 oz	0.96
Striped bass	3 oz	0.92
Atlantic salmon, wild	3 oz	0.88
Yellowfin tuna	3 oz	0.78
Chinook salmon	3 oz	0.77
Atlantic croaker	3 oz	0.73

RDA for adults in 8 mg for males and 18 mg for females

IRON

Greenland halibut	3 oz	0.72
Spanish mackerel	3 oz	0.63
Keta (chum) salmon	3 oz	0.60
Tilapia	3 oz	0.59
Florida pompano	3 oz	0.57
Yellowtail	3 oz	0.54
Coho salmon, wild	3 oz	0.52
Atlantic pollock	3 oz	0.50
Pollock	3 oz	0.48
Walleye pollock	3 oz	0.48
Atlantic cod	3 oz	0.42
Sockeye salmon	3 oz	0.42
Pink salmon	3 oz	0.38
Swordfish	3 oz	0.38
Whiting	3 oz	0.36
Coho salmon, farmed	3 oz	0.33
Rainbow trout, wild	3 oz	0.32
Alaskan halibut	3 oz	0.31
Rainbow trout, farmed	3 oz	0.31
Sea bass	3 oz	0.31
Catfish, wild	3 oz	0.30
Atlantic salmon, farmed	3 oz	0.29
Catfish, farmed	3 oz	0.24
Atlantic perch	3 oz	0.23
Flounder	3 oz	0.20
Snapper	3 oz	0.20
Haddock	3 oz	0.18
Atlantic halibut	3 oz	0.17
Pacific cod	3 oz	0.17

Fish, Shellfish, Cooked	Amount	Iron (mg)
Clams, breaded & fried	3 oz	11.82
Octopus	3 oz	8.11
Eastern oysters, farmed	3 oz	6.60
Eastern oysters, wild	3 oz	6.09
Oysters, breaded & fried	3 oz	5.91
Abalone	3 oz	3.23
Queen crab	3 oz	2.45
Clams, canned	3 oz	2.28
Shrimp, canned	3 oz	1.81
Shrimp, breaded & fried	3 oz	1.07
Blue crab cakes	3 oz	0.92
Squid, fried	3 oz	0.86
Crayfish	3 oz	0.71
Scallops, breaded & fried	3 oz	0.70

IRON

Alaskan king crab	3 oz	0.65
Blue crab, canned	3 oz	0.42
Blue crab	3 oz	0.42
Alaskan king crab, imitation	3 oz	0.33
Shrimp	3 oz	0.27
Northern lobster	3 oz	0.25

Fruit, Canned	Amount	Iron (mg)
Plums	1 cup	2.17
Pineapple	1 cup	0.97
Apricots	1 cup	0.77
Olives, black	5 large	0.73
Peaches	1 cup	0.71
Pears	1 cup	0.59
Applesauce, unsweetened	1 cup	0.56
Applesauce, sweetened	1 cup	0.31
Olives, green	5 large	0.07

Fruit, Dried	Amount	Iron (mg)
Peaches	1 cup	6.50
Cranberries	1 cup	6.00
Currants	1 cup	4.69
Pears	1 cup	3.78
Apricots	1 cup	3.46
Figs	1 cup	3.02
Apples	1 cup	1.20

Fruit, Frozen	Amount	Iron (mg)
Raspberries	1 cup	1.62
Blackberries	1 cup	1.21
Strawberries	1 cup	1.20
Peaches	1 cup	0.92
Blueberries	1 cup	0.90

Fruit, Raw	Amount	Iron (mg)
Raisins	1 cup	2.73
Mulberries	1 cup	2.59
Elderberries	1 cup	2.32
Black currants	1 cup	1.72
Prunes, uncooked, pitted	1 cup	1.62
Dates	1 cup	1.50
California avocado, pureed	1 cup	1.40
Stewed prunes	1 cup	1.02
Blackberries	1 cup	0.89

RDA for adults in 8 mg for males and 18 mg for females

IRON

Plantains	1 cup	0.89
Raspberries	1 cup	0.85
Strawberries	1 cup	0.68
Apricots	1 cup	0.64
Kiwi	1 cup	0.56
Cherries, no pits	1 cup	0.55
Grapes, red or green	1 cup	0.54
Pomegrenates	1 cup	0.52
Pineapple	1 cup	0.48
Blueberries	1 cup	0.41
Nectarine	1 cup	0.40
Florida avocado	1 cup	0.39
Peachs	1 cup	0.38
Papayas	1 cup	0.36
Water mellon	1 cup	0.36
Cantaloupe, cubes	1 cup	0.34
Honeydew	1 cup	0.29
Tangerine	1 cup	0.29
Plums	1 cup	0.28
Pears	1 cup	0.27
Mango	1 cup	0.26
Cranberries, whole	1 cup	0.25
Naval Oranges	1 cup	0.21
Grapefruit, pink or red, sections	1 cup	0.18
Oranges	1 cup	0.18
Florida Oranges	1 cup	0.17
Valencias oranges	1 cup	0.16
Apples	1 cup	0.15

Fruit, Raw	Amount	Iron (mg)
Plantains	1 fruit	1.07
Avocado, California	1 fruit	0.85
Pomegranates	1 fruit	0.85
Raisins	1 small box	0.81
Olives, Black	5 large	0.73
Chayote	1 fruit	0.69
Cherimoya	1 fruit	0.63
Persimmons, small native	1 fruit	0.62
Cantaloupe	1/2 fruit	0.58
Mango	1 fruit	0.54
Avocado, Florida	1 fruit	0.52
Prunes, uncooked	5 fruit	0.44
Dates	5 fruit	0.42
Papayas, small	1 fruit	0.39
Nectarine	1 fruit	0.38

RDA for adults in 8 mg for males and 18 mg for females

IRON

Bananas	1 medium	0.31
Cherries	10 fruit	0.30
Peaches	1 fruit	0.25
Pears	1 fruit	0.25
Persimmons, Japanese	1 fruit	0.25
Strawberries	5 fruit	0.25
Kiwi	1 fruit	0.24
Grapes	10 fruit	0.18
Naval Oranges	1 fruit	0.18
Apples	1 fruit	0.17
Figs, dried	1 fruit	0.17
Kumquats	1 fruit	0.16
Apricots	1 fruit	0.14
Pineapple, slices	1/2" x 3"	0.14
Florida Oranges	1 fruit	0.13
Tangerine	1 fruit	0.13
Plums	1 fruit	0.11
Valencias oranges	1 fruit	0.11
Grapefruit, pink or red	1/2 fruit	0.10
Star fruit, Carambola	1 fruit	0.07
Olives, Green	5 large	0.07
Pineapple guava, Feijoa	1 fruit	0.06

Game meat, Cooked	Amount	Iron (mg)
Squirrel	3 oz	5.79
Caribou	3 oz	5.24
Rabbit	3 oz	4.12
Deer	3 oz	3.80
Antelope	3 oz	3.57
Buffalo, steak, free range	3 oz	3.20
Elk	3 oz	3.09
Deer, ground	3 oz	2.85
Elk, ground	3 oz	2.84
Bison, ground	3 oz	2.62
Duck	3 oz	2.30
Wild boar	3 oz	0.95

Grains, Cooked	Amount	Iron (mg)
Amaranth	1 cup	5.17
Kamut	1 cup	3.46
Spelt	1 cup	3.24
White rice, long-grain, paraboiled	1 cup	3.17
White rice, long-grain, instant	1 cup	2.92
Quinoa	1 cup	2.76
Egg noodles	1 cup	2.35

RDA for adults in 8 mg for males and 18 mg for females

IRON

Continued

Oats, regular, unenriched	1 cup	2.11
Barley, pearled	1 cup	2.09
Oat bran	1 cup	1.93
White rice, long-grain, regular	1 cup	1.90
Macaroni	1 cup	1.79
Spaghetti	1 cup	1.79
Bulgur	1 cup	1.75
Egg & Spinach noodles	1 cup	1.74
Macaroni, Whole-Wheat	1 cup	1.48
Spaghetti, Whole-Wheat	1 cup	1.48
Spaghetti, spinach	1 cup	1.46
Buckwheat	1 cup	1.34
Millet	1 cup	1.10
Wild rice	1 cup	0.98
Brown rice	1 cup	0.82
Couscous	1 cup	0.60
Soba noodles	1 cup	0.55
Rice noodles	1 cup	0.25

Herbs & Spices	Amount	Iron (mg)
Thyme, dried	1 tsp	1.70
Cumin	1 tsp	1.39
Basil, dried & ground	1 tsp	1.26
Celery seeds	1 tsp	0.90
Onion powder	1 tsp	0.80
Turmeric, ground	1 tsp	0.80
Anise seed	1 tsp	0.78
Curry powder	1 tsp	0.59
Oregano	1 tsp	0.55
Tarragon, dried	1 tsp	0.52
Dill weed, dried	1 tsp	0.49
Chili powder	1 tsp	0.45
Paprika	1 tsp	0.44
Rosemary, dried	1 tsp	0.35
Caraway seeds	1 tsp	0.34
Coriander, seeds	1 tsp	0.29
Parsley, dried	1 tsp	0.29
Bay leaf, crumbled	1 tsp	0.26
Cloves	1 tsp	0.25
Coriander, dried	1 tsp	0.25
Ginger, ground	1 tsp	0.20
Pepper, black	1 tsp	0.20
Sage, ground	1 tsp	0.20
Chervil, dried	1 tsp	0.19
Cinnamon powder	1 tsp	0.19

RDA for adults in 8 mg for males and 18 mg for females

IRON

Continued

Garlic powder	1 tsp	0.16
All-spice, ground	1 tsp	0.13
Thyme, fresh	1 tsp	0.10
Saffron	1 tsp	0.08
Rosemary, fresh	1 tsp	0.05
Basil, fresh, chopped	1 tsp	0.03
Chives, raw	1 tsp	0.02

Juice	Amount	Iron (mg)
Prune	1 cup	3.02
Carrot	1 cup	1.09
Tomato	1 cup	1.04
Vegetable	1 cup	1.02
Pineapple	1 cup	0.78
Grape	1 cup	0.63
Orange juice, raw	1 cup	0.50
Apple	1 cup	0.30
Cranberry	1 cup	0.25
Pomegranate	1 cup	0.25
Lemon juice, raw	1 cup	0.20
Grapefruit juice, raw	1 cup	0.18

Lamb, Cooked	Amount	Iron (mg)
Cubed, for stew or kabob	3 oz	1.99
Rib, lean, trimmed to 1/4" fat	3 oz	1.88
Foreshank, trimmed to 1/8" fat	3 oz	1.82
Leg, whole, trimmed to 1/4" fat	3 oz	1.68
Chops, loin, lean, trimmed to 1/4" fat	3 oz	1.54
Ground	3 oz	1.52

Milk	Amount	Iron (mg)
Coconut milk, canned	1 cup	7.46
Soy milk, original, unfortified	1 cup	1.56
Canned, evaporated, nonfat	1 cup	0.74
Canned, condensed, sweetened	1 cup	0.58
Canned, evaporated	1 cup	0.48
Sheep milk	1 cup	0.24
Buttermilk, lowfat	1 cup	0.12
Goat milk	1 cup	0.12
Buttermilk, whole milk	1 cup	0.07
Dry, instant, nonfat	1/3 cup	0.07
Lowfat, 1%	1 cup	0.07
Nonfat, fat free or skim liquid milk	1 cup	0.07
Whole milk, 3.25%	1 cup	0.07

RDA for adults in 8 mg for males and 18 mg for females

Continued

Human milk	1 cup	0.07
Reduced fat, 2%	1 cup	0.05

Nuts & Seeds	Amount	Iron (mg)
Sesame seeds	1 oz	4.12
Tahini	1 oz	2.54
Pumpkin seeds	1 oz	2.50
Chia seeds	1 oz	2.19
Cashews	1 oz	1.89
Flaxseeds	1 oz	1.62
Pine nuts	1 oz	1.57
Sunflower seeds	1 oz	1.49
Hazelnuts	1 oz	1.33
Peanuts	1 oz	1.30
Pistachio	1 oz	1.11
Almonds	1 oz	1.05
Macadamia	1 oz	1.05
Mixed nuts, roasted with peanuts, no salt	1 oz	1.05
Trail mix, regular with chocolate chips	1 oz	0.96
Black walnuts	1 oz	0.88
Trail mix, regular, salted	1 oz	0.86
English walnuts	1 oz	0.82
Trail mix, tropical	1 oz	0.75
Pecans	1 oz	0.72
Brazilnuts	1 oz	0.69
Coconut, raw meat	1 oz	0.69
Peanut butter, smooth style	1 oz	0.53

Nuts & Seeds	Amount	Iron (mg)
Sesame seeds	1/4 cup	5.24
Pumpkin seeds	1/4 cup	2.84
Flaxseeds	1/4 cup	2.41
Pine nuts	1/4 cup	1.87
Sunflower seeds	1/4 cup	1.84
Peanuts	1/4 cup	1.67
Hazelnuts, chopped	1/4 cup	1.35
Almonds, whole	1/4 cup	1.33
Sesame seeds	1 tbsp	1.31
Mixed nuts, roasted with peanuts, no salt	1/4 cup	1.27
Peanut butter, smooth	1/4 cup	1.26
Macadamia	1/4 cup	1.24
Trail mix, regular with chocolate chips	1/4 cup	1.24
Pistachio	1/4 cup	1.21
Trail mix, regular, salted	1/4 cup	1.14
Black walnuts, chopped	1/4 cup	0.98

RDA for adults in 8 mg for males and 18 mg for females

IRON

Trail mix, tropical	1/4 cup	0.92
Brazilnuts, whole	1/4 cup	0.81
English walnuts, chopped	1/4 cup	0.73
Pecans, halves	1/4 cup	0.63
Flaxseeds	1 tbsp	0.59
Coconut meat, shredded	1/4 cup	0.49
Cashews	1/4 cup	x
Chia seeds	1/4 cup	x

Pork, Cooked	Amount	Iron (mg)
Braunschweiger	3 oz	9.52
Liverwurst spread	1/4 cup	4.87
Spareribs	3 oz	1.57
Bacon	3 oz	1.22
Italian sausage	3 oz	1.22
Polish sausage	3 oz	1.22
Sausage	3 oz	1.16
Tenderloin	3 oz	0.98
Chops, lean, pan-fried	3 oz	0.84
Cured ham, lean	3 oz	0.80
Chops, pan-fried	3 oz	0.79
Backribs	3 oz	0.78
Sirloin pork chops	3 oz	0.74
Cured ham	3 oz	0.74
Canadian-style bacon	3 oz	0.70
Center loin pork chops	3 oz	0.67
Chops, broiled	3 oz	0.67
Bratwurst	3 oz	0.45

Turkey, Cooked	Amount	Iron (mg)
Turkey bacon	3 oz	1.79
Ground turkey, 85% lean	3 oz	1.73
Turkey sausage, reduced fat	3 oz	1.53
Liver	3 oz	1.52
Ground turkey, 93% lean	3 oz	1.47
Breast meat	3 oz	1.30
Ground turkey	3 oz	1.29
Dark meat	3 oz	1.22
Ground turkey, fat free	3 oz	0.66
Light meat	3 oz	0.60

RDA for adults in 8 mg for males and 18 mg for females

IRON

Veal, Cooked	Amount	Iron (mg)
Leg, top round	3 oz	1.12
Foreshank	3 oz	1.06
Ground	3 oz	0.84
Rib	3 oz	0.82
Sirloin	3 oz	0.78
Loin	3 oz	0.74
Breast	3 oz	0.71

VEGETABLES

Vegetables, Canned	Amount	Iron (mg)
Spinach	1 cup	4.92
Asparagus	1 cup	4.43
Sauerkraut	1 cup	3.47
Pumpkin	1 cup	3.41
Stewed tomato	1 cup	3.39
Beets	1 cup	3.09
Tomato sauce	1 cup	2.50
Tomatoes	1 cup	2.33
Green peas	1 cup	2.07
Sweet potato	1 cup	1.86
Mushrooms	1 cup	1.23
Green beans	1 cup	1.17
Carrots	1 cup	0.93
Corn	1 cup	0.88

Vegetables, Cooked	Amount	Iron (mg)
Spinach	1 cup	6.43
Swiss chard	1 cup	3.95
Snow peas	1 cup	3.15
Beet greens	1 cup	2.74
White mushrooms	1 cup	2.71
Sweet Potato, mashed	1 cup	2.36
Collard greens	1 cup	2.20
Acorn squash	1 cup	1.91
Dandelion greens	1 cup	1.89
Brussels sprouts	1 cup	1.87
Bok-Choy	1 cup	1.77
Asparagus	1 cup	1.64
Tomatoes	1 cup	1.63
Mustard Spinach	1 cup	1.44
Pumpkin	1 cup	1.40
Beets	1 cup	1.34

RDA for adults in 8 mg for males and 18 mg for females

IRON

	Amount	Iron (mg)
Lambsquarters	1 cup	1.26
Butternut squash	1 cup	1.23
Kale	1 cup	1.17
Turnip greens	1 cup	1.15
Leeks	1 cup	1.14
Broccoli	1 cup	1.05
Artichokes	1 cup	1.02
Cabbage, Red	1 cup	0.99
Mustard greens	1 cup	0.98
Parsnips	1 cup	0.90
Rutabagas	1 cup	0.90
Winter squash	1 cup	0.90
Green beans	1 cup	0.81
Napa Cabbage	1 cup	0.81
Yams, cubed	1 cup	0.71
Corn	1 cup	0.67
Crookneck or Straighneck Squash, slices	1 cup	0.67
Kohlrabi	1 cup	0.66
Summer squash	1 cup	0.65
Shiitake mushrooms	1 cup	0.64
Celery	1 cup	0.63
Scallop or Pattypan Squash, slices	1 cup	0.59
Potatoes, mashed with whole milk	1 cup	0.57
Cabbage, Savoy	1 cup	0.55
Carrots	1 cup	0.53
Spaghetti squash	1 cup	0.53
Onions	1 cup	0.50
Okra	1 cup	0.45
Potatoes, flesh	1 cup	0.43
Zucchini	1 cup	0.42
Cauliflower	1 cup	0.40
Turnips	1 cup	0.28
Cabbage	1 cup	0.26
Eggplant	1 cup	0.25

Vegetables, Frozen	Amount	Iron (mg)
Spinach	1 cup	3.72
Turnip greens	1 cup	3.18
Green peas	1 cup	2.43
Collard greens	1 cup	1.90
Asparagus	1 cup	1.64
Kale	1 cup	1.22
Broccoli	1 cup	1.12
Okra	1 cup	0.96
Green beans	1 cup	0.89

RDA for adults in 8 mg for males and 18 mg for females

IRON

Carrots	1 cup	0.77
Yellow corn	1 cup	0.77
Brussels sprouts	1 cup	0.74
Cauliflower	1 cup	0.74
Rhubarb	1 cup	0.50

Vegetables, Raw	Amount	Iron (mg)
Mustard spinach	1 cup	2.25
Collards	1 cup	2.15
Snow peas	1 cup	2.04
Spirulina, dried	1 tbsp	2.00
Dandelion greens	1 cup	1.70
Green onions & scallions	1 cup	1.48
Kale	1 cup	1.14
Oyster mushrooms, sliced	1 cup	1.14
Butternut Winter Squash	1 cup	0.98
Broccoli, raab	1 cup	0.86
Purslane	1 cup	0.86
Yellow bell peppers	1 cup	0.86
Tomatillos	1 cup	0.82
Cabbage, Napa	1 cup	0.81
Spinach	1 cup	0.81
Enoki mushrooms	1 cup	0.75
Butterhead or boston lettuce	1 cup	0.68
Swiss chard	1 cup	0.65
Broccoli	1 cup	0.64
Red bell peppers	1 cup	0.64
Bok-Choy	1 cup	0.56
Red cabbage	1 cup	0.56
Romaine lettuce	1 cup	0.54
Cactus pads, Nopales	1 cup	0.51
Green bell peppers	1 cup	0.51
Tomatoes	1 cup	0.49
Green leaf lettuce	1 cup	0.48
Cauliflower	1 cup	0.42
Endive	1 cup	0.42
Zucchini	1 cup	0.42
Summer squash	1 cup	0.40
Tomatoes, cherry	1 cup	0.40
White mushrooms	1 cup	0.35
Onions	1 cup	0.34
Red leaf lettuce	1 cup	0.34
Cabbage	1 cup	0.33
Carrots	1 cup	0.33
Arugula	1 cup	0.29

RDA for adults in 8 mg for males and 18 mg for females

IRON

Continued

Cucumbers	1 cup	0.29
Savoy cabbage	1 cup	0.28
Portabella mushrooms	1 cup	0.27
Chicory greens	1 cup	0.26
Celery	1 cup	0.24
Iceburg lettuce	1 cup	0.23
Radicchio	1 cup	0.23
Belgian endive	1 cup	0.22
Watercress	1 cup	0.07
Shiitake mushrooms, dried	1 each	0.06

RDA for adults in 8 mg for males and 18 mg for females

Nutrient Data Collection Form

Food	Amount	Book Numbers	Multiply By	Estimated Nutrient Intake
Nutrient::	RDA:	Estimated:	% of RDA:	Total Estimated:

To download additional forms for free, go to www.TopNutrients4U.com

429

MAGNESIUM

Magnesium is a positive charged mineral needed daily in milligram (mg) quantities. It is found in the bones, brain, muscles, cells, and blood. It is needed for fat and carbohydrate metabolism, DNA and protein synthesis, cardiac muscle contractions, normal heart rhythms, and regulation of calcium, potassium, and sodium metabolism.

As much as 12% of all hospitalized patients have been reported deficient in magnesium. Deficiency is associated with asthma, diabetes, insomnia, and hypertension. Deficiency causes include alcoholic abuse, prolonged diarrhea, kidney diseases, diuretic therapy, and inadequate dietary habits for long periods of time. Deficiency symptoms include fatigue, muscle weakness, cramps and spasms, hypocalcemia, low potassium serum levels, anxiety, depression, personality changes, sensitivity to loud sounds, difficulty swallowing, and a feeling of lumps in the throat. Toxicity is extremely rare and usually found only with patients suffering from chronic kidney failure.

The recommended daily allowance (RDA) for magnesium is in milligram, mg, quantities.

Recommend Daily Intakes Levels for Magnesium

Children	Magnesium, mg
1 to 3 year olds	80
4 to 8 year olds	130

Males	
9 to 13 year olds	240
14 to 18 year olds	410
19 to 30 years	400
31 to 50 years	420
51 to 70 years	420
Over 70	420

Females	
9 to 13 year olds	240
14 to 18 year olds	360
19 to 30 years	310
31 to 50 years	320
51 to 70 years	320
Over 70	320
Pregnancy	350
Lactation	310

MAGNESIUM

Alcohol	Amount	Magnesium (mg)
Regular Beer	1 bottle	21
Light Beer	1 bottle	18
Red Wine	1 glass	18
White Wine	1 glass	15
Gin, Rum, Vodka, Whisky	1 shot	0

Beans, Canned	Amount	Magnesium (mg)
Great Northern	1 cup	134
White beans, mature	1 cup	134
Navy beans	1 cup	123
Lima beans	1 cup	94
Refried beans	1 cup	90
Cranberry beans	1 cup	83
Fava beans	1 cup	82
Pinto beans	1 cup	79
Kidney, red	1 cup	77
Baked beans, plain	1 cup	69
Black-eyed peas	1 cup	67
Garbanzo beans	1 cup	65
Yellow beans	1 cup	20
Green beans	1 cup	18

Beans, Cooked	Amount	Magnesium (mg)
Soybeans, mature, dry roasted	1 cup	212
Natto	1 cup	201
Mothbeans	1 cup	184
Hyacinath beans	1 cup	159
Soybeans, mature	1 cup	148
White beans, small	1 cup	122
Adzuki	1 cup	120
Black beans	1 cup	120
White beans, mature	1 cup	113
Soybeans, green	1 cup	108
Edamame	1 cup	99
Mung beans, mature seeds	1 cup	97
Navy beans	1 cup	96
Winged beans	1 cup	93
Black Turtle beans, mature	1 cup	91
Black-eyed peas	1 cup	91
Lupini beans	1 cup	90
Cranberry beans	1 cup	88
Great Northern	1 cup	88
Pinto beans	1 cup	86

MAGNESIUM

Lima beans	1 cup	81
Kidney beans	1 cup	80
Garbanzo beans	1 cup	79
Pigeon peas	1 cup	77
Fava beans	1 cup	73
Lentils	1 cup	71
Split peas	1 cup	71
Yardlong beans, Chinese long beans	1 cup	44
Yellow beans	1 cup	31
Green beans	1 cup	22

Beef, Cooked	Amount	Magnesium (mg)
Tri Tip steak, trim to 0" fat	3 oz	22
London Broil, top round	3 oz	22
Ribeye steak, lean, trim 0" fat	3 oz	21
Top sirloin, lean, trim to 1/8" fat	3 oz	21
Filet Mignon, trim to 0" fat	3 oz	20
Skirt Steak, trim to 0" fat	3 oz	20
Flank steak, lean, trim to 0" fat	3 oz	20
T-Bone steak, trim to 0" fat	3 oz	20
Brisket, lean, trim to 0" fat	3 oz	19
Ground beef, 90%	3 oz	19
Ground beef, 95%	3 oz	19
Porterhouse steak, trim to 0" fat	3 oz	19
Ground Beef 85%, broiled	3 oz	18
Beef ribs, trim to 1/8" fat	3 oz	17
Ground beef, 75%	3 oz	17
Ground beef, 80%	3 oz	17
Chuck roast, trim to 1/8" fat	3 oz	16

Beef, Cooked	Amount	Magnesium (mg)
Tri Tip steak, lean, trim to 0" fat	1 lb cooked	118
Skirt steak, trim to 0" fat	1 lb cooked	109
T-bone steak, trim to 0" fat	1 lb cooked	109
Flank steak, lean, trim to 0" fat	1 lb cooked	104
Brisket, lean, trim to 0" fat	1 lb cooked	100
Porterhouse steak, trim to 0" fat	1 lb cooked	100
Top Sirloin, trim to 1/8" fat	1 lb cooked	100
Beef ribs, trim to 1/8" fat	1 lb cooked	91
Flank steak, lean, trim to 0" fat	1 steak	88
Chuck roast, trim to 1/8" fat	1 lb cooked	86
Ribeye steak, boneless, trim to 0" fat	1 steak	52
Ribeye filet, lean, trim to 0" fat	1 filet	35
Top Sirloin, choice filet, trim to 0" fat	1 filet	35
Filet Mignon, tenderloin, trim to 0" fat	1 steak	21

RDA for adults is 320 mg for females and 420 mg for males

MAGNESIUM

Beef, Cooked	Amount	Magnesium (mg)
Ground beef, 90%	1/4 lb patty	18
Ground beef, 95%	1/4 lb patty	18
Ground beef, 85%	1/4 lb patty	16
Ground beef, 80%	1/4 lb patty	15
Ground beef, 75%	1/4 lb patty	14

Bread	Amount	Magnesium (mg)
Indian bread, Naan, whole wheat	1 piece	72
Bagel, wheat	4" bagel	50
Bagel, oat bran	4" bagel	33
Mexican roll, bollilo	1 roll	29
Bagels, cinnamon & raisen	4" bagel	25
Indian bread, Naan, plain	1 piece	24
Whole-Wheat	1 slice	23
Bagels, egg	4" bagel	22
Bagels, plain	4" bagel	20
Multi-Grain, and Whole-Grain	1 slice	20
Tortillas, corn	1 tortilla	19
Pumpernickle	1 slice	17
Frybread	5 inch bread	16
Pita, white	6 inch pita	16
Kaiser rolls	1 roll	15
English muffin	1 muffin	14
Cracked wheat	1 slice	13
Rye bread	1 slice	13
Cornbread	1 piece	12
Wheat	1 slice	12
Oatmeal bread	1 slice	10
Potato bread	1 slice	9
Croissants, butter	1 medium	9
Hamburger & Hotdog buns, plain	1 bun	9
Potato bread	1 slice	9
Reduced calorie wheat	1 slice	9
Egg bread	1 slice	8
Dinner Rolls, brown & serve	1 roll	7
French, italian, sourdough	1 slice	7
Raisin bread, enriched	1 slice	7
Tortillas, flour	1 tortilla	7
White	1 slice	6

MAGNESIUM

Butter	Amount	Magnesium (mg)
Regular dairy butter, salted	1 tbsp	0
Regular dairy whipped butter, salted	1 tbsp	0

Cereal, General Mills®	Amount	Magnesium (mg)
Multi-Bran CHEX	1 cup	53
Wheat Chex	1 cup	53
Raisin Nut Bran	1 cup	45
Wheaties	1 cup	39
Oatmeal Crisp, Crunchy Almond	1 cup	37
Basic 4	1 cup	32
Total Raisin Bran	1 cup	32
Total Whole Grain	1 cup	32
Total Cranberry Crunch	1 cup	26
Honey Nut Clusters	1 cup	24
Cocoa Puffs	1 cup	21
Lucky Charms	1 cup	21
Reese's Puffs	1 cup	21
Cinnamon Toast Crunch	1 cup	17
Kix	1 cup	12
Chocolate Chex	1 cup	11
Cinnamon Chex	1 cup	11
Cookie Crisp	1 cup	11
Dora The Explorer	1 cup	11
Golden Grahams	1 cup	11
Honey Nut Chex	1 cup	11
Corn Chex	1 cup	8
Rice Chex	1 cup	8
Trix	1 cup	8
Berry Berry Kix	1 cup	0

Cereal, General Mills Cheerios®	Amount	Magnesium (mg)
Original	1 cup	40
Apple Cinnamon	1 cup	32
Berry Burst	1 cup	32
Honey Nut	1 cup	32
Yogurt Burst, Strawberry	1 cup	32
Fruity	1 cup	30
Banana Nut	1 cup	21
Chocolate	1 cup	21
Crunch, Oat Clusters	1 cup	21
Frosted	1 cup	21
Multi Grain	1 cup	4

RDA for adults is 320 mg for females and 420 mg for males

MAGNESIUM

Cereal, General Mills Fiber One®	Amount	Magnesium (mg)
Frosted Shredded Wheat	1 cup	40
Original	1 cup	32
Caramel Delight	1 cup	32
Honey Clusters	1 cup	24
Raisin Bran Clusters	1 cup	24

Cereal, Kashi®	Amount	Magnesium (mg)
7-Whole Grain Nuggets	1 cup	97
Go Lean	1 cup	84
Heart to Heart, Oat Flakes & Blueberry Clusters	1 cup	80
Go Lean Crisp, Toasted Berry Crumble	1 cup	73
Go Lean Crunch, Honey Almond Flax	1 cup	63
Island Vanilla	27 biscuits	59
Berry Fruitful	29 biscuits	58
Go Lean Crisp, Cinnamon Crumble	1 cup	53
Go Lean Crunch	1 cup	53
Autumn Wheat	29 biscuits	44
7-Whole Grain Flakes	1 cup	38
Indigo Morning	1 cup	38
Simply Maize	1 cup	38
7-Whole Grain Honey Puffs	1 cup	34
7-Whole Grain Puffs	1 cup	29
Berry Blossom	1 cup	28
Strawberry Fields	1 cup	24
Honey Sunshine	1 cup	23
Heart to Heart, Warm Cinnamon	1 cup	12
Good Friends	1 cup	10
Heart to Heart, Honey Toasted Oat	1 cup	3
Blackberry Hills	1 cup	x
Cinnamon Harvest	28 biscuits	x
Go Lean Vanilla Graham	1 cup	x
Heart to Heart, Nutty Chia Flax	1 cup	x

Cereal, Kellogg's®	Amount	Magnesium (mg)
All-Bran Original	1 cup	224
All-Bran Bran Buds	1 cup	185
Cracklin' Oat Bran	1 cup	101
Raisin Bran	1 cup	77
All-Bran Complete Wheat Flakes	1 cup	74
MUESLIX	1 cup	73
Smart Start, Strong Heart, Toasted Oat	1 cup	65
Raisin Bran Extra	1 cup	61
Low Fat Granola with Raisins	1 cup	58

RDA for adults is 320 mg for females and 420 mg for males

MAGNESIUM

Continued

Frosted MINI-Wheats, Bite-Size	1 cup	57
Frosted MINI-Wheats, Big-Bite	1 cup	47
Raisin Bran Crunch	1 cup	47
Smart Start, Strong Heart, Antioxidants	1 cup	24
Fiberplus Berry Yogurt Crunch	1 cup	24
Honey Smacks	1 cup	21
Cocoa Krispies	1 cup	16
Product 19	1 cup	16
Apple Jacks	1 cup	11
Froot Loops	1 cup	11
Simply Cinnamon Corn Flakes	1 cup	11
Crunchy Nut Golden Honey Nut Flakes	1 cup	10
Rice Krispies Treats	1 cup	9
Smorz	1 cup	9
Frosted Rice Krispies	1 cup	9
Honey Crunch Corn Flakes	1 cup	9
Berry Rice Krispies	1 cup	9
Corn Pops	1 cup	8
Rice Krispies	1 cup	7
Crispix	1 cup	6
Fiberplus Cinnamon Oat Crunch	1 cup	5
CINNABON	1 cup	4
Corn Flakes	1 cup	3
Frosted Flakes	1 cup	3
Crunchy Nut Roasted Nut & Honey O's	1 cup	3

Cereal, Kellogg's Special-K®	Amount	Magnesium (mg)
Protein Plus	1 cup	91
Low Fat Granola	1 cup	78
Multigrain Oats & Honey	1 cup	34
Vanilla Almond	1 cup	29
Cinnamon Pecan	1 cup	27
Chocolately Delight	1 cup	25
Blueberry	1 cup	22
Fruit & Yogurt	1 cup	21
Red Berries	1 cup	17
Original	1 cup	4

Cereal, Post®	Amount	Magnesium (mg)
Grape-Nuts Cereal	1 cup	159
Raisin Bran	1 cup	93
Bran Flakes	1 cup	89
Shredded Wheat n' Bran, spoon-size	1 cup	82
Great Grains, Crunchy Pecan	1 cup	68
Shredded Wheat, Original, spoon-size	1 cup	65

RDA for adults is 320 mg for females and 420 mg for males

MAGNESIUM

Continued

Great Grains, Raisin, Date & Pecan	1 cup	64
Great Grains, Banana Nut Crunch	1 cup	57
Great Grains, Cranberry Almond Crunch	1 cup	57
Honey Nut Shredded Wheat	1 cup	55
Shredded Wheat, lightly frosted, spoon-size	1 cup	48
Grape-Nuts Flakes	1 cup	39
Shredded Wheat, Original, big-biscuit	1 biscuit	33
Alpha-Bits	1 cup	30
Blueberry Morning	1 cup	25
Golden Crisp	1 cup	21
Cocoa Pebbles	1 cup	12
Honeycomb	1 cup	10
Fruity Pebbles	1 cup	6

Post® Honey Bunches of Oats®	Amount	Magnesium (mg)
Just Bunches, Honey Roasted	1 cup	65
With Vanilla Bunches	1 cup	42
With Almonds	1 cup	26
Honey Roasted *	1 cup	20
With Strawberries	1 cup	19
With Cinnamon Bunches	1 cup	18
Pecan Bunches	1 cup	17

Cereal, Quaker®	Amount	Magnesium (mg)
Granola, Apple, Cranberry, & Almond	1 cup	104
Toasted Multigrain Crisp	1 cup	77
Oatmeal Squares	1 cup	65
Oatmeal Squares, Cinnamon	1 cup	65
Oatmeal Squares, Golden Maple	1 cup	64
LIFE Cereal, Original	1 cup	41
LIFE Cereal, Maple & Brown Sugar	1 cup	39
LIFE Cereal, Cinnamon	1 cup	38
CAP'N Crunch's Peanut Butter Crunches	1 cup	25
Corn Bran Crunch	1 cup	22
CAP'N Crunch	1 cup	20
Puffed Wheat	1 cup	20
CAP'N Crunch & Crunchberries	1 cup	19
CAP'N Crunch's OOPs! All Berries	1 cup	18
Honey Graham OH'S	1 cup	16
Puffed Rice	1 cup	6

MAGNESIUM

Cereal, Cooked	Amount	Magnesium (mg)
Oats, regular, unenriched	1 cup	63
Oats, instant, fortified	1 cup	61
White corn grits	1 cup	17
Farina	1 cup	17
CREAM OF WHEAT, regular	1 cup	13
Yellow corn grits	1 cup	12
Malt-o-Meal plain	1 serving	5

Cheese	Amount	Magnesium (mg)
Ricotta, part skim milk	1 cup	37
Ricotta, whole milk	1 cup	27
Cottage cheese, creamed, small curd	1 cup	18
Cottage cheese, lowfat, 2 %	1 cup	16
Cottage cheese, nonfat, uncreamed	1 cup	16
Cottage cheese, lowfat, 1 %	1 cup	11

Cheese	Amount	Magnesium (mg)
Goat cheese, hard	1 oz	15
Romano	1 oz	12
Parmesan, grated	1 oz	11
Swiss	1 oz	11
Gruyere	1 oz	10
Swiss, low fat	1 oz	10
Mozzarella, non fat	1 oz	9
Roquefort	1 oz	9
Cheddar	1 oz	8
Goat cheese, semisoft	1 oz	8
Gouda	1 oz	8
Monterey	1 oz	8
Monterey, low fat	1 oz	8
Muenster	1 oz	8
Muenster, low fat	1 oz	8
Provolone	1 oz	8
Provolone, reduced fat	1 oz	8
Blue cheese	1 oz	7
American, pasteurized process, fortified	1 oz	7
American, pasteurized process, low fat	1 oz	7
Colby	1 oz	7
Mozzarella, part skim milk, low moisture	1 oz	7
Brie	1 oz	6
Cream cheese, fat free	1 oz	6
Mozzarella, whole milk	1 oz	6
Cheddar, low fat	1 oz	5

RDA for adults is 320 mg for females and 420 mg for males

MAGNESIUM

Continued

Feta	1 oz	5
Goat cheese, soft	1 oz	5
Fotina	1 oz	4
American, pasteurized process, imitation	1 oz	3
Cream cheese	1 oz	3

Cheese, Mexican	Amount	Magnesium (mg)
Mexican, blend, reduced fat	1 oz	10
Queso anejo	1 oz	8
Mexican, blend	1 oz	7
Queso asadero	1 oz	7
Queso chihuahua	1 oz	7
Queso fresco	1 oz	7

Chicken, Cooked	Amount	Magnesium (mg)
Breast, with skin, fried in flour	1/2 breast	29
Breast, no skin, roasted	1/2 breast	25
Thigh, with skin, fried	1 thigh	18
Thigh, no skin, roasted	1 thigh	12
Drumstick, no skin, roasted	1 drumstick	11
Drumstick, with skin, fried	1 drumstick	11
Wing with skin, fried in batter	1 wing	8
Wing with skin, roasted	1 wing	6

Chicken, Cooked	Amount	Magnesium (mg)
Breast with skin, fried in flour	3 oz	26
Breast meat only, no skin, roasted	3 oz	25
Breast with skin, roasted	3 oz	23
Thigh with skin, fried in flour	3 oz	21
Drumstick meat only, no skin, roasted	3 oz	20
Drumstick with skin, fried in flour	3 oz	20
Drumstick with skin, roasted	3 oz	20
Thigh meat only, no skin, roasted	3 oz	20
Thigh with skin, roasted	3 oz	19
Wing meat only, no skin, roasted	3 oz	18
Cornish game hens, meat only	3 oz	16
Wing with skin, fried in flour	3 oz	16
Wing with skin, roasted	3 oz	16

Cream	Amount	Magnesium (mg)
Half & Half	1 tbsp	2
Sour Cream, reduced fat	1 tbsp	2
Heavy Cream	1 tbsp	1
Light Coffe cream	1 tbsp	1

RDA for adults is 320 mg for females and 420 mg for males

MAGNESIUM

Sour Cream, cultured	1 tbsp	1
Whipped Topping, pressurized	1 tbsp	0

Eggs	Amount	Magnesium (mg)
Egg whites, dried	1 ounce	25
Egg substitute, liquid, fat free	1/4 cup	9
Egg whole, scrambled	1 large	7
Egg whole, fried	1 large	6
Egg whole, poached	1 large	6
Egg whole, hard boiled	1 large	5
Egg whites, dried powder, stabilized	1 tbsp	5
Egg whites, raw	1 large	4
Egg yolk	1 large	1

Fish, Canned	Amount	Magnesium (mg)
Atlantic Sardines, in oil	3 oz	33
White (albacore) tuna, in oil	3 oz	29
White (albacore) tuna, in water	3 oz	28
Light tuna, in oil	3 oz	26
Light tuna, in water	3 oz	20

Fish, Cooked	Amount	Magnesium (mg)
Chinock salmon	3 oz	104
Atlantic mackerel	3 oz	82
Atlantic pollock	3 oz	73
Walleye pollock	3 oz	69
Bluefin tuna	3 oz	54
Sea bass	3 oz	45
Stripped bass	3 oz	43
Skipjack (aku) tuna	3 oz	37
Atlantic cod	3 oz	36
Atlantic croaker	3 oz	36
Yellowfin tuna	3 oz	36
King mackerel	3 oz	35
Northern pike	3 oz	34
Carp	3 oz	32
Freshwater bass	3 oz	32
Spanish mackerel	3 oz	32
Walley pike	3 oz	32
Yellowtail	3 oz	32
Atlantic salmon, wild	3 oz	31
Grouper	3 oz	31
Pacific & Jack mackerel	3 oz	31
Snapper	3 oz	31

RDA for adults is 320 mg for females and 420 mg for males

MAGNESIUM

Sockeye salmon	3 oz	31
Swordfish	3 oz	30
Coho salmon, farmed	3 oz	29
Tilapia	3 oz	29
Coho salmon, wild	3 oz	28
Greenland halibut	3 oz	28
Pink salmon	3 oz	27
Atlantic salmon, farmed	3 oz	26
Florida pompano	3 oz	26
Rainbow trout, farmed	3 oz	26
Rainbow trout, wild	3 oz	26
Alaskan halibut	3 oz	25
Atlantic & Pacific halibut	3 oz	24
Catfish, wild	3 oz	24
Halibut	3 oz	24
Keta (chum) salmon	3 oz	24
Atlantic perch	3 oz	23
Catfish, breaded & fried	3 oz	23
Whiting	3 oz	23
Haddock	3 oz	22
Catfish, farmed	3 oz	20
Pacific cod	3 oz	20
Flounder	3 oz	19
Orange roughy	3 oz	15
Atlantic herring, pickled	3 oz	7

Fish, Shellfish, Cooked	Amount	Magnesium (mg)
Alaskan king crab	3 oz	84
Queen crab	3 oz	54
Octopus	3 oz	51
Scallops, breaded & fried	3 oz	50
Oysters, breaded & fried	3 oz	49
Abalone	3 oz	48
Alaskan king crab, imitation	3 oz	37
Northern lobster	3 oz	37
Shrimp, breaded & fried	3 oz	34
Squid, fried	3 oz	32
Blue crab	3 oz	31
Blue crab, canned	3 oz	31
Shrimp	3 oz	31
Crab cakes	3 oz	28
Crayfish	3 oz	28
Eastern oysters, farmed	3 oz	28
Shrimp, canned	3 oz	28
Clams, canned	3 oz	27

MAGNESIUM

Eastern oysters, wild	3 oz	24
Clams, breaded & fried	3 oz	12

Fruit, Canned	Amount	Magnesium (mg)
Pineapple	1 cup	41
Apricots	1 cup	18
Peaches	1 cup	13
Plums	1 cup	13
Pears	1 cup	11
Applesauce, sweetened	1 cup	8
Applesauce, unsweetened	1 cup	7
Olives, black	5 large	1
Olives, green	5 large	1

Fruit, Dried	Amount	Magnesium (mg)
Figs	1 cup	101
Peaches	1 cup	67
Pears	1 cup	59
Currants	1 cup	59
Apricots	1 cup	42
Apples	1 cup	14
Cranberries	1 cup	6

Fruit, Frozen	Amount	Magnesium (mg)
Blackberries	1 cup	33
Raspberries	1 cup	32
Strawberries	1 cup	15
Peaches	1 cup	12
Blueberries	1 cup	5

Fruit, Raw	Amount	Magnesium (mg)
Prunes, uncooked, pitted	1 cup	71
Avocado, California, pureed	1 cup	67
Dates	1 cup	63
Avocado, Florida, pureed	1 cup	55
Plantains	1 cup	55
Raisins	1 cup	46
Stewed prunes	1 cup	45
Kiwi	1 cup	31
Papayas	1 cup	30
Blackberries	1 cup	29
Black currants	1 cup	27
Raspberries	1 cup	27
Mulberries	1 cup	25

RDA for adults is 320 mg for females and 420 mg for males

MAGNESIUM

Tangerine, sections	1 cup	23
Strawberries	1 cup	22
Pomegrenates	1 cup	21
Pineapple	1 cup	20
Cataloupe	1 cup	19
Florida Oranges	1 cup	18
Naval Oranges	1 cup	18
Valencias Oranges	1 cup	18
Cherries, pitted	1 cup	17
Honeydew	1 cup	17
Apricots	1 cup	16
Mango	1 cup	16
Water mellon	1 cup	15
Peachs, slices	1 cup	14
Nectarine	1 cup	13
Plums, sliced	1 cup	12
Grapes, green & red	1 cup	11
Pears	1 cup	11
Blueberries	1 cup	9
Elderberries	1 cup	7
Apples	1 cup	6

Fruit, Raw	Amount	Magnesium (mg)
Avocado, Florida	1 fruit	73
Plantains	1 fruit	66
Avocado, California	1 fruit	39
Pomegranates	1 fruit	34
Cantaloupe	1/2 fruit	33
Bananas	1 medium	32
Prunes, uncooked	5 prunes	19
Dates	5 dates	15
Naval Oranges	1 fruit	15
Florida Oranges	1 fruit	14
Kiwi	1 fruit	13
Nectarine	1 fruit	12
Pears	1 fruit	12
Valencias Oranges	1 fruit	12
Grapefruit, pink or red	1/2 fruit	11
Tangerine	1 fruit	10
Cherries	10 cherries	9
Peaches	1 fruit	9
Star fruit, Carambola	1 fruit	9
Strawberries	5 strawberries	8
Apples	1 fruit	7
Figs, dried	1 fruit	6

RDA for adults is 320 mg for females and 420 mg for males

MAGNESIUM

Pineapple	1/2" x 3" slice	6
Plums	1 fruit	5
Apricots	1 fruit	4
Kumquats	1 fruit	4
Pineapple guava, Feijoa	1 fruit	4
Raisins	1 packet	4
Olives, black	5 large	1
Olives, green	5 large	1

Game Meat, Cooked	Amount	Magnesium (mg)
Rabbit	3 oz	26
Antelope	3 oz	24
Squirrel	3 oz	24
Buffalo, steak, free range	3 oz	23
Caribou	3 oz	23
Wild boar	3 oz	23
Deer	3 oz	20
Deer, ground	3 oz	20
Elk	3 oz	20
Elk, ground	3 oz	20
Bison, ground	3 oz	19
Duck	3 oz	17

Grains, Cooked	Amount	Magnesium (mg)
Amaranth	1 cup	160
Quinoa	1 cup	118
Kamut	1 cup	96
Spelt	1 cup	95
Oat bran	1 cup	88
Spaghetti, spinach	1 cup	87
Buckwheat, groats	1 cup	86
Brown rice	1 cup	84
Millet	1 cup	77
Oats, regular, unenriched	1 cup	63
Bulgur	1 cup	58
Wild rice	1 cup	52
Macaroni, Whole-Wheat	1 cup	42
Spaghetti, Whole-Wheat	1 cup	42
Egg & Spinach noodles	1 cup	38
Barley, pearled	1 cup	35
Egg noodles	1 cup	34
Macaroni	1 cup	25
Spaghetti, enriched	1 cup	25
White rice, long-grain, regular	1 cup	19
White rice, long-grain, paraboiled	1 cup	16

RDA for adults is 320 mg for females and 420 mg for males

MAGNESIUM

Couscous	1 cup	13
Soba noodles	1 cup	10
White rice, long-grain, instant	1 cup	8
Rice noodles	1 cup	5

Herbs & Spices	Amount	Magnesium (mg)
Basil, dried, ground	1 tsp	10
Celery seeds	1 tsp	9
Coriander, seed	1 tsp	6
Parsley, dried	1 tsp	6
Tarragon, dried	1 tsp	6
Cloves, dried, ground	1 tsp	5
Caraway seeds	1 tsp	5
Curry powder	1 tsp	5
Dill weed, dried	1 tsp	5
Oregano, dreid, ground	1 tsp	5
Anise seed	1 tsp	4
Chili powder	1 tsp	4
Coriander, dried	1 tsp	4
Ginger, ground	1 tsp	4
Paprika	1 tsp	4
Pepper, black	1 tsp	4
Turmeric, ground	1 tsp	4
All-spice, ground	1 tsp	3
Onion powder	1 tsp	3
Rosemary, dried	1 tsp	3
Sage, ground	1 tsp	3
Spearmint, dried	1 tsp	3
Thyme, dried	1 tsp	3
Bay leaf, crumbled	1 tsp	2
Cinnamon powder	1 tsp	2
Garlic powder	1 tsp	2
Saffron	1 tsp	2
Rosemary, fresh	1 tsp	1
Thyme, fresh	1 tsp	1
Capers, canned	1 tsp	1
Chervil, dried	1 tsp	1
Chives, raw, chopped	1 tsp	0

Juice	Amount	Magnesium (mg)
Pomegranate	1 cup	36
Prune juice	1 cup	36
Carrot juice	1 cup	33
Pineapple juice	1 cup	30

RDA for adults is 320 mg for females and 420 mg for males

MAGNESIUM

Continued

Orange juice, raw	1 cup	27
Tomato juice	1 cup	27
Vegetable juice, cocktail	1 cup	27
Grape juice	1 cup	25
Grapefruit juice, raw	1 cup	21
Lemon juice, raw	1 cup	15
Apple juice	1 cup	12
Cranberry juice, cocktail	1 cup	3

Lamb, Cooked	Amount	Magnesium (mg)
Cubed, for stew or kabob	3 oz	26
Rib, lean, trim to 1/4" fat	3 oz	25
Chops, loin, lean, trim to 1/4" fat	3 oz	20
Ground	3 oz	20
Leg, whole, trim to 1/4" fat	3 oz	20
Foreshank, trim to 1/8" fat	3 oz	19

Milk	Amount	Magnesium (mg)
Coconut milk, canned	1 cup	104
Canned, condensed, sweetened	1 cup	80
Canned, evaporated, non fat	1 cup	69
Soy milk, original, unfortified	1 cup	61
Canned, evaporated	1 cup	60
Sheep milk	1 cup	44
Goat milk	1 cup	34
Dry, instant, non fat	1/3 cup	27
Buttermilk, low fat	1 cup	27
Lowfat, 1%	1 cup	27
Reduced fat, 2%	1 cup	27
Nonfat, fat free or skim liquid milk	1 cup	27
Buttermilk, whole milk	1 cup	24
Whole milk, 3.25%	1 cup	24
Human milk	1 cup	7

Nuts & Seeds	Amount	Magnesium (mg)
Pumpkin seeds	1 oz	168
Flaxseeds	1 oz	111
Brazilnuts	1 oz	107
Sesame seeds	1 oz	100
Chia seeds	1 oz	95
Sunflower seeds	1 oz	92
Cashews	1 oz	83
Almonds	1 oz	76
Pine nuts	1 oz	71

RDA for adults is 320 mg for females and 420 mg for males

MAGNESIUM

Continued

Mixed nuts, roasted with peanuts, no salt	1 oz	64
Black walnuts	1 oz	57
Peanuts	1 oz	48
Hazelnuts	1 oz	46
Trail mix, regular with chocolate chips	1 oz	46
English walnuts	1 oz	45
Trail mix, regular, salted	1 oz	45
Peanut butter, smooth style	1 oz	44
Macadamia	1 oz	37
Pecans	1 oz	34
Pistachio	1 oz	34
Tahini	1 oz	27
Trail mix, tropical	1 oz	27
Coconut, meat	1 oz	9

Nuts & Seeds	Amount	Magnesium (mg)
Pumpkin seeds	1/4 cup	191
Flaxseeds	1/4 cup	165
Sesame seeds	1/4 cup	126
Brazilnuts, whole	1/4 cup	125
Sunflower seeds	1/4 cup	114
Peanut butter, smooth	1/4 cup	99
Almonds, whole	1/4 cup	96
Pine nuts	1/4 cup	85
Mixed nuts, roasted with peanuts, no salt	1/4 cup	77
Black walnuts, chopped	1/4 cup	63
Peanuts	1/4 cup	61
Trail mix, regular with chocolate chips	1/4 cup	59
Trail mix, regular, salted	1/4 cup	59
Peanut butter, smooth	1 tbsp	49
Hazelnuts, chopped	1/4 cup	47
Macadamia	1/4 cup	44
English walnuts, chopped	1/4 cup	40
Flaxseeds	1 tbsp	40
Pistachio	1/4 cup	37
Trail mix, tropical	1/4 cup	34
Sesame seeds	1 tbsp	32
Pecans, halves	1/4 cup	30
Coconut meat, shredded	1/4 cup	6
Cashews	1/4 cup	x
Chia seeds	1/4 cup	x

RDA for adults is 320 mg for females and 420 mg for males

MAGNESIUM

Pork, Cooked	Amount	Magnesium (mg)
Bacon	3 oz	28
Tenderloin	3 oz	25
Sirloin pork chops	3 oz	23
Chops, broiled	3 oz	21
Center loin pork chops	3 oz	21
Spareribs	3 oz	20
Chops, pan-fried	3 oz	20
Chops, lean, pan-fried	3 oz	20
Cured ham, lean	3 oz	19
Bratwurst	3 oz	18
Canadian-style bacon	3 oz	18
Cured ham	3 oz	16
Italian sausage	3 oz	15
Backribs	3 oz	14
Sausage	3 oz	14
Polish sausage	3 oz	12
Braunschweiger	3 oz	9
Liverwurst spread	1/4 cup	7

Turkey, Cooked	Amount	Magnesium (mg)
Ground turkey, fat free	3 oz	30
Light meat	3 oz	27
Ground turkey	3 oz	26
Breast meat	3 oz	25
Turkey bacon	3 oz	25
Dark meat	3 oz	23
Liver	3 oz	22
Ground turkey, 93% lean	3 oz	21
Ground turkey, 85% lean	3 oz	21
Turkey sausage, reduced fat	3 oz	18

Veal, Cooked	Amount	Magnesium (mg)
Leg, top round	3 oz	25
Sirloin	3 oz	22
Foreshank	3 oz	21
Loin	3 oz	21
Ground	3 oz	20
Breast	3 oz	19
Rib	3 oz	19

RDA for adults is 320 mg for females and 420 mg for males

MAGNESIUM

Vegetables, Canned	Amount	Magnesium (mg)
Spinach	1 cup	163
Tomato paste	1 cup	110
Pumpkin	1 cup	56
Tomato pure	1 cup	55
Yellow sweet corn	1 cup	48
Tomato Sauce	1 cup	39
Green Peas	1 cup	31
Sauerkraut	1 cup	31
Stewed tomatoes	1 cup	31
Beets	1 cup	29
Tomatoes	1 cup	26
Sweet potato	1 cup	24
Asparagus	1 cup	24
Mushrooms	1 cup	23
Green beans	1 cup	18
Carrots	1 cup	12

Vegetables, Cooked	Amount	Magnesium (mg)
Chinese long beans	1 cup	168
Spinach	1 cup	157
Swiss chard	1 cup	150
Beet greens	1 cup	98
Acorn squash	1 cup	88
Artichokes	1 cup	71
Split peas	1 cup	71
Cactus pad, nopales	1 cup	70
Butternut squash	1 cup	59
Sweet potato, mashed	1 cup	59
Okra	1 cup	58
Parsnips	1 cup	45
Summer squash	1 cup	43
Snow peas	1 cup	42
Tarro	1 cup	40
Beets	1 cup	39
Rutabagas	1 cup	39
Yellow corn	1 cup	39
Collard greens	1 cup	38
Potatoes, mashed with whole milk	1 cup	38
Scallop or Pattypan Squash, slices	1 cup	34
Zucchini	1 cup	34
Broccoli	1 cup	33
Turnip greens	1 cup	32
Brussels sprouts	1 cup	31
Kohlrabi	1 cup	31

RDA for adults is 320 mg for females and 420 mg for males

MAGNESIUM

Potatoes, flesh	1 cup	30
Crookneck or Straighneck Squash, slices	1 cup	29
Winter squash	1 cup	27
Asparagus	1 cup	25
Dandelion greens	1 cup	25
Yams, cubed	1 cup	24
Cabbage	1 cup	23
Green beans	1 cup	23
Kale	1 cup	23
Onions	1 cup	23
Raab broccoli	1 cup	23
Pumpkin	1 cup	22
Tomatoes, red	1 cup	22
Mustard greens	1 cup	21
Shitake mushrooms	1 cup	20
Bok-Choy	1 cup	19
White mushrooms	1 cup	19
Cauliflower	1 cup	18
Celery	1 cup	18
Spaghetti squash	1 cup	17
Broccilini	1 cup	16
Carrots	1 cup	16
Leeks	1 cup	15
Turnips	1 cup	14
Mustard spinach	1 cup	13
Eggplant	1 cup	11
Napa cabbage	1 cup	9

Vegetables, Frozen	Amount	Magnesium (mg)
Spinach	1 cup	156
Okra	1 cup	74
Collard greens	1 cup	51
Corn	1 cup	46
Turnip Greens	1 cup	43
Green peas	1 cup	35
Rhubarb	1 cup	29
Brussels sprouts	1 cup	28
Green beans	1 cup	26
Broccoli	1 cup	24
Kale	1 cup	23
Butternut squash	1 cup	22
Carrots	1 cup	16
Cauliflower	1 cup	16
Asparagus	1 cup	18

RDA for adults is 320 mg for females and 420 mg for males

MAGNESIUM

Vegetables, Raw	Amount	Magnesium (mg)
Butternut squash	1 cup	48
Cactus pads, Nopales	1 cup	45
Swiss chard	1 cup	29
Tomatillos	1 cup	26
Snow peas	1 cup	24
Spinach	1 cup	24
Kale	1 cup	23
Yellow bell peppers	1 large	22
Dandelion greens	1 cup	20
Green onions & scallions	1 cup	20
Savoy cabbage	1 cup	20
Tomatoes	1 cup	20
Zucchini	1 cup	20
Summer squash	1 cup	19
Broccoli	1 cup	18
Red bell peppers	1 cup	18
Cauliflower	1 cup	16
Mustard spinach	1 cup	16
Onions	1 cup	16
Tomatoes, cherry	1 cup	16
Green bell peppers	1 cup	15
Cucumber	1 cup	14
Spirulina, dried	1 tbsp	14
Bok-Choy	1 cup	13
Carrots	1 cup	13
Celery	1 cup	13
Red cabbage	1 cup	11
Arugula	1 cup	9
Belgian endive	1 cup	9
Chicory greens	1 cup	9
Raab broccoli	1 cup	9
Cabbage	1 cup	8
Endive	1 cup	8
Romaine lettuce	1 cup	8
Butterhead & boston lettuce	1 cup	7
Green leaf lettuce	1 cup	7
Watercress	1 cup	7
White mushrooms	1 cup	6
Radicchio	1 cup	5
Shiitake mushrooms, dried	1 each	5
Iceburg lettuce	1 cup	4
Red leaf lettuce	1 cup	3

RDA for adults is 320 mg for females and 420 mg for males

MAGNESIUM

Yogurt	Amount	Magnesium (mg)
Plain yogurt, skim (non fat) milk	8 oz	43
Plain yogurt, low fat	8 oz	39
Plain yogurt, whole milk	8 oz	27
Plain greek yogurt, non fat	8 oz	25

RDA for adults is 320 mg for females and 420 mg for males

Nutrient Data Collection Form

Food	Amount	Book Numbers	Multiply By	Estimated Nutrient Intake
Nutrient::	RDA:	Estimated:	% of RDA:	Total Estimated:

To download additional forms for free, go to www.TopNutrients4U.com

455

Phosphorus & Kidney Disease

Phosphorus is an element on the periodic chart and humans are dependent on its dietary intake for survival. It is required by every cell in the human body and it plays a dominating role over nutrients, hormones, and human diseases. Knowing what phosphorus does in the human body is not important for the general public, but knowing what happens if you get too much or too little is.

A phosphorus deficiency is associated with impaired intestinal absorption found with Crohn's and Celiac disease, prolonged use of anti-acids, laxative abuse, and chronic diarrhea. But of course, the above health conditions would impair intestinal absorption of all essential nutrients and not just phosphorus, and would result in malnutrition.

Notwithstanding the above, it's very unlikely a deficiency would result from dietary intake because plenty of phosphorus is found naturally in all food. Additional amounts are added to ready-to-eat foods as preservatives and flavor enhancers. The additive forms of phosphorus amplify the negative effects of excessive phosphorus and represent a hidden burden on the human body that genetically programed human defense mechanisms did not anticipate.

The public's total and type of exposure, makes toxicity more common and a bigger concern than deficiencies. Complications from prolonged intake of excess phosphorus, is calcification of organs and most commonly the kidneys.

The deterioration of the human kidneys leads to the retention of many waste products, of which phosphorus may be the most important because it is the most destructive over time. In kidney disease and dialysis patients the therapeutic strategies aimed at controlling blood levels of phosphorus includes medical advice to restrict dietary intake between dialysis treatments and use of prescriptions.

In America, the amount of phosphorus absorbed daily from ingested food is larger than the amount of phosphorus that can be eliminated through a conventional 4-hr dialysis treatment. In response, pharmaceutical manufacturers have successfully created a line of drugs known as phosphorus binders. Binders react with the phosphorus in food, rendering the phosphorus unavailable to the human body.

Dialysis treatments and prescriptions have reduced human suffering for millions of Americans and have prolonged lives for years. Despite the advancements in technology only 50% of the dialysis population meets their targeted goal. In short, technology has not been able to completely offset the adverse effects of a phosphorus rich diet.

Historically, a barrier to balancing phosphorus has been blamed on the patient's inability to restrict dietary intake between dialysis treatments. Until now, patients have never been given the tools to do so.

The phosphorus in your blood is not the result of an infection, and it was not made by your body. It comes from the food you eat and the liquid you drink and from nowhere else. A dietary phosphorus intervention may be the missing link for better phosphorus control between dialysis treatments for the kidney diseased population.

When blood levels of phosphorus are too high relative to calcium, it bonds with calcium forming calcium-phosphate compounds. Salts of these compounds precipitate out of the blood, become localized, and attach to the soft tissues of vital organs. This is a condition known as calcification. Cells of tissues that will become calcified will be chemically transformed into bone-forming-like cells to accept the calcium deposits simultaneously while the body is losing calcium from bone. Although many tissues are known to become calcified the blood vessels, heart valves, and the kidneys seem particularly susceptible.

Calcification is an actively regulated process that takes place daily throughout a lifetime and the extent of calcification is influenced by the amount, type, and duration of dietary intake of phosphorus. It is known to start in an early age it is documented in young adults and progresses slowly and silently for many years at a subclinical level without any symptoms. Because of its slow evolution it has been referred to as "age-related" which means it's predictable. Reference of a disease to such a term as age-related may give a false impression that the diseases identified to be linked with calcification are unavoidable. Age-related does not mean that you are helpless and cannot prevent it. We're talking about normal body chemistry being changed in a negative way by diet with no infections being involved. Calcification is well documented in the scientific community and is expected to occur over time as a result of elevated phosphorus levels. It is believed to indicate activity of an ongoing disease. Calcification leads to a group of biochemical abnormalities commonly referred to as age-related diseases, such as bone disease, cardiovascular disease, and kidney disease. A common denominator found in all three of the above diseases is the existence of calcification deposits.

Normally, the kidneys keep levels of phosphorus in balance with excretion. When calcification strikes the kidneys, however, a level of blockage occurs. This blockage interferes with the kidney's ability to filter phosphorus at its initial normalized rate and excrete it from the body. Although small in the beginning, historically, the blockage has appeared to be permanent.

If phosphorus intake remains constant, while the kidney is losing its ability to filter phosphorus, each time the kidney's filtration rate drops a notch an incremental amount of phosphorus will be permanently retained by the body. This may take years or even decades, but it is sure to happen if daily intake of phosphorus is excessive.

Kidney damage will progressively intensify since the body requires less phosphorus to induce further damage after each drop in the filtration rate. Overtime, the decline in excretion will lead to a buildup of toxic levels of phosphorus in the blood, known as hyperphosphatemia.

To make things worse, critical functions of the body are totally dependent on blood levels of calcium being strictly maintained within a very narrow range. If calcium is dropped from the blood and deposited in tissues as calcification then blood concentrations may go to low levels and overtime could result in a condition known as hypocalcemia. Hyperphosphatemia is a documented cause of hypocalcemia, and when full blown hypocalcemia symptoms appear it will require emergency medical attention.

Elevated levels of phosphorus in addition to calcification, is known to inhibit the kidney's production of vitamin-D. A reduction in vitamin D reduces the absorption of calcium from food. This in turn reduces blood levels of calcium contributing to a mild hypocalcemia state that was already festering. This temporary mild hypocalcemia state will trigger the body to elevate its calcium-regulating hormones levels, known as the parathyroid hormones. This will take place within hours after each phosphorus rich meal and without noticeable changes in blood levels of phosphorus. Thus, more than one phosphorus rich meal during a day will create episodes of transient hypocalcemia states. And these overlapping episodes will cause the parathyroid hormones to linger in circulation longer than normal, during the day. But, may by morning, be returned back to the same levels as the previous morning. Therefore, daily and meal-to-meal phosphorus rich meals will result in persistent elevated levels of the parathyroid hormones, and a continuous slow erosion of bone.

The sole purpose of the parathyroid hormone is to prevent hypocalcemia by forcing bone to release calcium to replace any lost circulating calcium. Unfortunately, as genetically programed, the bone will continue to lose calcium as long as the parathyroid hormones stay elevated.

Overall, we have a loss of calcium circulating throughout the body due to calcification caused by excessive phosphorus. We cannot replenish the lost calcium with the food we eat because absorption of calcium has been shut down, due to a lack of vitamin-D, caused by excessive phosphorus. And we have a loss of calcium from bone due to the circulating parathyroid hormones caused by excessive phosphorus.

A compounding problem, in addition to excessive intake of phosphorus, is that blood levels of phosphorus considered to be clinically acceptable may be unsafe for the general public and an unreliable indicator of any existing or ensuing diseases.

First, as mentioned earlier a high dietary intake of phosphorus elevates the parathyroid hormones without changing blood concentrations of phosphorus, thus, blood levels of phosphorus will not reflect the damage being caused by dietary intake of phosphorus.

Second, since calcification precedes any clinical symptoms, the kidneys calcify before elevated levels of phosphorus can be detected in a laboratory.

Third, since hyperphosphatemia has no clinical symptoms of its own, its evolution and damage also goes unnoticed. Current clinical laboratory testing may not be sensitive enough to detect early stages of calcification and hyperphosphatemia.

 Fourth, in a study of 1077 males, averaging 69 years old, despite having kidney filtrations rates low enough to be defined as chronic kidney disease, over 50% of the study group had blood levels of phosphorus considered to be normal. In 2005, a study reported phosphorus levels on the high side but still within a normal range was associated with an increased risk of heart failure in patients with coronary disease. A study in 2007 demonstrated phosphorus levels above 3.5 milligrams per deciliter, although within the range deemed to be acceptable, were still associated with an increased risk of cardiovascular disease. This occurred in a community of men and women who had no prior cardiovascular disease or kidney disease. In 2008 and again in 2009 blood levels of phosphorus considered to be normal are associated with increased atherosclerosis and vascular calcification in the general population. Finally, in 2013, phosphorus levels are linked with increased mortality in healthy Americans.

 Fortunately, one study has suggested the possibility that calcification might be reversible with diet. In 2011, a study reported phosphorus concentrations at the lower end of the normal range appeared to correlate with a decline in artery calcification in individuals with normal renal functions.

 Strong clinical evidence exist that controlling dietary intake of phosphorus early in the course of kidney failure may greatly retard or even halt progression. Animal studies have shown dietary phosphorus restriction prevents calcification of the kidneys. And kidney patients who started their phosphorus management early after initial diagnosis had a more favorable outcome than those who failed to comply with dietary medical advice.

 In view of the frequency with which hyperphosphatemia and calcification deposits have been found in the kidney disease population, phosphorus's contribution to the destruction of the kidneys is beyond questioning. Hyperphosphatemia is a modifiable risk factor for kidney disease and maintaining blood levels of phosphorus within a narrow range is a standard of care in kidney disease patients.

Long-term intake of excessive phosphorus, even if it does not cause hyperphosphatemia, is still considered to be a risk factor for cardiovascular disease in the general population. One cardiology group studying lesions reported that phosphorus levels confer a cardiovascular risk similar to that of smoking and calcification has been implicated in the mechanical failure of transplanted heart valves.

Thus, dietary phosphorus is associated with cardiovascular disease in individuals who have no kidney disease, but cardiovascular disease appears to occur earlier in life, is more severe, and progresses more rapidly in those individuals who have kidney disease. The arteries of patients with kidney disease have more calcification deposits than the arteries of healthy individuals of the same age group.

Because dietary phosphorus is deemed to be a risk factor for cardiovascular disease in healthy persons as well as in the kidney disease population, the advice to restrict dietary intake of phosphorus obviously has been extended to include the general population.

On a final note, because phosphorus is a naturally occurring structural chemical component of all protein matter, phosphorus rich foods will naturally be rich in protein. It will be hard to find protein without any phosphorus. As a result, there has been concern that a strict phosphorus restriction with a proportional decline in protein could outweigh the benefits by leading to malnutrition. In order to ensure a phosphorus restriction does not compromise the nutritional protein intake, a dietary ratio of phosphorus / protein can be used to identify foods that are lowest in phosphorus but still high in protein. The lower the value of the phosphorus / protein ratio the more appropriate the food choice is for incorporating into a routine diet for dialysis and kidneys disease patients. And a dietary ratio of phosphorus/ protein equal to 10 mg / g or below has been considered for management of phosphorus.

To summarize all the above, blood levels of phosphorus will not reflect the damage being caused by dietary phosphorus, and high blood levels of phosphorus reduce blood levels of calcium by calcification, drive the initiation and progression of vascular calcification, is an independent determinant of severe coronary calcification, calcifies the kidneys and is a predictor of mortality in kidney disease patients, inhibits absorption of calcium, leaches calcium from bone, inhibits the body's synthesis of vitamin D, and elevates blood levels of the parathyroid hormones. Furthermore, phosphorus levels, has been associated with increased risk of atherosclerosis, cardiovascular disease, and mortality in healthy U.S. adults.

A diet taken from a variety of food groups consisting of low amounts of phosphorus can exert a protective effect against deterioration of the human kidneys. Likewise, increasing intake of foods with a low phosphorus / protein ratio, if incorporated into a life-style, could help in staying off all age-related diseases spawned by calcification.

Managing dietary intake of phosphorus should be initiated by all humans at an early age of life and practiced throughout a lifetime. There is nothing wrong with having your favorite phosphorus rich meal, the problem is in not knowing how much phosphorus is in your meal.

Because of this, any real effort to reduce intake of phosphorus must require cutting back on the consumption of processed, restaurant, and ready-to-eat foods because of their unknown amounts of phosphorus. In the future, manufactures would be wise to lists the amounts phosphorus on all food product labels and the phosphorus / protein ratio.

The phosphorus amounts in this chapter should help dialysis patients to better estimate and control a day-to-day and meal-to-meal intake of phosphorus between dialysis treatments. And, allow a comparison of nutrients between similar products. This chapter, list the values of phosphorus in milligrams (mg), and the phosphorus / protein ratio for food and beverages commonly consumed by Americans.

Bear in mind, blood levels of phosphorus may still become elevated enough over-time to stimulate bone-regulating hormone activity even when the total amount of phosphorus intake is seemingly modest if intake of phosphorus is excessive relative to intake of calcium.

A habitual low calcium / phosphorus dietary intake ratio is associated with an increased risk for bone disease in women. See the calcium / phosphorus ratio in the chapter on calcium.

Recommend Daily Intakes Levels for Phosphorus

Children	Phosphorus, mg
1 to 3 year olds	460
4 to 8 year olds	500

Males	
9 to 13 year olds	1250
14 to 18 year olds	1250
19 to 30 years	700
31 to 50 years	700
51 to 70 years	700
Over 70	700

Females	
9 to 13 years	1250
14 to 18 year	1250
19 to 30 years	700
31 to 50 years	700
51 to 70 years	700
Over 70	700

Pregnancy	
14 to 18 years	1250
19 to 30 years	700
31 to 50 years	700

Lactation	
14 to 18 year	1250
19 to 30 years	700
31 to 50 years	700

PHOSPHORUS

Alcohol	Amount	Phosphorus (mg)
Regular Beer	1 bottle	50
Light Beer	1 bottle	42
Red Wine	1 glass	34
White Wine	1 glass	26
Gin, Rum, Vodka, or Whisky	1 shot	2
Sake	1 fl oz	2

Beans, Canned	Amount	Phosphorus (mg)
Great Northern	1 cup	356
Navy beans	1 cup	351
Baked beans, with Pork & Tomato Sauce	1 cup	285
Kidney beans	1 cup	271
Refried beans	1 cup	264
White beans, mature	1 cup	238
Cranberry beans	1 cup	224
Pinto beans	1 cup	221
Fava beans	1 cup	202
Garbanzo beans	1 cup	192
Baked beans, plain	1 cup	188
Lima beans	1 cup	178
Black-eyed peas	1 cup	168
Yellow beans	1 cup	49
Green beans	1 cup	32

Beans, Cooked	Amount	Phosphorus (mg)
Soybeans, dry roasted	1 cup	604
Soybeans, mature	1 cup	421
Adzuki	1 cup	386
Lentils	1 cup	356
Natto	1 cup	304
White beans, small	1 cup	303
Great Northern	1 cup	292
Soybeans, green	1 cup	284
Black Turtle beans, mature	1 cup	281
Garbanzo beans	1 cup	276
Black-eyed peas	1 cup	268
Mothbeans	1 cup	266
Winged beans	1 cup	263
Edamame	1 cup	262
Navy beans	1 cup	262
Kidney beans	1 cup	251
Pinto beans	1 cup	251
Black beans	1 cup	241

PHOSPHORUS

Continued

Cranberry beans	1 cup	239
Hyacinth	1 cup	233
Fava beans	1 cup	212
Lupins	1 cup	212
Lima beans	1 cup	209
White beans, mature	1 cup	202
Mung beans, mature seeds	1 cup	200
Pigeon peas	1 cup	200
Split peas	1 cup	194
Yardlong beans, Chinese long beans	1 cup	59
Yellow beans	1 cup	49
Green beans	1 cup	36

Beef, Cooked	Amount	Phosphorus (mg)
Tri Tip steak, lean, trim to 0" fat	3 oz	232
Chuck roast, lean, trim to 0" fat	3 oz	200
Top sirloin, lean, trim to 1/8" fat	3 oz	198
Skirt steak, trim to 0" fat	3 oz	196
London Broil, top round, trim to 0" fat	3 oz	192
Ribeye steak, lean, trim 0" fat	3 oz	185
Flank steak, lean, trim to 0" fat	3 oz	184
Filet Mignon, tenderloin, trim to 0" fat	3 oz	180
Ground beef, 95%	3 oz	175
Brisket, lean, trim to 0" fat	3 oz	174
Flat Iron Steak	3 oz	173
Ground beef , 90%, (ground sirloin)	3 oz	172
T-Bone steak, trim 0" fat	3 oz	169
Chuck roast, trim to 1/8" fat	3 oz	168
Ground beef, 85%	3 oz	168
Ground beef, 80%	3 oz	165
Porterhouse steak, trim to 0" fat	3 oz	164
Ground beef, 75%	3 oz	161
Beef ribs, trim to 1/8" fat	3 oz	150

Beef, Cooked	Amount	Phosphorus (mg)
Tri Tip steak, lean, trim to 0" fat	1 lb	1234
Skirt steak, trim to 0" fat	1 lb	1043
Flank steak, lean, trim to 0" fat	1 lb	985
Top Sirloin, trim to 1/8" fat	1 lb	949
Brisket, lean, trim to 0" fat	1 lb	931
T-bone steak, trim to 0" fat	1 lb	903
Chuck roast, trim to 1/8" fat	1 lb	899
Porterhouse steak, trim to 0" fat	1 lb	875
Flank steak, lean, trim to 0" fat	1 steak	831
Beef ribs, trim to 1/8" fat	1 lb	804

RDA 700 mg for adults

PHOSPHORUS

Continued

London Broil, top round, trim to 0" fat	1 lb	590
Brisket, lean, trim to 0" fat	1 steak	554
Ribeye steak, boneless, trim to 0" fat	1 steak	460
Flat Iron Steak	1 steak	386
Top Sirloin, choice filet, trim to 0" fat	1 filet	316
Ribeye filet, lean, trim to 0" fat	1 filet	312
Filet Mignon, tenderloin, trim to 0" fat	1 steak	301

Beef, Ground, Cooked	Amount	Phosphorus (mg)
Ground beef, 95%	1/4 lb patty	169
Ground beef, 90%	1/4 lb patty	166
Ground beef, 85%	1/4 lb patty	152
Ground beef, 80%	1/4 lb patty	149
Ground beef, 75%	1/4 lb patty	132

Beverages	Amount	Phosphorus (mg)
Carnation Essential, Nutritional Drink	12 fl oz	548
Slimfast, High Protein Shake, 3-2-1 plan	1 bottle	401
Special-K Protein Shake	Serving	334
Chocolate Shake, all fast foods	12 fl oz	288
Nestle, Boost Plus, Nutritional Drink	1 bottle	273
Abbott Ensure Nutritional Drink	1 bottle	267
Vanilla Shake, all fast foods	12 fl oz	245
Abbott Ensure Plus	1 bottle	199
Hawaiian Punch Fruit Juicy	12 fl oz	173
Slimfast, High Protein Powder, 3-2-1 plan	1 scoop	146
Nestle, Cool Nesta Ice Tea, Lemon-flavored	12 fl oz	132
Coca-Cola® Classic	12 fl oz	62
Pepsico Quaker Gatorade, G Performance 2	1 bottle	61
Pepsi® One	12 fl oz	55
Pepsi® Twist	12 fl oz	54
Mountain Due, Code Red	12 fl oz	53
Pepsi® Cola	12 fl oz	53
Pepsi® Cola, Caffenine-Free	12 fl oz	53
RC Cola	12 fl oz	52
Slice Cola	12 fl oz	51
Dr. Pepper®	12 fl oz	45
Dr. Pepper®, Caffeine-Free	12 fl oz	45
Diet Dr. Pepper®	12 fl oz	44
Diet Pepsi® Vanilla	12 fl oz	43
Pepsi® Vanilla	12 fl oz	43
Diet Pepsi® Cola	12 fl oz	41
Diet Rite Cola	12 fl oz	41
Diet Pepsi® Twist	12 fl oz	41
Slice Cherry Spice	12 fl oz	34

RDA 700 mg for adults

PHOSPHORUS

Slice, Dr. Slice	12 fl oz	34
Nestea Sweetened	12 fl oz	32
Nestea Unsweetened	12 fl oz	32
Diet RC Cola	12 fl oz	31
Hire's® Diet Root Beer	12 fl oz	20
Hire's® Root Beer	12 fl oz	20
Coffee, regular ground, tap water	1 cup	7
Arizona Iced Tea, with Lemon Flavor	1 bottle	6
Coco-Cola Powerrade, lemon-lime	12 fl oz	4
Orange Soda	12 fl oz	4
Canada Dry Collins Mixer	12 fl oz	3
Ocean Spray, Cranberry Energy Juice Drink	1 bottle	2
7-Up®	12 fl oz	1
A&W® Root Beer	12 fl oz	1
Crush Orange	12 fl oz	1
Mug® Root Beer	12 fl oz	1
Squirt®	12 fl oz	1
Mountain Due®	12 fl oz	0
7-Up Diet	12 fl oz	0
A&W® Diet Root Beer	12 fl oz	0
Barg's® Root Beer	12 fl oz	0
Barg's® Diet Root Beer	12 fl oz	0
Canada Dry Club Soda	12 fl oz	0
Canada Dry Ginger Ale	12 fl oz	0
Club Soda	12 fl oz	0
Cream Soda	12 fl oz	0
Full Throttle Energy Drink	12 fl oz	0
Monster® Energy Drinks, Low Carb	12 fl oz	0
Nestea Diet Lemon	12 fl oz	0
Red Bull®	12 fl oz	0
Sprite®	12 fl oz	0
Sunkist® Orange	12 fl oz	0

Bologna	Amount	Phosphorus (mg)
Meat and Poultry	1 oz slice	70
Chicken, Pork, Beef	1 oz slice	64
Chicken, Pork	1 oz slice	62
Chicken, Turkey, Pork	1 oz slice	52
Beef and Pork, low fat	1 oz slice	51
Beef, low fat	1 oz slice	50
Beef	1 oz slice	46
Beef and Pork	1 oz slice	46
Pork	1 oz slice	39
Pork, Turkey and Beef	1 oz slice	36

RDA 700 mg for adults

Continued

| Turkey | 1 oz slice | 32 |
| Pork and Turkey, lite | 1 oz slice | 26 |

Bread	Amount	Phosphorus (mg)
Cornbread, drymix	1 piece	234
Indian bread, Naan, whole wheat	1 piece	199
Bagel, oat bran	4 1/2" bagel	144
Bagel, Wheat	4" bagel	139
Biscuits, refrigerated doug, baked	2-1/2" biscuit	138
Bagel, cinnamon-raisin	4 1/2" bagel	131
Potato bread	1 slice	118
Bagel, plain, enriched with calcium	4 1/2" bagel	114
Bagel, egg	4 1/2" bagel	110
Mexican roll, bollilo	1 roll	109
Biscuits, refrigerated doug, low fat, baked	2-1/4" biscuit	98
Indian bread, Naan, plain	1 piece	90
Tortillas, corn	1 tortilla	82
Croissants, butter	1 each	60
Multi-Grain, and Whole-Grain	1 slice	59
Pita, white	6-1/2" pita	58
Kaiser roll	1 slice	57
Pumpernickle	1 slice	57
Whole-Wheat	1 slice	57
English muffin, plain	1 muffin	52
Hamburger & hotdog buns, plain	1 bun	46
White	1 slice	45
Egg bread	1 slice	42
Rye bread	1 slice	40
Tortillas, flour	1 tortilla	40
Cracked wheat	1 slice	38
Wheat	1 slice	38
Dinner Rolls, brown & serve	1 roll	34
Oatmeal bread	1 slice	34
French and Sourdough	1 slice	29
Raisen bread	1 slice	28
Pita, white	4" pita	27
Italian	1 slice	21

Breakfast, Fast Foods	Amount	Phosphorus (mg)
McDonalds® Delux Breakfast	1 meal	907
McDonalds® Big Breakfast	1 meal	689
McDonalds® Sausage, Egg & Cheese, McGriddles	1 meal	611
McDonalds® Sausage Biscuit with Egg	1 meal	494

PHOSPHORUS

Continued

Taco Bell® Burrito Supreme with chicken	1 burrito	404
McDonalds® Sausage Biscuit	1 meal	378
McDonalds® Hot Cakes & Sausage	1 meal	328
Taco Bell® Burrito Supreme with steak	1 burrito	325
Taco Bell® Bean Burrito	1 burrito	302
Taco Bell® Burrito Supreme with beef	1 burrito	302
McDonalds® Sausage McMuffin with Egg	1 meal	282
Burger King® Croissan'Wich, Egg & Cheese	1 sandwich	274
McDonalds® Egg McMuffin	1 meal	252
Burger King® Croissan'Wich, Sausage, Egg & Cheese	1 sandwich	236
Burger King® Croissan'Wich, Sausage & Egg	1 sandwich	207
McDonalds® Sausage McMuffin	1 meal	187

Butter	Amount	Phosphorus (mg)
Sesame butter, tahini	1 tbsp	110
Sunflower seed butter, no salt	1 tbsp	107
Almond butter, plain, no salt	1 tbsp	81
Cashew butter, plain	1 tbsp	73
Peanut butter, smooth, with salt	1 tbsp	57
Regular dairy butter, salted	1 tbsp	3
Regular dairy whipped butter, salted	1 tbsp	2

Candies	Amount	Phosphorus (mg)
MARS® Almond Bar	1 bar	117
Milk Chocolate with Almonds	1 bar	108
SNICKERS®	1 bar	108
MR. Goodbar®	1 bar	80
5TH AVENUE®	1 bar	79
TWIX® Chocolate Bar	1 bar	75
Reese's® Peanut Butter Cups	1 pack of 2	72
M&M's Milk Chocolate	1 package	70
Hershey Kisses® Milk Chocolate with Almonds	5 pieces	66
Butterfinger® Bar	1 fun size	58
Hershey Kisses® Milk Chocolate	5 pieces	57
Kit Kat® Wafer Bar	1 bar	57
Almond Joy®	1 package	55
Hershey Kisses®Special Dark Chocolate	5 pieces	44
Milky Way® Bar	1 bar	39
100 Grand Bar®	1 bar	37
OH' Henry Bar	fun size	36
Skor Toffee®	1 bar	24
Tootsie Roll®	6 pieces	23
ROLO® Caramels in Milk Chocolate	5 pieces	21
3 Musketeers®	1 bar	19

RDA 700 mg for adults

PHOSPHORUS

Continued

Baby Ruth®	1 fun size	17
Milk Chocolate Coated Raisins	10 pieces	14
M&M's Milk Chocolate	10 pieces	10
Starburst®, Original fruit	5 pieces	10
Jellybeans	10 pieces	1
Jolly Ranchers®	4 pieces	1
Werther's Original	3 pieces	1
Butter Scotch	1 piece	0

CEREAL

General Mills®	Amount	Phosphorus (mg)
Multi-Bran CHEX	1 cup	200
Wheat Chex	1 cup	200
Raisin Nut Bran	1 cup	133
Total Whole Grain	1 cup	107
Wheaties	1 cup	107
Lucky Charms	1 cup	104
Basic 4	1 cup	100
Oatmeal Crisp, Hearty Raisin	1 cup	100
Total Raisin Bran	1 cup	100
Oatmeal Crisp, Crunchy Almond	1 cup	92
Cocoa Puffs	1 cup	80
Honey Nut Clusters	1 cup	80
Reese's Puffs	1 cup	80
Total Cranberry Crunch	1 cup	80
Cinnamon Toast Crunch	1 cup	66
Berry Berry Kix	1 cup	64
Trix	1 cup	60
Chocolate Chex	1 cup	57
Cookie Crisp	1 cup	53
Golden Grams	1 cup	53
Kix	1 cup	45
Corn Chex	1 cup	40
Rice Chex	1 cup	40
Cinnamon Chex	1 cup	27
Dora The Explorer	1 cup	27
Honey Nut Chex	1 cup	27

General Mills Cheerios®	Amount	Phosphorus (mg)
Original	1 cup	135
Honey Nut	1 cup	107
Honey Nut, Medley Crunch	1 cup	103
Frosted	1 cup	83
Apple Cinnamon	1 cup	80

PHOSPHORUS

Continued

Berry Burst, Triple Berry	1 cup	80
Fruity	1 cup	80
Multi Grain	1 cup	80
Oat Cluster Cheerios Crunch	1 cup	80
Yogurt Burst, Strawberry	1 cup	80
Banana Nut	1 cup	60
Chocolate	1 cup	53
Cinnamon Burst	1 cup	40

General Mills Fiber-One®	Amount	Phosphorus (mg)
Frosted Shreaded Wheat	1 cup	150
Original Bran Cereal	1 cup	120
80 Calorie Chocolate Squares	1 cup	107
80 Calorie Honey Squares	1 cup	107
Caramel Delight	1 cup	100
Raisin Bran Clusters	1 cup	80
Honey Clusters	1 cup	69
Nutty Clusters & almonds	1 cup	x

Kashi®	Amount	Phosphorus (mg)
7-Whole Grain Nuggets	1 cup	314
Go Lean	1 cup	247
Go Lean Crisp, Toasted Berry Crumble	1 cup	217
Go Lean Crunch, Honey Almond Flax	1 cup	167
Go Lean Crunch	1 cup	153
Island Vanilla	27 biscuits	151
Berry Fruitful	29 biscuits	133
Go Lean Crisp, Cinnamon Crumble	1 cup	133
Good Friends	1 cup	125
Autum Wheat	29 biscuits	122
Oat Flakes & Blueberry Clusters	1 cup	101
Simply Maize	1 cup	93
Indigo Morning	1 cup	92
7-Whole Grain Flakes	1 cup	87
7-Whole Grain Honey Puffs	1 cup	79
Berry Blossom	1 cup	58
Strawberry Fields	1 cup	54
7-Whole Grain Puffs	1 cup	46
Honey Sunshine	1 cup	45
Heart to Heart, Warm Cinnamon	1 cup	43
Heart to Heart, Honey Toasted Oat	1 cup	17
Blackberry Hills	1 cup	x
Cinnamon Harvest	28 biscuits	x
Go Lean Vanilla Graham	1 cup	x
Heart to Heart, Nutty Chia Flax	1 cup	x

RDA 700 mg for adults

PHOSPHORUS

Kellogg's®	Amount	Phosphorus (mg)
All-Bran Original	1 cup	713
All-Bran Bran Buds	1 cup	450
All-Bran Complete Wheat Flakes	1 cup	200
Cracklin' Oat Bran	1 cup	182
Frosted MINI-Wheats, Bite-Size	1 cup	162
Frosted MINI-Wheats, Big-Bite	1 cup	152
MUESLIX	1 cup	149
Raisin Bran Crunch	1 cup	119
Fiberplus Berry Yogurt Crunch	1 cup	100
Honey Smacks	1 cup	77
Smart Start, Strong heart, Antioxidants	1 cup	66
Cocoa Krispies	1 cup	42
Krave Chocolate	1 cup	42
Rice Krispies	1 cup	36
Frosted Rice Krispies	1 cup	32
Rice Krispies Treats	1 cup	32
Corn Flakes	1 cup	29
Crunchy Nut Golden Honey Nut Flakes	1 cup	26
Product 19	1 cup	26
Crispix	1 cup	25
Honey Crunch Corn Flakes	1 cup	24
Froot Loops	1 cup	21
Apple Jacks	1 cup	20
Frosted Flakes	1 cup	20
Smorz	1 cup	20
Raisin Bran	1 cup	18
CINNABON	1 cup	17
Corn Pops	1 cup	16
Crunchy Nut Roasted Nut & Honey O's	1 cup	15
Fiberplus Cinnamon Oat Crunch	1 cup	5

Kellogg's® Special-K®	Amount	Phosphorus (mg)
Low Fat Granola	1 cup	246
Protein Plus	1 cup	153
Multigrain Oats & Honey	1 cup	100
Vanilla Almond	1 cup	81
Cinnamon Pecan	1 cup	76
Chocolately Delight	1 cup	72
Fruit & Yogurt	1 cup	67
Blueberry	1 cup	66
Red Berries	1 cup	51
Original	1 cup	23

RDA 700 mg for adults

PHOSPHORUS

Post®	Amount	Phosphorus (mg)
Grape-Nuts Cereal	1 cup	397
Raisin Bran	1 cup	225
Bran Flakes	1 cup	212
Great Grains, Crunchy Pecan	1 cup	205
Shredded Wheat n' Bran, spoon-size	1 cup	197
Shredded Wheat, Original, spoon-size	1 cup	188
Great Grains, Raisin, Date & Pecan	1 cup	186
Great Grains, Banana Nut Crunch	1 cup	166
Great Grains, Cranberry Almond Crunch	1 cup	163
Honey Nut Shredded Wheat	1 cup	162
Shredded Wheat, lightly frosted, spoon-size	1 cup	144
Grape-Nuts Flakes	1 cup	108
Shredded Wheat, Original, big-biscuit	1 biscuit	92
Golden Crisp	1 cup	82
Blueberry Morning	1 cup	71
Alpha-Bits	1 cup	62
Cocoa Pebbles	1 cup	37
Honeycomb Cereal	1 cup	31
Fruity Pebbles	1 cup	26

Post® Honey Bunches of Oats®	Amount	Phosphorus (mg)
Just Bunches, Honey Roasted	1 cup	199
With Vanilla Bunches	1 cup	130
With Almonds	1 cup	73
Honey Roasted	1 cup	62
With Cinnamon Bunches	1 cup	60
Pecan Bunches	1 cup	57
With Strawberries	1 cup	57
Just Bunches Cinnamon	1 cup	x
Raisin Medley	1 cup	x

Quaker®	Amount	Phosphorus (mg)
Granola, Apple, Cranberry, & Almond	1 cup	327
Toasted Multigrain Crisp	1 cup	236
Oatmeal Squares	1 cup	208
Oatmeal Squares, Golden Maple	1 cup	208
Oatmeal Squares, Cinnamon	1 cup	207
LIFE Cereal, Original	1 cup	178
LIFE Cereal, Maple & Brown Sugar	1 cup	166
LIFE Cereal, Cinnamon	1 cup	164
CAP'N Crunch's Peanut Butter Crunch	1 cup	70
Corn Bran Crunch	1 cup	67
CAP'N Crunch	1 cup	60

RDA 700 mg for adults

PHOSPHORUS

Continued

CAP'N Crunch & Crunch Berries	1 cup	58
CAP'N Crunch's OOPs! All Berries	1 cup	54
Puffed Wheat	1 cup	50
Honey Graham OH'S	1 cup	49
Puffed Rice	1 cup	22

Cereal, Cooked	Amount	Phosphorus (mg)
Oats, instant	1 cup	180
Oats, regular, unenriched	1 cup	180
Farina	1 cup	88
Malt-o-Meal plain	1 serving	67
Corn grits, white	1 cup	48
CREAM OF WHEAT, regular	1 cup	38
Corn grits, yellow	1 cup	34

Cheese	Amount	Phosphorus (mg)
Ricotta, part skim milk	1 cup	450
Ricotta, whole milk	1 cup	389
Cottage cheese, 2%	1 cup	368
Cottage cheese, creamed, small curd	1 cup	334
Cottage cheese, 1%	1 cup	303
Cottage cheese, nonfat	1 cup	276

Cheese	Amount	Phosphorus (mg)
Velveeta, pasteurized process	1 oz	242
American, pasteurized process, low fat	1 oz	232
Cheez Whiz, pasteurized process	1 oz	226
Romano	1 oz	215
Goat cheese, hard type	1 oz	207
Parmesan, grated	1 oz	207
Mozzarella, nonfat	1 oz	186
American, pasteurized process, fortified	1 oz	182
Gruyere	1 oz	172
American, pasteurized process, imitation	1 oz	169
Swiss, low fat	1 oz	169
Swiss	1 oz	161
Gouda	1 oz	155
Mozzarella, part skim milk, low moisture	1 oz	149
Cream cheese, fat free	1 oz	148
Cheddar	1 oz	145
Provolone	1 oz	141
Provolone, reduced fat	1 oz	139
Cheddar, low fat	1 oz	137
Muenster	1 oz	133

PHOSPHORUS

Continued

Muenster, low fat	1 oz	131
Colby	1 oz	130
Monterey	1 oz	126
Monterey, low fat	1 oz	124
Roquefort	1 oz	111
Blue cheese	1 oz	110
Goat cheese, semisoft type	1 oz	106
Mozzarella, whole milk	1 oz	100
Fontina	1 oz	98
Feta cheese	1 oz	96
Goat cheese, soft type	1 oz	73
Cottage cheese, nonfat, uncreamed	1 oz	54
Brie	1 oz	53
Ricotta, part skim milk	1 oz	52
Cottage cheese, 2%	1 oz	46
Cottage cheese, creamed, small curd	1 oz	45
Ricotta, whole milk	1 oz	45
Cottage cheese, 1%	1 oz	38
Cream cheese	1 oz	30

Cheese, Mexican	Amount	Phosphorus (mg)
Mexican, blend, reduced fat	1 oz	163
Queso seco	1 oz	135
Queso blanco	1 oz	132
Queso anejo	1 oz	126
Queso asadero	1 oz	126
Queso chihuahua	1 oz	125
Mexican, blend	1 oz	123
Queso fresco	1 oz	109

Chicken, Cooked	Amount	Phosphorus (mg)
Breast, with skin, fried with flour	1 breast	228
Breast, with skin, roasted	1 breast	210
Breast, meat only, no skin, roasted	1 breast	196
Thigh, with skin, fried	1 thigh	133
Thigh, no skin, roasted	1 thigh	95
Drumstick, with skin, fried	1 drumstick	86
Drumstick, no skin, roasted	1 drumstick	81
Wing with skin, fried in batter	1 wing	59
Wing with skin, roasted	1 wing	51

PHOSPHORUS

Chicken, Cooked	Amount	Phosphorus (mg)
Breast meat only, no skin, roasted	3 oz	194
Breast with skin, fried in flour	3 oz	198
Breast with skin, roasted	3 oz	182
Cornish game hens, meat only	3 oz	127
Drumstick meat only, no skin, roasted	3 oz	170
Drumstick with skin, fried in flour	3 oz	150
Drumstick with skin, roasted	3 oz	165
Thigh meat only, no skin, roasted	3 oz	184
Thigh with skin, fried in flour	3 oz	159
Thigh with skin, roasted	3 oz	174
Wing meat only, no skin, roasted	3 oz	141
Wing with skin, fried in flour	3 oz	128
Wing with skin, roasted	3 oz	128

Chicken, Fast Food	Amount	Phosphorus (mg)
Kentucky Fried Chicken, Breast, Original	1 breast	458
Popeyes Fried Chicken, Breast, mild	1 breast	372
Kentucky Fried Chicken, Thigh, Original	1 thigh	307
Popeyes Fried Chicken, Thigh, mild	1 thigh	191
Kentucky Fried Chicken, Drumstick, Original	1 drumstick	158
Kentucky Fried Chicken, Wing, Original	1 wing	132
Popeyes Fried Chicken, Drumstick, mild	1 drumstick	130
Popeyes Fried Chicken, Wing, mild	1 wing	88

Chocolate	Amount	Phosphorus (mg)
Cocoa, dry powder, unsweetened	1 oz	208
Baking Chocolate	1 oz	113
Dark Chocolate, 70-85%, cacao solids	1 oz	87
Dark Chocolate, 60-69%, cacao solids	1 oz	74
Milk Chocolate	1 oz	59
Dark Chocolate, 45-59%, cacao solids	1 oz	58
White Chocolate	1 oz	50
Semisweet Chocolate	1 oz	37
Special Dark Chocolate	1 oz	14

Condiments	Amount	Phosphorus (mg)
Catsup	1 tbsp	5
Yellow Mustard	1 tsp	5
Sweet Pickel Relish	1 tbsp	2

PHOSPHORUS

Cookies	Amount	Phosphorus (mg)
Kebbler® Chips Delux, Chocolate Lovers	5 cookies	123
Mother's® Double Fudge Cream Sandwich	5 cookies	80
Kebbler® Chips Delux, Original Chocolate	5 cookies	71
Murray® Sugar Free, Chocolate Chip	5 cookies	59
Kebbler® Sardies, Pecan Shortbread	5 cookies	54
Mother's® Vanilla Sandwich	5 cookies	52
Mother's® Taffy Sandwich	5 cookies	47
Mother's® English Tea Sandwich	5 cookies	41
Famous Amos® Chocolate Chip Pecan	5 cookies	38
Girl Scouts, Thin Mints	5 cookies	30
Murray® Sugar Free, Vanilla Cream	5 cookies	25
Mother's® Iced Lemonade Cookies	5 cookies	22
Keebler® Iced Oatmeal Cookies	5 cookies	19
Famous Amos, Chocolate Chip	5 cookies	18
Mother's® Chocolate Chip	5 cookies	16
Mother's® Circus Animal Cookies	5 cookies	15
Mother's® Jungle Animal Cookies	5 cookies	15
Mother's® Iced Oatmeal Cookies	5 cookies	13

Crackers	Amount	Phosphorus (mg)
Kashi Original 7-Grain	1 serving	167
Kashi Fire Roasted Vegetable	1 serving	141
Kashi Toasted Asiago	1 serving	139
Kashi Honey Sesame	1 serving	100
Whole-Wheat, and Triscuits	1 serving	93
Wheat, regular, and Wheat-Thins	1 serving	80
Cheez-it, Low Sodium	1 serving	65
Special-K Sour Cream & Onion Chips	1 serving	61
Special-K Cracker Chips, Sea Salt	1 serving	57
Ritz crackers	1 serving	44
Special-K Cracker Chips, Cheddar	1 serving	36
Keebler Town House, Original	1 serving	32
Cheez-it, reduced fat	1 serving	31
Keebler Club, Original	1 serving	31
Melba toast, plain	1 serving	29
Special-K Multigrain Crackers	1 serving	29
Rye, crispbread, and Wasa	1 serving	27
Matzo, plain	1 serving	25
Cheez-It, hot & spicy	1 serving	22
Cheez-It, cheddar jack	1 serving	20
Cheez-it, original	1 serving	19
Saltines	1 serving	17
Graham crackers	1 serving	15
Keebler Town House, Flatbread, Sea Salt	1 serving	8

RDA 700 mg for adults

PHOSPHORUS

Cream & Nondairy Creamers	Amount	Phosphorus (mg)
CoffeeMate Original	1 tbsp	15
CoffeeMate French Vanilla	1 tbsp	15
CoffeeMate Hazelnut	1 tbsp	15
CoffeeMate Low-Fat Original	1 tbsp	15
International Delight, All Flavors	1 tbsp	15
Half & Half	1 tbsp	14
Sour Cream, cultured	1 tbsp	14
Sour Cream, reduced fat	1 tbsp	14
Light Coffe Cream	1 tbsp	12
CoffeeMate Fat Free French Vanilla	1 tbsp	12
Silk, All Flavors	1 tbsp	11
Heavy Cream	1 tbsp	9
Whipped Topping, pressurized	1 tbsp	3

Donuts	Amount	Phosphorus (mg)
Plain Cake-Type	1 donut	141
Glazed, twist	1 donut	105
Honeybun	1 donut	99
Chocolate Cake-Type	1 donut	97
Glazed, large	1 donut	74
Cream Filled	1 donut	65

Eggs	Amount	Phosphorus (mg)
Eggnog	1 cup	277
Egg whole, scrambled	1 large	101
Egg whole, fried	1 large	99
Egg whole, poached	1 large	99
Egg whole, hard boiled	1 large	86
Egg yolk	1 large	65
Egg substitute, liquid, fat free	1/4 cup	43
Egg whites, dried	1 ounce	31
Egg whites, dried powder, stabilized	1 tbsp	6
Egg whites	1 large	5

Fish, Canned	Amount	Phosphorus (mg)
Atlantic sardines, in oil	3 oz	417
Light tuna, in oil	3 oz	265
White (albacore) tuna, in oil	3 oz	227
White (albacore) tuna, in water	3 oz	184
Light tuna, in water	3 oz	118

PHOSPHORUS

Fish, Cooked	Amount	Phosphorus (mg)
Carp	3 oz	451
Chinook salmon	3 oz	315
Keta (chum) salmon	3 oz	309
Pacific cod	3 oz	293
Florida pompano	3 oz	290
Pink salmon	3 oz	286
Yellowfin tuna	3 oz	283
Coho salmon, farmed	3 oz	282
Bluefin tuna	3 oz	277
Coho salmon, wild	3 oz	274
King mackerel	3 oz	270
Sockeye salmon	3 oz	269
Flounder & Sole	3 oz	263
Catfish, wild	3 oz	258
Swordfish	3 oz	258
Atlantic perch	3 oz	255
Atlantic & Pacific Halibut	3 oz	244
Skipjack (aku) tuna	3 oz	242
Whiting	3 oz	242
Atlantic pollock	3 oz	241
Northern pike	3 oz	240
Surimi	3 oz	240
Atlantic mackerel	3 oz	236
Haddock	3 oz	236
Alaskan halibut	3 oz	234
Rainbow trout, farmed	3 oz	230
Spanish mackerel	3 oz	230
Rainbow trout, wild	3 oz	229
Walleye pike	3 oz	229
Alaskan pollock	3 oz	227
Walleye pollock	3 oz	227
Atlantic salmon, wild	3 oz	218
Freshwater bass	3 oz	218
Striped bass	3 oz	216
Atlantic salmon, farmed	3 oz	214
Pacific rockfish, mixed species	3 oz	211
Sea bass	3 oz	211
Catfish, farmed	3 oz	210
Striped mullet	3 oz	207
Atlantic croaker	3 oz	184
Cat fish, breaded & fried	3 oz	184
Greenland halibut	3 oz	178
Tilapia	3 oz	173
Snapper	3 oz	171

RDA 700 mg for adults

PHOSPHORUS

Continued

Yellowtail	3 oz	171
Chinook salmon, smoked	3 oz	139
Salmon, Lox	3 oz	139
Pacific & Jack mackerel	3 oz	136
Grouper	3 oz	122
Atlantic cod	3 oz	117
Orange roughy	3 oz	87
Atlantic herring, pickeled	3 oz	76

Fish, Shellfish, Cooked	Amount	Phosphorus (mg)
Clams, canned	3 oz	278
Shrimp, cooked	3 oz	260
Alaskan king crab, imitation	3 oz	240
Alaskan king crab	3 oz	238
Octopus	3 oz	237
Crayfish	3 oz	230
Squid, fried	3 oz	213
Scallops, breaded & fried	3 oz	201
Blue crab	3 oz	199
Blue crab, canned	3 oz	199
Shrimp, breaded & fried	3 oz	185
Abalone	3 oz	184
Blue crab cakes	3 oz	181
Shrimp, canned	3 oz	166
Clams, breaded & fried	3 oz	160
Northern lobster	3 oz	157
Oysters, breaded & fried	3 oz	135
Eastern oysters, wild	3 oz	128
Queen crab	3 oz	109
Eastern oysters, farmed	3 oz	98

Fruit, Canned	Amount	Phosphorus (mg)
Plums	1 cup	34
Apricots	1 cup	31
Peaches	1 cup	29
Pears	1 cup	19
Pineapple	1 cup	18
Applesauce, sweetened	1 cup	15
Applesauce, unsweetened	1 cup	12
Olives, black	5 large	1
Olives, green	5 large	1

PHOSPHORUS

Fruit, Dried	Amount	Phosphorus (mg)
Peaches	1 cup	190
Currants	1 cup	180
Pears	1 cup	106
Figs	1 cup	100
Apricots	1 cup	92
Apples	1 cup	33
Cranberries	1 cup	10

Fruit, Frozen	Amount	Phosphorus (mg)
Blackberries, unthawed	1 cup	45
Raspberries	1 cup	42
Strawberries	1 cup	33
Peaches	1 cup	28
Blueberries	1 cup	16

Fruit, Raw	Amount	Phosphorus (mg)
Raisins	1 cup	146
Avocado, California, pureed	1 cup	124
Prunes, uncooked	1 cup	120
Dates	1 cup	91
Stewed prunes	1 cup	74
Black currants	1 cup	66
Kiwi	1 cup	61
Elderberries	1 cup	57
Mulberries	1 cup	53
Plantains	1 cup	50
Grapefruit, pink or red, sections	1 cup	41
Strawberries	1 cup	40
Tangerine, sections	1 cup	39
Apricots	1 cup	38
Nectarine	1 cup	37
Raspberries	1 cup	36
Blackberries	1 cup	32
Cherries, pitted	1 cup	32
Grapes, red & green	1 cup	32
Pummelo, sections	1 cup	32
Peachs, slices	1 cup	31
Plums, sliced	1 cup	26
Oranges, sections	1 cup	25
Cataloupe, cubes	1 cup	24
Mango	1 cup	23

RDA 700 mg for adults

PHOSPHORUS

Continued

Honeydew	1 cup	19
Pears	1 cup	18
Blueberries	1 cup	17
Water mellon	1 cup	17
Apples	1 cup	14
Papayas	1 cup	14
Cranberries	1 cup	13
Pineapple	1 cup	13

Fruit, Raw	Amount	Phosphorus (mg)
Pummelo	1 fruit	104
Avocado, California	1 fruit	75
Cherimoya	1 fruit	61
Plantains	1 fruit	61
Avocado, Florida	1 fruit	55
Mango	1 fruit	47
Raisins	1 small box	43
Cantaloupe	1/2 fruit	41
Chayote	1 fruit	37
Nectarine	1 fruit	35
Persimmons, Japanese	1 fruit	29
Prunes, uncooked	5 prunes	29
Banana	1 fruit	26
Dates	5 dates	26
Kiwi	1 kiwi	26
Apples, Fugi, medium size	1 apple	25
Apples, Red Delicious, medium size	1 apple	25
Grapefruit, pink or red	1/2 fruit	22
Apples, Granny Smith, medium size	1 apple	20
Peaches	1 fruit	20
Apples, Gala, medium size	1 apple	19
Oranges	1 fruit	18
Pears	1 pear	18
Apples, Golden Delicious, medium	1 apple	17
Cherries	10 fruit	17
Tangerine	1 fruit	17
Papayas, small size	1 fruit	16
Strawberries	5 fruit	14
Plums	1 plum	11
Star fruit, Carambola	1 fruit	11
Apricots	1 fruit	8
Pineapple guava, Feijoa	1 fruit	8
Figs, dried	1 fruit	6

PHOSPHORUS

Continued

Persimmons, small native	1 fruit	6
Kumquats	1 fruit	4
Pineapple, slices	1/2"x 3"	4
Olives, black	5 large	1
Olives, green	5 large	1

Game Meat, Cooked	Amount	Phosphorus (mg)
Buffalo, steak, free range	3 oz	209
Rabbit	3 oz	204
Caribou	3 oz	198
Deer, ground	3 oz	194
Deer	3 oz	192
Elk, ground	3 oz	188
Squirrel	3 oz	179
Antelope	3 oz	178
Bison, ground	3 oz	174
Duck	3 oz	173
Elk	3 oz	153
Wild boar	3 oz	114

Grains, Cooked	Amount	Phosphorus (mg)
Amaranth	1 cup	364
Kamut	1 cup	304
Spelt	1 cup	291
Quinoa	1 cup	281
Oat bran	1 cup	261
Oats, regular, unenriched	1 cup	180
Millet	1 cup	174
Brown rice	1 cup	162
Spaghetti, spinach	1 cup	151
Wild rice	1 cup	134
Macaroni, whole-wheat	1 cup	125
Spaghetti, whole-wheat	1 cup	125
Egg noodles	1 cup	122
Buckwheat, groats	1 cup	118
Egg & Spinach noodles	1 cup	91
White rice, parboiled	1 cup	87
Barley, pearled	1 cup	85
Macaroni	1 cup	81
Spaghetti, enriched	1 cup	81
Bulgur	1 cup	73
White rice, long-grain, regular	1 cup	68
White rice, long-grain, instant	1 cup	61

RDA 700 mg for adults

PHOSPHORUS

Continued

Couscous	1 cup	35
Rice noodles	1 cup	35
Soba noodles	1 cup	28

Hamburgers, Fast Food	Amount	Phosphorus (mg)
Burger King, Whopper with Cheese	1 burger	357
McDonald's, Quarter Pounder with Cheese	1 burger	320
Wendy's Classic Hamburger with Cheese	1 burger	297
McDonald's, Big 'N Tasty with Cheese	1 burger	282
Burger King, Double Cheeseburger	1 burger	272
Burger King, Whopper no Cheese	1 burger	267
McDonald's, Big Mac	1 burger	267
McDonald's, Double Cheeseburger	1 burger	257
McDonald's, Big 'N Tasty no Cheese	1 burger	227
Wendy's Classic Hamburger no Cheese	1 burger	225
McDonald's, Quarter Pounder no Cheese	1 burger	212
Burger King, Cheeseburger	1 burger	190
Wendy's Jr. Hamburger with Cheese	1 burger	173
McDonald's, Cheeseburger	1 burger	167
Burger King, Hamburger	1 burger	125
Wendy's Jr. Hamburger no Cheese	1 burger	125
McDonald's, Hamburger no Cheese	1 burger	102

Herbs & Spices	Amount	Phosphorus (mg)
Garlic powder	1 tsp	13
Caraway seeds	1 tsp	12
Celery seeds	1 tsp	11
Fennel seed, whole	1 tsp	10
Anise seed	1 tsp	9
Chili powder	1 tsp	8
Onion powder	1 tsp	8
Coriander, seeds	1 tsp	7
Curry, powder	1 tsp	7
Paprika	1 tsp	7
Turmeric, ground	1 tsp	6
Dill weed, dried	1 tsp	5
Nutmeg, ground	1 tsp	5
Pepper, black, whole	1 tsp	5
Tarragon, dried, ground	1 tsp	5
Basil, dried & ground	1 tsp	4
Pepper, black, ground	1 tsp	4
Chervil, dried	1 tsp	3
Coriander, dried, leaves	1 tsp	3

PHOSPHORUS

Continued

Ginger, ground	1 tsp	3
Oregano, dried, ground	1 tsp	3
Thyme, dried, ground	1 tsp	3
All-spice, ground	1 tsp	2
Basil, dried leaves	1 tsp	2
Cilantro	1/4 cup	2
Cinnamon, ground	1 tsp	2
Cloves, ground	1 tsp	2
Mace, ground	1 tsp	2
Marjoram, dried	1 tsp	2
Parsley, dried	1 tsp	2
Saffron	1 tsp	2
Tarragon, dried, leaves	1 tsp	2
Thyme, dried, leaves	1 tsp	2
Bay leaf, crumbled	1 tsp	1
Chives, raw	1 tsp	1
Dill weed, fresh	1/4 cup	1
Oregano, dried, leaves	1 tsp	1
Rosemary, dried	1 tsp	1
Sage, ground	1 tsp	1
Spearmint, dried	1 tsp	1
Spearmint, fresh	1 tsp	1
Thyme, fresh	1 tsp	1
Capers, canned	1 tsp	0.3
Basil, fresh	1 tsp	0
Rosemary, fresh	1 tsp	0

Ice Cream	Amount	Phosphorus (mg)
Frozen yogurt, vanilla	1 cup	186
Chocolate ice cream	1 cup	170
Vanilla, Light	1 cup	156
Vanilla	1 cup	138
Strawberry	1 cup	132
Sherbet, Orange	1 cup	59

Juice	Amount	Phosphorus (mg)
Carrot	1 cup	99
Prune	1 cup	64
Tomato	1 cup	44
Orange, raw	1 cup	42
Grapefruit juice, raw	1 cup	41
Vegetable	1 cup	41
Grape	1 cup	35
Blackberry	1 cup	30
Pomegranate	1 cup	27

RDA 700 mg for adults

PHOSPHORUS

Continued

Acerola juice, raw	1 cup	22
Lemon juice, raw	1 cup	20
Pineapple	1 cup	20
Apple	1 cup	17
Cranberry	1 cup	3

Lamb, Cooked	Amount	Phosphorus (mg)
Cubed for stew or kabob	3 oz	190
Rib, lean, trim to 1/4" fat	3 oz	181
Ground	3 oz	171
Chops, loin, lean, trim to 1/4" fat	3 oz	167
Leg, whole	3 oz	162
Foreshank, trim to 1/8" fat	3 oz	141

Milk	Amount	Phosphorus (mg)
Canned, condensed, sweetened	1 cup	774
Canned, evaporated	1 cup	512
Canned, evaporated, nonfat	1 cup	499
Sheep milk	1 cup	387
Goat milk	1 cup	271
Chocolate Milk, lowfat	1 cup	258
Chocolate Milk, from whole milk	1 cup	253
Whole milk, dry powder	1/4 cup	248
Nonfat, fat free or skim liquid milk	1 cup	247
Lowfat,1%, added vitamin A & D	1 cup	232
Dry, instant, nonfat	1/3 cup	227
Reduced fat, 2%, added vitamins A & D	1 cup	224
Buttermilk, lowfat	1 cup	218
Coconut milk, canned	1 cup	217
Buttermilk, whole milk	1 cup	208
Whole milk, liquid, 3.25%	1 cup	205
Soy milk, original, unfortified	1 cup	126
Human milk	1 cup	34

Milk, Almond, Hemp & Oat	Amount	Phosphorus (mg)
Living Harvest Hempmilk, All Flavors	1 cup	400
Pacific Foods, Hemp Milk, Original	1 cup	300
Pacific Foods, Organic Oat Beverage	1 cup	270
Living Harvest Tempt Hempmilk	1 cup	200
Pacific Foods, Hazelnut	1 cup	195
Pacific Foods, All-Natural Hazelnut, Original	1 cup	195
Almond Breeze, Chocolate	1 cup	150
Almond Dream, Original	1 cup	150
Almond Breeze, Original	1 cup	100

PHOSPHORUS

Continued

Almond Breeze, Original, Unsweetened	1 cup	40
Pacific Foods, Almond Beverage, Plain	1 cup	28
Pacific Foods, Almond Beverage, Vanilla	1 cup	25
Pacific Foods, Unsweetened, Almond	1 cup	18

Milk, Rice	Amount	Phosphorus (mg)
Trader Joe's Rice Drink Vanilla, refrigerated	1 cup	200
Pacific Foods, Low Fat Rice, Plain & Vanilla	1 cup	175
Trader Joe's Rice Drink Original	1 cup	150
Good Kama Original Rice milk	1 cup	150
Rice Dream, Enriched, Original & Vanilla	1 cup	150
365 Organic Rice Milk, Original & Vanilla	1 cup	150
WestSoy Rice Drink, Plain & Vanilla	1 cup	100
Rice Dream Original	1 cup	57

Milk, Soy	Amount	Phosphorus (mg)
8th Continent Chocolate Soy Milk	1 cup	295
8th Continent Vanilla Soy Milk	1 cup	257
8th Continent Soy Milk, Original	1 cup	255
WestSoy Organic Plus, Plain & Vanilla	1 cup	250
WestSoy Soy Slender, Plain & Vanilla	1 cup	250
Vitasoy Lite Plus Vanilla, Beverage	1 cup	185
EdenSoy Chocolate	1 cup	150
EdenSoy Original	1 cup	150
Pacific Foods Organic Soy Beverage	1 cup	125
Organic Valley Soy Milk, Original	1 cup	106
EdenSoy Vanilla	1 cup	100
365 Organic Soymilk, Chocolate	1 cup	100
Silk Soymilk, Plain & Vanilla	1 cup	95
365® Organic Soymilk, Original, Plain & Vanilla	1 cup	80
Pacific Foods Ultra Soy Plain	1 cup	65

Nuts & Seeds, raw	Amount	Phosphorus (mg)
Pumpkin seeds, dried	1 oz	350
Chia seeds	1 oz	244
Tahini	1 oz	208
Brazilnuts	1 oz	206
Sunflower seeds, dried	1 oz	187
Flaxseeds	1 oz	182
Sesame seeds	1 oz	178
Cashews	1 oz	168
Pine nuts	1 oz	163
Black Walnuts	1 oz	145
Pistachio	1 oz	139

PHOSPHORUS

Continued

Almonds	1 oz	137
Mixed nuts, roasted with peanuts, no salt	1 oz	123
Trail mix, regular with chocolate chips	1 oz	110
Peanuts	1 oz	107
Peanut butter, smooth style	1 oz	101
English Walnuts	1 oz	98
Trail mix, regular, salted	1 oz	98
Hazlenut	1 oz	82
Pecans	1 oz	79
Macadamia	1 oz	53
Trail mix, tropical	1 oz	53
Coconut, raw meat	1 oz	32

Nuts & Seeds	Amount	Phosphorus (mg)
Pumpkin seeds, dried	1/4 cup	398
Flaxseeds	1/4 cup	270
Brazilnuts, whole	1/4 cup	241
Peanut butter, smooth, salted	1/4 cup	231
Sunflower seeds, dried	1/4 cup	231
Sesame seeds	1/4 cup	226
Pine nuts	1/4 cup	194
Almonds, whole	1/4 cup	173
Black walnuts, chopped	1/4 cup	160
Pistachio	1/4 cup	151
Mixed nuts, roasted with peanuts, no salt	1/4 cup	149
Trail mix, regular with chocolate chips	1/4 cup	141
Peanuts	1/4 cup	137
Trail mix, regular, salted	1/4 cup	129
Tahini	1 tbsp	110
English walnuts, chopped	1/4 cup	101
Hazelnuts, chopped	1/4 cup	83
Pecans, halves	1/4 cup	69
Flaxseeds	1 tbsp	66
Trail mix, tropical	1/4 cup	65
Macadamia	1/4 cup	63
Peanut butter, smooth, salted	1 tbsp	57
Sesame seeds	1 tbsp	53
Coconut meat, shredded	1/4 cup	23

PHOSPHORUS

Pies, commerically prepared	Amount	Phosphorus (mg)
Lemon Meringue	1 slice	119
Egg custard	1 slice	118
Pumpkin	1 slice	108
Cherry	1 slice	36
Apple	1 slice	30
Blueberry	1 slice	29

Pop Tarts® from Kelloggs®	Amount	Phosphorus (mg)
Blueberry	1 pastry	46
Frosted Blueberry	1 pastry	44
Frosted Cherry	1 pastry	42
Ginger Bread	1 pastry	40
S' mores	1 pastry	39
Brown Sugar Cinnamon	1 pastry	32
Strawberry	1 pastry	29
Frosted Brown Sugar	1 pastry	25
Frosted Wild Fruit Fussion	1 pastry	24
Frosted Wild Srawberry	1 pastry	24
Frosted Apple Strudel	1 pastry	22
Frosted Wild Berry	1 pastry	22
Frosted Cinnamon Roll	1 pastry	22
Frosted Wild Grape	1 pastry	22
Frosted Blueberry Muffin	1 pastry	22

Pizza, Frozen & baked	Amount	Phosphorus (mg)
Digiorno, Cheese, Stuffed Crust	1/4 pie	581
Digiorno, Pepperoni, Stuffed Crust	1/4 pie	483
Digiorno, Supreme, Rising Crust	1/4 pie	479
Digiorno, Pepperoni, Rising Crust	1/4 pie	466
Digiorno, Cheese, Rising Crust	1/4 pie	441
Digiorno, Cheese, Thin & Crisp Crust	1/4 pie	380
Digiorno, Pepperoni, Thin & Crisp Crust	1/4 pie	309
Digiorno, Supreme, Thin & Crisp Crust	1/4 pie	290

Pizza	Amount	Phosphorus (mg)
Domino's, Extravaganzza	1 slice	278
Pizza Hut, Cheese, Pan Crust	1 slice	242
Papa John's, Pepperoni, Original Crust	1 slice	242
Papa John's, Cheese, Original Crust	1 slice	238
Little Caesars, Pepperoni, Deep Dish	1 slice	224
Domino's, Cheese, hand tossed	1 slice	220
Pizza Hut, Pepperoni, Pan Crust	1 slice	218
Domino's, Pepperoni, hand tossed	1 slice	216

RDA 700 mg for adults

PHOSPHORUS

Continued

Little Caesars, Cheese	1 slice	206
Little Caesars, Pepperoni	1 slice	202
Little Caesars, Cheese, Thin Crust	1 slice	143

Pork, Cooked	Amount	Phosphorus (mg)
Bacon, cured, pre-sliced, pan-fried	3 oz	330
Polish sausage, 10 x 1 1/4 "	1 sausage	309
Canadian-style bacon	3 oz	252
Sirloin pork chops	3 oz	248
Pork chops, lean, pan-fried	3 oz	228
Tenderloin	3 oz	225
Spareribs	3 oz	222
Pork chops, pan-fried	3 oz	213
Cured ham, lean	3 oz	193
Ground Pork	3 oz	192
Center loin pork chops	3 oz	187
Pork chops, broiled	3 oz	187
Cured ham	3 oz	182
Bratwurst	3 oz	177
Italian sausage	3 oz	144
Braunschweiger	3 oz	143
Backribs	3 oz	140
Canadian-style bacon	2 slices	139
Bacon, cured, pre-sliced, pan-fried	3 slices	134
Sausage	3 oz	127
Liverwurst spread	1/4 cup	126
Polish sausage	3 oz	116
Sausage	1 patty	40
Sausage	1 link	34

AdvantEdge® Nutrition Bars	Amount	Phosphorus (mg)
Chocolate Carmel	1 bar	250
Double Chocolate	1 bar	250
Peanut Butter Caramel	1 bar	250

Atkins® Advantage® Protein Bars	Amount	Phosphorus (mg)
Almond Brownie	1 bar	250
Chocolate Coconut	1 bar	200
Chocolate Decadence	1 bar	200
Pralines 'n Cream	1 bar	200
Chocolate Peanut Butter	1 bar	150
Chocolate Chip Granola	1 bar	150
Carmel Fudge Brownie	1 bar	150
Golden Oats Granola	1 bar	150

PHOSPHORUS

Continued

Peanut Butter Granola	1 bar	100
Carmel Cookie Dough	1 bar	100
S 'Mores	1 bar	100

PowerBar® Protein Bars	Amount	Phosphorus (mg)
PowerBar® Protein Plus, all flavors	1 bar	350
PowerBar® Performance, all flavors	1 bar	350
PowerBar® Pria Complete, all flavors	1 bar	250
PowerBar® Harvest, all flavors	1 bar	200
PowerBar® Pria, all flavors	1 bar	150
PowerBar® Triple Threat	1 bar	150

Protein Bars	Amount	Phosphorus (mg)
Luna® Bars for Women, all flavors	1 bar	350
Genisoy Crispy Chocolate Mint	1 bar	250
Balance® Bars, all flavors	1 bar	150
ZonePerfect, all flavors	1 bar	150

Protein Powders	Amount	Phosphorus (mg)
Protein powder whey based	1 oz	375
Protein powder soy based	1 oz	265
ABBOTT whey protein powder	1 oz	182
Whey protein powder isolate	1 oz	165
ABBOTT soy protein powder	1 oz	125
Jay Robb's Whey protein powder	1 oz	70
Jay Robb's Egg White protein powder	1 oz	27
Egg whites, stabilized, dried powder	1 oz	25

Pudding ready-to-eat	Amount	Phosphorus (mg)
Rice	4 oz	93
Tapocia	4 oz	66
Chocolate	4 oz	60
Vanilla	4 oz	45

Salad Dressings	Amount	Phosphorus (mg)
Ranch, Reduced Fat	1 tbsp	29
Ranch, regular	1 tbsp	24
Blue cheese, Fat-Free	1 tbsp	18
Ranch, Fat-Free	1 tbsp	16
Italian, Fat-Free	1 tbsp	15
Blue cheese, regular	1 tbsp	11
Kraft, mayo light	1 tbsp	9
Blue cheese, light	1 tbsp	8

RDA 700 mg for adults

PHOSPHORUS

Continued

Honey Mustard, Fat-Free	1 tbsp	6
Caesar, Fat-Free	1 tbsp	5
Honey Mustard, regular	1 tbsp	4
Smart Balance, Omega Plus Light	1 tbsp	4
Thousand Island, regular	1 tbsp	4
Caesar, regular	1 tbsp	3
French, Reduced Fat	1 tbsp	3
French, regular	1 tbsp	3
Mayonnaise, regular	1 tbsp	3
Mayonnaise, soybean oil	1 tbsp	3
Russian, regular	1 tbsp	3
Italian, Reduced Fat	1 tbsp	2
Mayonnaise, light	1 tbsp	2
Italian, regular	1 tbsp	1
Balsamic Vinaigrette	1 tbsp	0
French, Fat-Free	1 tbsp	0
Thousand Island, Fat-Free	1 tbsp	0

Sauce, ready-to-serve	Amount	Phosphorus (mg)
Pasta, spaghetti / marinara sauce	1/2 cup	45
Teriyaki sauce	1 tbsp	28
Soy sauce, shoyu	1 tbsp	27
Soy sauce, tamari	1 tbsp	23
Worcestershire sauce	1 tbsp	10
Salsa Verde	1 tbsp	6
Hoisin sauce	1 tbsp	6
Plum sauce	1 tbsp	4
Tarter sauce	1 tbsp	3
Fish sauce	1 tbsp	1
Tobasco	1/4 tsp	0

Snacks	Amount	Phosphorus (mg)
Soft Pretzel	1 large	113
KRAFT Corn Nuts	1 oz	78
Tortilla Chips, Ranch-flavored	1 oz	71
Tortilla Chips, Low Fat, with olestra, cheese	1 oz	69
Tortilla Chips, Taco-flavored	1 oz	68
Fritolay Sunchips, Multigrain, Original	1 oz	63
Tortilla Chips, Plain, White Corn	1 oz	61
Potato Chips, Sour Cream & Onion	1 oz	50
Potato Chips, partially hydrogenated soybean	1 oz	47
Corn Based Chips,	1 oz	45
Potato Chips, Plain, Salted	1 oz	44
Potato Chips, Barbecue-flavored	1 oz	41
Popcorn, oil-popped, cheese-flavored	1 cup	40

PHOSPHORUS

Continued

Pretzel, Plain	1 oz	36
Pita Chips, plain	1 oz	35
Popcorn, air-popped, plain	1 cup	29
Popcorn, microwave, plain	1 cup	22
Popcorn, home prepared, oil-popped	1 cup	20

Soup, Canned & Condensed	Amount	Phosphorus (mg)
New England Clam Chowder	1 can	788
Mushroom Barley	1 can	152
Chicken with Dumplings	1 can	149
Tomato Bisque	1 can	147
Chicken Noodle	1 can	106
Vegetable Beef	1 can	98
Cream of Chicken	1 can	95
Cream of Celery	1 can	92
Tomato	1 can	91
Tomato, reduced sodium	1 can	88

Tofu	Amount	Phosphorus (mg)
Mori-Nu, Silken, firm	3 oz	173
Mori-Nu, Silken, extra firm	3 oz	154
Mori-Nu, Silken, soft	3 oz	103
Vitasoy USA, Nasoya Lite Silken	3 oz	84
Vitasoy USA, Nasoya Plus Firm	3 oz	78
Vitasoy USA, Nasoya Lite Firm	3 oz	72
Mori-Nu, Silken, lite extra firm	3 oz	69
Mori-Nu, Silken, lite firm	3 oz	54

Turkey, Cooked	Amount	Phosphorus (mg)
Turkey bacon	3 oz	391
Ground turkey, fat free	3 oz	224
Ground turkey	3 oz	216
Ground turkey, 85% lean	3 oz	200
Light meat	3 oz	196
Breast meat	3 oz	190
Dark meat	3 oz	180
Ground turkey, 93% lean	3 oz	178
Turkey sausage, reduced fat	3 oz	139

Veal, Cooked	Amount	Phosphorus (mg)
Leg, top round	3 oz	212
Foreshank	3 oz	191
Sirloin	3 oz	190
Ground	3 oz	184

RDA 700 mg for adults

PHOSPHORUS

Continued

Cubed for stew	3 oz	181
Loin	3 oz	180
Breast	3 oz	177
Rib	3 oz	167

VEGETABLES

Vegetables, Canned	Amount	Phosphorus (mg)
Tomato paste	1 cup	217
Tomato pure	1 cup	160
Corn	1 cup	134
Green peas	1 cup	117
Asparagus	1 cup	104
Mushrooms	1 cup	103
Spinach	1 cup	94
Pumpkin	1 cup	86
Tomato sauce	1 cup	64
Stewed tomatos	1 cup	51
Sweet potato	1 cup	49
Sauerkraut	1 cup	47
Tomatoes	1 cup	46
Carrots	1 cup	35
Beets	1 cup	29
Green beans	1 cup	28

Vegetables, Cooked	Amount	Phosphorus (mg)
Split peas	1 cup	194
White mushrooms	1 cup	136
Artichokes	1 cup	123
Corn	1 cup	115
Parsnips	1 cup	108
Broccoli	1 cup	105
Sweet potato, mashed	1 cup	105
Spinach,	1 cup	101
Taro, sliced	1 cup	100
Asparagus	1 cup	97
Potatoes, mashed, whole milk & butter	1 cup	97
Rutabagas	1 cup	95
Acorn squash	1 cup	92
Snow peas	1 cup	88
Brussels sprouts	1 cup	87
Kohlrabi	1 cup	74
Onions	1 cup	74
Pumpkin	1 cup	74

PHOSPHORUS

	Amount	Phosphorus (mg)
Summer squash	1 cup	70
Tomatoes	1 cup	67
Yams, cubed	1 cup	67
Zucchini	1 cup	67
Beets	1 cup	65
Cabbage, Red	1 cup	63
Potatoes, flesh	1 cup	61
Beet greens	1 cup	59
Swiss chard	1 cup	58
Collard greens	1 cup	57
Mustard greens	1 cup	57
Butternut squash	1 cup	55
Crookneck or Straighneck Squash	1 cup	52
Okra	1 cup	51
Cabbage	1 cup	50
Scallop or Pattypan Squash, slices	1 cup	50
Cabbage, Chinese, Bok-Choy	1 cup	49
Cabbage, Savoy	1 cup	48
Carrots	1 cup	47
Cabbage, Chinese, Pe-Tsai	1 cup	46
Dandelion greens	1 cup	44
Shiitake mushrooms	1 cup	42
Turnip greens	1 cup	42
Cabbage, Swamp	1 cup	41
Turnips	1 cup	41
Cauliflower	1 cup	40
Winter squash	1 cup	39
Celery	1 cup	38
Broccolini, chinese	1 cup	36
Green beans	1 cup	36
Kale	1 cup	36
Broccoli, raab	1 cup	29
Cactus pads, nopales	1 cup	24
Spaghetti winter squash	1 cup	22
Cabbage, Napa	1 cup	21
Leeks	1 cup	18
Eggplant	1 cup	15

Vegetables, Frozen	Amount	Phosphorus (mg)
Corn	1 cup	130
Green peas	1 cup	123
Spinach	1 cup	95
Broccoli	1 cup	90
Asparagus	1 cup	88
Brussels sprouts	1 cup	87

RDA 700 mg for adults

PHOSPHORUS

Okra	1 cup	68
Turnip greens	1 cup	56
Collard greens	1 cup	46
Carrots	1 cup	45
Cauliflower	1 cup	43
Green beans	1 cup	39
Kale	1 cup	36
Butternut squash, mashed	1 cup	34
Rhubarb, with sugar	1 cup	19

Vegetables, Raw	Amount	Phosphorus (mg)
Oyster mushrooms	1 cup	103
Portabella mushrooms	1 cup	93
Crimini mushrooms	1 cup	86
Enoki mushrooms, sliced	1 cup	68
White mushrooms	1 cup	60
Broccoli	1 cup	58
Snow peas	1 cup	52
Tomatillos	1 cup	51
Butternut squash	1 cup	46
Onions	1 cup	46
Cauliflower	1 cup	44
Summer squash	1 cup	43
Tomatoes	1 cup	43
Zucchini	1 cup	43
Carrots	1 cup	39
Red bell peppers	1 cup	39
Kale	1 cup	38
Green onions, scallions	1 cup	37
Dandelion greens	1 cup	36
Green beans	1 cup	36
Tomatoes, cherry	1 cup	36
Yellow bell peppers	1 cup	36
Green bell peppers	1 cup	30
Celery	1 cup	29
Raab broccoli	1 cup	29
Savoy Cabbage	1 cup	29
Bok-Choy	1 cup	26
Cucumber	1 cup	25
Belgian endive	1 cup	23
Red cabbage	1 cup	21
Shiitake mushrooms	1 whole	21
Watercress	1 cup	20
Butterhead or boston lettuce	1 cup	18
Cabbage	1 cup	18

PHOSPHORUS

Continued

Romaine lettuce	1 cup	17
Swiss chard	1 cup	17
Green leaf lettuce	1 cup	16
Radicchio	1 cup	16
Spinach	1 cup	15
Cactus pads, nopales	1 cup	14
Chicory greens	1 cup	14
Endive	1 cup	14
Iceburg lettuce	1 cup	11
Shiitake mushrooms, dried	1 each	11
Arugula	1 cup	10
Red leaf lettuce	1 cup	8
Spirulina, dried	1 tbsp	8

Yogurt	Amount	Phosphorus (mg)
Yoplait, Greek, Plain	6 oz	350
Yoplait, Greek, Flavored, all flavors	6 oz	300
Chobani, all flavors	6 oz	240
Stonyfield, all flavors	6 oz	200

RDA 700 mg for adults

Nutrient Data Collection Form

Food	Amount	Book Numbers	Multiply By	Estimated Nutrient Intake
Nutrient::	RDA:	Estimated:	% of RDA:	Total Estimated:

To download additional forms for free, go to www.TopNutrients4U.com

PHOSPHORUS TO PROTEIN RATIO

Alcohol	Amount	Phosphorus / Protein
Red Table Wine	1 glass	340
White Table Wine	1 glass	260
Light Beer	1 bottle	49
Regular Beer	1 bottle	31
Gin, Rum, Vodka, or Whisky	1 shot	2

Beans, Canned	Amount	Phosphorus / Protein
Refried beans	1 cup	21
Red Kidney beans	1 cup	20
Pinto beans	1 cup	20
Great Northern	1 cup	18
Navy beans	1 cup	18
Green beans	1 cup	17
Garbanzo beans	1 cup	16
Cranberry beans	1 cup	16
Baked beans, plain	1 cup	16
Lima beans	1 cup	15
Black-eyed peas	1 cup	15
Fava beans	1 cup	14
White beans, mature	1 cup	13

Beans, Cooked	Amount	Phosphorus / Protein
Adzuki	1 cup	22
Yardlong beans, chinese long beans	1 cup	22
Yellow beans	1 cup	21
Black-eyed peas	1 cup	20
Great Northern	1 cup	20
Lentils	1 cup	20
Black Turtle beans	1 cup	19
Garbanzo beans	1 cup	19
Mothbeans	1 cup	19
White beans, small	1 cup	19
Navy beans	1 cup	18
Pigeon peas	1 cup	18
Fava beans	1 cup	16
Soybeans, mature, dry roasted	1 cup	16
Kidney beans	1 cup	16
Pinto beans	1 cup	16
Black beans	1 cup	16
Edamame	1 cup	16
Green beans	1 cup	15
Hyacinath beans	1 cup	15
Soybeans, mature	1 cup	15

PHOSPHORUS TO PROTEIN RATIO

Continued

Cranberry beans	1 cup	15
Winged beans	1 cup	14
Lima beans	1 cup	14
Mung beans	1 cup	14
Soybeans, green	1 cup	13
White beans, mature	1 cup	12
Split peas	1 cup	12
Natto	1 cup	10
Lupins	1 cup	8

Beef, Cooked	Amount	Phosphorus / Protein
Skirt steak, trimmed to 0" fat	3 oz	8.9
Ribeye steak, lean, trimmed 0" fat	3 oz	8.8
Tri-tip sirloin steak, trimmed to 0" fat	3 oz	8.8
Porterhouse steak, trimmed to 0" fat	3 oz	8.2
Ground beef, 95%	3 oz	8.0
T-Bone steak, trimmed 0" fat	3 oz	8.0
Beef ribs, trimmed to 1/8" fat	3 oz	7.9
Top sirloin, lean, trimmed to 1/8" fat	3 oz	7.9
Filet mignon, trimmed to 0" fat	3 oz	7.8
Ground beef, 90%	3 oz	7.8
Flank steak, lean, trimmed to 0" fat	3 oz	7.7
Chuck roast, trimmed to 1/8" fat	3 oz	7.6
Ground beef, 85%	3 oz	7.6
Ground beef, 80%	3 oz	7.5
Ground beef, 75%	3 oz	7.3
Brisket, lean, trimmed to 0" fat	3 oz	6.2

Bread	Amount	Phosphorus / Protein
Tortillas, corn	1 tortilla	55
Cornbread, drymix	1 piece	53
White	1 slice	24
Pumpernickle	1 slice	20
Cracked wheat	1 slice	17
Multi-Grain, or Whole-Grain	1 slice	17
Whole-Wheat	1 slice	16
Rye bread	1 slice	15
Tortillas, flour	1 tortilla	15
Oatmeal bread	1 slice	15
Wheat	1 slice	14
Reduced calorie white	1 slice	14
Bagel, wheat	4" bagel	14
Raisen bread	1 slice	13
Croissants, butter	1 each	13
Italian	1 slice	12

PHOSPHORUS TO PROTEIN RATIO

Continued

Dinner Rolls, brown & serve	1 roll	11
Egg bread	1 slice	11
Hamburger & hotdog buns, plain	1 bun	11
Reduced calorie wheat	1 slice	11
Pita, white	6" pita	11
Bagel, oat bran	4" bagel	10
Bagel, cinnamon & raisens	4" bagel	10
English muffin, plain	1 muffin	10
Kaiser rolls	1 roll	10
French and sourdough	1 slice	10
Bagel, plain	4" bagel	9
Bagel, egg	4" bagel	8

Cereal, General Mills®	Amount	Phosphorus / Protein
Total Corn Flakes	1 cup	82
Trix	1 cup	43
Cocoa Puffs	1 cup	42
Cinnamon Toast Crunch	1 cup	41
Cookie Crisp	1 cup	41
Wheaties	1 cup	36
Whole Grain Total	1 cup	36
Total Raisin Bran	1 cup	35
Wheat Chex	1 cup	30
Raisin Nut Bran	1 cup	28
Reese's Puffs	1 cup	27
Total Cranberry Crunch	1 cup	27
Lucky Charms	1 cup	27
Apple Cinnamon Oatmeal Crisp	1 cup	25
Basic 4	1 cup	25
Multi-Bran CHEX	1 cup	25
Chocolate Chex	1 cup	23
Kix	1 cup	23
Berry Berry Kix	1 cup	22
Honey Nut Clusters	1 cup	20
Rice Chex	1 cup	20
Total Blueberry Pomegranate	1 cup	20
Corn Chex	1 cup	20
Crunchy Almond Oatmeal Crisp	1 cup	18
Golden Grams	1 cup	18
Cinnamon Chex	1 cup	14
Dora The Explorer	1 cup	14

PHOSPHORUS TO PROTEIN RATIO

Cereal, General Mills Cheerios®	Amount	Phosphorus / Protein
Fruity	1 cup	62
Multi Grain	1 cup	40
Honey Nut	1 cup	40
Original	1 cup	38
Banana Nut	1 cup	30
Apple Cinnamon	1 cup	30
Berry Burst	1 cup	30
Frosted	1 cup	30
Yogurt Burst, Strawberry	1 cup	27
Chocolate	1 cup	27
Crunch, Oat Clusters	1 cup	26

Cereal, General Mills Fiber One®	Amount	Phosphorus / Protein
80 Calories Chocolate Squares	1 cup	81
80 Calories Honey Squares	1 cup	60
Caramel Delight	1 cup	34
Frosted Shredded Wheat	1 cup	30
Original Bran	1 cup	30
Raisin Bran Clusters	1 cup	27
Nutty Clusters & Almonds	1 cup	25
Honey Clusters	1 cup	20

Cereal, Kashi®	Amount	Phosphorus / Protein
Granola Mountain Medley	1 cup	30
7-Whole Grain Honey Puffs	1 cup	26
Granola Cocoa Beach	1 cup	25
Organic Promise, Island Vanilla	1 cup	25
Golden Goodness	1 cup	25
Good Friends	1 cup	25
7-Whole Grain Flakes	1 cup	24
7-Whole Grain Puffs	1 cup	23
7-Whole Grain Nuggets	1 cup	22
Autumn Wheat	1 cup	19
Berry Blossom	1 cup	19
Go Lean Crisp, Toasted Berry Crumble	1 cup	18
Go Lean	1 cup	18
Heart to Heart, Wild Blueberry	1 cup	17
Honey Sunshine	1 cup	15
Go Lean Crunch	1 cup	13
Go Lean Crunch, Honey Almond Flax	1 cup	12
Heart to Heart, Honey Toasted Oat	1 cup	8
Heart to Heart, Warm Cinnamon	1 cup	7
Strawberry Fields	1 cup	6

PHOSPHORUS TO PROTEIN RATIO

Continued

Cereal, Kellogg's®	Amount	Phosphorus / Protein
All-Bran Original	1 cup	89
All-Bran Bran Buds	1 cup	71
All-Bran Complete Wheat Flakes	1 cup	49
Raisin Bran	1 cup	43
Raisin Bran Crunch	1 cup	43
Smart Start, Strong Heart, Toasted Oat	1 cup	42
Raisin Bran Extra	1 cup	40
All-Bran Strawberry Medley	1 cup	39
Frosted MINI-Wheats, Big-Bite	1 cup	33
Frosted MINI-Wheats, Bite-Size	1 cup	32
Honey Smacks	1 cup	31
Fiberplus Berry Yogurt Crunch	1 cup	29
Low Fat Granola with Raisins	1 cup	25
Smart Start, Strong Heart, Antioxidants	1 cup	23
Cocoa Krispies	1 cup	21
MUESLIX	1 cup	20
Berry Rice Krispies	1 cup	20
Frosted Rice Krispies	1 cup	19
Rice Krispies	1 cup	18
Product 19	1 cup	17
Rice Krispies Treats	1 cup	17
Froot Loops	1 cup	16
Apple Jacks	1 cup	16
Krave Chocolate	1 cup	15
Simply Cinnamon Corn Flakes	1 cup	15
Smorz	1 cup	14
Crispix	1 cup	13
Corn Pops	1 cup	12
CINNABON	1 cup	10
Frosted Flakes	1 cup	10
Crunchy Nut Golden Honey Nut Flakes	1 cup	10
Honey Crunch Corn Flakes	1 cup	9
Corn Flakes	1 cup	8
Crunchy Nut Roasted Nut & Honey O's	1 cup	7
Cracklin' Oat Bran	1 cup	5
Fiberplus Cinnamon Oat Crunch	1 cup	1

Cereal, Kellogg's Special-K®	Amount	Phosphorus / Protein
Multigrain Oats & Honey	1 cup	33
Vanilla Almond	1 cup	27
Red Berries	1 cup	26
Cinnamon Pecan	1 cup	25
Chocolately Delight	1 cup	24
Fruit & Yogurt	1 cup	22

PHOSPHORUS TO PROTEIN RATIO

Continued

Blueberry	1 cup	21
Protein Plus	1 cup	20
Low Fat Granola	1 cup	18
Original	1 cup	5

Cereal, Post	Amount	Phosphorus / Protein
100% Bran Cereal	1 cup	64
Raisin Bran	1 cup	47
Shredded Wheat, lightly frosted, spoon-size	1 cup	36
Crunchy Pecan	1 cup	35
Shredded Wheat, Sugar and Salt Free	1 cup	34
Honeynut Shredded Wheat	1 cup	32
Shredded Wheat n' Bran, spoon-size	1 cup	32
Golden Crisp	1 cup	32
Shredded Wheat, spoon-size	1 cup	31
Raisin, Date & Pecan	1 cup	31
Banana Nut Crunch	1 cup	31
Honeycomb Cereal	1 cup	31
Cranberry Almond Crunch	1 cup	29
Grape-Nuts Cereal	1 cup	28
Grape-Nuts Flakes	1 cup	27
Blueberry Morning	1 cup	24
OREO O's Cereal	1 cup	22
Cocoa Pebbles	1 cup	18
Fruity Pebbles	1 cup	13

Cereal, Quaker Cereal	Amount	Phosphorus / Protein
Honey Graham OH'S	1 cup	49
LIFE Cereal, Original	1 cup	45
LIFE Cereal, Maple & Brown Sugar	1 cup	42
LIFE Cereal, Cinnamon	1 cup	41
Granola, Apple, Cranberry, & Almond	1 cup	41
Oatmeal Squares	1 cup	35
Oatmeal Squares, Golden Maple	1 cup	35
Oatmeal Squares, Cinnamon	1 cup	35
Toasted Multigrain Crisp	1 cup	34
Corn Bran Crunch	1 cup	34
CAP'N Crunch	1 cup	30
CAP'N Crunch & Crunch Berries	1 cup	29
CAP'N Crunch's OOPs! All Berries	1 cup	27
Puffed Wheat	1 cup	25
CAP'N Crunch's Peanut Butter Crunch	1 cup	23
Puffed Rice	1 cup	22

PHOSPHORUS TO PROTEIN RATIO

Continued

Cereal, Cooked	Amount	Phosphorus / Protein
Oats, regular, unenriched	1 cup	31
Farina	1 cup	20
Malt-o-Meal plain	1 serving	19
Corn grits, white	1 cup	12
Corn grits, yellow	1 cup	11
CREAM OF WHEAT, regular	1 cup	11

Cheese	Amount	Phosphorus / Protein
Cheez Whiz, pasteurized process	1 oz	67
Velveeta, pasteurized process	1 oz	53
American, pasteurized process	1 oz	35
Cream cheese, fat free	1 oz	33
Goat cheese, hard type	1 oz	24
Romano	1 oz	24
Feta	1 oz	24
Gouda	1 oz	22
Swiss	1 oz	21
Swiss, low fat	1 oz	21
Mozzarella, nonfat	1 oz	21
Cheddar	1 oz	21
Mozzarella, part skim milk, low moisture	1 oz	20
Provolone, reduced fat	1 oz	20
Muenster	1 oz	20
Cheddar, low fat	1 oz	20
Provolone	1 oz	19
Colby	1 oz	19
Parmesan, grated	1 oz	19
Gruyere	1 oz	19
Muenster, low fat	1 oz	19
Roquefort	1 oz	18
Monterey	1 oz	18
Blue cheese	1 oz	18
Cream cheese	1 oz	18
Goat cheese, semisoft type	1 oz	17
Ricotta, part skim milk	1 oz	16
Mozzarella, whole milk	1 oz	16
Monterey, low fat	1 oz	16
Cottage cheese, creamed	1 oz	14
Ricotta, whole milk	1 oz	14
Goat cheese, soft type	1 oz	14
Fontina	1 oz	14
Brie	1 oz	9

PHOSPHORUS TO PROTEIN RATIO

Continued

Chicken, Cooked	Amount	Phosphorus / Protein
Breast, meat only, no skin, roasted	1/2 breast	7.35
Thigh, no skin, roasted	1 thigh	7.31
Breast with skin, roasted	1/2 breast	7.26
Breast, with skin, fried with flour	1/2 breast	7.24
Drumstick, with skin, fried	1 drumstick	7.17
Thigh, with skin, fried	1 thigh	7.00
Drumstick, no skin, roasted	1 drumstick	6.23
Wing with skin, fried in batter	1 wing	5.90
Wing with skin, roasted	1 wing	5.67

Chicken, Cooked	Amount	Phosphorus / Protein
Thigh with skin, roasted	3 oz	9
Thigh meat only, no skin, roasted	3 oz	9
Drumstick with skin, roasted	3 oz	9
Drumstick meat only, no skin, roasted	3 oz	9
Breast meat only, no skin, roasted	3 oz	7
Breast with skin, fried in flour	3 oz	7
Breast with skin, roasted	3 oz	7
Thigh with skin, fried in flour	3 oz	7
Drumstick with skin, fried in flour	3 oz	7
Cornish game hens, meat only	3 oz	6
Wing with skin, fried in flour	3 oz	6
Wing with skin, roasted	3 oz	6
Wing meat only, no skin, roasted	3 oz	5

Chocolate	Amount	Phosphorus / Protein
Dark Chocolate, 60-69%, cacao solids	1 oz	43
Dark Chocolate, 45-59%, cacao solids	1 oz	42
Dark Chocolate, 70-85%, cacao solids	1 oz	39
Cocoa, dry powder, unsweetened	1 oz	37
Semisweet Chocolate	1 oz	31
Baking Chocolate	1 oz	31
White Chocolate	1 oz	30
Milk Chocolate	1 oz	27
Special Dark Chocolate	1 oz	9

Crackers	Amount	Phosphorus / Protein
Kashi Original 7-Grain	1 serving	40
Keebler Town House, Original	1 serving	40
Kashi Fire Roasted Vegetable	1 serving	39
Kashi Honey Sesame	1 serving	38
Ritz crackers	1 serving	38
Kashi Toasted Asiago	1 serving	35

PHOSPHORUS TO PROTEIN RATIO

Continued

Rye, crispbread, and Wasa	1 serving	34
Whole-Wheat, and Triscuits	1 serving	31
Keebler Club, Original, crackers	1 serving	31
Wheat, regular, and Wheat-Thins	1 serving	29
Special-K Cracker Chips, Sea Salt	1 serving	28
Special-K Sour Cream & Onion Chips	1 serving	28
Matzo, Whole-Wheat	1 serving	23
Cheez-it, low sodium	1 serving	21
Special-K Cracker Chips, Cheddar	1 serving	19
Melba toast, plain	1 serving	16
Graham crackers	1 serving	16
Saltines	1 serving	12
Special-K Multigrain Crackers	1 serving	11
Matzo, plain	1 serving	9
Cheez-it, hot & spicy	1 serving	8.6
Cheez-it, reduced fat	1 serving	7.8
Cheez-it, cheddar jack	1 serving	6.8
Keebler Town House, Flatbread, Sea Salt	1 serving	6.6
Cheez-it, original	1 serving	5.5

Cream	Amount	Phosphorus / Protein
Sour cream, cultured	1 tbsp	56
Half & Half	1 tbsp	32
Sour cream, reduced fat	1 tbsp	32
Whipped topping, pressurized	1 tbsp	30
Light Coffe cream	1 tbsp	29
Heavy Cream	1 tbsp	29

Eggs	Amount	Phosphorus / Protein
Egg yolk	1 large	25
Egg whole, scrambled	1 large	17
Egg whole, fried	1 large	16
Egg whole, poached	1 large	16
Egg whole, hard boiled	1 large	14
Egg substitute, liquid, fat free	1/4 cup	7
Egg whites, dried	1 ounce	1.4
Egg whites, raw	1 large	1.4
Egg whites, dried powder, stabilized	1 tbsp	1

PHOSPHORUS TO PROTEIN RATIO

Fish, Canned	Amount	Phosphorus / Protein
Atlantic sardines, in oil	3 oz	20
Light tuna, in oil	3 oz	11
White (albacore) tuna, in oil	3 oz	10
White (albacore) tuna, in water	3 oz	9
Light tuna, in water	3 oz	7

Fish, Cooked	Amount	Phosphorus / Protein
Carp	3 oz	23
Flounder & Sole	3 oz	20
Surimi	3 oz	18
Pacific cod	3 oz	18
Catfish, wild	3 oz	16
Atlantic perch	3 oz	16
Chinook salmon	3 oz	14
Florida pompano	3 oz	14
Keta (chum) salmon	3 oz	14
Haddock	3 oz	14
Coho salmon, wild	3 oz	14
Coho salmon, farmed	3 oz	14
Catfish, farmed	3 oz	13
Swordfish	3 oz	13
Atlantic & Pacific Halibut	3 oz	13
Pink salmon	3 oz	13
Sockeye salmon	3 oz	13
Alaskan halibut	3 oz	12
King mackerel	3 oz	12
Whiting	3 oz	12
Atlantic croaker	3 oz	12
Cat fish, breaded & fried	3 oz	12
Rainbow trout, wild	3 oz	12
Atlantic mackerel	3 oz	12
Atlantic pollock	3 oz	11
Atlantic salmon, farmed	3 oz	11
Northern pike	3 oz	11
Rainbow trout, farmed	3 oz	11
Spanish mackerel	3 oz	11
Walleye pollock	3 oz	11
Yellowfin tuna	3 oz	11
Greenland halibut	3 oz	11
Striped bass	3 oz	11
Pacific rockfish	3 oz	11
Walleye pike	3 oz	11
Bluefin tuna	3 oz	11
Freshwater bass	3 oz	11

PHOSPHORUS TO PROTEIN RATIO

Continued

Atlantic salmon, wild	3 oz	10
Skipjack (aku) tuna	3 oz	10
Sea bass	3 oz	10
Striped mullet	3 oz	10
Chinook salmon, smoked	3 oz	9
Salmon, Lox	3 oz	9
Tilapia	3 oz	8
Snapper	3 oz	8
Yellowtail	3 oz	7
Atlantic herring, pickeled	3 oz	6
Pacific & Jack, mackerel	3 oz	6
Atlantic cod	3 oz	6
Grouper	3 oz	6
Orange roughy	3 oz	5

Fish, Shellfish, Cooked	Amount	Phosphorus / Protein
Alaskan king crab, imitation	3 oz	37
Oysters, breaded & fried	3 oz	18
Eastern oysters, wild	3 oz	17
Eastern oysters, farmed	3 oz	16
Crayfish	3 oz	16
Alaskan king crab	3 oz	14
Squid, fried	3 oz	14
Clams, canned	3 oz	14
Shrimp	3 oz	13
Clams, breaded & fried	3 oz	13
Blue crab	3 oz	13
Blue crab, canned	3 oz	13
Scallops, breaded & fried	3 oz	13
Abalone	3 oz	11
Blue crab, cakes	3 oz	11
Shrimp, breaded & fried	3 oz	10
Northern lobster	3 oz	10
Shrimp, canned	3 oz	10
Octopus	3 oz	9
Queen crab	3 oz	5

Fruit, Canned	Amount	Phosphorus / Protein
Plums	1 cup	37
Applesauce, sweetened	1 cup	37
Pears	1 cup	36
Applesauce, unsweetened	1 cup	29
Peaches	1 cup	25

PHOSPHORUS TO PROTEIN RATIO

Continued

Apricots	1 cup	23
Pineapple	1 cup	20
Olives, green	5 large	7
Olives, black	5 large	6

Fruit, Dried	Amount	Phosphorus / Protein
Cranberries	1 cup	125
Apples	1 cup	41
Peaches	1 cup	33
Pears	1 cup	32
Currants	1 cup	31
Apricots	1 cup	21
Figs	1 cup	20

Fruit, Frozen	Amount	Phosphorus / Protein
Blackberries, unthawed	1 cup	25
Strawberries	1 cup	24
Raspberries	1 cup	24
Peaches	1 cup	18
Blueberries	1 cup	17

Fruit, Raw	Amount	Phosphorus / Protein
Elderberries	1 cup	59
Apples	1 cup	44
Black currants	1 cup	42
Strawberries	1 cup	36
Cranberries	1 cup	33
Raisins	1 cup	33
Prunes, uncooked	1 cup	32
Stewed prunes	1 cup	31
Kiwi	1 cup	30
Pears	1 cup	30
Grapes, red & green	1 cup	28
Avocado, California, pureed	1 cup	28
Plantains	1 cup	26
Dates	1 cup	25
Tangerine, sections	1 cup	25
Nectarine	1 cup	24
Raspberries	1 cup	24
Grapefruit, pink or red, sections	1 cup	23
Plums, sliced	1 cup	23
Peachs, slices	1 cup	22

PHOSPHORUS TO PROTEIN RATIO

Continued

Honeydew	1 cup	21
Papayas	1 cup	21
Cherries, pitted	1 cup	20
Cantaloupe	1 cup	18
Water mellon	1 cup	17
Mango	1 cup	17
Apricots	1 cup	17
Blackberries	1 cup	16
Blueberries	1 cup	16
Oranges, sections	1 cup	15
Pineapple	1 cup	15

Game Meat, Cooked	Amount	Phosphorus / Protein
Duck	3 oz	9
Deer, ground	3 oz	9
Bison, ground	3 oz	9
Elk, ground	3 oz	8
Caribou	3 oz	8
Buffalo, steak, free range	3 oz	8
Deer	3 oz	8
Rabbit	3 oz	7
Antelope	3 oz	7
Squirrel	3 oz	7
Elk	3 oz	6
Wild boar	3 oz	5

Grains, Cooked	Amount	Phosphorus / Protein
Amaranth	1 cup	39
Oat bran	1 cup	37
Quinoa	1 cup	35
Brown rice	1 cup	32
Oats, regular, unenriched	1 cup	30
Millet	1 cup	29
Kamut	1 cup	27
Spelt	1 cup	27
Barley, pearled	1 cup	24
Spaghetti, spinach	1 cup	24
Rice noodles	1 cup	22
Buckwheat	1 cup	21
Wild rice	1 cup	21
Instant white rice	1 cup	17
Egg noodles	1 cup	17
Macaroni, whole-wheat	1 cup	17
Spaghetti, whole-wheat	1 cup	17
Bulgur	1 cup	14

PHOSPHORUS TO PROTEIN RATIO

Continued

White rice, regular	1 cup	13
Egg & Spinach noodles	1 cup	11
Macaroni	1 cup	10
Spaghetti	1 cup	10
Couscous	1 cup	6
Soba noodles	1 cup	5

Herbs & Spices	Amount	Phosphorus / Protein
Onion powder	1 tsp	36
Chives, raw	1 tsp	33
Coriander, seeds	1 tsp	32
Celery seeds	1 tsp	31
Turmeric, ground	1 tsp	30
Caraway seeds	1 tsp	29
Curry, powder	1 tsp	28
Garlic powder	1 tsp	25
Dill weed, dried	1 tsp	25
Saffron	1 tsp	25
Anise seed	1 tsp	24
Paprika	1 tsp	23
Coriander, dried	1 tsp	23
Thyme, dried, ground	1 tsp	23
Chili powder	1 tsp	22
Cinnamon, ground	1 tsp	22
Chervil, dried	1 tsp	21
Oregano, dried, ground	1 tsp	21
Bay leaf, crumbled	1 tsp	20
Pepper, black, ground	1 tsp	18
All-spice, ground	1 tsp	17
Rosemary, dried	1 tsp	17
Cloves, ground	1 tsp	15
Ginger, ground	1 tsp	15
Sage, ground	1 tsp	14
Tarragon, dried, ground	1 tsp	14
Basil, dried & ground	1 tsp	13
Thyme, fresh	1 tsp	10
Parsley, dried	1 tsp	6
Capers, canned	1 tsp	4

Juice	Amount	Phosphorus / Protein
Pomegranate	1 cup	73
Apple	1 cup	68
Carrot	1 cup	44
Prune	1 cup	41
Grape	1 cup	37

PHOSPHORUS TO PROTEIN RATIO

Continued

Vegetable	1 cup	27
Orange, raw	1 cup	24
Tomato	1 cup	24
Lemon juice, raw	1 cup	24
Grapefruit juice, raw	1 cup	23
Pineapple	1 cup	22

Lamb, Cooked	Amount	Phosphorus / Protein
Ground	3 oz	8.1
Cubed, for stew or kabob	3 oz	8.0
Rib, lean, trimmed to 1/4" fat	3 oz	7.7
Leg, whole, trimmed to 1/4" fat	3 oz	7.5
Chops, loin, lean, trimmed to 1/4" fat	3 oz	6.6
Foreshank, trimmed to 1/8" fat	3 oz	5.8

Milk	Amount	Phosphorus / Protein
Coconut milk, canned	1 cup	48
Canned, condensed, sweetened	1 cup	32
Goat milk	1 cup	31
Nonfat, fat free or skim liquid milk	1 cup	31
Canned, evaporated	1 cup	30
Lowfat, 1%	1 cup	28
Dry, instant, nonfat	1/3 cup	28
Lowfat, 2%	1 cup	27
Buttermilk, lowfat	1 cup	27
Whole milk, 3.25%	1 cup	27
Buttermilk, whole milk	1 cup	27
Sheep milk	1 cup	26
Canned, evaporated, nonfat	1 cup	26
Soy milk, original, unfortified	1 cup	16
Human milk	1 cup	13

Nuts & Seeds	Amount	Phosphorus / Protein
Chia seeds	1 oz	52
Brazil nuts	1 oz	51
Tahini	1 oz	43
Pine nuts	1 oz	42
Pumpkin seeds	1 oz	41
Sesame seeds	1 oz	35
Flaxseeds	1 oz	35
Coconut, raw meat	1 oz	34
Cashews	1 oz	33
Sunflower seeds	1 oz	32
Pecans	1 oz	30

PHOSPHORUS TO PROTEIN RATIO

Continued

Pistachio	1 oz	24
Macadamia	1 oz	24
Almonds	1 oz	23
English walnuts	1 oz	23
Black walnuts	1 oz	21
Hazlenut	1 oz	19
Peanut butter, smooth style	1 oz	14
Peanuts	1 oz	11

Pork, Cooked	Amount	Phosphorus / Protein
Liverwurst spread	1/4 cup	19
Bratwurst	3 oz	15
Bacon, pan-fried	3 oz	14
Canadian-style bacon	3 oz	12
Braunschweiger	3 oz	12
Tenderloin	3 oz	10
Cured ham	3 oz	10
Polish sausage	3 oz	10
Pork chops, lean, pan-fried	3 oz	9
Pork chops, pan-fried	3 oz	9
Cured ham, lean	3 oz	9
Spareribs	3 oz	9
Italian sausage	3 oz	9
Center loin chops	3 oz	9
Pork chops, broiled	3 oz	9
Sausage	3 oz	8
Backribs	3 oz	7
Sirloin chops	3 oz	6

Tofu	Amount	Phosphorus / Protein
Mori-Nu, Silken, firm	3 oz	30
Mori-Nu, Silken, soft	3 oz	26
Mori-Nu, Silken, extra firm	3 oz	25
Vitasoy USA, Nasoya Lite Silken	3 oz	14
Mori-Nu, Silken, lite extra firm	3 oz	12
Vitasoy USA, Nasoya Plus Firm	3 oz	11
Mori-Nu, Silken, lite firm	3 oz	10
Vitasoy USA, Nasoya Lite Firm	3 oz	10

Turkey, Cooked	Amount	Phosphorus / Protein
Turkey bacon	3 oz	16
Turkey sausage, reduced fat	3 oz	10
Ground turkey	3 oz	9
Ground turkey, 85% lean	3 oz	9

PHOSPHORUS TO PROTEIN RATIO

Continued

Ground turkey, fat free	3 oz	9
Ground turkey, 93% lean	3 oz	8
Light meat	3 oz	8
Dark meat	3 oz	8
Breast meat	3 oz	7

Veal, Cooked	Amount	Phosphorus / Protein
Cubed for stew	3 oz	11
Sirloin	3 oz	9
Ground	3 oz	9
Loin chops	3 oz	9
Rib	3 oz	8
Foreshank	3 oz	7
Leg, top round	3 oz	7
Breast	3 oz	7

Vegetables, Canned	Amount	Phosphorus / Protein
Tomato pure	1 cup	39
Carrots	1 cup	39
Mushrooms	1 cup	36
Pumpkin	1 cup	32
Corn	1 cup	26
Tomatoes	1 cup	24
Stewed tomatos	1 cup	22
Sauerkraut	1 cup	21
Asparagus	1 cup	20
Tomato sauce	1 cup	20
Sweet potato	1 cup	20
Tomato paste	1 cup	19
Beets	1 cup	18
Green beans	1 cup	18
Spinach	1 cup	16
Green peas	1 cup	15

Vegetables, Cooked	Amount	Phosphorus / Protein
Taro	1 cup	145
Parsnips	1 cup	52
Rutabagas	1 cup	43
Summer squash	1 cup	43
Beets	1 cup	42
Pumpkin	1 cup	42
Acorn squash	1 cup	40
White mushrooms	1 cup	40
Carrots	1 cup	39

PHOSPHORUS TO PROTEIN RATIO

Continued

Turnips	1 cup	37
Broccolini	1 cup	36
Yams, cubed	1 cup	33
Zucchini	1 cup	33
Butternut squash	1 cup	30
Celery	1 cup	30
Tomatoes	1 cup	29
Broccoli	1 cup	28
Cabbage	1 cup	26
Onions	1 cup	26
Potatoes, flesh	1 cup	26
Turnip greens	1 cup	26
Artichokes	1 cup	25
Kohlrabi	1 cup	25
Potatoes, mashed with whole milk	1 cup	24
Sweet potato, mashed	1 cup	23
Yellow sweet corn	1 cup	23
Brussels sprouts	1 cup	22
Spaghetti winter squash	1 cup	22
Dandelion greens	1 cup	21
Leeks	1 cup	21
Raab Broccoli	1 cup	21
Winter squash	1 cup	21
Shiitake mushrooms	1 cup	19
Spinach,	1 cup	19
Asparagus	1 cup	18
Bok-Choy	1 cup	18
Cauliflower	1 cup	18
Eggplant	1 cup	18
Mustard greens	1 cup	18
Swiss chard	1 cup	18
Napa cabbage	1 cup	17
Okra	1 cup	17
Snow peas	1 cup	17
Beet greens	1 cup	16
Green beans	1 cup	15
Kale	1 cup	15
Collard greens	1 cup	14
Prickly pear cactus pad, nopales	1 cup	12
Split peas	1 cup	12

Vegetables, Frozen	Amount	Phosphorus / Protein
Carrots	1 cup	56
Corn	1 cup	31
Okra	1 cup	23

PHOSPHORUS TO PROTEIN RATIO

Continued

Rhubarb	1 cup	21
Green beans	1 cup	20
Asparagus	1 cup	17
Broccoli	1 cup	16
Brussels sprouts	1 cup	16
Green peas	1 cup	15
Cauliflower	1 cup	15
Spinach	1 cup	13
Butternut squash	1 cup	11
Turnip greens	1 cup	10
Kale	1 cup	10
Collard greens	1 cup	9

Vegetables, Raw	Amount	Phosphorus / Protein
Portabella mushrooms, diced	1 cup	51
Shiitake mushrooms	1 whole	49
Chrimini mushrooms, sliced	1 cup	48
Tomatillos, chopped	1 cup	40
Enoki mushrooms, sliced	1 cup	39
Cucumber, slices with peel	1 cup	37
Oyster mushrooms, sliced	1 cup	36
Carrots	1 cup	35
Celery	1 cup	35
Butternut squash	1 cup	33
Shiitake mushrooms, dried	1 each	32
Summer squash, sliced	1 cup	31
Zucchini	1 cup	31
Yellow bell peppers	1 large	30
Chicory greens	1 cup	29
Belgian endive	1 cup	28
Radicchio	1 cup	28
White mushrooms	1 cup	28
Tomatoes, cherry	1 cup	27
Tomatoes, red	1 cup	27
Onions	1 cup	26
Red bell peppers	1 cup	26
Swiss chard	1 cup	26
Watercress	1 cup	26
Bok-Choy	1 cup	25
Romaine lettuce	1 cup	25
Butterhead or boston lettuce	1 cup	24
Dandelion greens	1 cup	24
Broccoli	1 cup	23
Endive, chopped	1 cup	23
Green bell peppers	1 cup	23

PHOSPHORUS TO PROTEIN RATIO

Continued

Green leaf lettuce	1 cup	23
Raab broccoli	1 cup	23
Iceburg lettuce	1 cup	22
Red leaf lettuce	1 cup	22
Cauliflower	1 cup	21
Red cabbage	1 cup	21
Savoy Cabbage	1 cup	21
Cabbage, shredded	1 cup	20
Green onions, scallions	1 cup	20
Arugula	1 cup	19
Snow peas	1 cup	19
Kale	1 cup	17
Spinach	1 cup	17
Green beans	1 cup	15
Spirulina, dried	1 tbsp	2

Yogurt	Amount	Phosphorus / Protein
Yogurt, plain skim milk	8 ounces	27
Yogurt, plain low fat	8 ounces	27
Yogurt, plain whole milk	8 ounces	27
Yogurt, plain greek, non-fat	8 ounces	13

Potassium is a water soluble mineral needed daily in large quantities. It is popularly known as an alkaline electrolyte. Potassium is needed for the transmission of nerve impulses, muscle contractions, cardiac functions, and acid-base balance.

Deficiency associations include diuretic therapy, diarrhea, chronic use of laxatives, inadequate dietary intake, and high sodium diets. Deficiency is linked with cardiovascular mortality, osteoporosis, and hypertension. Some deficiency symptoms include irritability, fatigue, weak leg muscles, leg cramps, nausea, vomiting, intestinal problems like constipation, and weak and irregular heart pulse.

Recommend Daily Intakes Levels for Phosphorus

Children	Potassium, mg
1 to 3 year olds	3000
4 to 8 year olds	3800

Males	
9 to 13 year olds	4500
14 to 18 year olds	4700
19 to 30 years	4700
31 to 50 years	4700
51 to 70 years	4700
Over 70	4700

Females	
9 to 13 year olds	4500
14 to 18 year olds	4700
19 to 30 years	4700
31 to 50 years	4700
51 to 70 years	4700
Over 70	4700
Pregnancy	4700
Lactation	5100

NOTES

POTASSIUM

Alcohol	Amount	Potassium (mg)
White Wine	1 glass	187
Red Wine	1 glass	104
Beer, regular all types	1 bottle	96
Beer, light	1 bottle	74
Gin, Rum, Vodka, Whisky	1 shot	1

Beans, Canned	Amount	Potassium (mg)
White beans, mature	1 cup	1189
Great Northern	1 cup	920
Refried beans	1 cup	800
Navy beans	1 cup	755
Cranberry beans	1 cup	676
Kidney beans	1 cup	666
Pinto beans	1 cup	662
Fava beans	1 cup	620
Baked beans, plain	1 cup	569
Lima beans	1 cup	530
Black-eyed peas	1 cup	413
Garbanzo beans	1 cup	346
Yellow beans	1 cup	167
Green beans	1 cup	162

Beans, Cooked	Amount	Potassium (mg)
Natto	1 cup	1276
Soybeans, matured, dry roasted	1 cup	1269
Adzuki	1 cup	1224
White beans, mature	1 cup	1004
Soybeans, green	1 cup	970
Lima beans	1 cup	955
Soybeans, matured	1 cup	886
White beans, small	1 cup	829
Black Turtle beans, mature	1 cup	801
Pinto beans	1 cup	746
Lentils	1 cup	731
Kidney beans	1 cup	713
Split peas	1 cup	710
Navy beans	1 cup	708
Great Northern	1 cup	692
Cranberry beans	1 cup	685
Edamame	1 cup	676
Hyacinth beans	1 cup	654
Pigeon peas	1 cup	645
Black beans	1 cup	611

RDA is 4700 mg for adults

POTASSIUM

Mothbeans	1 cup	538
Mung beans, mature seeds	1 cup	537
Winged beans	1 cup	482
Garbanzo beans, chickpeas	1 cup	477
Black-eyed peas	1 cup	475
Fava beans	1 cup	456
Lupini beans	1 cup	407
Yellow beans	1 cup	374
Yardlong beans, Chinese long beans	1 cup	302
Green beans	1 cup	182

Beef, Cooked	Amount	Potassium (mg)
Tri Tip steak, lean, trimmed to 0" fat	3 oz	382
Top sirloin, lean, trimmed to 1/8" fat	3 oz	320
Flank steak, lean, trimmed to 0" fat	3 oz	298
Ground beef, 95%	3 oz	296
Ribeye steak, lean, trimmed 0" fat	3 oz	295
Filet Mignon, trimmed to 0" fat	3 oz	290
London Broil, top round	3 oz	284
Ground beef, 90%,	3 oz	283
Ground beef, 85%,	3 oz	270
Beef ribs, trimmed to 1/8" fat	3 oz	259
Ground beef, 80%,	3 oz	258
T-Bone steak, trimmed 0" fat	3 oz	257
Porterhouse steak, trimmed to 0" fat	3 oz	254
Ground beef, 75%	3 oz	246
Skirt Steak, trimmed to 0" fat	3 oz	246
Brisket, lean, trimmed to 0" fat	3 oz	227
Chuck roast, trimmed to 1/8" fat	3 oz	196

Beef, Cooked	Amount	Potassium (mg)
Tri Tip steak, lean, trimmed to 0" fat	1 lb	1982
Flank steak, lean, trimmed to 0" fat	1 lb	1589
Top Sirloin, trimmed to 1/8" fat	1 lb	1525
Beef ribs, trimmed to 1/8" fat	1 lb	1385
T-bone steak, trimmed to 0" fat	1 lb	1370
Porterhouse steak, trimmed to 0" fat	1 lb	1356
Flank steak, lean, trimmed to 0" fat	1 steak	1340
Skirt steak, trimmed to 0" fat	1 lb	1311
Brisket, lean, trimmed to 0" fat	1 lb	1212
Chuck roast, trimmed to 1/8" fat	1 lb	1044
Ribeye steak, boneless, trimmed to 0" fat	1 steak	734
Brisket, lean, trimmed to 0" fat	1 steak	721
Ribeye filet, lean, trimmed to 0" fat	1 filet	494

RDA is 4700 mg for adults

POTASSIUM

Continued

Top Sirloin, choice filet, trimmed to 0" fat	1 filet	490
Filet Mignon, tenderloin, trimmed to 0" fat	1 steak	410

Beef, Cooked	Amount	Potassium (mg)
Ground beef, 95%	1/4 lb patty	285
Ground beef, 90%	1/4 lb patty	273
Ground beef, 85%	1/4 lb patty	245
Ground beef, 80%	1/4 lb patty	234
Ground beef, 75%	1/4 lb patty	202

Bread	Amount	Potassium (mg)
Potato bread	1 slice	230
Bagel, Wheat	4" bagel	162
Bagel, cinnamon & raisens	4" bagel	132
Mexican roll, bollilo	1 roll	128
Indian bread, Naan, plain	1 piece	112
Indian bread, Naan, whole wheat	1 piece	196
Bagel, oat bran	4" bagel	121
Egg bread	1 slice	96
Cornbread, drymix	1 piece	77
Pita, white	6" pita	72
Whole-Wheat	1 slice	69
Bagel plain	4" bagel	67
Croissants, butter	1 medium	67
Pumpernickle	1 slice	67
French and Sourdough	1 slice	64
English Muffin, plain	1 muffin	62
Kaiser rolls	1 roll	62
Bagel, egg	4" bagel	61
Multi-Grain, or Whole-Grain	1 slice	60
Raisen bread	1 slice	59
Rye bread	1 slice	53
Tortillas, flour	1 tortilla	50
Tortillas, corn	1 tortilla	48
Wheat	1 slice	46
Cracked wheat	1 slice	44
Hamburger & Hotdog buns, plain	1 bun	40
Dinner Rolls, brown & serve	1 roll	39
Oatmeal bread	1 slice	38
Reduced calorie wheat	1 slice	28
White	1 slice	25
Reduced calorie rye	1 slice	23
Italian	1 slice	22
Reduced calorie white	1 slice	17

RDA is 4700 mg for adults

POTASSIUM

Butter	Amount	Potassium (mg)
Regular dairy butter, salted	1 tbsp	3
Regular dairy whipped butter, salted	1 tbsp	2

Cereal, Arrowhead	Amount	Potassium (mg)
Oat Bran Flakes	1 cup	140
Kamut Flakes	1 cup	135
Spelt Flakes	1 cup	135
Amaranth Flakes	1 cup	120
Maple Buckwheat Flakes	1 cup	100
Sweetened Rice Flakes	1 cup	85

Cereal, Barbara's Organic	Amount	Potassium (mg)
High Fiber Flax & Granola	1 cup	220
High Fiber Cranberry	1 cup	190
Shredded Oats Original	1 cup	184
High Fiber Original	1 cup	180
Shredded Minis Blueberry Burst	1 cup	180
Shredded Spoonfuls Multigrain	1 cup	167
Shredded Wheat	2 biscuits	160
Shredded Oats Cinnamon Crunch	1 cup	150
Shredded Oats Vanilla Almond	1 cup	150
Puffins Peanut Butter	1 cup	140
Corn Flakes	1 cup	133
Brown Rice Crisps	1 cup	127
Puffins Original	1 cup	113
Puffins Puffs Crunchy Cocoa	1 cup	113
Hole 'n Oats Honey Nut	1 cup	107
Hole 'n Oats: Fruit Juice Sweetened	1 cup	107
Puffins Peanut Butter & Chocolate	1 cup	93
Puffins Puffs Fruit Medley	1 cup	93
Puffins Honey Rice	1 cup	87
Puffins Multigrain	1 cup	87
Puffins Cinnamon	1 cup	68

Cereal, Cascadian Farm	Amount	Potassium (mg)
Raisin bran	1 cup	x
Hearty Morning	1 cup	280
Dark Chocolate Almond Granola	1 cup	213
Purel O's	1 cup	190
Fruit & Nut Granola	1 cup	187
Multi Gain Squares	1 cup	113
Chocolate O's	1 cup	93
Honey Nut O's	1 cup	75

RDA is 4700 mg for adults

POTASSIUM

Continued

Fruit Ful O's	1 cup	73
Cinnamon Crunch	1 cup	65

Cereal, Ezekiel	Amount	Potassium (mg)
Sprouted Grain Almond, 4:9	1 cup	440
Sprouted Grain Original, 4:9	1 cup	400
Sprouted Grain Golden Flax, 4:9	1 cup	380
Sprouted Grain Cinnamon Flax, 4:9	1 cup	320

Cereal, General Mills®	Amount	Potassium (mg)
Total Raisin Bran	1 cup	280
Multi-Bran CHEX	1 cup	240
Wheat Chex	1 cup	227
Raisin Nut Bran	1 cup	191
Oatmeal Crisp, Crunchy Almond	1 cup	177
Basic 4	1 cup	157
Total Whole Grain	1 cup	120
Wheaties	1 cup	120
Total Cranberry Crunch	1 cup	112
Honey Nut Clusters	1 cup	105
Reese's Puffs	1 cup	87
Cocoa Puffs	1 cup	80
Golden Grams	1 cup	80
Cookie Crisp	1 cup	67
Dora The Explorer	1 cup	67
Honey Nut Chex	1 cup	67
Cinnamon Toast Crunch	1 cup	63
Corn Chex	1 cup	60
Berry Berry Kix	1 cup	56
Lucky Charms	1 cup	55
Chocolate Chex	1 cup	53
Cinnamon Chex	1 cup	50
Trix	1 cup	50
Kix	1 cup	48
Rice Chex	1 cup	45

Cereal, General Mills Cheerios®	Amount	Potassium (mg)
Apple Cinnamon	1 cup	183
Original	1 cup	170
Honey Nut	1 cup	153
Chocolate	1 cup	105
Banana Nut	1 cup	94
Multi Grain	1 cup	85
Berry Burst	1 cup	80

RDA is 4700 mg for adults

POTASSIUM

Continued

Crunch, Oat Clusters	1 cup	80
Fruity	1 cup	80
Yogurt Burst, Strawberry	1 cup	80
Frosted	1 cup	73

Cereal, General Mills Fiber One®	Amount	Potassium (mg)
Original	1 cup	360
Raisin Bran Clusters	1 cup	206
Frosted Shredded Wheat	1 cup	183
Honey Clusters	1 cup	165
Caramel Delight	1 cup	130

Cereal, Kashi®	Amount	Potassium (mg)
7-Whole Grain Nuggets	1 cup	x
Go Lean® Cereal	1 cup	482
Go Lean Crunch, Honey Almond Flax	1 cup	354
Go Lean Vanilla Graham	1 cup	350
Go Lean Crisp, Toasted Berry Crumble	1 cup	334
Go Lean Crunch	1 cup	290
Go Lean Crisp, Cinnamon Crumble	1 cup	248
Good Friends	1 cup	194
Autum Wheat	29 biscuits	185
Cinnamon Harvest	28 biscuits	174
Berry Fruitful	29 biscuits	172
Island Vanilla	27 biscuits	172
Heart to Heart, Honey Toasted Oat	1 cup	136
Heart to Heart, Warm Cinnamon	1 cup	130
7-Whole Grain Flakes	1 cup	122
Heart to Heart, Oat Flakes & Blueberry Clusters	1 cup	112
Honey Sunshine	1 cup	112
Berry Blossom	1 cup	106
Indigo Morning	1 cup	104
Simply Maize	1 cup	91
Blackberry Hills	1 cup	90
Heart to Heart, Nutty Chia Flax	1 cup	80
Strawberry Fields	1 cup	68
7-Whole Grain Honey Puffs	1 cup	67
7-Whole Grain Puffs	1 cup	53

Cereal, Kellogg's®	Amount	Potassium (mg)
All- Bran Bran Buds	1 cup	901
All-Bran Original	1 cup	632
MUESLIX	1 cup	358
All-Bran Strawberry Medley	1 cup	351

RDA is 4700 mg for adults

POTASSIUM

Continued

Smart Start, Strong Heart, Toasted Oat	1 cup	303
Cacklin' Oat Bran	1 cup	294
Raisin Bran	1 cup	258
All-Bran Complete Wheat Flakes	1 cup	228
Raisin Bran Crunch	1 cup	213
Frosted MINI-Wheats, Bite Size	1 cup	209
Raisin Bran Extra	1 cup	184
Frosted MINI-Wheats, Big Bite	1 cup	180
Low fat Granola with Raisins	1 cup	176
Fiberplus Berry Yogurt Crunch	1 cup	122
Smart Start, Strong Heart, Antioxidants	1 cup	90
Cocoa Krispies	1 cup	81
Fiberplus Cinnamon Oat Crunch	1 cup	61
Crunchy Nut Golden Honey Nut Flakes	1 cup	56
Honey Smacks	1 cup	54
Product 19	1 cup	50
Simply Cinnamon Corn Flakes	1 cup	47
Corn Pops	1 cup	46
Honey Crunch Corn Flakes	1 cup	41
Crispix	1 cup	39
CINNABON	1 cup	39
Apple Jacks	1 cup	36
Froot Loops	1 cup	34
Crunchy Nut Roasted Nut & Honey O's	1 cup	34
Rice Krispies Treats	1 cup	31
Berry Rice Krispies	1 cup	30
Smorz	1 cup	29
Frosted Flakes	1 cup	28
Corn Flakes	1 cup	25
Rice Krispies	1 cup	25
Frosted Rice Krispies	1 cup	24

Cereal, Kellogg's Special-K®	Amount	Potassium (mg)
Protein Plus	1 cup	430
Low fat Granola	1 cup	230
Chocolately Delight	1 cup	111
Cinnamon Pecan	1 cup	106
Multigrain Oats & Honey	1 cup	105
Vanilla Almond	1 cup	100
Blueberry	1 cup	79
Fruit & Yogurt	1 cup	79
Red Berries	1 cup	69
Original	1 cup	20

RDA is 4700 mg for adults

POTASSIUM

Cereal, Post®	Amount	Potassium, mg
Grape-Nuts Cereal	1 cup	464
Raisin Bran	1 cup	317
Great Grains, Raisin, Date & Pecan	1 cup	277
Great Grains, Crunchy Pecan	1 cup	234
Bran Flakes	1 cup	221
Great Grains, Banana Nut Crunch	1 cup	206
Honey Nut Shredded Wheat	1 cup	206
Great Grains, Cranberry Almond Crunch	1 cup	197
Shredded Wheat, Original, spoon-size	1 cup	190
Shredded Wheat n' Bran, spoon-size	1 cup	185
Shredded Wheat, frosted, spoon-size	1 cup	170
Grape-Nuts Flakes	1 cup	130
Shredded Wheat, Original, big-biscuit	1 biscuit	94
Blueberry Morning	1 cup	86
Alpha-Bits	1 cup	80
Cocoa Pebbles	1 cup	75
Golden Crisp	1 cup	63
Honeycomb Cereal	1 cup	33
Fruity Pebbles	1 cup	26

Post® Honey Bunches of Oats®	Amount	Potassium (mg)
Just Bunches Honey Roasted	1 cup	216
With Vanilla Bunches	1 cup	147
With Strawberries	1 cup	91
With Almonds	1 cup	90
Honey Roasted	1 cup	84
With Cinnamon Bunches	1 cup	74
Pecan Bunches	1 cup	67

Cereal, Quaker®	Amount	Potassium (mg)
Granola Apple Cranberry Almond	1 cup	435
Oatmeal Squares, Cinnamon	1 cup	204
Oatmeal Squares	1 cup	203
Oatmeal Squares, Golden Maple	1 cup	200
Toasted Multigrain Crisp	1 cup	200
LIFE Cereal, Original	1 cup	119
LIFE Cereal, Maple & Brown Sugar	1 cup	112
LIFE Cereal, Cinnamon	1 cup	109
Corn Bran Crunch	1 cup	86
CAP'N Crunch's Peanut Butter Crunch	1 cup	85
CAP'N Crunch	1 cup	67
CAP'N Crunch & Crunchberries	1 cup	65
CAP'N Crunch's OOPs! All Berries		60

RDA is 4700 mg for adults

POTASSIUM

Continued

Honey Grahan OH'S	1 cup	59
Puffed Wheat	1 cup	55
Puffed Rice	1 cup	22

Cereal, Uncle Sam	Amount	Potassium (mg)
Wheat Berry & Flaxseed, Original	1 cup	333
Wheat Berry & Flaxseed, & Strawberry	1 cup	140
Wheat Berry & Flaxseed, Honey Almond	1 cup	100
Skinners Raisin Bran	1 cup	x

Cereal, Cooked	Amount	Potassium (mg)
Oats, regular, unenriched	1 cup	164
Oats, instant, fortified, plain	1 packet	108
White corn grits	1 cup	65
Farina	1 cup	55
Malt-o-Meal plain	1 serving	54
Yellow corn grits	1 cup	53
CREAM OF WHEAT, regular	1 cup	40

Cheese	Amount	Potassium (mg)
Ricotta, part skim milk	1 cup	308
Ricotta, whole milk	1 cup	258
Cottage cheese, creamed, small curd	1 cup	234
Cottage cheese, nonfat	1 cup	199
Cottage cheese, 1 %	1 cup	194
Cottage cheese, 2 %	1 cup	190

Cheese	Amount	Potassium (mg)
Cream cheese, fat free	1 oz	79
Blue cheese	1 oz	73
American, pasteurized process, low fat	1 oz	50
Goat cheese, semisoft type	1 oz	45
Brie	1 oz	43
Cream cheese	1 oz	39
Provolone	1 oz	39
Provolone, reduced fat	1 oz	39
Muenster	1 oz	38
Muenster, low fat	1 oz	38
American, pasteurized process, fortified	1 oz	37
American, pasteurized process, imitation	1 oz	36
Colby	1 oz	36
Parmesan, grated	1 oz	35
Gouda	1 oz	34
Swiss, low fat	1 oz	31

RDA is 4700 mg for adults

POTASSIUM

Mozzarella, non fat	1 oz	30
Cheddar	1 oz	28
Mozzarella, part skim milk, low moisture	1 oz	27
Roquefort	1 oz	26
Romano	1 oz	24
Gruyere	1 oz	23
Monterey	1 oz	23
Monterey, low fat	1 oz	23
Mozzarella, whole milk	1 oz	22
Swiss	1 oz	22
Cheddar, low fat	1 oz	19
Feta	1 oz	18
Fontina	1 oz	18
Goat cheese, hard type	1 oz	14
Goat cheese, soft type	1 oz	7

Cheese, Mexican	Amount	Potassium (mg)
Queso fresco	1 oz	37
Queso blanco	1 oz	36
Queso seco	1 oz	33
Mexican, blend, reduced fat	1 oz	26
Queso anejo	1 oz	25
Mexican, blend	1 oz	24
Queso asadero	1 oz	24
Queso chihuahua	1 oz	15

Chicken, Cooked	Amount	Potassium (mg)
Breast, skin, fried with flour	1/2 breast	254
Breast, no skin, roasted	1/2 breast	220
Thigh, with skin, fried	1 thigh	165
Thigh, no skin, roasted	1 thigh	124
Drumstick, with skin, fried	1 drumstick	112
Drumstick, no skin, roasted	1 drumstick	108

Chicken, Cooked	Amount	Potassium (mg)
Thigh meat only, no skin, roasted	3 oz	235
Drumstick meat only, no skin, roasted	3 oz	225
Thigh with skin, roasted	3 oz	221
Breast with skin, fried in flour	3 oz	220
Breast meat only, no skin, roasted	3 oz	218
Drumstick with skin, roasted	3 oz	218
Cornish game hens, meat only	3 oz	212
Breast with skin, roasted	3 oz	208

RDA is 4700 mg for adults

POTASSIUM

Thigh with skin, fried in flour	3 oz	201
Drumstick with skin, fried in flour	3 oz	195
Wing meat only, no skin, roasted	3 oz	178
Wing with skin, roasted	3 oz	156
Wing with skin, fried in flour	3 oz	150

Cream	Amount	Potassium (mg)
Half & Half	1 tbsp	20
Sour Cream, reduced fat	1 tbsp	19
Light Coffe Cream	1 tbsp	18
Sour Cream, cultured	1 tbsp	17
Heavy Cream	1 tbsp	11
Whipped Topping, pressurized	1 tbsp	4

Eggs	Amount	Potassium (mg)
Egg whites, dried	1 ounce	319
Egg substitute, liquid, fat free	1/4 cup	128
Egg whole, scrambled	1 large	81
Egg whites, dried powder, stabilized	1 tbsp	78
Egg whole, fried	1 large	70
Egg whole, poached	1 large	69
Egg whole, hard-boiled	1 large	63
Egg whites	1 large	54
Egg yolk	1 large	18

Fish, Canned	Amount	Potassium (mg)
White (albacore) tuna, in oil	3 oz	463
Atlantic sardines, in oil	3 oz	338
White (albacore) tuna, in water	3 oz	201
Light tuna, canned in oil	3 oz	176
Light tuna, in water	3 oz	152

Fish, Cooked	Amount	Potassium (mg)
Florida pompano	3 oz	541
Atlantic salmon, wild	3 oz	534
King mackerel	3 oz	474
Spanish mackerel	3 oz	471
Keta (chum) salmon	3 oz	468
Yellowtail	3 oz	457
Atlantic & Pacific halibut	3 oz	449
Halibut	3 oz	449
Yellowfin tuna	3 oz	448
Skipjack (aku) tuna	3 oz	444
Snapper	3 oz	444

POTASSIUM

Continued

Pacific mackerel	3 oz	443
Chinook salmon	3 oz	429
Alaskan halibut	3 oz	426
Swordfish	3 oz	424
Walleye pike	3 oz	424
Grouper	3 oz	404
Coho salmon, farmed	3 oz	391
Atlantic pollock	3 oz	388
Freshwater bass	3 oz	388
Rainbow trout, farmed	3 oz	382
Rainbow trout, wild	3 oz	381
Pink salmon	3 oz	373
Coho salmon, wild	3 oz	369
Pollock	3 oz	366
Walleye pollock	3 oz	366
Carp	3 oz	363
Catfish, wild	3 oz	356
Sockeye salmon	3 oz	347
Atlantic mackerel	3 oz	341
Atlantic salmon, farmed	3 oz	326
Tilapia	3 oz	323
Catfish, farmed	3 oz	311
Haddock	3 oz	298
Greenland halibut	3 oz	292
Atlantic croaker	3 oz	289
Catfish, breaded & fried	3 oz	289
Northern pike	3 oz	281
Sea bass	3 oz	279
Striped bass	3 oz	279
Bluefin tuna, fresh	3 oz	275
Pacific cod	3 oz	246
Atlantic cod	3 oz	207
Atlantic perch	3 oz	192
Flounder & Sole	3 oz	167
Orange roughy	3 oz	154
Chinock salmon, smoked	3 oz	149
Atlantic herring, pickled	3 oz	59

Fish, Shellfish, Cooked	Amount	Potassium (mg)
Octopus	3 oz	536
Clams, canned	3 oz	534
Scallops, breaded & fried	3 oz	283
Clams, breaded & fried	3 oz	277
Blue crab cakes	3 oz	275
Crayfish	3 oz	252

RDA is 4700 mg for adults

POTASSIUM

Continued

Abalone	3 oz	241
Squid, fried	3 oz	237
Alaskan king crab	3 oz	223
Blue crab	3 oz	220
Blue crab, canned	3 oz	220
Oysters, breaded & fried	3 oz	207
Eastern oysters, wild	3 oz	206
Northern lobster	3 oz	196
Shrimp, breaded & fried	3 oz	191
Queen crab	3 oz	170
Shrimp	3 oz	144
Eastern oysters, farmed	3 oz	129
Alaskan king crab, imitation	3 oz	76
Shrimp, canned	3 oz	68

Fruit, Canned	Amount	Potassium (mg)
Apricots	1 cup	361
Pineapple	1 cup	264
Peaches	1 cup	241
Plums	1 cup	235
Applesauce, sweetened	1 cup	191
Applesauce, unsweetened	1 cup	181
Pears	1 cup	173
Olives, green	5 large	6
Olives, black	5 large	2

Fruit, Dried	Amount	Potassium (mg)
Peaches	1 cup	1594
Apricots	1 cup	1511
Currants	1 cup	1284
Figs	1 cup	1013
Pears	1 cup	959
Apples	1 cup	387
Cranberries	1 cup	48

Fruit, Frozen	Amount	Potassium (mg)
Peaches	1 cup	325
Raspberries	1 cup	285
Strawberries	1 cup	250
Blueberries	1 cup	230
Blackberries, unthawed	1 cup	211

RDA is 4700 mg for adults

POTASSIUM

Fruit, Raw	Amount	Potassium (mg)
Prunes, uncooked	1 cup	1274
Dates	1 cup	1168
Avocado, California, pureed	1 cup	1166
Raisins	1 cup	1086
Avocado, Florida, pureed	1 cup	807
Stewed prunes	1 cup	796
Plantains	1 cup	739
Kiwi	1 cup	562
Apricots	1 cup	427
Cantaloupe	1 cup	427
Pomegranates	1 cup	411
Elderberries	1 cup	406
Honeydew	1 cup	388
Black currants	1 cup	361
Cherries, pitted	1 cup	342
Tangerine, sections	1 cup	324
Valcenias oranges	1 cup	322
Florida Oranges	1 cup	313
Grapefruit, pink or red	1 cup	310
Grapes, red & green	1 cup	306
Peachs, slices	1 cup	293
Nectarine	1 cup	287
Mango	1 cup	277
Navel Oranges	1 cup	274
Mulberries	1 cup	272
Plums, sliced	1 cup	259
Papayas	1 cup	255
Strawberries	1 cup	254
Blackberries	1 cup	233
Pears	1 cup	192
Raspberries	1 cup	186
Pineapple	1 cup	180
Water mellon	1 cup	170
Apples	1 cup	134
Blueberries	1 cup	112
Cranberries	1 cup	85

Fruit, Raw	Amount	Potassium (mg)
Pummelo	1 fruit	1315
Avocado, Florida	1 fruit	1067
Plantains	1 fruit	893
Avocado, California	1 fruit	690
Cherimoya	1 fruit	674
Pomegranates	1 fruit	666

RDA is 4700 mg for adults

POTASSIUM

Continued

Mango	1 fruit	564
Bananas	1 fruit	422
Prunes, uncooked	5 prunes	348
Raisins	1 small box	322
Papayas	1 fruit	286
Nectarine	1 fruit	273
Persimmons, Japanese	1 fruit	270
Chayote	1 fruit	254
Florida Oranges	1 fruit	238
Kiwi	1 fruit	237
Dates	5 dates	233
Navel Oranges	1 fruit	232
Valcenias Oranges	1 fruit	217
Peaches	1 fruit	186
Cherries	10 fruit	182
Pears	1 fruit	176
Grapefruit, pink or red	1/2 fruit	166
Apples	1 fruit	148
Tangerine	1 fruit	139
Star fruit, Carambola	1 fruit	121
Plums	1 fruit	104
Strawberries	5 fruit	92
Apricots	1 fruit	91
Persimmons, small native	1 fruit	78
Pineapple guava, Feijoa	1 fruit	72
Figs, dried	1 fruit	57
Pineapple, slices	1/2" x 3"	54
Kumquats	1 fruit	35

Game Meat, Cooked	Amount	Potassium (mg)
Wild boar	3 oz	337
Buffalo, steak, free range	3 oz	320
Antelope	3 oz	316
Deer, ground	3 oz	309
Elk, ground	3 oz	301
Squirrel	3 oz	299
Rabbit	3 oz	292
Bison, ground	3 oz	290
Deer	3 oz	285
Elk	3 oz	279
Caribou	3 oz	264
Duck	3 oz	214

RDA is 4700 mg for adults

POTASSIUM

Grains, Cooked	Amount	Potassium (mg)
Kamut	1 cup	347
Amaranth	1 cup	332
Quinoa	1 cup	318
Spelt	1 cup	277
Oat bran	1 cup	201
Oats, regular, unenriched	1 cup	180
Wild rice	1 cup	166
Buckwheat, groats	1 cup	148
Barley, pearled	1 cup	146
Bulgur	1 cup	124
Millet	1 cup	108
Couscous	1 cup	91
White rice, long-grain, paraboiled	1 cup	88
Brown rice	1 cup	84
Spaghetti, spinach	1 cup	81
Macaroni	1 cup	62
Macaroni, Whole-Wheat	1 cup	62
Spaghetti, enriched	1 cup	62
Spaghetti, Whole-Wheat	1 cup	62
Egg noodles	1 cup	61
Egg & Spinach noodles	1 cup	59
White rice, long-grain, regular	1 cup	55
Soba noodles	1 cup	40
White rice, long-grain, instant	1 cup	15
Rice noodles	1 cup	7

Herbs & Spices	Amount	Potassium (mg)
Turmeric, ground	1 tsp	56
Chili powder	1 tsp	53
Paprika	1 tsp	52
Tarragon, dried, ground	1 tsp	48
Cumin	1 tsp	38
Basil, dried, ground	1 tsp	37
Garlic powder	1 tsp	37
Dill weed, dried	1 tsp	33
Curry powder	1 tsp	31
Pepper, black, ground	1 tsp	31
Anise seed	1 tsp	30
Caraway seeds	1 tsp	28
Celery seeds	1 tsp	28
Chervil, dried	1 tsp	28
Coriander leaf, dried	1 tsp	27
Ginger, ground	1 tsp	24
Onion powder	1 tsp	24

RDA is 4700 mg for adults

POTASSIUM

Continued

Coriander seed	1 tsp	23
Oregano, dried	1 tsp	23
Cloves, dried	1 tsp	21
All-spice, ground	1 tsp	20
Parsley, dried	1 tsp	13
Saffron	1 tsp	12
Cinnamon powder	1 tsp	11
Rosemary, dreid	1 tsp	11
Thyme, dried, ground	1 tsp	11
Sage, ground	1 tsp	7
Bay leaf, crumbled	1 tsp	3
Chives, chopped	1 tsp	3
Thyme, fresh	1 tsp	2
Cappers	1 tsp	1

Juice	Amount	Potassium (mg)
Prune	1 cup	707
Carrot	1 cup	689
Tomato	1 cup	556
Pomegranate	1 cup	533
Orange juice, raw	1 cup	496
Vegetable	1 cup	467
Pineapple, unsweetened	1 cup	325
Grapefruit juice, raw	1 cup	310
Grape, unsweetened	1 cup	263
Lemon juice, raw	1 cup	251
Apple	1 cup	250
Cranberry	1 cup	35

Lamb, Cooked	Amount	Potassium (mg)
Ground	3 oz	288
Cubed for stew or kabob	3 oz	285
Chops, loin, lean, trimmed to 1/4" fat	3 oz	278
Leg, whole, trimmed to 1/4" fat	3 oz	266
Rib, lean, trimmed to 1/4" fat	3 oz	266
Foreshank, trimmed to 1/8" fat	3 oz	218

Milk	Amount	Potassium (mg)
Canned, condensed, sweet	1 cup	1135
Canned, evaporated, nonfat	1 cup	850
Canned, evaporated	1 cup	764
Goat milk	1 cup	498
Coconut milk, canned	1 cup	497
Dry, instant, nonfat	1/3 cup	392

RDA is 4700 mg for adults

POTASSIUM

Continued

Nonfat, fat free or skim liquid milk	1 cup	382
Buttermilk, lowfat	1 cup	370
Lowfat, 1%	1 cup	366
Reduced fat, 2%	1 cup	342
Sheep milk	1 cup	336
Buttermilk, whole milk	1 cup	331
Whole milk, 3.25%	1 cup	322
Soy milk, original, unfortified	1 cup	287
Human milk	1 cup	125

Nuts & Seeds	Amount	Potassium (mg)
Pistachio nuts	1 oz	291
Flaxseeds	1 oz	230
Pumpkin seeds	1 oz	229
Trail mix, tropical	1 oz	201
Almonds	1 oz	200
Peanuts	1 oz	200
Trail mix, regular, salted	1 oz	194
Hazelnuts	1 oz	193
Brazilnuts	1 oz	187
Cashews	1 oz	187
Peanut butter, smooth style	1 oz	184
Trail mix, regular with chocolate chips	1 oz	184
Sunflower seeds	1 oz	183
Pine nuts	1 oz	169
Mixed nuts, roasted with peanuts, no salt	1 oz	169
Black walnuts	1 oz	148
Sesame seeds	1 oz	133
English walnuts	1 oz	125
Tahini	1 oz	117
Pecans	1 oz	116
Chia seeds	1 oz	115
Macadamia	1 oz	104
Coconut, raw meat	1 oz	101

Nuts & Seeds	Amount	Potassium (mg)
Peanut butter, smooth	1/4 cup	419
Flaxseeds	1/4 cup	341
Pistachio	1/4 cup	315
Pumpkin seeds	1/4 cup	261
Peanuts	1/4 cup	257
Trail mix, regular, salted	1/4 cup	257
Almonds, whole	1/4 cup	252
Trail mix, tropical	1/4 cup	248
Trail mix, regular with chocolate chips	1/4 cup	237

RDA is 4700 mg for adults

POTASSIUM

Continued

Sunflower seeds	1/4 cup	226
Brazilnuts, whole	1/4 cup	219
Peanut butter, smooth	1 tbsp	208
Mixed nuts, roasted with peanuts, no salt	1/4 cup	204
Pine nuts	1/4 cup	201
Hazelnuts, chopped	1/4 cup	196
Sesame seeds	1/4 cup	168
Black walnuts, chopped	1/4 cup	163
Macadamia	1/4 cup	123
English walnuts, chopped	1/4 cup	110
Pecans, halves	1/4 cup	101
Flaxseeds	1 tbsp	84
Coconut meat, shredded	1/4 cup	71
Sesame seeds	1 tbsp	42
Cashews	1/4 cup	x
Chia seeds	1/4 cup	x

Pork, Cooked	Amount	Potassium (mg)
Sirloin pork chops	3 oz	357
Tenderloin	3 oz	356
Canadian-style bacon	3 oz	332
Pork chops, lean, pan-fried	3 oz	321
Pork chops, pan-fried	3 oz	300
Bratwurst	3 oz	296
Pork chops, broiled	3 oz	292
Center loin pork chops	3 oz	292
Spareribs	3 oz	272
Cured ham, lean	3 oz	269
Italian sausage	3 oz	258
Cured ham	3 oz	243
Backribs	3 oz	204
Polish sausage	3 oz	202
Canadian-style bacon	2 slices	181
Braunschweiger	3 oz	169
Bacon	3 slices	107
Sausage	1 patty	79
Sausage	2 links	70

Turkey, Cooked	Amount	Potassium (mg)
Turkey bacon	3 oz	336
Ground turkey, fat free	3 oz	288
Ground turkey	3 oz	250
Breast meat	3 oz	248
Light meat	3 oz	212
Ground turkey, 93% lean	3 oz	210

RDA is 4700 mg for adults

POTASSIUM

Continued

Ground turkey, 85% lean	3 oz	206
Dark meat	3 oz	193
Turkey sausage, reduced fat	3 oz	176

Veal, Cooked	Amount	Potassium (mg)
Leg, top round	3 oz	326
Sirloin	3 oz	298
Ground	3 oz	286
Loin	3 oz	276
Foreshank	3 oz	259
Rib	3 oz	251
Breast	3 oz	246

Vegetables, Canned	Amount	Potassium (mg)
Tomato paste	1 cup	2657
Tomato sauce	1 cup	811
Spinach	1 cup	740
Stewed tomatos	1 cup	528
Pumpkin	1 cup	505
Tomatoes	1 cup	451
Asparagus	1 cup	416
Sauerkraut	1 cup	401
Yellow sweet corn	1 cup	391
Sweet potato	1 cup	378
Carrots	1 cup	261
Beets	1 cup	252
Mushrooms	1 cup	201
Green peas	1 cup	180
Green beans	1 cup	143

Vegetables, Cooked	Amount	Potassium (mg)
Swiss chard	1 cup	961
Yams, cubed	1 cup	911
Acorn squash	1 cup	896
Spinach	1 cup	839
Sweet potato, mashed	1 cup	754
Split peas	1 cup	710
Bok-Choy	1 cup	631
Potatoes, mashed with whole milk	1 cup	622
Pumpkin	1 cup	564
White mushrooms	1 cup	555
Rutabagas	1 cup	554
Beets	1 cup	519
Brussels sprouts	1 cup	495

RDA is 4700 mg for adults

POTASSIUM

Winter squash	1 cup	494
Artichokes	1 cup	480
Potatoes, flesh, baked	1 cup	477
Zucchini	1 cup	475
Broccoli	1 cup	457
Celery	1 cup	426
Carrots	1 cup	367
Onions	1 cup	349
Summer squash	1 cup	346
Corn	1 cup	325
Asparagus	1 cup	310
Kale	1 cup	296
Cabbage	1 cup	294
Turnip greens	1 cup	292
Mustard greens	1 cup	283
Turnips	1 cup	276
Dandelion greens	1 cup	244
Collard greens	1 cup	220
Okra	1 cup	216
Cauliflower	1 cup	176
Shiitake mushrooms	1 cup	170
Eggplant	1 cup	122
Napa cabbage	1 cup	95
Leeks	1 cup	90

Vegetables, Frozen	Amount	Potassium (mg)
Spinach	1 cup	574
Brussels sprouts	1 cup	450
Collard greens	1 cup	427
Yellow sweet corn	1 cup	382
Turnip greens	1 cup	367
Asparagus	1 cup	310
Carrots	1 cup	280
Broccoli	1 cup	261
Rhubarb	1 cup	230
Green peas	1 cup	176

Vegetables, Raw	Amount	Potassium (mg)
Mustard spinach	1 cup	674
Butternut squash	1 cup	493
Tomatoes	1 cup	427
Yellow bell peppers	1 large	394
Tomattillos	1 cup	354
Tomatoes, cherry	1 cup	353
Carrots	1 cup	352

POTASSIUM

Continued

Cauliflower	1 cup	320
Red bell peppers	1 cup	314
Kale	1 cup	299
Summer squash	1 cup	296
Zucchini	1 cup	295
Broccoli	1 cup	278
Green onions & scallions	1 cup	276
Celery	1 cup	263
Green bell peppers	1 cup	261
Onions	1 cup	234
White mushrooms	1 cup	223
Prickley pear cactus pads, nopales	1 cup	221
Dandelion greens	1 cup	218
Snow peas	1 cup	196
Belgian endive	1 cup	190
Bok-Choy	1 cup	176
Red cabbage	1 cup	170
Spinach	1 cup	167
Savoy cabbage	1 cup	161
Cucumbers	1 cup	153
Romaine lettuce	1 cup	138
Swiss chard	1 cup	136
Butterhead or boston lettuce	1 cup	131
Chicory greens	1 cup	122
Radicchio	1 cup	121
Cabbage	1 cup	119
Watercress	1 cup	112
Green leaf lettuce	1 cup	109
Spirulina, dried	1 tbsp	95
Iceburg lettuce	1 cup	78
Raab broccoli	1 cup	78
Arugula	1 cup	74
Shiitake mushrooms, dried	1 each	55
Red leaf lettuce	1 cup	52

Yogurt	Amount	Potassium (mg)
Plain yogurt, skim milk	8 oz	579
Plain yogurt, low fat milk	8 oz	531
Plain yogurt, whole milk	8 oz	352
Plain Greek Yogurt, non fat	6 oz	240

RDA is 4700 mg for adults

Nutrient Data Collection Form

Food	Amount	Book Numbers	Multiply By	Estimated Nutrient Intake
Nutrient::	RDA:	Estimated:	% of RDA:	Total Estimated:

NOTES

When one thinks of the human skeleton what comes to mind is calcium. Few are aware that protein makes up 1/3 of the weight of the human skeleton and 1/2 of its volume.

Protein and calcium interact with each other constructively to form structures which are incorporated into and become a permanent part of the bones architecture. This structure, known as the protein matrix, is a primary constituent of bone; thus, the interrelationships between protein, calcium, and bone are of primary concern. Protein is as essential for healthy bone as is calcium and vitamin D.

For many years a high protein diet, especially animal protein, was generally considered to be detrimental to skeletal bone.

It has been known for 80 years that as the intake of protein increases so does the amount of urinary calcium and this appears to be normal for humans. At that time it was felt that skeletal bone was the source of urinary calcium.

The explanation proposed was that the amino acids containing the element sulfur created acidic conditions in the body. In response to the acid, the bones would release alkalizing calcium to neutralize the increased acidity. The prevailing view that emerged from this was a habitual intake of a high protein diet would eventually lead to a lower bone mineral density and an increased risk of osteoporosis. At odds with the acid hypothesis, studies have shown a high protein diet is, in fact, associated with a higher bone mineral density and not a lower one.

Studies revealed that a high protein diet is typically accompanied with increased absorption of dietary calcium sufficient enough to compensate for the loss urinary calcium. Further, since laboratory tests failed to identify bio markers of calcium's mobilization from bone, it was reasonable to assume the calcium excreted was not of bone origin.

If in fact, acidity from protein is responsible for the increased urinary calcium, then neutralizing the acid should result in a change of urinary calcium. In an experiment on healthy volunteers adding alkalizing potassium salts to a high protein diet did result in neutralizing the acid, but it did not prevent or decrease the amount of calcium excreted. Findings like this, indicate the greater amount of urinary calcium observed in a high protein diet is not due to an acid load and is not coming from bone but appears to be coming from the additional calcium being absorbed.

Nevertheless, animal protein does increase the acidity in humans and has been associated with negative effects. From a pure chemical point of view, however, it appears that the increase in acidity from a high protein diet is not of sufficient magnitude to chemically drive a significant loss of calcium from bones. Thus, the detrimental effect of acidity on bone is relatively small, but of course this small effect could have a large impact over a lifetime if one consumes only acid forming foods.

What negative effects have been associated with acidity may reflect more of an inadequate intake of fruits and vegetables rather than overconsumption of animal protein since the dominating dietary source for alkalizing nutrients such as potassium is fruits and vegetables.

A study of non-smoking, postmenopausal women given a high protein intake was associated with higher bone mineral density when in the presence of adequate dietary calcium. What adverse effects had been noticed in some high protein studies were observed only among individuals who consumed inadequate amounts of calcium.

Current research no longer supports a theory that a high protein diet's induced increase in urinary calcium reflects a leaching of calcium from bones and will eventually lead to osteoporosis. In fact, experimental and clinical intervention studies indicate a high protein intake, compared with a medium intake, is associated with increased bone mineral mass and density.

In contrast to the above, a low protein diet is associated with a lower bone mineral density and loss of muscle. In healthy elderly women after 10 weeks of being fed a protein diet at 1/2 the RDA the women experienced a significant loss of lean tissue and muscle function.

An intervention study of healthy young women reported the short term effects of dietary protein intake at three different levels. This study consisted of a well-controlled diet that had been weighed and balanced in all other nutrients.

As expected, there was a rise in calcium excretion as protein intake increased. What was unanticipated was within one week on the lowest protein intake, all subjects abruptly developed elevated levels of the parathyroid hormones. The parathyroid hormone is the dominating hormone which signals the body to release calcium from bones. As long as the parathyroid hormones remain elevated the amount of calcium in bone will continue to decline.

Another study using the same diet, directly measured the absorption of calcium at the different protein intakes. The protein intake at the lower amounts impaired calcium absorption and again elevated the parathyroid hormones. This group provided direct evidence that impaired absorption of calcium explains the elevated levels of the parathyroid hormones when protein intake is restricted.

When all other dietary factors and nutrients are controlled and held constant individuals who consume the lowest protein diets do appear to have the lowest bone mineral density. A study of 1800 women 50 years old and older, after adjustment for age and body weight, reported a low protein intake was associated with a lower bone mineral density in the hips. A second group of 615 subjects participated in an osteoporosis study for a four year period. In this group the lower levels of protein intake again was associated with lower bone mineral densities at both the hip and spine in both elderly men and women.

Based on the above, protein intake just below the RDA has been associated with a reduction of calcium absorption sufficient to cause elevated levels of the parathyroid hormones. Protein intake at 1/2 the RDA resulted in a decline in skeletal muscle mass and function in healthy elderly women.

Although, no optimal value of protein intake exists for the elderly population, there is a general agreement that moderately increasing protein intake beyond the current RDA of .8 g / Kg / day may enhance both bone and muscle health.

In summary, a high rate of bone loss is significantly associated with low levels of protein intake in premenopausal women, postmenopausal women, and elderly men.

The recommended daily allowance, RDA, is in gram quantities. To calculate your protein intake for adults based on the RDA take your body weight and divide it by 2.2 and then multiply the answer by point eight (.8). Daily protein intake = (body weight in pounds / 2.2) x (.8). This chapter lists protein in grams (g) and in total percent of calories from protein.

Individuals	Grams / Day	Grams / Kg Body wt.	% of Calories
1 to 3 year olds	13	1.1	5-20
4 to 8 year olds	19	.95	10-30
9 to 13 year olds	34	.95	10-30
14 to 18 year olds	52	.85	10-30
Over 18, males	56	.80	10-35
Over 18, females	46	.80	10-35
Pregnancy & Lactation	71	1.1	10-35

PROTEIN

Alcohol	Amount	Protein (g)
Regular Beer, all types	1 bottle	1.63
Light Beer, all types	1 bottle	0.85
Red Wine	1 glass	0.1
White Wine	1 glass	0.1
Gin, Rum, Vodka, Whisky	1 shot	0

Beans, Canned	Amount	Protein (g)
Navy beans	1 cup	20
Great Northern	1 cup	19
White beans, mature	1 cup	19
Cranberry beans	1 cup	14
Fava beans	1 cup	14
Kidney bean	1 cup	13
Refried beans	1 cup	13
Baked beans, plain	1 cup	12
Lima beans	1 cup	12
Garbanzo beans	1 cup	12
Black-eyed peas	1 cup	11
Pinto beans	1 cup	11
Yellow beans	1 cup	2
Green beans	1 cup	2

Beans, Cooked	Amount	Protein (g)
Soybeans, dry roasted	1 cup	37
Natto	1 cup	31
Soybeans, mature	1 cup	29
Lupins, mature	1 cup	26
Soybeans, green	1 cup	22
Winged beans	1 cup	18
Lentils	1 cup	18
White beans, mature	1 cup	17
Adzuki	1 cup	17
Edamame	1 cup	17
Cranberry beans	1 cup	17
Split peas	1 cup	16
White beans, small	1 cup	16
Hyacinth beans	1 cup	16
Pinto beans	1 cup	15
Kidney beans	1 cup	15
Black beans	1 cup	15
Black Turtle beans, mature	1 cup	15
Navy beans	1 cup	15
Great Northern	1 cup	15

PROTEIN

Continued

Lima beans	1 cup	15
Garbanzo beans	1 cup	15
Mothbeans	1 cup	14
Mung beans, mature seeds	1 cup	14
Black-eyed peas	1 cup	13
Fava beans	1 cup	13
Pigeon peas	1 cup	11
Yardlong beans, Chinese long beans	1 cup	3
Green beans	1 cup	2
Yellow beans	1 cup	2

Beef, Cooked	Amount	Protein (g)
Beef ribs, trim to 1/8" fat	3 oz	19
Brisket, lean, trim to 0" fat	3 oz	28
Chuck roast, trim to 1/8" fat	3 oz	22
Filet Mignon, trim to 0" fat	3 oz	26
Flank steak, lean, trim to 0" fat	3 oz	24
Flat-Iron steak	3 oz	21
Ground beef, 75%, broiled	3 oz	22
Ground beef, 80%	3 oz	22
Ground beef, 85%	3 oz	22
Ground beef, 90%	3 oz	22
Ground beef, 95%,	3 oz	22
London Broil, top round, trim to 0" fat	3 oz	30
Porterhouse steak, trim to 0" fat	3 oz	20
Ribeye steak, lean, trim 0" fat	3 oz	21
Skirt Steak, trim to 0" fat	3 oz	22
T-Bone steak, trim 0" fat	3 oz	21
Top Sirloin, lean, trim to 1/8" fat	3 oz	25
Tri Tip steak, lean, trim to 0" fat	3 oz	26

Beef, Cooked	Amount	Protein (g)
Tri Tip steak, lean, trim to 0" fat	1 lb	139
Skirt steak, trim to 0" fat	1 lb	119
T-bone steak, trim to 0" fat	1 lb	110
Porterhouse steak, trim to 0" fat	1 lb	109
Flank steak, lean, trim to 0" fat	1 steak	107
Brisket, lean, trim to 0" fat	1 steak	90
Top Sirloin, trim to 1/8" fat	1 lb	83
Chuck roast, trim to 1/8" fat	1 lb	65
Ribeye steak, boneless, trim to 0" fat	1 steak	52
Flat-Iron steak	1 steak	47
Ribeye filet, lean, trim to 0" fat	1 filet	38
Top Sirloin, choice filet, trim to 0" fat	1 filet	38
Filet Mignon, tenderloin, trim to 0" fat	1 steak	36

PROTEIN

Beef, Ground, Cooked	Amount	Protein (g)
Ground beef, 95%	1/4 lb patty	21.6
Ground beef, 90%	1/4 lb patty	21.4
Ground beef, 85%	1/4 lb patty	20.0
Ground beef, 80%	1/4 lb patty	19.8
Ground beef, 75%	1/4 lb patty	17.9

Bread	Amount	Protein (g)
Bagel, oat bran	4" bagel	11.2
Indian bread, Naan, whole wheat	1 piece	10.8
Mexican roll, bollilo	1 roll	10.4
Bagel, wheat	4" bagel	10.0
Bagel, egg	4" bagel	9.4
Bagel, plain	4" bagel	8.9
Bagel, cinnamon & raisins	4" bagel	8.7
Indian bread, Naan, plain	1 piece	8.6
Kaiser rolls	1 roll	5.6
Pita, white	6" pita	5.5
English Muffin, plain	1 muffin	5.1
Croissants, butter	1 medium	4.7
Cornbread, drymix	1 piece	4.3
Hamburger & Hotdog buns, plain	1 bun	4.1
Potato bread	1 slice	4.0
Egg bread	1 slice	3.8
Whole-Wheat	1 slice	3.6
Multi-Grain, or Whole-Grain	1 slice	3.5
Dinner Rolls, brown & serve	1 roll	3.0
Italian bread, Oroweat Premium	1 slice	3.0
French and Sourdough	1 slice	2.9
Pumpernickle	1 slice	2.8
Wheat	1 slice	2.7
Rye bread	1 slice	2.7
Tortillas, flour	1 tortilla	2.7
Oatmeal bread	1 slice	2.3
Cracked Wheat	1 slice	2.2
Raisen bread	1 slice	2.1
White	1 slice	1.9
Tortillas, corn	1 tortilla	1.5

Butter	Amount	Protein (g)
Regular dairy butter, salted	1 tbsp	0.1
Regular dairy whipped butter, salted	1 tbsp	0.1

PROTEIN

CEREAL

Arrowhead Mills®	Amount	Protein (g)
Shredded Wheat, Bite-Size	1 cup	6
Oat Bran Flakes	1 cup	5
Sweetened Shredded Wheat	1 cup	5
Spelt Flakes	1 cup	4
Maple Buckwheat Flakes	1 cup	4
Kamut Flakes	1 cup	4
Amaranth Flakes	1 cup	4
Sprouted Multigrain Flakes	1 cup	4
Sweetened Rice Flakes	1 cup	3

Barbara's	Amount	Protein (g)
Shredded Oats Vanilla Almond	1 cup	7
Shredded Oats Cinnamon Crunch	1 cup	6
Shredded Minis Blueberry Burst	1 cup	6
Hole 'n Oats: Fruit Juice Sweetened	1 cup	5
Shredded Spoonfuls Multigrain	1 cup	5
Shredded Oats Original	1 cup	5
High Fiber Original	1 cup	5
High Fiber Flax & Granola	1 cup	5
High Fiber Cranberry	1 cup	5
Shredded Wheat	2 biscuits	4
Hole 'n Oats Honey Nut	1 cup	4
Puffins Peanut Butter	1 cup	4
Puffins Cinnamon	1 cup	3
Corn Flakes	1 cup	3
Brown Rice Crisps	1 cup	3
Puffins Peanut Butter & Chocolate	1 cup	3
Puffins Multigrain	1 cup	3
Puffins Original	1 cup	3
Puffins Honey Rice	1 cup	3
Puffins Puffs Crunchy Cocoa	1 cup	3
Puffins Puffs Fruit Medley	1 cup	3

Bear Naked®	Amount	Protein (g)
Peak Protein, Original Granola	1 cup	24
Vanila Almond Crucnh Granola	1 cup	16
Banana Nut Granola	1 cup	12
Fruit & Nut Ganola	1 cup	12
Nut Cluster Crunch Cereal	1 cup	5

PROTEIN

Cereal, Cadia	Amount	Protein (g)
Crunch	1 cup	9
All Natural Raisin Bran	1 cup	4
Honey Kissed Cadi-O's	1 cup	4
Whole Grain Cadi-O's Toasted Oats	1 cup	4

Cereal, Cascadian Farms	Amount	Protein (g)
Cinnamon Raisin Granola	1 cup	8
Maple Brown Sugar Granola	1 cup	8
Oats & Honey Granola	1 cup	8
Hearty Morning	1 cup	7
French Vanilla Almond Granola	1 cup	5
Dark Chocolate Almond Granola	1 cup	5
Fruit & Nut Granola	1 cup	5
Raisin bran	1 cup	4
Multi Grain Squares	1 cup	4
Purely O's	1 cup	3
Chocolate O's	1 cup	3
Fruit Ful O's	1 cup	3
Cinnamon Crunch	1 cup	2
Honey Nut O's	1 cup	2

Cereal, Erewhon Organic	Amount	Protein (g)
Raisin Bran	1 cup	6
Corn Flakes	1 cup	4
Cocoa Crispy Brown Rice	1 cup	3
Rice Twice	1 cup	3
Crispy Brown Rice, Strawberry Crisp	1 cup	3
Crispy Brown Rice, Original	1 cup	2
Crispy Brown Rice, Gluten Free	1 cup	2
Crispy Brown Rice, Mixed Berries	1 cup	2

Ezekiel	Amount	Protein (g)
Sprouted Grain Original, 4:9	1 cup	16
Sprouted Grain Golden Flax, 4:9	1 cup	16
Sprouted Grain Almond, 4:9	1 cup	16
Sprouted Grain Cinnamon Flax, 4:9	1 cup	14

General Mills®	Amount	Protein (g)
Multi-Bran CHEX	1 cup	8.0
Wheat Chex	1 cup	6.7
Oatmeal Crisp, Crunchy Almond	1 cup	5.0
Apple Cinnamon Oatmeal Crisp	1 cup	4.0

PROTEIN

Continued

Honey Nut Clusters	1 cup	4.0
Raisin Nut Bran	1 cup	4.0
Basic 4	1 cup	3.9
Golden Grams	1 cup	3.0
Honey Nut Chex	1 cup	3.0
Reese's Puffs	1 cup	3.0
Total Cranberry Crunch	1 cup	3.0
Total Raisin Bran	1 cup	3.0
Total Whole Grain	1 cup	3.0
Wheaties	1 cup	2.8
Chocolate Chex	1 cup	2.3
Lucky Charms	1 cup	2.1
Kix	1 cup	2.0
Cinnamon Chex	1 cup	2.0
Corn Chex	1 cup	2.0
Dora The Explorer	1 cup	2.0
Rice Chex	1 cup	2.0
Berry Berry Kix	1 cup	1.6
Cinnamon Toast Crunch	1 cup	1.6
Cocoa Puffs	1 cup	1.6
Trix	1 cup	1.4
Cookie Crisp	1 cup	1.3

General Mills Cheerios®	Amount	Protein (g)
Original	1 cup	3.2
Crunch, Oat Clusters	1 cup	3.1
Yogurt Burst, Strawberry	1 cup	3.0
Apple Cinnamon	1 cup	2.7
Berry Burst	1 cup	2.7
Frosted	1 cup	2.7
Honey Nut	1 cup	2.7
Dulce de leche	1 cup	2.6
Multi Grain Peanut Butter	1 cup	2.6
Chocolate	1 cup	2.0
Banana Nut	1 cup	2.0
Cinnamon Burst	1 cup	2.0
Multi Grain	1 cup	2.0
Fruity	1 cup	1.3

General Mills Fiber One®	Amount	Protein (g)
Frosted Shredded Wheat	1 cup	5
Honey Clusters & Almonds	1 cup	4
Original Bran Cereal	1 cup	4
Caramel Delight	1 cup	3
Honey Clusters	1 cup	3

PROTEIN

Continued

Raisin Bran Clusters	1 cup	3
80 Calories, Honey Squares	1 cup	2
80 Calories, Chocolate Squares	1 cup	1

Glutino®	Amount	Protein (g)
Honey Nut Cereal	1 cup	2
Apple & Cinnamon Rings	1 cup	2
Corn Rice Flakes	1 cup	2
Berry Sensible Beginning	1 cup	2
Frosted Corn & Rice Flakes	1 cup	2
Corn Rice Flakes with Strawberries	1 cup	2

Cereal, Health Valley	Amount	Protein (g)
Oat Bran Almond Crunch	1 cup	12
Heart Wise	1 cup	11
Low Fat Date, Almond Flavor Granola	1 cup	8
Low Fat Raisin Cinnamon Granola	1 cup	8
Golden Flax	1 cup	6
Fiber 7	1 cup	6
Oat Bran Flakes	1 cup	5
Amaranth Flakes	1 cup	5
Oat Bran Flakes & Raisins	1 cup	5
Cranberry Crunch	1 cup	5
Multigrain Maple, Honey, Nut Squares	1 cup	4
Multigrain Apple Cinnamon Squares	1 cup	4
Rice Crunch-EMS	1 cup	2
Corn Crunch-EMS	1 cup	2

Kashi®	Amount	Protein (g)
Go Lean	1 cup	13
Go Lean Crisp, Cinnamon Crumble	1 cup	13
Go Lean Crisp, Toasted Berry Crumble	1 cup	12
Go Lean Vanilla Graham	1 cup	11
Go Lean Crunch	1 cup	9
Go Lean Crunch, Honey Almond Flax	1 cup	9
7-Whole Grain Flakes	1 cup	6
7-Whole Grain Nuggets	1 cup	6
Autum Wheat	29 biscuits	6
Berry Fruitful	29 biscuits	6
Cinnamon Harvest	28 biscuits	6
Heart to Heart, Oat Flakes & Blueberry Clusters	1 cup	6
Island Vanilla	27 biscuits	6
Heart to Heart, Warm Cinnamon	1 cup	5
Heart to Heart, Honey Toasted Oat	1 cup	5

PROTEIN

Continued

Strawberry Fields	1 cup	5
Good Friends	1 cup	5
Blackberry Hills	1 cup	4
Heart to Heart, Nutty Chia Flax	1 cup	4
7-Whole Grain Honey Puffs	1 cup	3
Berry Blossom	1 cup	3
Honey Sunshine	1 cup	3
Indigo Morning	1 cup	3
Simply Maize	1 cup	3
7-Whole Grain Puffs	1 cup	2

Kellogg's®	Amount	Protein (g)
All-Bran Original	1 cup	8
Low Fat Granola with Raisins	1 cup	8
MUESLIX	1 cup	7
All-Bran Bran Buds	1 cup	6
All-Bran Strawberry Medley	1 cup	6
Raisin Bran	1 cup	5
Cracklin' Oat Bran	1 cup	5
Frosted MINI-Wheats, Bite-Size	1 cup	5
Smart Start, Strong Heart, Toasted Oat	1 cup	5
Frosted MINI-Wheats, Big-Bite	1 cup	5
Fiberplus Berry Yogurt Crunch	1 cup	4
Fiberplus Cinnamon Oat Crunch	1 cup	4
Raisin Bran Extra	1 cup	4
Smart Start, Strong Heart, Antioxidants	1 cup	4
All-Bran Complete Wheat Flakes	1 cup	4
Crunchy Nut Golden Honey Nut Flakes	1 cup	3
Honey Crunch Corn Flakes	1 cup	3
Krave Chocolate	1 cup	3
Raisin Bran Crunch	1 cup	3
Product 19	1 cup	2
Berry Rice Krispies	1 cup	2
CINNABON	1 cup	2
Cocoa Krispies	1 cup	2
Crunchy Nut Roasted Nut & Honey O's	1 cup	2
Frosted Flakes	1 cup	2
Frosted Rice Krispies	1 cup	2
Honey Smacks	1 cup	2
Rice Krispies	1 cup	2
Rice Krispies Treats	1 cup	2
Simply Cinnamon Corn Flakes	1 cup	2
Crispix	1 cup	2
Corn Flakes	1 cup	2
Froot Loops	1 cup	2

PROTEIN

Continued

Apple Jacks	1 cup	2
Smorz	1 cup	1
Corn Pops	1 cup	1

Kellogg's Special-K®	Amount	Protein (g)
Low Fat Granola	1 cup	14
Protein Plus	1 cup	13
Original	1 cup	6
Multigrain Oats & Honey	1 cup	3
Vanilla Almond	1 cup	3
Cinnamon Pecan	1 cup	3
Fruit & Yogurt	1 cup	3
Blueberry	1 cup	3
Chocolately Delight	1 cup	3
Red Berries	1 cup	2

Mom's Best Naturals	Amount	Protein (g)
Raisin Bran	1 cup	5.0
Sweetened Wheat Fuls	1 cup	5.0
Blue Pom Wheat Fuls	1 cup	5.0
Oats & Honey Blend	1 cup	2.6
Honey Ful Wheats	1 cup	2.6
Honey Nut Toastey O's	1 cup	2.0
Mallow Oats	1 cup	2.0
Toasted Cinnamon Squares	1 cup	1.3
Honey Graham	1 cup	1.3
Crispy Cocoa Rice	1 cup	1.3

Nature's Path™	Amount	Protein (g)
Optimum Banana Almond	1 cup	13.3
Optimum Power Blueberry Cinnamon	1 cup	12.0
Peanut Butter Granola	1 cup	9.3
Optimum Slim Low Fat Vanilla	1 cup	9.0
AGAVE Plus Granola	1 cup	8.0
Flax Plus Maple Pecan Crunch	1 cup	8.0
Flax Plus Pumpkin Flax Granola	1 cup	8.0
Flax Plus Pumpkin Raisin Crunch	1 cup	8.0
Flax Plus Raisin Bran Flakes	1 cup	8.0
Flax Plus Redberry Crunch	1 cup	8.0
Flax Plus Vanilla Almond Granola	1 cup	8.0
Hemp Plus Granola	1 cup	8.0
Heritage Crunch	1 cup	8.0
Acai Apple Granola	1 cup	6.7
Optimum Cranberry Ginger	1 cup	6.7

PROTEIN

Continued

Pomegran Cherry Granola	1 cup	6.7
Pomegran Plus Granola	1 cup	6.7
Smart Bran	1 cup	6.0
Flax Plus Multibran Flakes	1 cup	5.3
Heritage Flakes	1 cup	5.3
Organic Millet Rice	1 cup	5.3
Heritage Heirloom Whole Grain	1 cup	4.0
Mesa Sunrise, Gluten Free	1 cup	4.0
Multigrain Oat bran	1 cup	4.0
OATY BITES Whole Grain	1 cup	4.0
Crunchy Maple Sunrise, Gluten Free	1 cup	3.0
Crunchy Vanilla Sunrise	1 cup	3.0
Whole O's	1 cup	3.0
Honeyed Corn Flakes, Gluten Free	1 cup	2.7

Peace All Natural	Amount	Protein (g)
Wild Berry Clusters & Flakes	1 cup	9
Golden Honey Granola	1 cup	9
Walnut Spice Clusters & Flakes	1 cup	8
Cherry Almond Clusters & Flakes	1 cup	8
Vanilla Almond Clusters & Flakes	1 cup	5
Maple Pecan	1 cup	5
Mango Peach Passion Clusters & Flakes	1 cup	4

Post®	Amount	Protein, g
Grape-Nuts Cereal	1 cup	13
Great Grains, Crunchy Pecan	1 cup	6
Great Grains, Raisin, Date & Pecan	1 cup	6
Shredded Wheat, Original, spoon-size	1 cup	6
Shredded Wheat n' Bran	1 cup	5
Great Grains, Banana Nut Crunch	1 cup	5
Honey Nut Shredded Wheat	1 cup	5
Great Grains, Cranberry Almond Crunch	1 cup	5
Raisin Bran	1 cup	5
Shredded Wheat, frosted, spoon-size	1 cup	4
Bran Flakes	1 cup	4
Grape-Nuts Flakes	1 cup	4
Alpha-Bits	1 cup	3
Shredded Wheat, Original, big-biscuit	1 biscuit	3
Blueberry Morning	1 cup	3
Golden Crisp	1 cup	2
Cocoa Pebbles	1 cup	2
Fruity Pebbles	1 cup	2
Honeycomb Cereal	1 cup	1

PROTEIN

Post® Honey Bunches of Oats®	Amount	Protein, g
Just Bunches, Cinnamonn	1 cup	8
Just Bunches, Honey roasted	1 cup	8
With Vanilla Bunches	1 cup	4
Honey Roasted	1 cup	3
Pecan Bunches	1 cup	3
Raisin Medley	1 cup	3
With Almonds	1 cup	3
With Cinnamon Bunches	1 cup	3
With Peaches	1 cup	3
With Strawberries	1 cup	3

Quaker®	Amount	Protein (g)
Granola Oats, Honey & Almonds	1 cup	10
Granola Apple Cranberry Almond	1 cup	8
Toasted Multigrain Crisp	1 cup	7
Oatmeal Squares, Golden Maple	1 cup	6
Oatmeal Squares, Brown Sugar	1 cup	6
Oatmeal Squares, Cinnamon	1 cup	6
LIFE Cereal, Original	1 cup	4
LIFE Cereal, Maple & Brown Sugar	1 cup	4
LIFE Cereal, Cinnamon	1 cup	4
CAP'N Crunch's Peanut Butter Crunch	1 cup	3
Corn Bran Crunch	1 cup	2
CAP'N Crunch	1 cup	2
CAP'N Crunch with Crunch Berries	1 cup	2
CAP'N Crunch's OOPs! All Berries	1 cup	2
Puffed Wheat	1 cup	2
Honey Graham OH'S	1 cup	1
Puffed Rice	1 cup	1

Cereal, Uncle Sam	Amount	Protein (g)
Flaxseed, Original	1 cup	9
Flaxseed, & Strawberry	1 cup	9
Flaxseed, Honey Almond	1 cup	8
Skinners Raisin Bran	1 cup	6

Cereal, Wild Harvest	Amount	Protein (g)
Golden Honey & Flax Granola	1 cup	9
Crunchy Vanilla Almond Granola	1 cup	8
Cherry Vanilla Granola	1 cup	7
Blueberry Flax Granola	1 cup	6
Wholesome Raisin Bran	1 cup	5
Maple Pecan Flakes & Clusters	1 cup	4

PROTEIN

Wild Berry Crisp	1 cup	4
Cranberry Almond	1 cup	3
Mango Crisp	1 cup	3

Cereal, Cooked	Amount	Protein (g)
Oats, regular, unenriched	1 cup	5.9
Farina	1 cup	4.4
Corn grits, white	1 cup	4.1
WHEATENA	1 cup	4.9
Malt-o-Meal plain	1 serving	3.6
CREAM OF WHEAT, regular	1 cup	3.6
Corn grits, yellow	1 cup	3.0

Cheese	Amount	Protein (g)
Parmesan, grated	1 oz	10.9
Gruyere	1 oz	9.2
Mozzarella, non fat	1 oz	9.0
Romano	1 oz	9.0
Goat cheese, hard type	1 oz	8.7
Swiss, low fat	1 oz	8.0
Monterey, low fat	1 oz	7.9
Swiss	1 oz	7.5
Mozzarella, skim milk, low moisture	1 oz	7.4
Fontina	1 oz	7.3
Provolone	1 oz	7.3
Gouda	1 oz	7.1
Cheddar	1 oz	7.0
Dubliner	1 oz	7.0
Muenster, low fat	1 oz	7.0
Cheddar, low fat	1 oz	6.9
Monterey	1 oz	6.9
Provolone, reduced fat	1 oz	6.9
American, pasteurized process, low fat	1 oz	6.9
Colby	1 oz	6.7
Muenster	1 oz	6.6
Mozzarella, whole milk	1 oz	6.3
Blue cheese	1 oz	6.1
Goat cheese, semisoft type	1 oz	6.1
Roquefort	1 oz	6.1
Pepper Jack, Red & Green Jalapenos	1 oz	6.0
Brie	1 oz	5.9
Goat cheese, soft type	1 oz	5.3
American, pasteurized process, fortified	1 oz	5.1
Velveeta, pasteurized process	1 oz	4.6
Cream cheese, fat free	1 oz	4.5

PROTEIN

Continued

Feta	1 oz	4.0
Cottage cheese, low fat, 1 %	1 oz	3.5
Cheez Whiz, pasteurized process	1 oz	3.4
Cottage cheese, low fat, 2 %	1 oz	3.3
Ricotta cheese whole milk	1 oz	3.2
Ricotta cheese, part skim milk	1 oz	3.2
Cottage cheese, creamed, large & small curd	1 oz	3.1
Cottage cheese, non fat, uncreamed	1 oz	2.9
Cream cheese	1 oz	1.7
American, pasteurized process, imitation	1 oz	1.2

Chicken, Cooked	Amount	Protein (g)
Breast, fried with flour	1/2 breast	31.2
Breast, roasted	1/2 breast	29.0
Breast, no skin, roasted	1/2 breast	26.7
Thigh, with skin, fried	1 thigh	18.6
Thigh, no skin, roasted	1 thigh	13.5
Drumstick, fried in flower	1 drumstick	13.2
Drumstick, no skin, roasted	1 drumstick	12.5
Wing with skin, fried in batter	1 wing	10.0
Wing with skin, roasted	1 wing	9.0

Chicken, Cooked	Amount	Protein (g)
Breast with skin, fried in flour	3 oz	27.1
Breast meat only, no skin, roasted	3 oz	26.4
Wing meat only, no skin, roasted	3 oz	25.9
Breast with skin, roasted	3 oz	25.3
Drumstick with skin, fried in flour	3 oz	22.9
Wing with skin, roasted	3 oz	22.8
Wing with skin, fried in flour	3 oz	22.2
Thigh with skin, fried in flour	3 oz	22.7
Thigh meat only, no skin, roasted	3 oz	20.4
Drumstick meat only, no skin, roasted	3 oz	19.9
Cornish game hens, meat only	3 oz	19.8
Drumstick with skin, roasted	3 oz	19.2
Thigh with skin, roasted	3 oz	19.2

CHILI

Chili, Amy's Organic	Amount	Protein (g)
Light in Sodium Medium Chili	1 can	30
Light in Sodium Spicy Chili	1 can	30
Medium Chili	1 can	30
Spicy Chili	1 can	30

PROTEIN

Continued

Black Bean Chili	1 can	26
Southwestern Black Bean Chili	1 can	24
Medium Chili with Vegetables	1 can	20

Chili, Campbell's® Chunky	Amount	Protein (g)
Beef Chili no Beans	1 can	44
Chili with Beans Roadhouse	1 can	32
Chili with Beans Firehouse	1 can	32
Chili with Beans Grilled Steak	1 can	32

Chili, Cattle Drive®	Amount	Protein (g)
Cattle Drive Golden Chili with beans	1 can	40

Chili, Dennison®	Amount	Protein (g)
Hot Chili Con Carne with Beans	1 can	41
Chili Con Carne with Beans	1 can	40
Original Chili Con Carne with Beans	1 can	40
Chunky Chili Con Carne with Beans	1 can	40
Hot & Chunky Chili with Beans	1 can	40
Turkey Chili with Beans	1 can	32
Vegetarian Chili with Beans	1 can	18

Chili, Eden Organic	Amount	Protein (g)
Kidney Bean & Kamut Chili	1 can	28
Pinto Bean & Spelt Chili	1 can	22
Black Bean & Quinoa Chili	1 can	20
Great Northern Bean & Barley Chili	1 can	18

Chili, Hardy Jack's	Amount	Protein (g)
Chili with beans	1 can	24
Chili no beans	1 can	22

Chili, Healthy Valley	Amount	Protein (g)
Black Bean Mole Chili	1 can	22
Three Bean Chipotle Chili	1 can	22
No salt Added Tame Tomato Chili	1 can	20
Santa Fe White Bean Chili	1 can	20
Spicy Tomato Chili	1 can	20
Black Bean Mango Chili	1 can	18

PROTEIN

Chili, Hormel®	Amount	Protein (g)
Turkey Chili no Beans	1 can	46
Cook- off White Chicken Chili	1 can	38
Turkey Chili with Beans	1 can	34
Cook-off Chipotle Chicken Chili	1 can	34
Chili with Beans	1 can	32
Chili no Beans	1 can	32
Chunky Chili with Beans	1 can	32
Hot Chili with beans	1 can	32
Less Sodium Chili no Beans	1 can	32
Less Sodium Chili with Beans	1 can	32
Cook-off Roasted Tomato Chili	1 can	28
Vegetarian Chili & Beans 99% Fat Free	1 can	22

Chili, Nalley's®	Amount	Protein (g)
Thick Chili with beans	1 can	34
Original Chili with beans	1 can	34
Jalapeno Hot Chili with beans	1 can	34
Turkey Chili with beans	1 can	32

Chili, Stagg®	Amount	Protein (g)
Turkey Ranchero Chili with Beans	1 can	44
Laredo Chili with Beans, and Jalapno	1 can	36
Classi Chili with beans	1 can	34
Silverado Beef Chili with Beans	1 can	34
Steak House Chili no Beans	1 can	34
Ranch House Chicken Chili with Beans	1 can	34
White Chicken Chili with Beans	1 can	34
Dynamite Hot Chili with Beans	1 can	34
Chunkero Chili with Beans	1 can	32
Country Brand Chili with Beans	1 can	30
Country Brand Chili & Sweet Peppers	1 can	30
Fiesta Grille Chili with Beans	1 can	30
Vegetarian Garden Four Bean Chili	1 can	20

Chili, Wolf Brand	Amount	Protein (g)
Turkey Chili no Beans	1 can	48
Lean Beaf no Beans	1 can	46
Turkey Chili with Beans	1 can	46
Lean Beaf with Beans	1 can	40
Chili no Beans	1 can	38
Hot Chili no Beans	1 can	38

PROTEIN

Continued

Chili with Beans	1 can	36
Homestyle Chili with Beans	1 can	30
Spicy Chili with Beans	1 can	26

Cream	Amount	Protein (g)
Half & Half	1 tbsp	0.44
Sour Cream, reduced fat	1 tbsp	0.44
Light Coffe cream	1 tbsp	0.41
Heavy Cream	1 tbsp	0.31
Sour Cream, cultured	1 tbsp	0.25
Whipped Topping, pressurized	1 tbsp	0.10

Eggs	Amount	Protein (g)
Egg whites, dried	1 ounce	22.90
Egg whole, hard-boiled	1 large	6.29
Egg whole, fried	1 large	6.26
Egg whole, poached	1 large	6.26
Egg whole, scrambled	1 large	6.09
Egg substitute, liquid, fat free	1/4 cup	6.00
Egg whites, dried powder, stabilized	1 tbsp	5.77
Egg whites, raw	1 large	3.64
Egg yolk	1 large	2.63

FISH

Fish, Canned	Amount	Protein (g)
Light tuna, in oil	3 oz	24.9
European anchovy, in oil	3 oz	24.6
White (albacore) tuna, in oil	3 oz	22.6
Atlantic sardines, in oil	3 oz	20.9
White (albacore) tuna, in water	3 oz	20.1
Atlantic cod	3 oz	19.4
Pacific sardines, in tomato sauce	3 oz	17.7
Sockeye salmon	3 oz	17.4
Pink salmon	3 oz	16.8
Light tuna, in water	3 oz	16.5

Fish, Cooked	Amount	Protein (g)
Bluefin tuna	3 oz	25
Yellowtail	3 oz	25
Yellowfin tuna	3 oz	25
Skipjack (aku) tuna	3 oz	24
Snapper	3 oz	22

PROTEIN

Continued

Tilapia	3 oz	22
King mackerel	3 oz	22
Keta (chum) salmon	3 oz	22
Pacific & Jack mackerel	3 oz	22
Chinook salmon	3 oz	22
Atlantic salmon, wild	3 oz	22
Sockeye salmon	3 oz	22
Atlantic pollock	3 oz	21
Grouper	3 oz	21
Sea bass	3 oz	21
Northern pike	3 oz	21
Pink salmon	3 oz	21
Walleye pike	3 oz	21
Coho salmon, farmed	3 oz	21
Freshwater bass	3 oz	21
Atlantic mackerel	3 oz	20
Rainbow trout, farmed	3 oz	20
Florida pompano	3 oz	20
Spanish mackerel	3 oz	20
Walleye pollock	3 oz	20
Whiting	3 oz	20
Coho salmon, wild	3 oz	20
Swordfish	3 oz	20
Rainbow trout, wild	3 oz	19
Carp	3 oz	19
Atlantic cod	3 oz	19
Striped bass	3 oz	19
Orange roughy	3 oz	19
Halibut, Atlantic & Pacific	3 oz	19
Halibut, Alaskan	3 oz	19
Atlantic salmon, farmed	3 oz	19
Haddock	3 oz	17
Pacific cod	3 oz	16
Atlantic perch	3 oz	16
Catfish, wild	3 oz	16
Catfish, farmed	3 oz	16
Halibut, Greenland	3 oz	16
Chinook salmon, smoked	3 oz	16
Atlantic croaker	3 oz	15
Catfish, breaded & fried	3 oz	15
Flounder & Sole	3 oz	13
Atlantic herring, pickeled	3 oz	12

PROTEIN

Fish, Shellfish, Cooked	Amount	Protein (g)
Octopus	3 oz	25.4
Clams, canned	3 oz	20.6
Queen crab	3 oz	20.2
Shrimp	3 oz	19.4
Shrimp, breaded & fried	3 oz	18.2
Scallops, bay & sea, steamed	3 oz	17.5
Shrimp, canned	3 oz	17.4
Blue crab cakes	3 oz	17.2
Abalone	3 oz	16.7
Alaskan king crab	3 oz	16.5
Northern lobster	3 oz	16.2
Scallops, breaded & fried	3 oz	15.4
Squid, fried	3 oz	15.3
Blue crab	3 oz	15.2
Blue crab, canned	3 oz	15.2
Crayfish	3 oz	14.3
Clams, breaded & fried	3 oz	12.1
Eastern oysters, wild	3 oz	7.5
Oysters, breaded & fried	3 oz	7.5
Alaskan king crab, imitation	3 oz	6.5
Eastern oysters, farmed	3 oz	6.0

FRUIT

Fruit, Canned	Amount	Protein (g)
Apricoit	1 cup	1.37
Peaches	1 cup	1.18
Plums	1 cup	0.93
Pineapple	1 cup	0.89
Pears,	1 cup	0.53
Applesauce, sweetened	1 cup	0.41
Applesauce, unsweetened	1 cup	0.41
Olives, black	5 large	0.18
Olives, green	5 large	0.14

Fruit, Dried	Amount	Protein (g)
Currants	1 cup	5.88
Peaches	1 cup	5.78
Figs	1 cup	4.92
Apricots	1 cup	4.41
Pears	1 cup	3.37
Apples	1 cup	0.80
Cranberries	1 cup	0.08

PROTEIN

Fruit, Frozen	Amount	Protein (g)
Blackberries, unthawed	1 cup	1.78
Raspberries	1 cup	1.75
Peaches	1 cup	1.58
Strawberries	1 cup	1.35
Blueberries	1 cup	0.92

Fruit, Raw	Amount	Protein (g)
Avocado, Florida, pureed	1 cup	5.13
Avocado, California, pureed	1 cup	4.51
Raisins	1 cup	4.45
Prunes, uncooked	1 cup	3.79
Dates	1 cup	3.60
Pomegranates	1 cup	2.91
Stewed prunes	1 cup	2.38
Apricots	1 cup	2.31
Kiwi	1 cup	2.05
Blackberries	1 cup	2.00
Plantains	1 cup	1.92
Grapefruit, pink & red, sections	1 cup	1.77
Valencias oranges	1 cup	1.69
Cherries, pitted	1 cup	1.63
Sweet cheeries	1 cup	1.63
Tangerine, sections	1 cup	1.58
Black curramts	1 cup	1.57
Nectarines	1 cup	1.52
Naval oranges, sections	1 cup	1.50
Raspberries	1 cup	1.48
Sweet cheeries	1 cup	1.46
Pummelo, sections	1 cup	1.44
Peachs, slices	1 cup	1.40
Mango	1 cup	1.35
Cataloupe	1 cup	1.34
Florida oranges	1 cup	1.30
Grapes, red & green	1 cup	1.15
Plums, sliced	1 cup	1.15
Strawberries	1 cup	1.11
Chayote, 1" pieces	1 cup	1.08
Blueberries	1 cup	1.07
Water mellon	1 cup	0.98
Elderberries	1 cup	0.96
Jicama	1 cup	0.94
Honeydew	1 cup	0.92
Pineapple	1 cup	0.89
Papayas	1 cup	0.68

PROTEIN

Pears	1 cup	0.61
Cranberries	1 cup	0.39
Apples	1 cup	0.32

Fruit, Raw	Amount	Protein (g)
Avocado, Florida	1 fruit	6.78
Pomegranates	1 fruit	4.71
Cherimoya	1 fruit	3.69
Cantaloupe	1/2 fruit	3.44
Avocado, California	1 fruit	2.67
Plantains	1 fruit	2.33
Chayote	1 fruit	1.66
Nectarine	1 fruit	1.44
Bananas	1 fruit	1.29
Naval Oranges	1 fruit	1.27
Valencias oranges	1 fruit	1.26
Prunes, uncooked	5 fruit	1.04
Dates	5 fruit	1.02
Florida oranges	1 fruit	0.99
Persimmons, Japanese	1 fruit	0.97
Grapefruit, pink or red	1/2 fruit	0.95
Star fruit, Carambola	1 fruit	0.95
Star fruit, Carambola	1 fruit	0.95
Peaches	1 fruit	0.89
Kiwi	1 fruit	0.87
Sweet Cherries	10 fruit	0.87
Tangerine	1 fruit	0.68
Pears	1 fruit	0.56
Apricots	1 fruit	0.49
Plums	1 fruit	0.46
Raisins	1 packet	0.43
Pineapple guava, Feijoa	1 fruit	0.41
Strawberries	5 fruit	0.40
Apples	1 fruit	0.36
Kumquats	1 fruit	0.36
Figs, dried	1 fruit	0.28
Pineapple	1/2" x 3" slice	0.27
Persimmons, small natives	1 fruit	0.20

Game Meat, Cooked	Amount	Protein (g)
Rabbit	3 oz	28.1
Buffalo, steak, free range	3 oz	27.6
Squirrel	3 oz	26.2
Deer	3 oz	25.7
Elk	3 oz	25.7

PROTEIN

Continued

Caribou	3 oz	25.3
Antelope	3 oz	25.0
Wild boar	3 oz	24.1
Elk, ground	3 oz	22.6
Deer, ground	3 oz	22.5
Bison, ground	3 oz	20.2
Duck	3 oz	20.0

Grains, Cooked	Amount	Protein (g)
Kamut	1 cup	11
Spelt	1 cup	11
Amaranth	1 cup	9
Egg & Spinach noodles	1 cup	8
Macaroni	1 cup	8
Quinoa	1 cup	8
Spaghetti	1 cup	8
Egg noodles	1 cup	7
Oat bran	1 cup	7
Whole-Wheat macaroni	1 cup	7
Whole-Wheat spaghetti	1 cup	7
Wild rice	1 cup	7
Buckwheat	1 cup	6
Bulgur	1 cup	6
Couscous	1 cup	6
Millet	1 cup	6
Soba noodles	1 cup	6
Spinach spaghetti	1 cup	6
Brown rice	1 cup	5
Barley, pearled	1 cup	4
White rice, long-grain, regular	1 cup	4.3
White rice, long grain, instant	1 cup	3.6
Barley, pearled	1 cup	3.6
Rice noodles	1 cup	1.6

Herbs & Spices	Amount	Protein (g)
Garlic powder	1 tsp	0.51
Caraway seeds	1 tsp	0.42
Anise seed	1 tsp	0.37
Celery seeds	1 tsp	0.36
Chili powder	1 tsp	0.36
Tarragon, dried, ground	1 tsp	0.36
Parsley, dried	1 tsp	0.35
Basil, dried & ground	1 tsp	0.32
Paprika	1 tsp	0.30
Curry powder	1 tsp	0.25

PROTEIN

Continued

Coriander, seeds	1 tsp	0.22
Onion powder	1 tsp	0.22
Pepper, black	1 tsp	0.22
Dill weed, dried	1 tsp	0.20
Ginger, ground	1 tsp	0.20
Turmeric, ground	1 tsp	0.20
Chervil, dried	1 tsp	0.14
Oregano	1 tsp	0.14
Cloves, ground	1 tsp	0.13
Coriander, dried leafs	1 tsp	0.13
Thyme, dried, ground	1 tsp	0.13
All-spice, ground	1 tsp	0.12
Thyme, fresh	1 tsp	0.10
Cinnamon, ground	1 tsp	0.09
Saffron	1 tsp	0.08
Capers, canned	1 tsp	0.07
Sage, ground	1 tsp	0.07
Rosemary, dried	1 tsp	0.06
Bay leaf, crumbled	1 tsp	0.05
Basil, fresh, chopped	1 tsp	0.03
Chives, raw, chopped	1 tsp	0.03
Rosemary, fresh	1 tsp	0.02

Juice	Amount	Protein (g)
Carrot	1 cup	2.24
Tomato	1 cup	1.85
Grapefruit juice, raw	1 cup	1.77
Orange, raw	1 cup	1.74
Prune	1 cup	1.56
Vegetable	1 cup	1.52
Grape	1 cup	0.94
Pineapple	1 cup	0.90
Lemon juice, raw	1 cup	0.85
Pomegranate	1 cup	0.37
Apple	1 cup	0.25
Cranberry	1 cup	0

Lamb, Cooked	Amount	Protein (g)
Loin chops, lean, trim to 1/4" fat	3 oz	25.5
Foreshank, trim to 1/8" fat	3 oz	24.1
Cubed, lean, for stew or kabob	3 oz	23.9
Rib, lean, trim to 1/4" fat	3 oz	23.6
Leg, whole, trim to 1/4" fat	3 oz	21.7
Ground	3 oz	21.0

PROTEIN

Milk	Amount	Protein (g)
Canned, condensed, sweetened	1 cup	24.2
Canned, evaporated, non fat	1 cup	19.3
Canned, evaporated	1 cup	17.2
Sheep milk	1 cup	14.7
Goat milk	1 cup	8.7
Whole milk, dry powder	1 cup	8.4
Non fat, fat free or skim liquid milk	1 cup	8.3
Lowfat, 1%	1 cup	8.2
Buttermilk, low fat	1 cup	8.1
Dry, instant, nonfat	1/3 cup	8.1
Reduced fat, 2%	1 cup	8.1
Soy milk, original, unfortified	1 cup	8.0
Buttermilk, whole milk	1 cup	7.9
Whole milk, liquid, 3.25%	1 cup	7.7
Coconut milk, canned	1 cup	4.6
Human milk	1 cup	2.2

Nuts & Seeds	Amount	Protein (g)
Peanuts	1 oz	9.42
Pumpkin seeds	1 oz	8.57
Peanut butter, smooth style	1 oz	7.11
Black walnuts	1 oz	6.82
Almonds	1 oz	6.02
Sunflower seeds	1 oz	5.89
Pistachio	1 oz	5.75
Flaxseed	1 oz	5.19
Cashews	1 oz	5.17
Sesame seeds	1 oz	5.03
Mixed nuts, roasted with peanuts, no salt	1 oz	4.90
Tahini	1 oz	4.82
Chia seeds	1 oz	4.69
English walnuts	1 oz	4.32
Hazelnuts	1 oz	4.24
Brazilnuts	1 oz	4.06
Trail mix, regular with chocolate chips	1 oz	4.03
Trail mix, regular, salted	1 oz	3.91
Pine nuts	1 oz	3.88
Pecans	1 oz	2.60
Macadamia	1 oz	2.24
Trail mix, tropical	1 oz	1.79
Coconut, raw meat	1 oz	0.94

PROTEIN

Pork, Cooked	Amount	Protein (g)
Sirloin chops	3 oz	44.8
Bacon, pan-fried	3 oz	31.5
Pork chops, lean, pan-fried	3 oz	25.1
Spareribs	3 oz	24.7
Pork chops, pan-fried	3 oz	23.5
Tenderloin	3 oz	22.1
Ground pork	3 oz	21.8
Center loin chops	3 oz	21.8
Pork chops, broiled	3 oz	21.8
Cured ham, lean	3 oz	21.3
Canadian-style bacon	3 oz	20.6
Backribs	3 oz	19.6
Cured ham	3 oz	18.3
Sausage	3 oz	16.5
Italian sausage	3 oz	16.3
Braunschweiger	3 oz	12.3
Polish sausage	3 oz	12.0
Bratwurst	3 oz	11.7
Bacon, pan-fried	3 slices	7.0
Liverwurst spread	1/4 cup	6.8
Sausage	1 patty	5.3
Sausage	2 links	5.1

Tofu	Amount	Protein (g)
House Foods Premium Firm	3 oz	8.4
House Foods Premium Soft	3 oz	5.0
Mori-Nu, Silken, Extra Firm	3 oz	6.2
Mori-Nu, Silken, Firm	3 oz	5.8
Mori-Nu, Silken, Lite Extra Firm	3 oz	5.8
Mori-Nu, Silken, Lite Firm	3 oz	5.3

Turkey, Cooked	Amount	Protein (g)
Light meat	3 oz	25.6
Breast meat	3 oz	25.6
Turkey bacon	3 oz	25.2
Ground turkey, fat free	3 oz	24.6
Dark meat	3 oz	23.6
Ground turkey	3 oz	23.3
Ground turkey, 85% lean	3 oz	22.0
Ground turkey, 93% lean	3 oz	22.0
Turkey sausage, reduced fat	3 oz	14.5

PROTEIN

Veal, Cooked	Amount	Protein (g)
Leg, top round	3 oz	30.7
Foreshank	3 oz	26.8
Breast	3 oz	25.8
Sirloin	3 oz	21.4
Loin	3 oz	21.1
Ground	3 oz	20.7
Rib	3 oz	20.4
Cubed for stew	3 oz	17.2

VEGETABLES

Vegetables, Canned	Amount	Protein (g)
Tomato paste	1 cup	11.3
Green peas	1 cup	7.6
Spinach	1 cup	6.0
Asparagus	1 cup	5.2
Corn	1 cup	5.1
Tomato pure	1 cup	4.1
Tomato sauce	1 cup	3.2
Mushrooms	1 cup	2.9
Pumpkin	1 cup	2.7
Sweet potato	1 cup	2.5
Stewed tomatos	1 cup	2.3
Sauerkraut	1 cup	2.2
Tomatoes	1 cup	1.9
Green beans	1 cup	1.6
Beets	1 cup	1.6
Carrots	1 cup	0.9

Vegetables, Cooked	Amount	Protein (g)
Split peas	1 cup	16.4
Yardlong beans	1 cup	14.2
Spinach	1 cup	5.4
Snow peas	1 cup	5.2
Hubbard squash	1 cup	5.1
Corn	1 cup	5.1
Artichokes	1 cup	4.9
Sweet potato, mashed	1 cup	4.5
Asparagus	1 cup	4.3
Collard greens	1 cup	4.0
Potatoes, mashed with whole milk	1 cup	4.0
Brussels sprouts	1 cup	4.0
Broccoli	1 cup	3.7

PROTEIN

Continued

Beet greens	1 cup	3.7
White mushrooms	1 cup	3.4
Swiss chard	1 cup	3.3
Broccoli raab	1 cup	3.3
Mustard greens	1 cup	3.2
Okra	1 cup	3.0
Kohlrabi	1 cup	3.0
Onions	1 cup	2.9
Bok-Choy	1 cup	2.7
Kale	1 cup	2.5
Potatoes, flesh	1 cup	2.4
Green beans	1 cup	2.4
Acorn squash, baked, cubes	1 cup	2.3
Cauliflower	1 cup	2.3
Tomatoes	1 cup	2.3
Shitake mushrooms	1 cup	2.3
Rutabagas	1 cup	2.2
Dandelion greens	1 cup	2.1
Parsnips	1 cup	2.1
Zucchini	1 cup	2.1
Yams, cubed	1 cup	2.0
Prickly pear cactus pad, nopales	1 cup	2.0
Cabbage	1 cup	1.9
Crookneck and Straightneck squash	1 cup	1.9
Scallop or Pattypan squash, sliced	1 cup	1.9
Butternut squash, baked, cubes	1 cup	1.8
Winter squash	1 cup	1.8
Pumpkin	1 cup	1.8
Summer squash	1 cup	1.6
Turnip greens	1 cup	1.6
Beets	1 cup	1.6
Celery	1 cup	1.3
Napa cabbage	1 cup	1.2
Carrots	1 cup	1.2
Turnips	1 cup	1.1
Broccolini	1 cup	1.0
Spaghetti squash, baked	1 cup	1.0
Leaks	1 cup	0.8
Eggplant	1 cup	0.8

Vegetables, Frozen	Amount	Protein (g)
Green peas	1 cup	8.2
Spinach	1 cup	7.6
Broccoli	1 cup	5.7
Brussels sprouts	1 cup	5.6

PROTEIN

Continued

Turnip greens	1 cup	5.5
Asparagus	1 cup	5.3
Collard greens	1 cup	5.1
Corn	1 cup	4.2
Kale	1 cup	3.7
Okra	1 cup	3.0
Butternut squash	1 cup	3.0
Cauliflower	1 cup	2.9
Green beans	1 cup	2.0
Rhubarb	1 cup	0.9
Carrots	1 cup	0.8

Vegetables, Raw	Amount	Protein (g)
Cabbage, Napa	1 cup	x
Spirulina, dried	1 tbsp	4.0
Oyster mushrooms	1 cup	2.9
Snow peas	1 cup	2.7
Broccoli	1 cup	2.5
Kale	1 cup	2.2
White mushrooms, sliced	1 cup	2.2
Cauliflower, chopped	1 cup	2.1
Green onions & scallions	1 cup	1.8
Portabella mushrooms, diced	1 cup	1.8
Chrimini mushrooms, sliced	1 cup	1.8
Onions	1 cup	1.8
Enoki mushrooms, sliced	1 cup	1.7
Tomatoes, red, chopped	1 cup	1.6
Yellow bell pepper	1 cup	1.5
Dandelion greens	1 cup	1.5
Red bell peppers, chopped	1 cup	1.5
Butternut squash, cubes	1 cup	1.4
Cabbage, Mustard	1 cup	1.4
Cabbage, Savoy	1 cup	1.4
Summer squash, sliced	1 cup	1.4
Zucchini, sliced	1 cup	1.4
Tomatoes, cherry	1 cup	1.3
Green bell peppers	1 cup	1.3
Broccoli, Raab	1 cup	1.3
Tomatillos, chopped	1 cup	1.3
Cactus pads, nopales	1 cup	1.1
Carrots	1 cup	1.1
Cabbage, Chinese, Bok-Choy	1 cup	1.1
Cabbage, Red	1 cup	1.0
Cabbage	1 cup	0.9
Cabbage, Chinese, Pe-Tsai	1 cup	0.9

PROTEIN

Continued

Spinach	1 cup	0.9
Celery	1 cup	0.8
Belgian endive	1 cup	0.8
Cabbage, Danish	1 cup	0.8
Watercress,chopped	1 cup	0.8
Butterhead, bibb or boston lettuce	1 cup	0.7
Green leaf lettuce	1 cup	0.7
Romaine lettuce	1 cup	0.7
Cucumber, slices	1 cup	0.7
Swiss chard	1 cup	0.7
Endive, chopped	1 cup	0.6
Radicchio, shredded	1 cup	0.6
Arugula	1 cup	0.5
Iceburg lettuce	1 cup	0.5
Chicory greens	1 cup	0.5
Shiitake mushrooms	1 whole	0.4
Red leaf lettuce	1 cup	0.4
Shiitake mushrooms, dried	1 each	0.3

Nutrient Data Collection Form

Food	Amount	Book Numbers	Multiply By	Estimated Nutrient Intake
Nutrient::	RDA:	Estimated:	% of RDA:	Total Estimated:

To download additional forms for free, go to www.TopNutrients4U.com

% OF TOTAL CALORIES FROM PROTEIN

Alcohol	Amount	% of Total Calories from Protein
Beer, regular all types	1 bottle	4
Beer, light all types	1 bottle	3
Red Wine	1 glass	0
White Wine	1 glass	0
Gin, Rum, Vodka, Whisky	1 shot	0

Beans, Canned	Amount	% of Total Calories from Protein
Fava beans	1 cup	31
Navy beans	1 cup	27
Cranberry beans	1 cup	26
Yellow beans	1 cup	26
Great Northern	1 cup	25
Kidney bean	1 cup	25
Lima beans	1 cup	25
White beans, mature	1 cup	25
Black-eyed peas	1 cup	24
Refried beans	1 cup	24
Garbanzo beans	1 cup	23
Pinto beans	1 cup	22
Green beans	1 cup	21
Baked beans, plain	1 cup	20

Beans, Cooked	Amount	% of Total Calories from Protein
Lupini beans	1 cup	53
Soybeans, mature, dry roasted	1 cup	50
Soybeans, mature	1 cup	46
Edamame	1 cup	36
Black Turtle beans, mature	1 cup	33
Natto	1 cup	33
Lentils	1 cup	31
Great Northern	1 cup	29
Cranberry beans	1 cup	28
Fava beans	1 cup	28
Hyacinath beans	1 cup	28
Lima beans	1 cup	28
Split peas	1 cup	28
Winged beans	1 cup	28
Yardlong beans, Chinese long beans	1 cup	28
Kidney beans	1 cup	27
White beans, mature	1 cup	27

% OF TOTAL CALORIES FROM PROTEIN

Continued

Black beans	1 cup	26
Black-eyed peas	1 cup	26
Mothbeans	1 cup	26
Mung beans, mature seeds	1 cup	26
Pinto beans	1 cup	25
White beans, small	1 cup	25
Navy beans	1 cup	24
Adzuki	1 cup	23
Garbanzo beans	1 cup	22
Pigeon peas	1 cup	22
Soybeans, green	1 cup	21
Green beans	1 cup	19
Yellow beans	1 cup	18

Beef, Cooked	Amount	% of Total Calories from Protein
Top sirloin, trimmed to 1/8" fat	3 oz	66
Brisket, lean, trimmed to 0" fat	3 oz	64
Flank steak, lean, trimmed to 0" fat	3 oz	61
Ground beef, 95%	3 oz	61
Filet Mignon, trimmed to 0" fat	3 oz	50
Ground beef, 90%	3 oz	49
Skirt steak, trimmed to 0" fat	3 oz	48
Ground beef, 85%	3 oz	41
Ribeye steak, boneless, trim to 0" fat	3 oz	41
T-bone steak, trimmed to 0" fat	3 oz	40
Ground beef, 80%	3 oz	38
Ground beef, 75%	3 oz	37
Porterhouse steak, trimmed to 0" fat	3 oz	34
Chuck roast, trimmed to 1/8" fat	3 oz	29
Beef ribs, trimmed to 1/8" fat	3 oz	26

Bread, Baked	Amount	% of Total Calories from Protein
Whole-Wheat	1 slice	21
Multi-Grain, or Whole-Grain	1 slice	20
Potato bread	1 slice	19
Reduced calorie wheat	1 slice	19
Potato bread	1 slice	19
Bagel, oat bran	4" bagel	17
Bagel, plain	4" bagel	16
Bagel, wheat	4" bagel	16
English Muffin, plain	1 muffin	16
French and Sourdough	1 slice	16
Wheat bread	1 slice	16

% OF TOTAL CALORIES FROM PROTEIN

Continued

Bagel, egg	4" bagel	15
Bagel, cinnamon & raisins	4" bagel	14
Cracked Wheat	1 slice	14
Dinner Rolls, brown & serve	1 roll	14
Hamburger & Hotdog buns, plain	1 bun	14
Pumpernickle	1 slice	14
Egg bread	1 slice	13
Kaiser rolls	1 roll	13
Oatmeal bread	1 slice	13
Pita, white	6" pita	13
Rye bread	1 slice	13
Raisen bread	1 slice	12
White bread	1 slice	12
Tortillas, corn	1 tortilla	11
Tortillas, flour	1 tortilla	11
Cornbread, drymix	1 piece	9
Croissants, butter	1 medium	8
Italian, medium slice	1 slice	3

Cereal, Arrowhead Mills	Amount	% of Total Calories from Protein
Shredded Wheat, Bite-Size	1 cup	16
Oat Bran Flakes	1 cup	14
Kamut Flakes	1 cup	13
Spelt Flakes	1 cup	13
Sprouted Multigrain Flakes	1 cup	13
Amaranth Flakes	1 cup	11
Sweetened Shredded Wheat	1 cup	10
Maple Buckwheat Flakes	1 cup	9
Sweetened Rice Flakes	1 cup	7

Cereal, Barbara's	Amount	% of Total Calories from Protein
Hole 'n Oats: Fruit Juice Sweetened	1 cup	13
Puffins Peanut Butter	1 cup	13
Shredded Oats Vanilla Almond	1 cup	13
Shredded Spoonfuls Multigrain	1 cup	13
High Fiber Cranberry	1 cup	11
High Fiber Original	1 cup	11
Shredded Minis Blueberry Burst	1 cup	11
Shredded Oats Original	1 cup	11
Shredded Wheat	2 biscuits	11
High Fiber Flax & Granola	1 cup	10
Hole 'n Oats Honey Nut	1 cup	10
Puffins Original	1 cup	10

% OF TOTAL CALORIES FROM PROTEIN

Continued

Shredded Oats Cinnamon Crunch	1 cup	10
Puffins Cinnamon	1 cup	9
Brown Rice Crisps	1 cup	8
Corn Flakes	1 cup	8
Puffins Honey Rice	1 cup	8
Puffins Multigrain	1 cup	8
Puffins Peanut Butter & Chocolate	1 cup	8
Puffins Puffs Crunchy Cocoa	1 cup	8
Puffins Puffs Fruit Medley	1 cup	8

Cereal, Bear Naked®	Amount	% of Total Calories from Protein
Peak Protein, Original Granola	1 cup	17
Vanila Almond Crucnh Granola	1 cup	13
Nut Cluster Crunch Cereal	1 cup	10
Banana Nut Granola	1 cup	9
Fruit & Nut Ganola	1 cup	9

Cereal, Cadia	Amount	% of Total Calories from Protein
Crunch	1 cup	19
Honey Kissed Cadi-O's	1 cup	11
Whole Grain Cadi-O's Toasted Oats	1 cup	11
All Natural Raisin Bran	1 cup	8

Cereal, Cascadian Farms	Amount	% of Total Calories from Protein
Hearty Morning	1 cup	11
Multi Grain Squares	1 cup	11
Purely O's	1 cup	11
Maple Brown Sugar Granola	1 cup	10
Chocolate O's	1 cup	9
Fruit Ful O's	1 cup	8
Cinnamon Crunch	1 cup	7
Dark Chocolate Almond Granola	1 cup	7
French Vanilla Almond Granola	1 cup	7
Fruit & Nut Granola	1 cup	7
Honey Nut O's	1 cup	7
Cinnamon Raisin Granola	1 cup	5
Oats & Honey Granola	1 cup	5
Raisin bran	1 cup	4

% OF TOTAL CALORIES FROM PROTEIN

Cereal, Erewhon Organic	Amount	% of Total Calories from Protein
Raisin Bran	1 cup	14
Corn Flakes	1 cup	9
Crispy Brown Rice, Strawberry Crisp	1 cup	8
Rice Twice	1 cup	8
Crispy Brown Rice, Gluten Free	1 cup	7
Crispy Brown Rice, Mixed Berries	1 cup	7
Crispy Brown Rice, Original	1 cup	7
Cocoa Crispy Brown Rice	1 cup	6

Cereal, Ezekiel	Amount	% of Total Calories from Protein
Sprouted Grain Golden Flax, 4:9	1 cup	17
Sprouted Grain Almond, 4:9	1 cup	17
Sprouted Grain Original, 4:9	1 cup	16
Sprouted Grain Cinnamon Flax, 4:9	1 cup	16

Cereal, General Mills®	Amount	% of Total Calories from Protein
Multi-Bran CHEX	1 cup	15
Wheat Chex	1 cup	13
Wheaties	1 cup	11
Oatmeal Crisp, Crunchy Almond	1 cup	9
Kix	1 cup	9
Total Whole Grain	1 cup	9
Raisin Nut Bran	1 cup	8
Rice Chex	1 cup	8
Basic 4	1 cup	8
Total Cranberry Crunch	1 cup	8
Honey Nut Clusters	1 cup	8
Oatmeal Crisp, Apple Cinnamon	1 cup	8
Golden Grams	1 cup	8
Honey Nut Chex	1 cup	8
Reese's Puffs	1 cup	7
Total Raisin Bran	1 cup	7
Berry Berry Kix	1 cup	7
Corn Chex	1 cup	7
Lucky Charms	1 cup	7
Dora The Explorer	1 cup	6
Chocolate Chex	1 cup	5
Cinnamon Chex	1 cup	5
Cocoa Puffs	1 cup	5
Trix	1 cup	5

% OF TOTAL CALORIES FROM PROTEIN

Continued

Cookie Crisp	1 cup	4
Cinnamon Toast Crunch	1 cup	4

Cereal, General Mills Cheerios®	Amount	% of Total Calories from Protein
Original	1 cup	13
Crunch, Oat Clusters	1 cup	9
Berry Burst	1 cup	8
Dulce de leche	1 cup	8
Yogurt Burst, Strawberry	1 cup	8
Frosted	1 cup	7
Honey Nut	1 cup	7
Cinnamon Burst	1 cup	7
Multi Grain	1 cup	7
Multi Grain Peanut Butter	1 cup	7
Apple Cinnamon	1 cup	7
Chocolate	1 cup	6
Banana Nut	1 cup	6
Fruity	1 cup	4

Cereal, General Mills Fiber One®	Amount	% of Total Calories from Protein
Original	1 cup	13
Frosted Shredded Wheat	1 cup	10
Nuty Clusters & Almond	1 cup	9
Honey Clusters	1 cup	8
Caramel Delight	1 cup	7
Raisin Bran Clusters	1 cup	7
80 Calorie Honey Squares	1 cup	5

Cereal, Glutino® Gluten Free	Amount	% of Total Calories from Protein
Corn Rice Flakes	1 cup	7
Berry Sensible Beginning	1 cup	7
Frosted Corn & Rice Flakes	1 cup	7
Corn Rice Flakes with Strawberries	1 cup	7
Honey Nut Cereal	1 cup	3
Apple & Cinnamon Rings	1 cup	3

Cereal, Health Valley	Amount	% of Total Calories from Protein
Heart Wise	1 cup	22
Fiber 7	1 cup	15
Golden Flax	1 cup	13

% OF TOTAL CALORIES FROM PROTEIN

Continued

Oat Bran Almond Crunch	1 cup	12
Amaranth Flakes	1 cup	12
Low Fat Date, Almond Flavor Granola	1 cup	11
Low Fat Raisin Cinnamon Granola	1 cup	11
Oat Bran Flakes	1 cup	11
Multigrain Maple, Honey, Nut Squares	1 cup	10
Oat Bran Flakes & Raisins	1 cup	10
Multigrain Apple Cinnamon Squares	1 cup	10
Rice Crunch-EMS	1 cup	9
Cranberry Crunch	1 cup	8
Corn Crunch-EMS	1 cup	7

Cereal, Kashi®	Amount	% of Total Calories from Protein
Go Lean	1 cup	38
Go Lean Crunch	1 cup	20
Go Lean Crisp, Toasted Berry Crumble	1 cup	20
7-Whole Grain Puffs	1 cup	19
Go Lean Crunch, Honey Almond Flax	1 cup	17
Heart to Heart, Warm Cinnamon	1 cup	15
Organic Promise, Autumn Wheat	1 cup	14
7-Whole Grain Nuggets	1 cup	14
Heart to Heart, Honey Toasted Oat	1 cup	14
Cinnamon Harvest	1 cup	13
Good Friends	1 cup	13
7-Whole Grain Flakes	1 cup	13
Golden Goodness	1 cup	12
Island Vanilla	1 cup	12
7-Whole Grain Honey Puffs	1 cup	11
Heart to Heart, Wild Blueberry	1 cup	11
Granola Mountain Medley	1 cup	10
Granola Cocoa Beach	1 cup	10
Berry Blossom	1 cup	9
Honey Sunshine	1 cup	9
Strawberry Fields	1 cup	9

Cereal, Kellogg's®	Amount	% of Total Calories from Protein
All-Bran Original	1 cup	20
Low Fat Granola with Raisins	1 cup	20
Smart Start, Strong Heart, Antioxidants	1 cup	17
Smart Start, Strong Heart, Toasted Oat	1 cup	17
All-Bran Strawberry Medley	1 cup	14
All-Bran Complete Wheat Flakes	1 cup	13

% OF TOTAL CALORIES FROM PROTEIN

Continued

All-Bran Bran Buds	1 cup	11
Fiberplus Cinnamon Oat Crunch	1 cup	11
Frosted MINI-Wheats, Bite-Size	1 cup	11
Fiberplus Berry Yogurt Crunch	1 cup	10
Frosted MINI-Wheats, Big-Bite	1 cup	10
MUESLIX	1 cup	10
Raisin Bran	1 cup	10
Raisin Bran Extra	1 cup	10
Krave Chocolate	1 cup	9
Corn Flakes	1 cup	8
Crunchy Nut Golden Honey Nut Flakes	1 cup	8
Product 19	1 cup	8
Apple Jacks	1 cup	7
Berry Rice Krispies	1 cup	7
CINNABON	1 cup	7
Cracklin' Oat Bran	1 cup	7
Crispix	1 cup	7
Froot Loops	1 cup	7
Rice Krispies	1 cup	7
Simply Cinnamon Corn Flakes	1 cup	7
Crunchy Nut Roasted Nut & Honey O's	1 cup	6
Frosted Flakes	1 cup	6
Raisin Bran Crunch	1 cup	6
Cocoa Krispies	1 cup	5
Frosted Rice Krispies	1 cup	5
Honey Smacks	1 cup	5
Rice Krispies Treats	1 cup	5
Honey Crunch Corn Flakes	1 cup	4
Corn Pops	1 cup	3
Smorz	1 cup	3

Cereal, Kellogg's Special-K®	Amount	% of Total Calories from Protein
Protein Plus	1 cup	39
Original	1 cup	21
Low Fat Granola	1 cup	15
Blueberry	1 cup	8
Cinnamon Pecan	1 cup	8
Fruit & Yogurt	1 cup	8
Multigrain Oats & Honey	1 cup	8
Vanilla Almond	1 cup	8
Chocolately Delight	1 cup	7
Red Berries	1 cup	7

% OF TOTAL CALORIES FROM PROTEIN

Cereal, Mom's Best Naturals	Amount	% of Total Calories from Protein
Blue Pom Wheat Fuls	1 cup	10
Sweetened Wheat Fuls	1 cup	10
Raisin Bran	1 cup	9
Honey Ful Wheats	1 cup	7
Honey Nut Toastey O's	1 cup	7
Mallow Oats	1 cup	7
Oats & Honey Blend	1 cup	7
Crispy Cocoa Rice	1 cup	3
Honey Graham	1 cup	3
Toasted Cinnamon Squares	1 cup	3

Cereal, Nature's Path	Amount	% of Total Calories from Protein
Optimum Banana Almond	1 cup	21
Optimum Power Blueberry Cinnamon	1 cup	18
Optimum Slim Low Fat Vanilla	1 cup	18
Smart Bran	1 cup	15
Flax Plus Multibran Flakes	1 cup	14
Flax Plus Raisin Bran Flakes	1 cup	13
Organic Millet Rice	1 cup	13
Flax Plus Maple Pecan Crunch	1 cup	11
Flax Plus Pumpkin Raisin Crunch	1 cup	11
Flax Plus Redberry Crunch	1 cup	11
Heritage Flakes	1 cup	11
Heritage Heirloom Whole Grain	1 cup	11
Multigrain Oat bran	1 cup	11
OATY BITES Whole Grain	1 cup	11
Optimum Cranberry Ginger	1 cup	11
Peanut Butter Granola	1 cup	11
AGAVE Plus Granola	1 cup	10
Flax Plus Vanilla Almond Granola	1 cup	10
Heritage Crunch	1 cup	10
Mesa Sunrise, Gluten Free	1 cup	10
Flax Plus Pumpkin Flax Granola	1 cup	9
Hemp Plus Granola	1 cup	9
Acai Apple Granola	1 cup	8
Pomegran Cherry Granola	1 cup	8
Pomegran Plus Granola	1 cup	8
Crunchy Maple Sunrise, Gluten Free	1 cup	7
Crunchy Vanilla Sunrise	1 cup	7
Honeyed Corn Flakes, Gluten Free	1 cup	7
Whole O's	1 cup	7

% OF TOTAL CALORIES FROM PROTEIN

Cereal, Peace All Natural	Amount	% of Total Calories from Protein
Golden Honey Granola	1 cup	10
Wild Berry Clusters & Flakes	1 cup	10
Cherry Almond Clusters & Flakes	1 cup	9
Walnut Spice Clusters & Flakes	1 cup	9
Maple Pecan	1 cup	8
Vanilla Almond Clusters & Flakes	1 cup	8
Mango Peach Passion Clusters & Flakes	1 cup	7

Cereal, Post®	Amount	% of Total Calories from Protein
100% Bran Cereal	1 cup	18
Grape-Nuts Cereal	1 cup	14
Shredded Wheat, Original, spoon-size	1 cup	14
Shredded Wheat, Sugar and Salt Free	1 cup	13
Shredded Wheat n' Bran	1 cup	12
Grape-Nuts Flakes	1 cup	11
Raisin Bran	1 cup	11
Great Grains, Crunchy Pecan	1 cup	9
Great Grains, Raisin, Date & Pecan	1 cup	9
Honeynut Shredded Wheat	1 cup	9
Shredded Wheat, frosted, spoon-size	1 cup	9
Banana Nut Crunch	1 cup	8
Cranberry Almond Crunch	1 cup	8
Blueberry Morning	1 cup	7
Golden Crisp	1 cup	6
Cocoa Pebbles	1 cup	5
Fruity Pebbles	1 cup	5
Honeycomb Cereal	1 cup	5
OREO O's Cereal	1 cup	5

Cereal, Honey Bunches of Oats®	Amount	% of Total Calories from Protein
Just Bunches Cinnamonn	1 cup	8.4
Just Bunches Honey roasted	1 cup	8.4
Cinnamon Bunches	1 cup	7.5
Honey Roasted	1 cup	7.5
Pecan Bunches	1 cup	7.5
With Peaches	1 cup	7.5
With Strawberries	1 cup	7.5
Vanilla Bunches	1 cup	7.3
With Almonds	1 cup	6.9
Raisin Medley	1 cup	6

% OF TOTAL CALORIES FROM PROTEIN

Cereal, Uncle Sam	Amount	% of Total Calories from Protein
Flaxseed, Original	1 cup	14
Skinners Raisin Bran	1 cup	13
Flaxseed, & Strawberry	1 cup	11
Flaxseed, Honey Almond	1 cup	10

Cereal, Wild Harvest	Amount	% of Total Calories from Protein
Wholesome Raisin Bran	1 cup	11
Golden Honey & Flax Granola	1 cup	10
Wild Berry Crisp	1 cup	10
Crunchy Vanilla Almond Granola	1 cup	9
Cherry Vanilla Granola	1 cup	8
Maple Pecan Flakes & Clusters	1 cup	7
Blueberry Flax Granola	1 cup	6
Cranberry Almond	1 cup	6
Mango Crisp	1 cup	5

Cereal, Cooked	Amount	% of Total Calories from Protein
WHEATENA	1 cup	15
Oats, regular, unenriched	1 cup	14
Malt-o-Meal plain	1 serving	14
CREAM OF WHEAT, regular	1 cup	13
Farina	1 cup	12
White corn grits	1 cup	9
Yellow corn grits	1 cup	8

Cheese	Amount	% of Total Calories from Protein
Cottage cheese, low fat, 1%	1 cup	69
Cottage cheese, non fat, uncreamed	1 cup	58
Cottage cheese, low fat, 2%	1 cup	55
Cottage cheese, creamed, small curd	1 cup	49
Ricotta cheese, part skim milk	1 cup	33
Ricotta cheese, whole milk	1 cup	26

Cheese	Amount	% of Total Calories from Protein
Mozzarella, non fat	1 oz	90
Cottage cheese, low fat, 1%	1 oz	70
Swiss, low fat	1 oz	65

% OF TOTAL CALORIES FROM PROTEIN

Continued

Cream cheese, fat free	1 oz	59
Cottage cheese, non fat, uncreamed	1 oz	58
Cheddar, low fat	1 oz	56
American, pasturized process, low fat	1 oz	55
Cottage cheese, low fat, 2%	1 oz	55
Cottage cheese, creamed, large & small curd	1 oz	45
Muenster, low fat	1 oz	37
Monterey, low fat	1 oz	36
Parmesan, grated	1 oz	36
Provolone, reduced fat	1 oz	36
Mozzarella, skim milk, low moisture	1 oz	35
Ricotta cheese, part skim milk	1 oz	33
Romano	1 oz	33
Gruyere	1 oz	31
Mozzarella, whole milk	1 oz	30
Provolone	1 oz	29
Gouda	1 oz	28
Swiss	1 oz	28
Goat cheese, soft type	1 oz	28
Goat cheese, hard type	1 oz	27
Fontina	1 oz	27
Monterey	1 oz	26
Muenster	1 oz	26
Ricotta cheese whole milk	1 oz	26
Dubliner	1 oz	25
Brie	1 oz	25
Cheddar	1 oz	25
Colby	1 oz	25
Blue cheese	1 oz	24
Goat cheese, semisoft type	1 oz	24
Roquefort	1 oz	23
Pepper Jack, Red & Green Jalapenos	1 oz	22
Feta	1 oz	21
Velveeta, pasteurized process	1 oz	21
American, pasturized process, fortified, D	1 oz	20
Cheez Whiz, pasteurized process	1 oz	17
Cream cheese	1 oz	7
American, pasturized process, imitation	1 oz	6

Cheese, Mexican	Amount	% of Total Calories from Protein
Mexican, blend, reduced fat	1 oz	35
Queso seco	1 oz	30
Mexican, blend	1 oz	26
Queso asadero	1 oz	26

Continued

Queso blanco	1 oz	26
Queso freso	1 oz	24
Queso anejo	1 oz	23
Queso chihuahua	1 oz	23

Chicken, Cooked	Amount	% of Total Calories from Protein
Breast meat only, no skin, roasted	3 oz	75
Cornish game hens, meat only	3 oz	70
Drumstick meat only, no skin, roasted	3 oz	62
Breast with skin, roasted	3 oz	61
Wing meat only, no skin, roasted	3 oz	60
Breast with skin, fried in flour	3 oz	57
Thigh meat only, no skin, roasted	3 oz	54
Drumstick with skin, roasted	3 oz	49
Drumstick with skin, fried in flour	3 oz	44
Thigh with skin, fried in flour	3 oz	41
Thigh with skin, roasted	3 oz	40
Wing with skin, roasted	3 oz	37
Wing with skin, fried in flour	3 oz	33

Chili, Amy's Organic	Amount	% of Total Calories from Protein
Black Bean Chili	1 can	26
Light in Sodium Medium Chili	1 can	21
Light in Sodium Spicy Chili	1 can	21
Medium Chili	1 can	21
Spicy Chili	1 can	21
Southwestern Black Bean Chili	1 can	20
Medium Chili with Vegetables	1 can	17

Chili, Campbell's® Chunky	Amount	% of Total Calories from Protein
Beef Chili no Beans	1 can	40
Chili with Beans Firehouse	1 can	29
Chili with Beans Grilled Steak	1 can	29
Chili with Beans Roadhouse	1 can	29

Chili, Cattle Drive®	Amount	% of Total Calories from Protein
Cattle Drive Golden Chili with beans	1 can	28

% OF TOTAL CALORIES FROM PROTEIN

Chili, Dennison®	Amount	% of Total Calories from Protein
Turkey Chili with Beans	1 can	30
Chunky Chili Con Carne with Beans	1 can	27
Hot & Chunky Chili with Beans	1 can	27
Hot Chili Con Carne with Beans	1 can	23
Original Chili Con Carne with Beans	1 can	22
Vegetarian Chili with Beans	1 can	19

Chili, Eden Organic	Amount	% of Total Calories from Protein
Kidney Bean & Kamut Chili	1 can	23
Black Bean & Quinoa Chili	1 can	21
Pinto Bean & Spelt Chili	1 can	20
Great Northern Bean & Barley Chili	1 can	18

Chili, Hardy Jack's	Amount	% of Total Calories from Protein
Chili with beans	1 can	15
Chili no beans	1 can	13

Chili, Healthy Valley	Amount	% of Total Calories from Protein
Three Bean Chipotle Chili	1 can	22
Spicy Tomato Chili	1 can	21
Black Bean Mole Chili	1 can	20
Santa Fe White Bean Chili	1 can	20
No Salt Added Tame Tomato Chili	1 can	19
Black Bean Mango Chili	1 can	17

Chili, Hormel®	Amount	% of Total Calories from Protein
Turkey Chili no Beans	1 can	48
Cook-off White Chicken Chili	1 can	35
Turkey Chili with Beans	1 can	32
Chili no Beans	1 can	29
Less Sodium Chili no Beans	1 can	29
Cook-off Chipotle Chicken Chili	1 can	28
Chili with Beans	1 can	25
Chunky Chili with Beans	1 can	25
Cook-off Roasted Tomato Chili	1 can	25
Hot Chili with beans	1 can	25
Less Sodium Chili with Beans	1 can	25
Chili with Beans 99% Fat Free	1 can	23

% OF TOTAL CALORIES FROM PROTEIN

Chili, Nalley's	Amount	% of Total Calories from Protein
Turkey Chili with beans	1 can	28
Jalapeno Hot Chili with beans	1 can	26
Original Chili with beans	1 can	26
Thick Chili with beans	1 can	25

Chili, Stagg®	Amount	% of Total Calories from Protein
Turkey Ranchero Chili with Beans	1 can	37
Ranch House Chicken Chili with Beans	1 can	28
Silverado Beef Chili with Beans	1 can	27
White Chicken Chili with Beans	1 can	26
Fiesta Grille Chili with Beans	1 can	24
Laredo Chili with Beans, and Jalapno	1 can	23
Classi Chili with beans	1 can	21
Steak House Chili no Beans	1 can	21
Chunkero Chili with Beans	1 can	20
Dynamite Hot Chili with Beans	1 can	20
Vegetarian Garden Four Bean Chili	1 can	20
Country Brand Chili with Beans	1 can	19
Country Brand Chili & Sweet Peppers	1 can	18

Chili, Wolf Brand	Amount	% of Total Calories from Protein
Turkey Chili no Beans	1 can	53
Lean Beaf no Beans	1 can	44
Turkey Chili with Beans	1 can	40
Lean Beaf with Beans	1 can	32
Homestyle Chili with Beans	1 can	21
Chili with Beans	1 can	20
Chili no Beans	1 can	19
Hot Chili no Beans	1 can	19
Spicy Chili with Beans	1 can	16

Cream	Amount	% of Total Calories from Protein
Half & Half	1 tbsp	9
Sour Cream, reduced fat	1 tbsp	9
Light Coffe cream	1 tbsp	6
Whipped Topping, pressurized	1 tbsp	5
Sour Cream, cultured	1 tbsp	4
Heavy Cream	1 tbsp	2

% OF TOTAL CALORIES FROM PROTEIN

Eggs	Amount	% of Total Calories from Protein
Egg whites, dried powder, stabilized	1 tbsp	89
Egg whites	1 large	86
Egg whites, dried	1 ounce	85
Egg substitute, liquid, fat free	1/4 cup	83
Egg whole, poached	1 large	36
Egg whole, hard-boiled	1 large	33
Egg whole, fried	1 large	28
Egg whole, scrambled	1 large	27
Egg yolk	1 large	20

Fish, Canned	Amount	% of Total Calories from Protein
Light tuna, in water	3 oz	90
White (albacore) tuna, in water	3 oz	74
Light tuna, in oil	3 oz	59
White (albacore) tuna, in oil	3 oz	58
Atlantic sardines, in oil	3 oz	48

Fish, Cooked	Amount	% of Total Calories from Protein
Yellowfin tuna	3 oz	90
Haddock	3 oz	89
Northern pike	3 oz	88
Pacific cod	3 oz	88
Atlantic cod	3 oz	87
Orange roughy	3 oz	86
Skipjack (aku) tuna	3 oz	86
Atlantic pollock	3 oz	85
Walleye pollock	3 oz	85
Mahi Mahi	3 oz	84
Grouper	3 oz	84
Walleye pike	3 oz	83
Atlantic & Pacific halibut	3 oz	82
Pacific rockfish	3 oz	82
Snapper	3 oz	82
Tilapia	3 oz	81
Whiting	3 oz	81
Sea bass	3 oz	80
Alaskan halibut	3 oz	78
King mackerel	3 oz	78
Atlantic perch	3 oz	77
Striped bass	3 oz	73

% OF TOTAL CALORIES FROM PROTEIN

Continued

Catfish, wild	3 oz	71
Flounder & Sole	3 oz	71
Coho salmon, wild	3 oz	67
Keta (chum) salmon	3 oz	67
Freshwater bass	3 oz	66
Striped mullet	3 oz	66
Bluefin tuna, fresh	3 oz	65
Lox	3 oz	65
Pink salmon	3 oz	64
Chinook salmon, smoked	3 oz	63
Yellowtail	3 oz	63
Surimi	3 oz	62
Rainbow trout, wild	3 oz	61
Spanish mackerel	3 oz	60
Sockeye salmon	3 oz	58
Rainbow trout, farmed	3 oz	57
Atlantic salmon, wild	3 oz	56
Carp	3 oz	56
Coho salmon, farmed	3 oz	55
Swordfish	3 oz	54
Catfish, farmed	3 oz	51
Pacific & Jack mackerel	3 oz	51
Chinook salmon	3 oz	45
Florida pompano	3 oz	45
Atlantic salmon, farmed	3 oz	43
Atlantic mackerel	3 oz	36
Atlantic croaker	3 oz	33
Catfish, breaded & fried	3 oz	32
Greenland halibut	3 oz	31
Sablefish, smoked	3 oz	28
Atlantic herring, pickeled	3 oz	22

Fish, Shellfish, Cooked	Amount	% of Total Calories from Protein
Blue crab	3 oz	86
Blue crab, canned	3 oz	86
Northern lobster	3 oz	85
Crayfish	3 oz	82
Queen crab	3 oz	82
Shrimp, canned	3 oz	81
Alaskan king crab	3 oz	80
Shrimp	3 oz	77
Octopus	3 oz	73
Clams, canned	3 oz	69
Blue crab cakes	3 oz	52

% OF TOTAL CALORIES FROM PROTEIN

Continued

Eastern oysters, wild	3 oz	45
Abalone	3 oz	41
Squid, fried	3 oz	41
Eastern oysters, farmed	3 oz	36
Shrimp, breaded & fried	3 oz	35
Alaskan king crab, imitation	3 oz	33
Scallops, breaded & fried	3 oz	33
Clams, breaded & fried	3 oz	28
Oysters, breaded & fried	3 oz	18

Fruit, Canned	Amount	% of Total Calories from Protein
Olives, black	5 large	3
Olives, green	5 large	3
Apricoit	1 cup	3
Peaches	1 cup	2
Pineapple	1 cup	2
Applesauce, unsweetened	1 cup	2
Plums	1 cup	2
Pears,	1 cup	1
Applesauce, sweetened	1 cup	1

Fruit, Dried	Amount	% of Total Calories from Protein
Peaches	1 cup	6
Currants	1 cup	6
Apricots	1 cup	6
Figs	1 cup	5
Pears	1 cup	3
Apples	1 cup	2
Cranberries	1 cup	0.1

Fruit, Frozen	Amount	% of Total Calories from Protein
Blackberries, unthawed	1 cup	7
Peaches	1 cup	3
Raspberries	1 cup	3
Strawberries	1 cup	2
Blueberries	1 cup	2

PROTEIN

Fruit, Raw	Amount	% of Total Calories from Protein
Chayote, 1" pieces"	1 cup	17
Blackberries	1 cup	13
Apricots	1 cup	12
Cataloupe	1 cup	10
Nectarines	1 cup	10
Raspberries	1 cup	9
Black currants	1 cup	9
Peachs, slices	1 cup	9
Water mellon	1 cup	9
Strawberries	1 cup	8
Pomegranates	1 cup	8
Pomelo, sections	1 cup	8
Valencias oranges	1 cup	8
Jicama	1 cup	8
Kiwi	1 cup	8
Avocado, Florida, pureed	1 cup	7
Naval oranges, sections	1 cup	7
Sweet cheeries	1 cup	7
Grapefruit, pink & red, sections	1 cup	7
Cherries, pitted	1 cup	7
Florida oranges	1 cup	6
Plums, sliced	1 cup	6
Tangerine, sections	1 cup	6
Honeydew	1 cup	6
Sweet cheeries	1 cup	6
Mango	1 cup	5
Blueberries	1 cup	5
Avocado, California, pureed	1 cup	5
Papayas	1 cup	4
Pineapple	1 cup	4
Plantains	1 cup	4
Grapes, red & green	1 cup	4
Raisins	1 cup	4
Elderberries	1 cup	4
Prunes, uncooked	1 cup	4
Stewed prunes	1 cup	4
Dates	1 cup	4
Cranberries	1 cup	3
Pears	1 cup	3
Apples	1 cup	2

% OF TOTAL CALORIES FROM PROTEIN

Fruit, Raw	Amount	% of Total Calories from Protein
Apricots	1 fruit	12
Kumquats	1 fruit	11
Cantaloupe	1/2 fruit	10
Nectarine	1 fruit	10
Peaches	1 fruit	9
Valencias oranges	1 fruit	9
Strawberries	5 fruit	8
Pomegranates	1 fruit	8
Kiwi	1 fruit	8
Avocado, Florida	1 fruit	7
Naval oranges	1 fruit	7
Grapefruit, pink or red	1/2 fruit	7
Sweet Cherries	10 fruit	7
Plums	1 fruit	6
Florida oranges	1 fruit	6
Tangerine	1 fruit	6
Figs, dried	1 fruit	5
Banana	1 fruit	5
Avocado, California	1 fruit	5
Pineapple	1/2" x 3" slice	4
Plantains	1 fruit	4
Dates	5 fruit	4
Prunes, uncooked	5 fruit	4
Pears	1 fruit	2
Apples	1 fruit	2
Raisins	1 packet	1

Game Meat, Cooked	Amount	% of Total Calories from Protein
Buffalo, steak, frce range	3 oz	89
Elk	3 oz	83
Antelope	3 oz	78
Deer	3 oz	77
Rabbit	3 oz	76
Caribou	3 oz	71
Squirrel	3 oz	71
Wild boar	3 oz	71
Deer, ground	3 oz	57
Elk, ground	3 oz	55
Duck	3 oz	47
Bison, ground	3 oz	40

% OF TOTAL CALORIES FROM PROTEIN

Grains, Cooked	Amount	% of Total Calories from Protein
Oat bran	1 cup	32
Soba noodles	1 cup	20
Kamut	1 cup	18
Spelt	1 cup	17
Whole-Wheat spaghetti	1 cup	17
Whole-Wheat macaroni	1 cup	17
Wild rice	1 cup	16
Egg & Spinach noodles	1 cup	15
Amaranth	1 cup	15
Bulgur	1 cup	15
Buckwheat	1 cup	15
Macaroni	1 cup	15
Spaghetti	1 cup	15
Quinoa	1 cup	15
Spinach spaghetti	1 cup	14
Couscous	1 cup	14
Egg noodles	1 cup	13
Millet	1 cup	12
Brown rice	1 cup	9
White rice, long-grain, regular	1 cup	8
Barley, pearled	1 cup	7
Rice noodles	1 cup	3

Herbs & Spices	Amount	% of Total Calories from Protein
Chervil, dried	1 tsp	56
Basil, dried & ground	1 tsp	43
Capers, canned	1 tsp	40
Thyme, fresh	1 tsp	40
Tarragon, dried, ground	1 tsp	36
Parsley, dried	1 tsp	35
Dill weed, dried	1 tsp	27
Coriander, dried leafs	1 tsp	26
Caraway seeds	1 tsp	24
Anise seed	1 tsp	21
Chili powder	1 tsp	21
Garlic powder	1 tsp	20
Paprika	1 tsp	20
Celery seeds	1 tsp	18
Coriander, seeds	1 tsp	18
Pepper, black	1 tsp	18
Thyme, dried, ground	1 tsp	17
Saffron	1 tsp	16

% OF TOTAL CALORIES FROM PROTEIN

Continued

Curry powder	1 tsp	14
Oregano	1 tsp	14
Sage, ground	1 tsp	14
Ginger, ground	1 tsp	13
Onion powder	1 tsp	13
Turmeric, ground	1 tsp	11
Bay leaf, crumbled	1 tsp	10
All-spice, ground	1 tsp	10
Rosemary, fresh	1 tsp	8
Cloves, ground	1 tsp	7
Cinnamon, ground	1 tsp	6
Rosemary, dried	1 tsp	6

Juice	Amount	% of Total Calories from Protein
Tomato	1 cup	18
Vegetable	1 cup	13
Carrot	1 cup	10
Lemon juice, raw	1 cup	6
Grapefruit juice, raw	1 cup	6
Orange, raw	1 cup	6
Prune	1 cup	3
Blackberry	1 cup	3
Pineapple	1 cup	3
Grape	1 cup	3
Pomegranate	1 cup	1
Apple	1 cup	1
Cranberry	1 cup	0

Lamb, Cooked	Amount	% of Total Calories from Protein
Cubed, lean, for stew or kabob	3 oz	60
Foreshank, trimmed to 1/8" fat	3 oz	47
Rib, lean, trimmed to 1/4" fat	3 oz	47
Leg, whole, trimmed to 1/4" fat	3 oz	40
Loin chops, lean, trimmed to 1/4" fat	3 oz	38
Ground	3 oz	35

Milk	Amount	% of Total Calories from Protein
Non Fat, fat free or skim milk	1 cup	40
Canned, evaporated, non fat	1 cup	39
Dry, instant, non fat	1/3 cup	39
Buttermilk, low fat	1 cup	33

% OF TOTAL CALORIES FROM PROTEIN

Continued

Low fat milk, 1%	1 cup	32
Reduced fat, 2%	1 cup	26
Soymilk, original, unfortified	1 cup	24
Sheep milk	1 cup	22
Goat milk	1 cup	21
Whole milk, 3.25%	1 cup	21
Canned, evaporated	1 cup	20
Canned, condensed, sweet	1 cup	10
Human milk	1 cup	6
Coconut milk, canned	1 cup	4

Nuts & Seeds	Amount	% of Total Calories from Protein
Pumpkin seeds	1/4 cup	22
Peanuts	1/4 cup	18
Peanut butter, smooth style	1/4 cup	17
Peanut butter, smooth style	1 tbsp	17
Black walnuts, chopped	1/4 cup	16
Almonds	1/4 cup	15
Pistachio nuts	1/4 cup	14
Sunflower seeds	1/4 cup	14
Flaxseeds	1/4 cup	14
Flaxseeds	1 tbsp	14
Chia	1/4 cup	14
Cashews	1/4 cup	13
Sesame seeds	1/4 cup	12
Sesame seeds	1 tbsp	12
Hazelnuts	1/4 cup	10
English walnuts	1/4 cup	9
Brazilnuts	1/4 cup	9
Pine nuts	1/4 cup	8
Pecans, halves	1/4 cup	5
Macadamia	1/4 cup	4
Coconut meat, shredded	1/4 cup	4

Pork, Cooked	Amount	% of Total Calories from Protein
Tenderloin	3 oz	71
Sirloin chops	3 oz	67
Cured ham, lean	3 oz	64
Chops, lean, pan-fried	3 oz	61
Canadian-style bacon	3 oz	52
Center loin chops	3 oz	49
Chops, broiled	3 oz	49
Chops, pan-fried	3 oz	47

% OF TOTAL CALORIES FROM PROTEIN

Continued

Cured ham	3 oz	35
Backribs	3 oz	32
Spareribs	3 oz	29
Bacon, pan-fried	3 oz	27
Sausage	3 oz	23
Italian sausage	3 oz	22
Braunschweiger	3 oz	18
Polish sausage	3 oz	17
Bratwurst	3 oz	16

Amy's Organic Soup	Amount	% of Total Calories from Protein
Split Pea Soup	1 can	28
Chunky Vegetable	1 can	20
Lentil Soup	1 can	18
Lentil Vegetable Soup	1 can	18
Black Bean Vegetable Soup	1 can	17
Black Bean, Low Fat, Vegetable Soup	1 can	17
Minestrone	1 can	13
Southwest Vegetable Soup	1 can	11
Vegetable Barley	1 can	11
Butternut Squash	1 can	8

Andersen's Soup	Amount	% of Total Calories from Protein
Creamy Split Pea with Bacon Soup	1 can	29
Creamy Split Pea Soup	1 can	28
Creamy Lentil Soup	1 can	22
Creamy Tomato Soup	1 can	6

Campbell's® Chunky Soup	Amount	% of Total Calories from Protein
Roasted Beef, Mushrooms & Vegetables	1 can	27
Sirloin Burger & Country Vegetable	1 can	27
Split Pea & Ham	1 can	26
Hearty Beef Noodle	1 can	25
Grilled Sirloin Steak & Vegetables	1 can	24
Hearty Bean & Ham	1 can	24
Beef with White Wild Rice	1 can	23
Classic Chicken Noodle	1 can	23
Heart Italian Style Wedding	1 can	23
Hearty Beef Barley	1 can	23
Old Fashioned Vegetable Beef	1 can	23
Savory Pot Roast	1 can	23

% OF TOTAL CALORIES FROM PROTEIN

Continued

Steak"N" Potato Soup"	1 can	23
Beef with Country Vegetables	1 can	22
Grilled Chicken with vegetables & Pasta	1 can	22
Hearty Chicken with Vegetables	1 can	22
Grilled Chicken Sausage Gumbo	1 can	19
Creamy Chicken & Dumplings	1 can	18
Fajita Chicken with Rice & Beans	1 can	18
Savory Chicken & White Wild Rice	1 can	18
Chicken Broccoli, Cheese & Potato	1 can	15
Baked Potato with Cheddar & Bacon Bits	1 can	14
Chicken Corn Chowder	1 can	13
Potato Ham Chowder	1 can	13
New England Clam Chowder	1 can	11
Savory Vegetable	1 can	11

Campbell's® Chunky Healthy Request	Amount	% of Total Calories from Protein
Beef with Country Vegetables	1 can	25
Classic Chicken Noodle Soup	1 can	25
Sirloin Burger & Country Vegetable	1 can	24
Old Fashioned Vegetable Beef	1 can	23
Roasted Chicken & Country Vegetables	1 can	22
Hearty Italian Style Wedding	1 can	18
Italian Style Wedding	1 can	18
Chicken Corn Chowder Soup	1 can	17
Grilled Chicken & Sausage Gumbo Soup	1 can	17
New England Clam Chowder	1 can	15
Split Pea & Ham	1 can	12
Savory Vegetable	1 can	10

Campbell's® Kettle Style Soup	Amount	% of Total Calories from Protein
Tuscan Style Chicken & White Beans	1 can	34
Southwest Style Chicken Chili	1 can	32
Burgurdy Beef Stew	1 can	28
Portobello Mushroom & Maderia Bisque	1 can	10
Tomato with Sweet Basil	1 can	6

Campbell's® Microwavable Soup	Amount	% of Total Calories from Protein
Chunky Sirloin Burger & Country Vegetables	1 can	27
Chunky Classic Chicken Noodle	1 can	25
Chunky Beef & Country Vegetables	1 can	22
Chunky Grilled Chicken & Sausage Gumbo	1 can	20

% OF TOTAL CALORIES FROM PROTEIN

Continued

Homestyle Chicken Noodle	1 can	17
Original Chicken Noodle	1 can	17
Chunky New England Clam Chowder	1 can	12
Creamy Tomato	1 can	8

Campbell's® 100% Natural	Amount	% of Total Calories from Protein
Chicken & Egg Noodle	1 can	27
Chicken Tuscany	1 can	27
Carmelized French Onion	1 can	24
Italian Style Wedding	1 can	24
Creamy Gouda Bisque with Chicken	1 can	23
Southwestern White Chicken Chili	1 can	23
Creole-Style Chicken & Red Beans & Rice	1 can	22
Mexican-Style Chicken Tortilla	1 can	22
Savory Chicken & Long Grain Rice	1 can	18
98% Light New England Clam Chowder	1 can	17
Southwestern Style Vegetables	1 can	13
Harvest Tomato with Basil	1 can	12
New England Clam Chowder	1 can	11
Nesty Tomato Bisque	1 can	10
Creamy Potato & Roasted Garlic	1 can	9
Potato Broccoli & Cheese	1 can	8
Butternut Squash Bisque	1 can	4

Campbell's® 100% Natural Healthy Request	Amount	% of Total Calories from Protein
Chicken & Whole Grain Pasta	1 can	28
Italian Style Wedding	1 can	20
Mexican Style Chicken Tortilla	1 can	20
Whole-Grain Pasta Fagioli	1 can	18
Harvest Tomato with Basil	1 can	12

Campbell's® Soup at Hand Soup	Amount	% of Total Calories from Protein
Chicken with Mini Noodles	1 container	10
Chicken with Mini Noodles, 25% Less Sodium	1 container	10
Chicken & Stars	1 container	9
Vegetable Beef, 70 Calories	1 container	9
Classic Tomato	1 container	4
Classic Tomato, 25% Less Sodium	1 container	4
Cream of Broccoli	1 container	4
Creamy Chicken	1 container	4
Creamy Tomato Parmesan Bisque	1 container	4

% OF TOTAL CALORIES FROM PROTEIN

New England Clam Chowder	1 container	4
Vegetable with Mini Round Noodles	1 container	4
Creamy Tomato	1 container	3

Campbell's® V8 Soup	Amount	% of Total Calories from Protein
Garden Vegetable	1 can	17
Garden Broccoli	1 can	13
Tomato Herb	1 can	13
Potato Leek	1 can	12
Sweet Red Pepper	1 can	10
Golden ButterNut Squash	1 can	9
South West Corn	1 can	9

Healthy Choice Microwavable	Amount	% of Total Calories from Protein
Chicken Noodles	1 can	36
Mediterranean Style Chicken with Orzo	1 can	31
Chicken with Rice	1 can	27
Chicken Tortilla	1 can	26
Thai Style Chicken Brown Rice	1 can	25
Beef Pot Roast	1 can	22
Country Vegetable	1 can	16
Cheese Tortellini	1 can	13
Hearty Vegetable Barley	1 can	11
Tomato Basil	1 can	7
Butternut Squash	1 can	4

Healthy Valley Organic Soup	Amount	% of Total Calories from Protein
Lentil & Carrots, Less Sodium	1 can	29
Split Pea, 40% Less Sodium	1 can	28
Lentil, No Salt Added	1 can	26
Chicken Noodle, No Salt Added	1 can	25
Split Pea & Carrots, Less Sodium	1 can	23
Split Pea, No Salt Added	1 can	23
Black Bean Vegetable, Less Sodium	1 can	22
Italian Minestrone, Less Sodium	1 can	22
5 Bean Vegetable, Less Sodium	1 can	20
Black Bean, No Salt Added	1 can	20
Chicken Noodle	1 can	20
Chicken Rice	1 can	18
Minestrone, No Salt Added	1 can	18
Tomato Vegetable, Less Sodium	1 can	17

% OF TOTAL CALORIES FROM PROTEIN

Continued

14 Garden Vegetable, 40% Less Sodium	1 can	15
Vegetable Barley, Less Sodium	1 can	13
Corn & Vegetable, Less Sodium	1 can	12
Vegetable, 40% Less Sodium	1 can	12
Vegetable, No Salt Added	1 can	12
Cream of Chicken	1 can	11
Rice Primavera, No Salt Added	1 can	11
Cream of Celery	1 can	9
Mushroom Barley, No Salt Added	1 can	9
Cream of Mushroom	1 can	8
Potato Leek, 40% Less Sodium	1 can	8
Potato Leek, No Salt Added	1 can	8
Tomato, No Salt Added	1 can	4

Imagine Natural Creation Soup	Amount	% of Total Calories from Protein
Meatball with Orzo	1 can	24
Split Pea	1 can	20
Tuscan White Bean	1 can	20
Cuban Black Bean Bisque	1 can	19
Chicken Pot Pie	1 can	18
Creamy Chicken	1 can	17
Moroccan Chick Pea Bisque	1 can	17
Chicken & Wild Rice	1 can	16
Savory Lentil Apple	1 can	16
Creamy Broccoli	1 can	13
Creamy Tomato Basil	1 can	13
Minestrone	1 can	13
Southwestern Tortilla	1 can	13
Corn Chipotle Bisque	1 can	12
Portobellow Mushroom	1 can	11
Creamy Corn & Lemon Grass	1 can	10
Creamy Garden Tomato, 50% Less	1 can	10
Creamy Tomato	1 can	10
Creamy Potato Leek	1 can	8
Creamy Sweet Potato	1 can	7
Creamy Sweet Potato, 50% Less	1 can	7
Fire Roasted Tomato Bisque	1 can	7
Roasted Garlic Potato	1 can	7
Creamy Acorn Squash & Mango	1 can	6
Creamy Butternut Squash	1 can	2

% OF TOTAL CALORIES FROM PROTEIN

Juanita's Mexican Gourmet Soup	Amount	% of Total Calories from Protein
Beef & Vegetable	1 can	24
Chicken Chipotle	1 can	22
Chicken Tortilla	1 can	18
Fiesta Chicken & Vegetable	1 can	22
Zesty Vegetable & Pasta	1 can	11

Muir Glen's Organic Soup	Amount	% of Total Calories from Protein
Homestyle Split Pea	1 can	20
South West Black Bean	1 can	14
Chicken Tortilla	1 can	12
Savory Lentil	1 can	12
Beef & Vegetable	1 can	10
Beef Barley	1 can	10
Tomato Basil	1 can	10
Cajun Style Chicken Gumbo	1 can	8
Classic Minestrone	1 can	8
Creamy Tomato Bisque	1 can	8
Organic Chicken & Wild Rice	1 can	8
Organic Chicken Noodle	1 can	8
Reduced Sodium Chicken Noodle	1 can	8
Garden Vegetable	1 can	6
Reduced Sodium Garden Vegetable	1 can	6

Pacific Natural Organic Soup	Amount	% of Total Calories from Protein
Chicken Noodle	1 can	22
Vegetable Lentil & Roasted R. Pepper	1 can	21
Creamy Tomato	1 can	20
Creamy Tomato, 50% Less sodium	1 can	20
Spicy Black Bean Soup	1 can	20
Chicken & Wild Rice	1 can	18
Minestrone with Chicken Meatballs	1 can	18
Roasted Red Pepper & Tomato	1 can	18
Roasted Red Pepper & Tomato, 50 % Less sodium	1 can	18
Santa Fe Style Chicken	1 can	17
Chicken Spinach Penne	1 can	15
Curried Red Lentil Soup	1 can	14
French Onion	1 can	13
Roasted Garlic Mushroom Lentil	1 can	13
Creamy Butternut Squash	1 can	9

% OF TOTAL CALORIES FROM PROTEIN

Continued

Creamy Butternut Squash, 50% Less sodium	1 can	9
Thai Sweet Potatos	1 can	8
Butter Nut Squash Bisque	1 can	7
Chipotle Sweet Potatoes	1 can	7
Poblano Pepper & Corn Chowder	1 can	6
Hearty Tomato Bisque	1 can	5
Cashew Carrot Ginger	1 can	3
Rosmary Potato Chowder	1 can	2

Progresso® High Fiber Soup	Amount	% of Total Calories from Protein
Chicken Tuscany	1 can	25
Three Bean Chili with Beef	1 can	20
Hearty Vegetable & Noodle	1 can	18
Homestyle Minestrone	1 can	18
Creamy Tomato Basil	1 can	6

Progresso® Light Soup	Amount	% of Total Calories from Protein
Beef Pot Roast	1 can	35
Chicken Noodle	1 can	29
Chicken Vegetable Rotini	1 can	29
Roasted Chicken & Vegetable	1 can	29
Chicken & Dumplings	1 can	25
Zesty Santa Fee Style Chicken	1 can	25
Vegetable & Noodle	1 can	20
Zesty Southwestern Style Vegetable	1 can	20
Italian Style Vegetable	1 can	17
Italian Style Meatball	1 can	15
Homestyle Vegetable & Rice	1 can	13
Reduced Vegetable	1 can	13
Savory Vegetable Barley	1 can	13
Vegetable	1 can	13
New England Clam Chowder	1 can	12

Progresso® Reduced Sodium Soup	Amount	% of Total Calories from Protein
Chicken Noodle	1 can	27
Beef & Vegetable	1 can	25
Chicken Gumbo	1 can	25
Tomato Parmesan	1 can	25
Chicken & Wild Rice	1 can	20
Italian Style Wedding	1 can	20

% OF TOTAL CALORIES FROM PROTEIN

Continued

Minestrone	1 can	17
Garden Vegetable	1 can	12

Progresso® Rich & Hearty Soup	Amount	% of Total Calories from Protein
Steak & Homestyle Noodles	1 can	29
Savory Beef Barley Vegetable	1 can	28
Beef Pot Roast & Country Vegetables	1 can	27
Slow Cooked Vegetable Beef	1 can	26
Chicken Home Style Noodle	1 can	25
Steak & Roasted Russet Potatoes	1 can	25
Steak & Vegetables	1 can	25
Steak Burger & County Vegetables	1 can	21
Creamy Roasted Chicken Wild Rice	1 can	20
Hearty Roasted Chicken Pot Pie	1 can	19
Roasted Chicken Pot Pies	1 can	19
Chicken Corn Chowder with Bacon Flavor	1 can	14
New England Clam Choder	1 can	11
Loaded Potato with Bacon	1 can	9

Progresso® Traditional Soup	Amount	% of Total Calories from Protein
Chicken Barley	1 can	35
Chicken & Orzo with Lemon	1 can	28
Chicken Noodle	1 can	28
Chicken Vegetable & Pearl Pasta	1 can	28
Hearty Chicken & Rotini	1 can	28
Roasted Chicken Primavera	1 can	28
Roasted Garlic Chicken	1 can	28
Beef & Vegetables	1 can	27
Beef Barley	1 can	27
Chicken Noodle, 99% Fat Free	1 can	27
Roasted Chicken with Garlic & Penne	1 can	27
Split Pea & Ham	1 can	26
Chickarima with Meat Balls	1 can	25
Roasted Chicken Rotini	1 can	25
Turkey Noodle	1 can	25
Chicken & Wild Rice	1 can	24
Beef Barley, 99% Fat Free	1 can	23
Italian Style Wedding	1 can	23
Chicken Rice & Vegetables	1 can	22
Chicken & Herb Dumplings	1 can	20
Southwestern Chicken Chowder	1 can	20

% OF TOTAL CALORIES FROM PROTEIN

Continued

Chicken Cheese Enchilada	1 can	19
Chicken & Sausage Gumbo	1 can	18
New England Clam Chowder 99% Fat Free	1 can	15
New England Clam Chowder	1 can	13
Manhattan Clam Chowder	1 can	12
Potato Broccoli & Cheese Chowder	1 can	10

Progresso® Vegetable Classic Soup	Amount	% of Total Calories from Protein
Vegetable	1 can	25
Green Split Pea with Bacon	1 can	23
Lentil	1 can	23
Lentil, 99% Fat Free	1 can	23
Hearty Black Bean	1 can	20
Macaroni & Bean	1 can	20
Minestrone, 99% Fat Free	1 can	20
French Onion	1 can	16
Minestrone	1 can	16
Vegetable Italiano	1 can	16
Hearty Penne in Chicken Broth	1 can	15
Vegetarian Vegetable with Barley	1 can	15
Garden Vegetable	1 can	13
Tomato Rotini	1 can	12
Hearty Tomato	1 can	11
Tomato Basil	1 can	8
Creamy Mushroom	1 can	5

Progresso® World Recipes Soup	Amount	% of Total Calories from Protein
Caldo de Pollo	1 can	22
Progresso Tortilla y Pollo	1 can	22
Albondigas (Meatballs & Rice)	1 can	15
Progresso Frijoles Negros y Jalapeno	1 can	15

Wolfgang Puck's Organic Soup	Amount	% of Total Calories from Protein
Chicken & Egg Noodles	1 can	22
Thick Lentil & Vegetable	1 can	19
Chicken & White & Wild Rice	1 can	18
Black Bean	1 can	17
Classic Minestrone	1 can	17
Chicken & Dumplings	1 can	14
Tortilla	1 can	13
Thick Hearty Vegetable	1 can	9

% OF TOTAL CALORIES FROM PROTEIN

Continued

Vegetble Barley	1 can	8
Hearty Garden Vegetable	1 can	6
Classic Tomato with Basil	1 can	5
Creamy Butternut Squash	1 can	3

TOFU	Amount	% of Total Calories from Protein
Mori-Nu, Silken, Lite Extra Firm Tofu	3 oz	74
Vitasoy USA, Nasoya Lite Silken Tofu	3 oz	73
Mori-Nu, Silken, Lite Firm Tofu	3 oz	68
Vitasoy USA, Nasoya Lite Firm Tofu	3 oz	63
Mori-Nu, Silken, Extra Firm Tofu	3 oz	54
House Foods Premium Firm	3 oz	46
Mori-Nu, Silken, Firm Tofu	3 oz	45
Vitasoy USA, Nasoya Plus Firm Tofu	3 oz	45
Vitasoy USA, Nasoya Firm Tofu	3 oz	43
Vitasoy USA, Azumaya Extra Firm Tofu	3 oz	42
Vitasoy USA, Azumaya Silken Tofu	3 oz	42
Vitasoy USA, Nasoya Silken Tofu	3 oz	42
Vitasoy USA, Nasoya Extra Firm Tofu	· 3 oz	41
House Foods Premium Soft	3 oz	40
Vitasoy USA, Azumaya Firm Tofu	3 oz	40
Mori-Nu, Silken, Soft Tofu	3 oz	35

Turkey, Cooked	Amount	% of Total Calories from Protein
Breast meat	3 oz	89
Ground turkey, fat free	3 oz	84
Light meat	3 oz	82
Dark meat	3 oz	64
Turkey bacon	3 oz	63
Ground turkey	3 oz	54
Ground turkey, 93% lean	3 oz	50
Ground turkey, 85% lean	3 oz	42
Turkey sausage, reduced fat	3 oz	33
Liver	3 oz	28

Veal, Cooked	Amount	% of Total Calories from Protein
Leg, top round	3 oz	69
Foreshank	3 oz	66
Ground	3 oz	57
Breast	3 oz	56
Sirloin	3 oz	50

Continued

Loin	3 oz	46
Rib	3 oz	42

Vegetables, Canned	Amount	% of Total Calories from Protein
Spinach	1 cup	49
Asparagus	1 cup	45
Mushrooms	1 cup	30
Green peas	1 cup	26
Tomato sauce	1 cup	22
Green beans	1 cup	21
Tomato paste	1 cup	21
Sauerkraut	1 cup	20
Tomatoes	1 cup	19
Tomato pure	1 cup	17
Stewed tomatos	1 cup	14
Pumpkin	1 cup	13
Beets	1 cup	12
Corn	1 cup	12
Carrots	1 cup	10
Sweet potato	1 cup	5

Vegetables, Cooked	Amount	% of Total Calories from Protein
Mustard greens	1 cup	60
Bok-Choy	1 cup	53
Broccoli raab	1 cup	47
Asparagus	1 cup	43
Beet greens	1 cup	38
Swiss chard	1 cup	38
Napa cabbage	1 cup	37
Prickly pear cactus pad, nopales	1 cup	37
Okra	1 cup	34
Cauliflower	1 cup	33
Collard greens	1 cup	33
Snow peas	1 cup	31
White mushrooms	1 cup	31
Zucchini	1 cup	30
Brussels sprouts	1 cup	28
Split peas	1 cup	28
Broccoli	1 cup	27
Kale	1 cup	27
Scallop or Pattypan squash	1 cup	26
Kohlrabi	1 cup	25
Dandelion greens	1 cup	24

% OF TOTAL CALORIES FROM PROTEIN

Continued

Turnip greens	1 cup	23
Artichokes	1 cup	22
Cabbage, shredded	1 cup	22
Crookneck and Straightneck squash	1 cup	22
Broccoli, Chinese, Broccolini	1 cup	21
Green beans	1 cup	21
Tomatoes, red, ripe	1 cup	21
Hubbard squash	1 cup	20
Celery, diced	1 cup	19
Summer squash	1 cup	18
Corn, yellow	1 cup	14
Pumpkin, mashed	1 cup	14
Rutabagas, cubes	1 cup	13
Turnips, cubes	1 cup	13
Onions	1 cup	12
Leeks, chopped	1 cup	11
Shitake mushrooms	1 cup	11
Spaghetti squash	1 cup	10
Spaghetti winter squash	1 cup	10
Winter squash	1 cup	10
Butternut squash	1 cup	9
Carrots, sliced	1 cup	9
Eggplant	1 cup	9
Acorn squash, cubes	1 cup	8
Beets	1 cup	8
Potatoes, flesh, baked	1 cup	8
Parsnips	1 cup	7
Potatoes, mashed with whole milk & butter	1 cup	7
Sweet potato, mashed	1 cup	7
Spinach	1 cup	5
Yams, cubed	1 cup	5
Taro, sliced	1 cup	1

Vegetables, Frozen	Amount	% of Total Calories from Protein
Asparagus	1 cup	66
Spinach	1 cup	48
Turnip greens	1 cup	47
Broccoli	1 cup	44
Kale	1 cup	38
Brussels sprouts	1 cup	34
Cauliflower	1 cup	34
Collard greens	1 cup	33
Green peas	1 cup	26
Okra	1 cup	23

% OF TOTAL CALORIES FROM PROTEIN

Continued

Green beans	1 cup	21
Yellow sweet corn	1 cup	13
Carrots	1 cup	6
Rhubarb	1 cup	1

Vegetables, Raw	Amount	% of Total Calories from Protein
Watercress	1 cup	83
Spirulina, dried	1 tbsp	80
White mushrooms, sliced	1 cup	58
Raab Broccoli, chopped	1 cup	56
Spinach	1 cup	49
Bok-Choy	1 cup	47
Crimini mushrooms, sliced	1 cup	45
Arugula	1 cup	42
Butterhead, bibb or boston lettuce	1 cup	42
Oyster mushrooms, sliced	1 cup	41
Portabella mushrooms, diced	1 cup	38
Red leaf lettuce	1 cup	37
Swiss chard	1 cup	37
Green leaf lettuce	1 cup	35
Broccoli, chopped	1 cup	33
Prickley pear cactus pads, nopales	1 cup	33
Endive	1 cup	31
Cauliflower, chopped	1 cup	30
Summer squash, sliced	1 cup	30
Savoy cabbage, shredded	1 cup	29
Shiitake mushrooms	1 whole	29
Zucchini, sliced	1 cup	29
Chicory greens, chopped	1 cup	28
Romaine lettuce	1 cup	28
Snow peas, chopped	1 cup	27
Kale, chopped	1 cup	26
Iceberg lettuce	1 cup	25
Radicchio	1 cup	25
Dandelion greens	1 cup	24
Green onions & scallions, chopped	1 cup	23
Belgian endive	1 cup	22
Cabbage, shredded	1 cup	20
Tomatoes, chopped	1 cup	20
Tomatoes, cherry	1 cup	19
Red cabbage, shredded	1 cup	18
Celery, chopped	1 cup	17
Cucumbers, slices	1 cup	17
Green bell peppers, chopped	1 cup	17

% OF TOTAL CALORIES FROM PROTEIN

Continued

Yellow bell peppers	1 cup	15
Red bell peppers, chopped	1 cup	13
Shiitake mushrooms, dried	1 each	12
Tomatillos, chopped	1 cup	12
Onions, chopped	1 cup	11
Butternut squash, cubes	1 cup	9
Carrots, sliced	1 cup	9

Blueberry Yogurt	Amount	% of Total Calories from Protein
Yoplait Fiber One Blueberry	6.0 oz	27
Cascade Fat Free Blueberry	6.0 oz	25
Dannon Light & Fit Blueberry	6.0 oz	25
Activia Light Blueberry	6.0 oz	23
Emmi Swiss Low Fat Blueberry	6.0 oz	21
Brown Cow, Non Fat, Creamy Blueberry	6.0 oz	20
Wallaby Low Fat Blueberry	6.0 oz	20
Yoplait Light Blueberry	6.0 oz	20
Noosa Blueberry Yogurt with Fruit	6.0 oz	17
Clover Low Fat Blueberry	6.0 oz	17
Dannon Blueberry with Fruit Bottom	6.0 oz	17
Brown Cow, Low Fat Blueberry & Fruit	6.0 oz	16
Activia Blueberry	6.0 oz	13
Yoplait Original Blueberry	6.0 oz	12
Clover Blueberry with Cream on Top	6.0 oz	11
Liberte Mediterranee Blueberry	6.0 oz	9

Blueberry Greek Yogurt	Amount	% of Total Calories from Protein
Fage Total 0% Blueberry	6.0 oz	43
Stoneyfield Organic Oikos Blueberry	5.3 oz	43
Voskos Organic Blueberry	5.3 oz	43
Chobani Blueberry	6.0 oz	40
Dannon Oikos, Non Fat, Blueberry	5.3 oz	37
Athenos Blueberry	5.3 oz	36
Yoplait Blueberry	6.0 oz	35
Fage Total 2% Blueberry	5.3 oz	34
Activia Selects Creamy Blueberry	6.0 oz	25
Fage Total Blueberry	5.3 oz	17

Blueberry Specility Yogurt	Amount	% of Total Calories from Protein
Green Valley Lactose Free Blueberry Yogurt	6.0 oz	20
Redwood Hill Farms Blueberry Goat Yogurt	6.0 oz	17

% OF TOTAL CALORIES FROM PROTEIN

Continued

Whole Soy Blueberry Soy Yogurt	6.0 oz	14
Amande Blueberry Almond Milk Yogurt	6.0 oz	8
So Delicious Blueberry Coconut Milk Yogurt	6.0 oz	3

Cherry Yogurt	Amount	% of Total Calories from Protein
Stoneyfield Creamy 0% Fat Black Cherry	6.0 oz	28
Cascade Fat Free Cherry Vanilla	6.0 oz	25
Dannon Light & Fit Cherry	6.0 oz	25
Yoplait Light Vanilla Cherry Yogurt	6.0 oz	24
Activia Light Cherry	6.0 oz	23
Cascade Low Fat Cherry	6.0 oz	23
Emmi Swiss Low Fat Black Cherry Yogurt	6.0 oz	21
Wallaby Organic Low Fat Black Cherry	6.0 oz	20
Dannon Cherry with Fruit on the Bottom	6.0 oz	17
Brown Cow Low Fat Black Cherry with Fruit	6.0 oz	16
Activia Black Cherry	6.0 oz	15
Yoplait Original Cherry	6.0 oz	12
Brown Cow Cherry Vanilla with Fruit	6.0 oz	11
Liberte Mediterranee Black Cherry	6.0 oz	9

Peach Yogurt	Amount	% of Total Calories from Protein
Stoneyfield Creamy 0% Fat Peach Yogurt	6.0 oz	28
Yoplait Fiber One Peach	6.0 oz	27
Cascade Fat Free Peach	6.0 oz	25
Dannon Light & Fit Peach	6.0 oz	25
Activia Light Peach	6.0 oz	23
Cascade Low Fat Peach	6.0 oz	23
Yoplait Light Harvest Peach	6.0 oz	20
Brown Cow Low Fat Creamy Peach	6.0 oz	19
Clover Organic Low Fat Peach	6.0 oz	18
Wallaby Organic Low Fat Peach	6.0 oz	17
Dannon Peach with Fruit Bottom	6.0 oz	16
Activia Peach	6.0 oz	13
Activia Fiber Peach	6.0 oz	12
Clover Organic Peach & Cream on Top	6.0 oz	12
Yoplait Original Peach	6.0 oz	12
Brown Cow Peach with Fruit	6.0 oz	11
Liberte Mediterranee Peach & Passion Fruit	6.0 oz	9

% OF TOTAL CALORIES FROM PROTEIN

Peach Greek Yogurt	Amount	% of Total Calories from Protein
Athenos Peach Greek	5.3 oz	40
Chobani Peach Greek	6.0 oz	40
Stonyfield Oikos Peach Mango Greek	5.3 oz	40
Dannon Oikos Non Fat Peach Greek	5.3 oz	37
Yoplait Peach Greek	6.0 oz	35
Fage Total 2% Peach	5.3 oz	34
Fage Total Peach	5.3 oz	17

Pomegranate Yogurt	Amount	% of Total Calories from Protein
Chobani Pomegranate Greek Yogurt	6.0 oz	40
Fage Total 0% Cherry & Pomegranate Greek	5.3 oz	40
Stoneyfield Creamy 0% Fat Pomegranate	6.0 oz	28
Dannon Light & Fit Pomegranate	6.0 oz	25
Activia Selects Creamy Pomegranate Greek	6.0 oz	24
Emmi Swiss Low Fat Pomegranate	6.0 oz	21
The Greek Gods Pomegranate	6.0 oz	10

Plain Yogurt	Amount	% of Total Calories from Protein
Cascade, Fat Free, Plain Yogurt	6.0 oz	50
Horizon Organic Fat Free Plain	6.0 oz	40
Mountain High Fat Free Plain Yogurt	6.0 oz	40
Nancy's Organic Non Fat Plain	6.0 oz	40
Stoneyfield Creamy 0% Fat Plain	6.0 oz	40
Wallaby Organic Low Fat Plain	6.0 oz	32
Clover Organic Low Fat Plain	6.0 oz	31
Mountain High Low Fat Plain	6.0 oz	30
Nancy's Organic Low Fat Plain	6.0 oz	29
Horizon Organic Whole Milk Plain	6.0 oz	27
Nancy's Organic Whole Milk Plain	6.0 oz	25
Emmi Swiss Low Fat Plain Yogurt	6.0 oz	24
Mountain High Original Style Plain	6.0 oz	24
Clover Organic Plain with Cream on Top	6.0 oz	18
Brown Cow Creamy Plain	6.0 oz	15

% OF TOTAL CALORIES FROM PROTEIN

Plain Greek Yogurt	Amount	% of Total Calories from Protein
Brown Cow Plain Greek	5.3 oz	75
Dannon Oikos Non Fat Plain	5.3 oz	75
Stonyfield Organic Oikos Plain	5.3 oz	75
Chobani Plain Greek Yogurt	6.0 oz	72
Fage Total 0% Plain	6.0 oz	72
Voskos Nonfat Plain Greek Yogurt	6.0 oz	69
Voskos Organic Plain	5.3 oz	67
Yoplait Plain	6.0 oz	57
Athenos Plain	6.0 oz	53
Fage Total 2% Plain	6.0 oz	53
Fage Total Plain	6.0 oz	24

Plain Specility Yogurt	Amount	% of Total Calories from Protein
Green Valley, Lactose Free Plain Yogurt	6.0 oz	32
Redwood Hill Farms Plain Goat Milk Yogurt	6.0 oz	28
Wildwood Organic Plain Soy Milk Yogurt	6.0 oz	22
Amande Plain Almond Milk Yogurt	8.0 oz	21
Whole Soy Plain Soy Milk Yogurt	6.0 oz	21
So Delicious Plain Coconut Milk Yogurt	5.3 oz	3

Raspberry Yogurt	Amount	% of Total Calories from Protein
Chobani Raspberry Greek	6.0 oz	40
Dannon Raspberry with Fruit Bottom	6.0 oz	30
Cascade Fat Free Raspberry	6.0 oz	25
Activia Light Raspberry Yogurt	6.0 oz	23
Cascade Low Fat Raspberry	6.0 oz	23
Emmi Swiss Low Fat Raspberry	6.0 oz	21
Yoplait Light Raspberry	6.0 oz	20
Wildwood Organic Raspberry Soy Milk Yogurt	6.0 oz	13
Brown Cow Raspberry with Fruit	6.0 oz	12
Yoplait Original Raspberry	6.0 oz	12

Strawberry Yogurt	Amount	% of Total Calories from Protein
Stoneyfield Creamy 0% Fat Strawberry	6.0 oz	28
Mountain High Fat Free Strawberry Yogurt	6.0 oz	27
Yoplait Fiber One Strawberry	6.0 oz	27
Dannon Light & Fit Strawberry	6.0 oz	25
Activia Light Strawberry	6.0 oz	23
Cascade Low Fat Strawberry	6.0 oz	23

% OF TOTAL CALORIES FROM PROTEIN

Continued

Emmi Swiss Low Fat Strawberry	6.0 oz	21
Wallaby Organic Low Fat Strawberry	6.0 oz	20
Yoplait Light Strawberry	6.0 oz	20
Brown Cow Non Fat Strawberry with Fruit	6.0 oz	18
Clover Organic Low Fat Strawberry	6.0 oz	17
LALA Nonfat Strawberry Yogurt	6.0 oz	16
Brown Cow Low Fat Strawberry with Fruit	6.0 oz	16
Dannon Strawberry Banana & Fruit	6.0 oz	16
Dannon Strawberry with Fruit Bottom	6.0 oz	16
Activia Strawberry	6.0 oz	13
Activia Fiber Strawberry	6.0 oz	12
Yoplait Original Strawberry	6.0 oz	12
Brown Cow Strawberry with Fruit	6.0 oz	11
Clover Strawberry & Cream Top	6.0 oz	11
Liberte Mediterranee Strawberry	6.0 oz	9

Strawberry Greek Yogurt	Amount	% of Total Calories from Protein
Stonyfield Organic Oikos Strawberry Greek	5.3 oz	47
Fage Total 0% Strawberry Greek	6.0 oz	43
Voskos Organic Wild Strawberry	5.3 oz	43
Athenos Strawberry Greek Yogurt	5.3 0z	40
Chobani Strawberry Greek Yogurt	6.0 oz	40
Dannon Oikos Non Fat Strawberry	5.3 oz	40
Yoplait Strawberry Greek	6.0 oz	35
Fage Total 2% Strawberry	5.3 oz	34
Activia Selects Creamy Strawberry	6.0 oz	25
Fage Total Peach Greek Yogurt	5.3 oz	17

Strawberry Specility Yogurt	Amount	% of Total Calories from Protein
Green Valley Lactose Free Strawberry Yogurt	6.0 oz	20
Redwood Hill's Farms Goat Milk Yogurt	6.0 oz	16
Whole Soy Strawberry Soy Yogurt	6.0 oz	15
Wildwood Organic Strawberry Soy Milk	6.0 oz	13
Amande Strawberry Almond Milk Yogurt	6.0 oz	8
So Delicious Strawberry Coconut Milk Yogurt	6.0 oz	3

Vanilla Yogurt	Amount	% of Total Calories from Protein
Activia Light Vanilla	6.0 oz	30
Mountain High Fat Free Vanilla	6.0 oz	30
Mountain High Low Fat Plain	6.0 oz	30
Stoneyfield Creamy 0% Fat French Vanilla	6.0 oz	28

% OF TOTAL CALORIES FROM PROTEIN

Continued

Yoplait Fiber One Vanilla	6.0 oz	27
Cascade Fat Free Vanilla	6.0 oz	25
Dannon Light & Fit Vanilla	6.0 oz	25
Clover Organic Low Fat Vanilla	6.0 oz	23
Brown Cow Non Fat Creamy Vanilla	6.0 oz	22
Horizon Organic Fat Free Vanilla	6.0 oz	22
Yoplait Light Very Vanilla	6.0 oz	22
Emmi Swiss Low Fat Vanilla Bean	6.0 oz	21
Mountain High Original Style Vanilla	6.0 oz	21
Wallaby Organic Low Fat Vanilla	6.0 oz	17
Brown Cow Low Fat Vanilla Bean & Fruit	6.0 oz	16
Horizon Organic Whole Milk Vanilla	6.0 oz	15
Activia Fiber Vanilla	6.0 oz	12
Yoplait Original French Vanilla	6.0 oz	12
Activia Vanilla	6.0 oz	9

Vanilla Greek Yogurt	Amount	% of Total Calories from Protein
Stonyfield Organic Oikos Vanilla	5.3 oz	55
Chobani Vanilla Greek Yogurt	6.0 oz	53
Brown Cow Vanilla	5.3 oz	51
Dannon Oikos Non Fat	5.3 oz	40
Trader Joe's Non Fat Greek Vanilla Bean	5.3 oz	37
Voskos Organic Vanilla Bean	5.3 oz	37
Yoplait Honey Vanilla	6.0 oz	37
Activia Selects Creamy Vanilla	6.0 oz	25
Greek Gods Reduced Fat	6.0 oz	16

Vanilla Specility Yogurt	Amount	% of Total Calories from Protein
Green Valley Lactose Free Vanilla	6.0 oz	23
Redwood Hill Farms Vanilla Goat Milk	6.0 oz	20
Wildwood Organic Vanilla Soy Milk	6.0 oz	18
Whole Soy Vanilla Soy Milk	6.0 oz	13
Amande Vanilla Almond Milk Yogurt	8.0 oz	7

SODIUM

It is acknowledged that Americans consume more sodium than needed. Evidence has clearly established a link between sodium intake and high blood pressure. Further, the relation between high blood pressure and cardiovascular disease is equally documented. Fortunately, high blood pressure can be lowered by lowering dietary intake of sodium.

Sodium dietary guidelines for American adults are currently being met by less than 1% of the population. It is estimated that 25% of adults have hypertension, and 50% of adults have some stage of high blood pressure.

In 1984 the FDA added sodium to the list of nutrients required on food labels. It was the FDA's intentions to provide consumers with nutritional information about a food product relative to their overall diet. However, the food industries use of different serving sizes on labels of similar foods makes a side-by-side comparison of food labels impractical for making informed dietary choices.

Americans are consuming more sodium than recommended primarily because, although they are aware of its harmful effects, they are unable to judge whether the amount of sodium in their daily diet is acceptable. Bear in mind that 1 teaspoon of table salt contains 2,325 mg of sodium and 1 dash approximately 155 mg.

Recommend Daily Intakes Levels for Sodium

Children	Sodium, mg
1 to 3 year olds	1000
4 to 8 year olds	1200

Males	
9 to 13 year olds	1500
14 to 18 year olds	1500
19 to 30 years	1500
31 to 50 years	1500
51 to 70 years	1300
Over 70	1200

Females	
9 to 13 year olds	1500
14 to 18 year olds	1500
19 to 30 years	1500
31 to 50 years	1500
51 to 70 years	1300
Over 70	1200
Pregnancy & Lactation	1500

SODIUM

Continued

Alcohol	Amount	Sodium (mg)
Beer, light, all types	1 bottle	14
Beer, regular, all types	1 bottle	14
White Wine	1 glass	7
Red Wine	1 glass	6
Gin, Rum, Vodka, Whisky	1 shot	0

Beans, Canned	Amount	Sodium (mg)
Navy beans	1 cup	1174
Fava beans	1 cup	1160
Refried beans	1 cup	1069
Baked beans, plain	1 cup	871
Cranberry beans	1 cup	863
Lima beans, mature	1 cup	810
Black-eyed peas	1 cup	718
Pinto beans	1 cup	643
Garbanzo beans	1 cup	622
Kidney beans, rinsed	1 cup	329
White beans	1 cup	13
Great Northern	1 cup	10
Green beans, no salt added	1 cup	3
Yellow beans, no salt added	1 cup	3

Beans, Cooked, no salt added	Amount	Sodium (mg)
Soybeans, green	1 cup	25
Winged beans	1 cup	22
Adzuki	1 cup	18
Moth beans	1 cup	18
Hyacinth beans	1 cup	14
Natto	1 cup	12
Garbanzo beans	1 cup	11
White beans, mature	1 cup	11
Edamame	1 cup	9
Fava beans	1 cup	8
Pigeon peas	1 cup	8
Black-eyed peas	1 cup	7
Lupini	1 cup	7
Black Turtle beans, mature	1 cup	6
Great Northern beans	1 cup	4
Kidney beans	1 cup	4
Lentils	1 cup	4
Lima beans	1 cup	4
Mung beans, mature seeds	1 cup	4
Split Pea	1 cup	4

Daily Adequate Intake is 1500 mg for adults

SODIUM

White beans, small	1 cup	4
Yardlong, Chinese long beans	1 cup	4
Yellow beans	1 cup	4
Black beans	1 cup	2
Cranberry beans	1 cup	2
Pinto beans	1 cup	2
Soybeans, dryroasted	1 cup	2
Soybeans, mature	1 cup	2
Green beans	1 cup	1
Navy beans	1 cup	0

Beef, Cooked	Amount	Sodium (mg)
Ribeye steak, lean, trim 0" fat	3 oz	72
Ground beef, 75%	3 oz	66
Ground beef, 80%	3 oz	64
Skirt Steak, trim to 0" fat	3 oz	64
Tri Tip steak, lean, trim to 0" fat	3 oz	62
Ground beef, 85%	3 oz	61
Ground beef, 90%	3 oz	58
T-Bone steak, trim 0" fat	3 oz	57
Ground beef, 95%	3 oz	55
Porterhouse steak, trim to 0" fat	3 oz	55
Beef ribs, trim to 1/8" fat	3 oz	54
Chuck roast, trim to 1/8" fat	3 oz	54
Top sirloin, lean, trim to 1/8" fat	3 oz	52
Filet Mignon, trim to 0" fat	3 oz	48
Flank steak, lean, trim to 0" fat	3 oz	48
Brisket, lean, trim to 0" fat	3 oz	46
London Broil, top round	3 oz	38

Beef, Cooked	Amount	Sodium (mg)
Skirt steak, trim to 0" fat	1 lb cooked	340
Tri Tip steak, lean, trim to 0" fat	1 lb cooked	327
T-bone steak, trim to 0" fat	1 lb cooked	304
Porterhouse steak, trim to 0" fat	1 lb cooked	295
Beef ribs, trim to 1/8" fat	1 lb cooked	291
Chuck roast, trim to 1/8" fat	1 lb cooked	291
Flank steak, lean, trim to 0" fat	1 lb cooked	259
Top Sirloin, trim to 1/8" fat	1 lb cooked	254
Brisket, lean, trim to 0" fat	1 lb cooked	245
Flank steak, lean, trim to 0" fat	1 steak	218
Ribeye steak, boneless, trim to 0" fat	1 steak	180
Ribeye filet, lean, trim to 0" fat	1 filet	112
Top Sirloin, choice filet, trim to 0" fat	1 filet	73
Filet Mignon, tenderloin, trim to 0" fat	1 steak	67

Daily Adequate Intake is 1500 mg for adults

SODIUM

Beef, Cooked	Amount	Sodium (mg)
Ground beef, 75%	1/4 lb patty	55
Ground beef, 80%	1/4 lb patty	58
Ground beef, 85%	1/4 lb patty	55
Ground beef, 90%	1/4 lb patty	56
Ground beef, 95%	1/4 lb patty	53

Bread	Amount	Sodium (mg)
Bagel, oat bran	4" bagel	620
Mexican roll, bollilo	1 roll	496
Indian bread, Naan, whole wheat	1 piece	495
Cornbread, drymix	1 piece	467
Bagel, plain	4" bagel	460
Bagel, egg	4" bagel	449
Bagel, wheat	4" bagel	430
Indian bread, Naan, plain	1 piece	418
Bagel, cinnamon & raisins	4" bagel	385
Pita, white	6" pita	322
Kaiser rolls	1 roll	310
French and Sourdough	1 slice	256
Egg bread	1 slice	230
Pumpernickle	1 slice	215
Rye bread	1 slice	211
English Muffin, plain	1 muffin	206
Hamburger & Hotdog buns	1 bun	206
Tortillas, flour	1 tortilla	204
Dinner rolls, brown & serve	1 roll	150
Cracked Wheat	1 slice	135
Whole-Wheat	1 slice	132
Wheat	1 slice	130
White	1 slice	128
Oatmeal bread	1 slice	127
Potato bread	1 slice	120
Italian	1 slice	117
Multi-Grain, includes Whole-Grain	1 slice	109
Raisin bread	1 slice	81
Tortillas, corn	1 tortilla	12

Butter	Amount	Sodium (mg)
Regular dairy butter, salted	1 tbsp	91
Regular dairy whipped butter, salted	1 tbsp	62

Daily Adequate Intake is 1500 mg for adults

SODIUM

CEREAL

Albertsons® Brand Cereal	Amount	Sodium (mg)
Nutty Nuggets	1 cup	580
Honey Gram Crunch	1 cup	360
Low Fat Granola & Almonds	1 cup	333
Low Fat Granola, Raisin & Almond	1 cup	316
Muesli, Raisin, Dates, Almond	1 cup	285
Wheat Bran Flakes	1 cup	280
Golden Corn Nuggets	1 cup	270
Crispy Crunchy Berry	1 cup	253
Honey Oats & Flakes with Strawberry	1 cup	253
Crispy Rice	1 cup	240
Crunch Rice Squares	1 cup	240
Raisin Bran	1 cup	230
Honey Oats & Flakes	1 cup	226
Cocoa Crispy Rice	1 cup	200
Cinni-Mini Crunches	1 cup	186
Crunchy Oat Squares	1 cup	186
Honey Nut Toasted Oats	1 cup	186
Corn Flakes	1 cup	180
Raisin Bran Crunch Granola	1 cup	180
Frosted Flakes	1 cup	160
Toasted Oats	1 cup	160
Apple Crunchies	1 cup	150
Frosted Fruit O's	1 cup	150
Good Day with Strawberry	1 cup	150
Cocoa Comets	1 cup	146
Multigrain	1 cup	120
Golden Wheat Puffs	1 cup	86

Arrowhead Mills®	Amount	Sodium (mg)
Maple Buckwheat Flakes	1 cup	190
Sweetened Rice Flakes	1 cup	190
Spelt Flakes	1 cup	100
Sprouted Wheat Bran & Quinoa	1 cup	85
Oat Bran Flakes	1 cup	80
Sprouted Corn Flakes	80	75
Kamut Flakes	1 cup	70
Shredded Wheat, Bite Size	1 cup	5
Amaranth Flakes	1 cup	0
Sprouted Multigrain Flakes	1 cup	0
Sweetened Shredded Wheat	1 cup	0

Daily Adequate Intake is 1500 mg for adults

SODIUM

Barbara's®	Amount	Sodium (mg)
Puffins Peanut Butter	1 cup	307
Shredded Spoonfuls Multigrain	1 cup	267
Multigrain Spoonfuls, Original	1 cup	266
Puffins Original	1 cup	253
Toasted Oatmeal Flakes	1 cup	253
Morning Oat Crunch, Original	1 cup	250
Puffins Cinnamon	1 cup	227
Morning Oat Crunch, Cinnamon	1 cup	220
Shredded Oats Cinnamon Crunch	1 cup	220
Morning Oat Crunch, Vanilla & Almonds	1 cup	210
Shredded Oats Vanilla Almond	1 cup	210
Shredded Oats Original	1 cup	208
Multigrain Squarefuls, Maple Brown Sugar	1 cup	190
Graham Crunch*	1 cup	187
Honey Nut O's	1 cup	170
Morning Oat Crunch, Vanilla	1 cup	150
High Fiber Medley Cranberry	1 cup	140
High Fiber Medley Flax & Granola	1 cup	140
High Fiber Original	1 cup	140
Morning Oat Crunch, Blueberry	1 cup	140
Puffins Peanut Butter & Chocolate	1 cup	140
Shredded Minis Blueberry Burst	1 cup	140
Honest O's, Honey Nut	1 cup	107
Hole 'n Oats Honey Nut	1 cup	107
Hole 'n Oats: Fruit Juice Sweetened	1 cup	107
Puffins Honey Rice	1 cup	107
Puffins Multigrain	1 cup	107
Puffins Puffs Crunchy Cocoa	1 cup	107
Puffins Puffs Fruit Medley	1 cup	107
Brown Rice Crisps	1 cup	80
Corn Flakes	1 cup	80
Honest O's, Original	1 cup	80
Honest O's, Multigrain	1 cup	20
Shredded Wheat	2 biscuits	0

Cascadian Farm®	Amount	Sodium (mg)
Cinnamon Raisin Granola	1 cup	345
Dark Chocolate Almond Granola	1 cup	270
Raisin bran	1 cup	240
Hearty Morning	1 cup	200
Maple Brown Sugar Granola	1 cup	196
Multi Gain Squares	1 cup	190
Graham Crunch	1 cup	187
Fruitful O's	1 cup	173

Daily Adequate Intake is 1500 mg for adults

SODIUM

Continued

Honey Nut O's	1 cup	170
Purely O's	1 cup	160
Oats & Honey Granola	1 cup	157
French Vanilla Almond Granola	1 cup	150
Fruit & Nut Granola	1 cup	142
Berry Cobbler Granola	1 cup	140
Cinnamon Crunch	1 cup	140
Chocolate O's	1 cup	127

Cadia®	Amount	Sodium (mg)
Honey Kissed Cadi-O's	1 cup	200
Crunch	1 cup	100
All Natural Raisin Bran	1 cup	90
Whole Grain Cadi-O's Toasted Oats	1 cup	80
High Fiber Tripple Bran	1 cup	46

Erewhon®	Amount	Sodium (mg)
Buckwheat & Hemp	1 cup	210
Cocoa Crispy Brown Rice	1 cup	190
Quinoa & Chia	1 cup	190
Crispy Brown Rice, Original	1 cup	180
Strawberry Crisp	1 cup	167
Crispy Brown Rice	1 cup	160
Honey Crispy Brown Rice, Mixed Berries	1 cup	100
Raisin Bran	1 cup	100
Corn Flakes	1 cup	80
Honey Rice Twice	1 cup	80
Rice Twice	1 cup	80
Crispy Brown Rice, no salt added	1 cup	10

Ezekiel 4:9	Amount	Sodium (mg)
Original	1 cup	400
Almond	1 cup	380
Golden Flax	1 cup	380
Cinnamon Flax	1 cup	320
Cinnamon Raisin	1 cup	320

General Mills®	Amount	Sodium (mg)
Multi-Bran CHEX	1 cup	360
Wheat Chex	1 cup	360
Golden Grams	1 cup	320
Raisin Nut Bran	1 cup	306
Honey Nut Clusters	1 cup	290
Basic 4	1 cup	280

Daily Adequate Intake is 1500 mg for adults

SODIUM

Continued

Oatmeal Crisp, Hearty Raisin	1 cup	270
Honey Nut Chex	1 cup	267
Chocolate Chex	1 cup	266
Vanilla Chex	1 cup	253
Cinnamon Chex	1 cup	240
Cinnamon Toast Crunch	1 cup	240
Corn Chex	1 cup	240
Rice Chex	1 cup	240
Total Raisin Bran	1 cup	239
Lucky Charms	1 cup	226
Wheaties	1 cup	221
Dora The Explorer	1 cup	219
Reese's Puffs	1 cup	213
Chocolate Lucky Charms	1 cup	200
Cocoa Puffs	1 cup	200
Trix	1 cup	200
Total Whole Grain	1 cup	186
Hersheys Cookies "N" Cream	1 cup	166
Cookie Crisp	1 cup	160
Total Cranberry Crunch	1 cup	152
Kix	1 cup	144
Berry Berry Kix	1 cup	136
Oatmeal Crisp, Crunchy Almond	1 cup	114

General Mills Cheerios®	Amount	Sodium (mg)
Berry Burst	1 cup	227
Yogurt Burst	1 cup	227
Frosted	1 cup	226
Protein	1 cup	224
Banana Nut	1 cup	213
Honey Nut	1 cup	213
Chocolate	1 cup	200
Dulce de leche	1 cup	180
Fruity	1 cup	180
Multi Grain Peanut Butter	1 cup	173
Crunch, Oat Clusters	1 cup	172
Multi Grain Dark Chocolate Crunch	1 cup	166
Honey Nut Medley Crunch	1 cup	160
Apple Cinnamon	1 cup	153
Original	1 cup	140
Cinnamon Burst	1 cup	125
Multi Grain	1 cup	120

Daily Adequate Intake is 1500 mg for adults

SODIUM

General Mills Fiber-One®	Amount	Sodium (mg)
Caramel Delight	1 cup	226
Honey Clusters	1 cup	220
Raisin Bran Clusters	1 cup	211
Nuty Cluster & Almonds	1 cup	210
Original	1 cup	210
80 Calories, Chocolate Squares	1 cup	173
80 Calories, Chocolate	1 cup	173
Protein, Maple Brown Sugar	1 cup	150
Protein	1 cup	150
Protein, Cranberry Almond	1 cup	140
80 Calories, Honey Squares	1 cup	X
Frosted Shredded Wheat	1 cup	X

Glutino®	Amount	Sodium (mg)
Apple & Cinnamon Rings	1 cup	240
Honey Nut Cereal	1 cup	240
Berry Sensible Beginning	1 cup	230
Corn Rice Flakes	1 cup	130
Corn Rice Flakes with Strawberries	1 cup	125
Frosted Corn & Rice Flakes	1 cup	120
Honey Nut Rings	1 cup	113

Health Valley	Amount	Sodium (mg)
Oat Bran Flakes	1 cup	190
Oat Bran Almond Crunch	1 cup	180
Corn Crunch-EMS	1 cup	160
Oat Bran Flakes & Raisins	1 cup	160
Amaranth Flakes	1 cup	152
Heart Wise	1 cup	140
Low fat Date & Almond Flavored Granola	1 cup	136
Low fat Raisin Cinnamon Granola	1 cup	136
Cranberry Crunch	1 cup	133
Rice Crunch-EMS	1 cup	120
Fiber 7	1 cup	100
Multigrain Apple Cinnamon Squares	1 cup	100
Multigrain Maple, Honey, Nut Squares	1 cup	100
Golden Flax	1 cup	65

Kashi®	Amount	Sodium (mg)
7-Whole Grain Nuggets	1 cup	520
Strawberry Fields	1 cup	190
Raisin Vineyard	1 cup	186
Honey Sunshine	1 cup	180

Daily Adequate Intake is 1500 mg for adults

SODIUM

Continued

Berry Blossom	1 cup	166
Go Lean Crisp, Cinnamon Crumble	1 cup	166
Go Lean Crisp, Toasted Berry Crumble	1 cup	166
Indigo Morning	1 cup	166
Blackberry Hills	1 cup	160
7-Whole Grain Flakes	1 cup	150
Simply Maize	1 cup	146
Go Lean Crunch, Honey Almond Flax	1 cup	140
Heart to Heart, Oat Flakes & Blueberry Clusters	1 cup	135
Go Lean Crunch	1 cup	133
Heart to Heart, Honey Toasted Oat	1 cup	120
Heart to Heart, Warm Cinnamon	1 cup	113
Good Friends	1 cup	110
Go Lean	1 cup	90
Go Lean Vanilla Cream	1 cup	85
Heart to Heart, Nuty Chia Flax	1 cup	80
Island Vanilla	27 biscuits	5
7-Whole Grain Honey Puffs	1 cup	0
7-Whole Grain Puffs	1 cup	0
Autum Wheat	29 biscuits	0
Berry Fruitful	29 biscuits	0
Cinnamon Harvest	28 biscuits	0

Kellogg's®	Amount	Sodium (mg)
All-Bran Bran Buds	1 cup	630
Raisin Bran Extra	1 cup	307
Honey Crunch Corn Flakes	1 cup	280
All-Bran Complete Wheat Flakes	1 cup	276
Smart Start, Strong Heart Antioxidants	1 cup	275
MUESLIX	1 cup	254
All-Bran Strawberry Medley	1 cup	228
Rice Krispies Treats	1 cup	222
Berry Rice Krispies	1 cup	218
Low fat Granola with Raisins	1 cup	216
Crunchy Nut Golden Honey Nut Flakes	1 cup	215
Simply Cinnamon Corn Flakes	1 cup	211
Product 19	1 cup	207
Corn Flakes	1 cup	200
Fiberplus Berry Yogurt Crunch	1 cup	200
Raisin Bran Crunch	1 cup	200
Raisin Bran	1 cup	190
Rocky Mountain Chocolate Factory	1 cup	190
Fiberplus Cinnamon Oat Crunch	1 cup	186
Frosted Flakes	1 cup	186
Cracklin' Oat Bran	1 cup	180

Daily Adequate Intake is 1500 mg for adults

SODIUM

Continued

Crispix	1 cup	180
Cocoa Krispies	1 cup	173
Crunchy Nut Roasted Nut & Honey O's	1 cup	167
All-Bran Original	1 cup	160
Rice Krispies	1 cup	152
Frosted Rice Krispies	1 cup	148
Smorz	1 cup	137
Froot Loops	1 cup	135
Krave Chocolate	1 cup	133
Apple Jacks	1 cup	129
Krave Double Chocolate	1 cup	126
Cinnamon Jacks	1 cup	125
CINNABON	1 cup	116
Smart Start, Strong Heart Toasted Oat	1 cup	112
Corn Pops	1 cup	104
Honey Smacks	1 cup	53
Frosted MINI-Wheats, Big-Bite	1 cup	5
Frosted MINI-Wheats, Bite-Size	1 cup	3
Frosted MINI-Wheats, Little Bites, Original	1 cup	0
Frosted MINI-Wheats, Original	1 cup	0

Kellogg's® Special-K®	Amount	Sodium (mg)
Cinnamon Pecan	1 cup	253
Protein	1 cup	253
Chocolately Delight	1 cup	240
Chocolately Strawberry	1 cup	240
Low Fat Granola	1 cup	230
Chocolate Almond	1 cup	225
Original	1 cup	220
Multigrain Oats & Honey	1 cup	215
Vanilla Almond	1 cup	213
Oats & Honey	1 cup	210
Fruit & Yogurt	1 cup	195
Multigrain	1 cup	190
Red Berries	1 cup	190
Blueberry	1 cup	188

Mom's Best Naturals®	Amount	Sodium (mg)
Honey Grahams	1 cup	360
Raisin Bran	1 cup	340
Honey Nut Toasty O's	1 cup	210
Crispy Coco Rice	1 cup	200
Mallow Oats	1 cup	200
Oats & Honey Blend	1 cup	200
Toasted Cinnamon Squares	1 cup	187

SODIUM

Safari Cocoa Crunch	1 cup	147
Honey-Ful Wheats	1 cup	87
Blue Pom Wheat-Fuls	1 cup	10
Sweetened Wheat-Fuls	1 cup	10
Toasted Wheat Fuls	1 cup	10

Natures Path®	Amount	Sodium (mg)
Optimum Power Blueberry Cinnamon	1 cup	307
Blueberry Cinnamon Flax	1 cup	306
Optimum Slim Low Fat Vanilla	1 cup	290
Heritage Crunch	1 cup	280
Multigrain Spoonfuls	1 cup	267
Smart Bran	1 cup	260
Flax Plus Maple Pecan Crunch	1 cup	253
Flax Plus Raisin Bran	1 cup	253
Flax Plus Redberry Crunch	1 cup	213
Crispy Rice	1 cup	213
Sunrise, Crunchy Vanilla	1 cup	202
Flax Plus Pumpkin Raisin Crunch	1 cup	200
Sunrise, Crunchy Maple	1 cup	197
Optimum Banana Almond	1 cup	187
Flax Plus Multibran Flakes	1 cup	180
Heritage Flakes	1 cup	173
Whole O's	1 cup	173
Corn Flakes & Fruit Juice	1 cup	166
Mesa Sunrise, Gluten Free	1 cup	166
OATY BITES Whole Grain	1 cup	153
Organic Millet Rice	1 cup	153
Millet	1 cup	153
Multigrain Oat bran	1 cup	147
Honeyed Corn Flakes	1 cup	140
AGAVE Plus Granola	1 cup	127
Optimum Cranberry Ginger	1 cup	127
Flax Plus Vanilla Almond Granola	1 cup	107
Peanut Butter Granola	1 cup	100
Acai Apple Granola	1 cup	93
Pomegran Cherry Granola	1 cup	80
Pomegran Plus Granola	1 cup	80
Coconut Chia Granola	1 cup	67
Chia Plus Coconut Chia Granola	1 cup	67
Flax Plus Pumpkin Flax Granola	1 cup	60
Hemp Plus Granola	1 cup	60

Daily Adequate Intake is 1500 mg for adults

SODIUM

Peace Cereal®	Amount	Sodium (mg)
Ancient Grain Blend	1 cup	450
Wild Berry	1 cup	330
Maple Pecan	1 cup	220
Vanilla Almond	1 cup	210
Goji Berry & Chia	1 cup	190
Golden Honey Granola	1 cup	180
Blueberry Walnut	1 cup	157
Coconut Chia Almond	1 cup	142
Cherry Almond	1 cup	113
Blueberry Pomegranate	1 cup	27

Post®	Amount	Sodium (mg)
Grape-Nuts	1 cup	588
100% Bran Cereal	1 cup	363
Cocoa Pebbles	1 cup	253
Fruity Pebbles	1 cup	252
Raisin Bran	1 cup	250
Crunchy Pecan Cereal	1 cup	200
Raisin, Date & Pecan	1 cup	180
OREO O's Cereal	1 cup	171
Blueberry Morning	1 cup	168
Grape-Nuts Flakes	1 cup	167
Blueberry Morning	1 cup	165
Banana Nut Crunch	1 cup	140
Cranberry Almond Crunch	1 cup	140
Honeycomb Cereal	1 cup	115
Shredded Wheat, Honey Nut	1 cup	60
Golden Crisp	1 cup	34
Shredded Wheat, Frosted, spoon-size	1 cup	10
Shredded Wheat, Sugar and Salt Free	2 biscuits	3
Shredded Wheat n' Bran	1 cup	1
Shredded Wheat, spoon-size	1 cup	1
Shredded Wheat Original	2 biscuits	0

Post® Honey Bunches Of Oats®	Amount	Sodium (mg)
Cinnamon Bunches	1 cup	200
Raisin Medley	1 cup	200
Honey Roasted	1 cup	187
Pecan Bunches	1 cup	187
With Almonds	1 cup	180
With Vanilla Bunches	1 cup	170

Daily Adequate Intake is 1500 mg for adults

SODIUM

Continued

With Strawberries	1 cup	167
With Peaches	1 cup	160
Just Bunches, Honey Roasted	1 cup	121

Quaker®	Amount	Sodium (mg)
Corn Bran Crunch	1 cup	312
CAP'N Crunch	1 cup	271
CAP'N Crunch & Crunchberries	1 cup	251
Honey Graham OH'S	1 cup	220
LIFE Cereal, Original	1 cup	213
CAP'N Crunch's OOPs! All Berries	1 cup	204
LIFE Cereal, Cinnamon	1 cup	204
LIFE Cereal, Maple & Brown Sugar	1 cup	200
Oatmeal Squares	1 cup	193
Toasted Multigrain Crisp	1 cup	193
Oatmeal Squares, Brown Sugar	1 cup	190
Oatmeal Squares, Cinnamon	1 cup	190
Oatmeal Squares, Golden Maple	1 cup	190
Oatmeal Squares, Honey Nut	1 cup	190
Real Medley, Peach, Apple, Walnut	1 cup	60
Simply Granola, Oats, Honey, Raisin & Almond	1 cup	60
Real Medley, Cherry, Almond, Pecan	1 cup	54
Simply Granola, Oats, Honey & Almond	1 cup	50

Ralphs® Kroger® Brand Cereal	Amount	Sodium (mg)
Corn Flakes	1 cup	240
Bran Flakes	1 cup	226
Chocolate Toasted Oats	1 cup	226
Vanilla Flavored Flakes with Almond	1 cup	200
Cinnamon Swirls	1 cup	186
Honey Nut Bitz	1 cup	186
Honey Nut Toasted Oats	1 cup	186
Crunchy Raisin Bran	1 cup	180
Toasted Flakes Fruit with Yogurt	1 cup	173
Peanut Butter Multigrain Toasted Oats	1 cup	166
Frosted Flakes	1 cup	160
Honey Crisp Medley & Almond	1 cup	160
Crispy Rice	1 cup	144
Crispy Berry Crunch	1 cup	140
Fruity Rings	1 cup	135
Cocoa Crispy Rice	1 cup	133
Multigrain Toasted Oats	1 cup	110
Blueberry Frosted Shredded Wheat	1 cup	10

Daily Adequate Intake is 1500 mg for adults

SODIUM

Stater Brothers® Cereal	Amount	Sodium (mg)
Nutty Nuggets	1 cup	580
Banana Nut Medley	1 cup	465
Toasted Wheat	1 cup	440
Fruit & Crips, Raisin, Date, Pecan	1 cup	373
Honey Gram Crunch	1 cup	360
Cranberry Almond Crunch	1 cup	340
Toasted Rice	1 cup	240
Raisin Bran	1 cup	230
Bran Flakes	1 cup	226
Magic Stars	1 cup	213
Fiber Advantage	1 cup	210
Gini Mini Crunch	1 cup	186
Honey Nut Squares	1 cup	186
Honey Nut Toasted Oats	1 cup	186
Simple Living Oat	1 cup	186
Cocoa Crunchies	1 cup	180
Crunchy Raisin Bran	1 cup	180
Honey Oats & Flakes	1 cup	180
Koo Kies	1 cup	173
Apple Cinnamon Toasted Oats	1 cup	160
Corn Flakes	1 cup	160
Frosted Flakes	1 cup	160
Honey Oats & Flakes with Almonds	1 cup	160
Toasted Oats	1 cup	160
Freaky Fruits	1 cup	140
Cocoa Crispy Rice	1 cup	133
Multigrain Tasteeos'	1 cup	120
Frosted Shredded Wheat	1 cup	0
Shredded Wheat	1 cup	0

Target® Brand Cereal	Amount	Sodium (mg)
Toasted Cinnamon Squares	1 cup	280
Honey & Nut Toasted Oats	1 cup	253
Honey & Oat Mixers with Almonds	1 cup	240
Raisin Bran	1 cup	230
Frosted Bites with Marshmallows	1 cup	200
Honey & Oat Mixers	1 cup	187
Cinnamon Oat Bites	1 cup	180
Corn Flakes	1 cup	180
Toasted Oats	1 cup	160
Sugar Frosted Flakes	1 cup	153
Crispy Flakes with Red berries	1 cup	150
Toasted Rice	1 cup	144

Daily Adequate Intake is 1500 mg for adults

SODIUM

Trader Joe's® Brand Cereal	Amount	Sodium (mg)
Bran Flakes*	1 cup	293
Corn Flakes	1 cup	280
Toasted Oatmeal Flakes	1 cup	253
Crispy Rice	1 cup	250
Triple Berry O's*	1 cup	240
Honey Nut O's*	1 cup	213
Organic Raisin Bran Clusters	1 cup	170
Raisin Bran Clusters	1 cup	170
Frosted Flakes*	1 cup	166
Joes O's	1 cup	160
Banana Nut Clusters	1 cup	140
Maple Pecan Clusters	1 cup	140
Super Nutty Toffe Clusters	1 cup	140
Very Berry Clusters	1 cup	140
MuitiGrain O's	1 cup	135
Strawberry Yogurt Cereal*	1 cup	127
Vanilla Almond Clusters	1 cup	115
High Fiber Cereal	1 cup	105
Fruity O's	1 cup	95
Organic High Fiber O's	1 cup	88
Puffed Wheat	1 cup	0

Uncle Sam®	Amount	Sodium (mg)
Original	1 cup	180
Strawberry	1 cup	160
Honey Almond	1 cup	140
Skinners Raisin Bran	1 cup	120

Vons® Safeway® Brand Cereal	Amount	Sodium (mg)
Raisin Bran	1 cup	280
Honey Nut & Toasted Oats	1 cup	253
Rice Pockets	1 cup	240
Toasted Oats	1 cup	210
Cinnamon Crunch	1 cup	186
Live It Up	1 cup	186
Cinnamon Live it Up	1 cup	180
Crunchy Granola Raisin Bran	1 cup	180
Oats & More with Honey	1 cup	180
Corn Flakes	1 cup	160
Oats & More with Almond	1 cup	160
Apple Orbits	1 cup	150
Frosted Shredded Wheat, Bit Size	1 cup	10

Daily Adequate Intake is 1500 mg for adults

SODIUM

Vons® Eating Right® Cereal	Amount	Sodium (mg)
Cranberry Almond Multigrain	1 cup	340
Granola Cereal	1 cup	303
Granola Cereal & Raisins	1 cup	288
Toasted Rice, Wheat Flakes & Strawberry	1 cup	150

Wall Mart® Cereal	Amount	Sodium (mg)
Raisin Bran	1 cup	350
Extra Raisin Raisin Bran	1 cup	290
Cinnamon Crunch	1 cup	280
Toasted Whole-Grain	1 cup	269
Sugar Frosted Flakes	1 cup	267
Honey Nut	1 cup	253
Honey Nut Spins	1 cup	253
Crunchy Honey Oats with Almonds	1 cup	240
Toasted Rice	1 cup	240
Toasted Wheat	1 cup	240
Toasted Corn	1 cup	230
Berry Crunch	1 cup	226
Bran Flakes	1 cup	226
Crunchy Honey Oats	1 cup	226
Strawberry Awake	1 cup	220
Vanilla Almond Awake	1 cup	200
Crunchy Raisin Bran	1 cup	180
Corn Flakes	1 cup	160
Apple Blast	1 cup	150
Crispy Rice	1 cup	144
Fruit Spins	1 cup	135
Frosted Shredded Wheats	1 cup	0

Whole Foods® 365 Brand Cereal	Amount	Sodium (mg)
Cinnamon Raisin	1 cup	320
Wheat Waffles	1 cup	226
Morning O's	1 cup	160
Honey Flakes & Oat Clusters	1 cup	140
Multi-Grain Morning O's	1 cup	135
Bran Flakes	1 cup	133
Berry Flax Protein & Fiber Crunch	1 cup	120
Cocoa Rice Crisps	1 cup	120
Raisin Bran	1 cup	120
High Fiber Morning O's	1 cup	110
Protein & Fiber	1 cup	100
Brown Rice Crisp	1 cup	85
Corn Flakes	1 cup	80

Daily Adequate Intake is 1500 mg for adults

SODIUM

Frosted Flakes	1 cup	65
Wheat Squares	1 cup	0
Whole Wheat Flakes	1 cup	0

Wild Harvest®	Amount	Sodium (mg)
Wild Berry Crisp	1 cup	320
Maple Pecan Flakes	1 cup	210
Cranberry Almond	1 cup	190
Golden Honey Flax Granola	1 cup	180
Raisin Bran	1 cup	150
Crunchy Vanilla Almond Granola	1 cup	105
Blueberry Flax Granola	1 cup	90

Cereal, Cooked	Amount	Sodium (mg)
Farina	1 cup	43
CREAM OF WHEAT, regular	1 cup	15
Oats, regular, unenriched	1 cup	9
Malt-o-Meal, plain	1 serving	8
White corn grits	1 cup	5
Yellow corn grits	1 cup	5
WHEATENA	1 cup	5

Cheese	Amount	Sodium (mg)
Roquefort	1 oz	513
American, pasteurized process, fortified	1 oz	474
Parmesan, grated	1 oz	433
American, pasteurized process, low fat	1 oz	400
Blue cheese	1 oz	395
American, pasteurized process, imitation	1 oz	368
Romano	1 oz	340
Feta	1 oz	316
Provolone	1 oz	248
Provolone, reduced fat	1 oz	245
Gouda	1 oz	232
Cream cheese, fat free	1 oz	199
Pepper Jack, Red & Green Jalapenos	1 oz	190
Mozzarella, part skim milk, low moisture	1 oz	185
Brie	1 oz	178
Mozzarella, whole milk	1 oz	178
Muenster	1 oz	178
Cheddar	1 oz	175
Cheddar, low fat	1 oz	174
Colby	1 oz	171
Muenster, low fat	1 oz	168

SODIUM

Monterey, low fat	1 oz	158
Goat cheese, semisoft type	1 oz	146
Goat cheese, soft type	1 oz	104
Goat cheese, hard type	1 oz	98
Gruyere	1 oz	95
Cream cheese	1 oz	91
Swiss, low fat	1 oz	73
Swiss	1 oz	54

Cheese, Mexican	Amount	Sodium (mg)
Queso anejo	1 oz	321
Mexican, blend, reduced	1 oz	220
Queso fresco	1 oz	213
Mexican, blend	1 oz	195
Queso asadero	1 oz	186
Queso chihuahua	1 oz	175

Chicken, Cooked	Amount	Sodium (mg)
Thigh, with skin, fried	1 thigh	248
Breast, with skin, fried with flour	1/2 breast	74
Breast, no skin, roasted	1/2 breast	64
Thigh, no skin, roasted	1 thigh	46
Drumstick, with skin, fried	1 drumstick	44
Drumstick, no skin, roasted	1 drumstick	42

Chicken, Cooked	Amount	Sodium (mg)
Drumstick meat only, no skin, roasted	3 oz	100
Wing meat only, no skin, roasted	3 oz	78
Drumstick with skin, fried in flour	3 oz	76
Thigh with skin, fried in flour	3 oz	75
Thigh meat only, no skin, roasted	3 oz	74
Thigh with skin, roasted	3 oz	73
Wing with skin, fried in flour	3 oz	65
Breast meat only, no skin, roasted	3 oz	63
Breast with skin, roasted	3 oz	60

CHILI

Chili, Amy's Organic	Amount	Sodium (mg)
Cattle Drive Golden Chili with beans	1 can	1640
Black Bean Chili	1 can	1360
Medium Chili	1 can	1360
Southwestern Black Bean Chili	1 can	1360

Daily Adequate Intake is 1500 mg for adults

SODIUM

Continued

Spicy Chili	1 can	1360
Medium Chili with Vegetables	1 can	1180
Light in Sodium Medium Chili	1 can	680
Light in Sodium Spicy Chili	1 can	680

Chili, Campbell's® Chunky	Amount	Sodium (mg)
Chunky Chili with Beans Roadhouse	1 can	1740
Chunky Chili with Beans Firehouse	1 can	1740
Chunky Chili with Beans Grilled Steak	1 can	1740
Chunky Chili no Beans	1 can	1540

Chili, Dennison's®	Amount	Sodium (mg)
Chili Con Carne no Beans	1 can	2220
Chunky Chili Con Carne with Beans	1 can	2040
Hot & Spicy Chili Con Carne with Beans	1 can	1960
Original Chili Con Carne with Beans	1 can	1880
Hot & Chunky Chili with Beans	1 can	1860
Turkey Chili with Beans	1 can	1700
Vegetarian Chili with Beans	1 can	1600

Chili, Eden's	Amount	Sodium (mg)
Great Northern Bean & Barley Chili	1 can	980
Kidney Bean & Kamut Chili	1 can	920
Pinto Bean & Spelt Chili	1 can	920

Chili, Hardy Jack's	Amount	Sodium (mg)
Chili with beans	1 can	2400

Chili, Healthy Valley	Amount	Sodium (mg)
No salt Added Tame Tomato Chili	1 can	940
Santa Fe White Bean Chili	1 can	940
Vegetarian Black Bean Mole Chili	1 can	940
Vegetarian Three Bean Chipotle Chili	1 can	940

Chili, Hormel®	Amount	Sodium (mg)
Hot Chili with beans	1 can	2120
Cook- off White Chicken Chili	1 can	1980
Cook-off Roasted Tomato Chili	1 can	1980
Chili no Beans	1 can	1940
Cook-off Chipotle Chicken Chili	1 can	1940
Vegetarian Chili with Beans 99% fat free	1 can	1560
Less Sodium Chili no Beans	1 can	1440

Daily Adequate Intake is 1500 mg for adults

SODIUM

Chili, Nalley's	Amount	Sodium (mg)
Lean Beaf with Beans	1 can	2500
Turkey Chili no Beans	1 can	2470
Original Chili Con Carne with beans	1 can	2280
Steak House Chili no Beans	1 can	2160
Turkey Chili with Beans	1 can	2160
White Chicken Chili with Beans	1 can	2020
Fiesta Grille Chili with Beans	1 can	1900
Silverado Beef Chili with Beans	1 can	1720
Chunkero Chili with Beans	1 can	1700
Classi Chili with beans	1 can	1640
Dynamite Hot Chili with Beans	1 can	1600
Ranch House Chicken Chili with Beans	1 can	1560

Crackers	Amount	Sodium (mg)
Milton Gourmet, Original Whole Grain	1 cracker	52
Brenton, Original	1 cracker	37
Keebler Club, Original	1 cracker	31
Saltines	1 cracker	27
Keebler Town House, Original	1 cracker	26
Triscuits, Original	1 cracker	26
Carr's Table Water Crackers	1 cracker	20
Melba Rounds	1 cracker	16
Wheat Thins, Original	1 cracker	14
Cheez-It. Original	1 cracker	9
Ritz, Original	1 cracker	6

Cream	Amount	Sodium (mg)
Sour Cream, cultured	1 tbsp	10
Half & Half	1 tbsp	6
Heavy Cream	1 tbsp	6
Light Coffe cream	1 tbsp	6
Sour Cream, reduced fat	1 tbsp	6
Whipping Cream, pressurized	1 tbsp	4

Eggs	Amount	Sodium (mg)
Egg whites, dried	1 ounce	363
Egg substitute, liquid, fat free	1/4 cup	119
Egg whole, fried	1 large	95
Egg whole, scrambled	1 large	88
Egg whites, dried powder, stabilized	1 tbsp	87
Egg whole, hard-boiled	1 large	62
Egg whites	1 large	55
Egg yolk	1 large	8

Daily Adequate Intake is 1500 mg for adults

SODIUM

Fish, Canned	Amount	Sodium (mg)
White tuna, in oil	3 oz	337
White tuna, in water	3 oz	320
Light tuna, in water	3 oz	210
Light tuna, in oil	3 oz	30

Fish, Cooked	Amount	Sodium (mg)
Atlantic hearing, pickled	3 oz	740
Chinock salmon, smoked	3 oz	666
Whiting	3 oz	369
Walley pollock	3 oz	356
Pacific cod	3 oz	316
Flounder & Sole	3 oz	309
Atlantic croaker	3 oz	296
Atlantic perch	3 oz	295
Cat fish, breaded & fried	3 oz	238
Haddock	3 oz	222
King mackerel	3 oz	173
Sockeye salmon	3 oz	114
Cat fish, farmed	3 oz	101
Atlantic pollock	3 oz	94
Pacific mackerel	3 oz	94
Greenland halibut	3 oz	88
Swordfish	3 oz	82
Freshwater bass	3 oz	76
Pink salmon	3 oz	76
Striped bass	3 oz	75
Sea bass	3 oz	74
Alaskan halibut	3 oz	73
Atlantic mackerel	3 oz	71
Atlantic & Pacific halibut	3 oz	70
Halibut	3 oz	70
Atlantic cod	3 oz	66
Florida pompano	3 oz	65
Orange roughy	3 oz	59
Spanish mackerel	3 oz	56
Walleye pike	3 oz	55
Carp	3 oz	54
Keta (chum) salmon	3 oz	54
Atlantic salmon, farmed	3 oz	52
Rainbow trout, farmed	3 oz	52
King, chinook salmon	3 oz	51

SODIUM

Continued

Coho salmon, wild	3 oz	49
Atlantic salmon, wild	3 oz	48
Rainbow trout, wild	3 oz	48
Snapper	3 oz	48
Tilapia	3 oz	48
Yellowfin tuna	3 oz	46
Grouper	3 oz	45
Coho salmon, farmed	3 oz	44
Bluefin tuna	3 oz	42
Cat fish, wild	3 oz	42
Northern pike	3 oz	42
Yellowtail	3 oz	42
Skipjack (aku) tuna	3 oz	40

Fish, Shellfish, Cooked	Amount	Sodium (mg)
Alaskan king crab	3 oz	911
Shrimp	3 oz	805
Alaskan king crab, imitation	3 oz	715
Shrimp, canned	3 oz	660
Queen crab	3 oz	587
Abalone	3 oz	502
Scallops, breaded & fried	6 large	432
Northern lobster	3 oz	413
Octopus	3 oz	391
Oysters, breaded & fried	3 oz	354
Blue crab	3 oz	336
Blue crab, canned	3 oz	336
Clams, breaded & fried	3 oz	309
Shrimp, breaded & fried	3 oz	292
Blue crab cakes	3 oz	280
Squid, fried	3 oz	260
Eastern oysters, wild	3 oz	206
Eastern oysters, farmed	3 oz	139
Crayfish	3 oz	80

Daily Adequate Intake is 1500 mg for adults

SODIUM

FRUIT

Fruit, Canned	Amount	Sodium (mg)
Olives, green	5 large	210
Olives, black	5 large	162
Plums	1 cup	49
Peaches	1 cup	16
Pears	1 cup	13
Apricots	1 cup	10
Applesauce, sweetened	1 cup	5
Pineapple	1 cup	3

Fruit, Dried	Amount	Sodium (mg)
Apples	1 cup	75
Figs	1 cup	15
Apricots	1 cup	13
Currants	1 cup	12
Peaches	1 cup	11
Pears	1 cup	11

Fruit, Frozen	Amount	Sodium (mg)
Peaches	1 cup	15
Strawberries	1 cup	8
Blackberries	1 cup	2
Blueberries	1 cup	2

Fruit, Raw	Amount	Sodium (mg)
Honeydew	1 cup	31
Cataloupe	1 cup	26
Avocado, California	1 cup	18
Raisins	1 cup	16
Papayas	1 cup	12
Elderberries	1 cup	9
Plantains	1 cup	7
Pineapple	1 cup	6
Jicama	1 cup	5
Tangerine	1 cup	4
Dates	1 cup	3
Grapes, green & red	1 cup	3
Prunes, uncooked	1 cup	3
Apricots	1 cup	2
Black currants	1 cup	2
Cranberries	1 cup	2

Daily Adequate Intake is 1500 mg for adults

SODIUM

Mango	1 cup	2
Pears	1 cup	2
Strawberries	1 cup	2
Water mellon	1 cup	2
Apples	1 cup	1
Blackberries	1 cup	1
Raspberries	1 cup	1
Cherries	1 cup	0
Nectarine	1 cup	0
Oranges	1 cup	0
Peachs	1 cup	0
Plums	1 cup	0

Fruit, Raw	Amount	Sodium (mg)
Avocado, California	1 fruit	10
Avocado, Florida	1 fruit	5
Kiwi	1 fruit	2
Tangerine	1 fruit	2
Apples	1 fruit	1
Banana	1 fruit	1
Dates	5 fruit	1
Figs, dried	1 fruit	1
Prunes, uncooked	5 fruit	1
Strawberries	5 fruit	1
Apricots	1 fruit	0
Cherries	10 fruit	0
Nectarine	1 fruit	0
Oranges	1 fruit	0
Pineapple	1/2" x 3" slice	0
Plums	1 fruit	0

Game Meat	Amount	Sodium (mg)
Elk, ground	3 oz	72
Deer, ground	3 oz	66
Bison, ground	3 oz	62
Duck	3 oz	55
Elk	3 oz	52
Antelope	3 oz	46
Deer	3 oz	46
Rabbit	3 oz	38

Daily Adequate Intake is 1500 mg for adults

SODIUM

Grains	Amount	Sodium (mg)
Spaghetti, enriched	1 cup	183
Soba noodles	1 cup	68
Rice noodles	1 cup	33
Spaghetti, spinach	1 cup	20
Egg & Spinach noodles	1 cup	19
Amaranth	1 cup	15
Quinoa	1 cup	13
Brown rice	1 cup	10
Bulgur	1 cup	9
Oats, regular, unenriched	1 cup	9
Couscous	1 cup	8
Egg noodles	1 cup	8
Buckwheat, groats	1 cup	7
White rice, instant	1 cup	7
Macaroni, Whole-Wheat	1 cup	4
Spaghetti, Whole-Wheat	1 cup	4
White rice, paraboiled	1 cup	3
Oat bran	1 cup	2
White rice, regular	1 cup	2
Macaroni	1 cup	1

Herbs & Spices	Amount	Sodium (mg)
Table salt	1 tsp	2325
Chili powder	1 tsp	43.0
Parsley, dried	1 tsp	6.0
Cloves, dried	1 tsp	4.9
Cumin	1 tsp	4.0
Celery seeds	1 tsp	3.0
Garlic powder	1 tsp	2.0
Onion powder	1 tsp	2.0
All-spice, ground	1 tsp	1.3
Basil, dried & ground	1 tsp	1.0
Curry powder	1 tsp	1.0
Paprika	1 tsp	1.0
Saffron	1 tsp	1.0
Tarragon, dried	1 tsp	0.9
Turmeric, ground	1 tsp	0.8
Thyme, dried	1 tsp	0.7
Ginger, ground	1 tsp	0.6
Coriander, seeds	1 tsp	0.6
Chervil, dried	1 tsp	0.5
Rosemary, dried	1 tsp	0.5
Rosemary, fresh	1 tsp	0.4
Anise seed	1 tsp	0.3

Daily Adequate Intake is 1500 mg for adults

SODIUM

Bay leaf, crumbled	1 tsp	0.1
Thyme, fresh	1 tsp	0.1
Chives, raw	1 tsp	0
Cinnamon powder	1 tsp	0
Oregano	1 tsp	0
Pepper, black	1 tsp	0

Juice	Amount	Sodium (mg)
Tomato, canned with salt	1 cup	654
Vegetable	1 cup	479
V8 Original Vegetable, 5.5 fl oz	1 small can	450
Carrot	1 cup	156
Pomegranate	1 cup	22
Grape, unsweetened	1 cup	13
Apple, unsweetened	1 cup	10
Prune	1 cup	10
Pineapple, unsweetened	1 cup	5
Lemon juice, raw	1 cup	2
Orange juice, raw	1 cup	2

Lamb, Cooked	Amount	Sodium (mg)
Rib, lean, trim to 1/4" fat	3 oz	72
Ground	3 oz	69
Chops, loin, lean, trim to 1/4" fat	3 oz	65
Cubed, for stew or kabob	3 oz	65
Foreshank, trim to 1/8" fat	3 oz	61
Leg, whole, trim to1/4" fat	3 oz	56

Milk	Amount	Sodium (mg)
Canned, condensed, sweetened	1 cup	389
Canned, evaporated, non fat	1 cup	294
Canned, evaporated	1 cup	267
Dry, instant, non fat	1/3 cup	126
Soy milk, original, unfortified	1 cup	124
Sheep milk	1 cup	108
Lowfat,1%	1 cup	107
Whole milk, 3.25%	1 cup	105
Nonfat, fat free or skim liquid milk	1 cup	103
Human milk	1 cup	42
Coconut milk, canned	1 cup	29

Daily Adequate Intake is 1500 mg for adults

SODIUM

Nuts & Seeds	Amount	Sodium (mg)
Peanuts, roasted with salt	1 oz	192
Cashews, roasted with salt	1 oz	181
Sunflower seeds, roasted with salt	1 oz	116
Pecans, roasted with salt	1 oz	109
Almonds, roasted with salt	1 oz	96
Macadamia, roasted with salt	1 oz	75
Flaxseeds	1 oz	9
Coconut, raw meat	1 oz	6
Chia seeds	1 oz	5
Peanuts	1 oz	5
Pumpkin seeds, roasted no salt	1 oz	5
Cashews, raw	1 oz	3
Sunflower seeds	1 oz	3
Pumpkin seeds	1 oz	2
Black Walnuts	1 oz	1
Brazilnuts	1 oz	1
English Walnuts	1 oz	1
Macadamia, raw	1 oz	1
Pine nuts	1 oz	1
Almonds, raw	1 oz	0
Hazelnuts	1 oz	0

Pork, Cooked	Amount	Sodium (mg)
Bacon	3 oz	1964
Canadian-style bacon	3 oz	1314
Cured ham, lean	3 oz	1128
Italian sausage	3 oz	1026
Cured ham	3 oz	1009
Braunschweiger	3 oz	830
Polish sausage	3 oz	745
Bratwurst	3 oz	719
Canadian-style bacon	2 slices	719
Sausage	3 oz	637
Bacon	3 slices	439
Liverwurst spread	1/4 cup	385
Pork chops, lean, pan fried	3 oz	84
Backribs	3 oz	80
Pork chops, pan fried	3 oz	80
Ground pork	3 oz	62
Sirloin pork chops	3 oz	55
Tenderloin	3 oz	48
Pork chops, broiled	3 oz	47

Daily Adequate Intake is 1500 mg for adults

SALAD DRESSING

Albertsons® Brand Dressings	Amount	Sodium (mg)
Zesty French	2 tbsp	380
Thousand Island, Reduced Fat	2 tbsp	350
Italian	2 tbsp	340
Italian, reduced Fat	2 tbsp	340
Caesar	2 tbsp	290
Balsamic Vinaigrette	2 tbsp	290
Buttermilk Ranch	2 tbsp	290
Thousand Island	2 tbsp	270
Blue Cheese	2 tbsp	270
Creamy Ranch	2 tbsp	260
French	2 tbsp	230

Annies's® Organic Dressing	Amount	Sodium (mg)
Thousand Island	2 tbsp	360
Creamy Asiago Cheese	2 tbsp	330
Goddnes	2 tbsp	320
Woodstock	2 tbsp	310
Artichoke Parmesan	2 tbsp	290
Asian Sesame	2 tbsp	290
Buttermilk Dressing	2 tbsp	250
Cowgirl Ranch	2 tbsp	250
Sesame Ginger Vinaigrette	2 tbsp	250
Tuscany Italian	2 tbsp	250
Caesar	2 tbsp	240
Roasted Red Pepper	2 tbsp	240
Oil & Vinegar	2 tbsp	220
Roasted Garlic Vinaigrette	2 tbsp	220
French Dressing	2 tbsp	200
Pomegranate Vinaigrette	2 tbsp	200
Redwine & Olive Oil	2 tbsp	190
Papaya Poppy Seed	2 tbsp	180
Green Garlic	2 tbsp	170
Lemon Chive	2 tbsp	170
Balsamic Vinaigrette	2 tbsp	55
Raspberry Balsamic, Fat-Free	2 tbsp	10
Mango Fat Free	2 tbsp	5

Annies's® Lite Dressing	Amount	Sodium (mg)
Gingerly Lite	2 tbsp	280
Goodness	2 tbsp	240
Herb Balsamic	2 tbsp	230

SODIUM

Continued

Italian	2 tbsp	230
Poppy Seed	2 tbsp	210
Honey Mustard	2 tbsp	125
Raspberry	2 tbsp	55

Archer Farms® from Target®	Amount	Sodium (mg)
House Italian	2 tbsp	460
Basil Parmesan	2 tbsp	350
Chipolte Caesar	2 tbsp	300
Roasted Garlic Bacon Ranch	2 tbsp	280
Three Cheese Ranch	2 tbsp	260
Raspberry Balsamic	2 tbsp	230

Bernstein's® Dressing	Amount	Sodium (mg)
Cheese Fantastico	2 tbsp	440
Basil Parmesan	2 tbsp	400
Cheese & Garlic Italian	2 tbsp	400
Cheese & Garlic Italian, Fat Free	2 tbsp	400
Light Fantastic Cheese Fantastico	2 tbsp	370
Restaurant Recipe Italian	2 tbsp	370
Italian & Marinade	2 tbsp	360
Light Parmesan Garlic Ranch	2 tbsp	330
Light Roasted Garlic Balsamic	2 tbsp	320
Roasted Garlic Balsamic	2 tbsp	280
Herb Garden French	2 tbsp	260
Balsamic Italian	2 tbsp	250
Redwine & Garlic Italian	2 tbsp	250
Creamy Caesar	2 tbsp	230
Chunky Blue Chees	2 tbsp	180

Best Food® Mayonnaise Dressing	Amount	Sodium (mg)
Low Fat Mayonnaise	2 tbsp	260
Mayonnaise with Olive Oil	2 tbsp	260
Light Mayonnaise	2 tbsp	250
Canola Cholesterol Free Mayonnaise	2 tbsp	230
Real Mayonnaise	2 tbsp	180
Mayonesa Con Jugo De Lemon	2 tbsp	180

Bob's Big-Boy® Dressing	Amount	Sodium (mg)
Roquefort	2 tbsp	240
Blue Cheese	2 tbsp	190
Thousand Island	2 tbsp	180
Ranch	2 tbsp	160

Daily Adequate Intake is 1500 mg for adults

SODIUM

Bolthouse® Farms Desssing	Amount	Sodium (mg)
Asian Ginger & Olive Oil Vinaigrettes	2 tbsp	310
Classic Ranch Yogurt Dressing	2 tbsp	280
Zesty French Yogurt	2 tbsp	220
Cilantro Avocado Yogurt Dressing	2 tbsp	210
Mango Chipotle	2 tbsp	210
Salsa Ranch Yogurt Dressing	2 tbsp	210
Miso Ginger	2 tbsp	190
Thousand Island Yogurt Dressing	2 tbsp	180
Caesar Parmigino Yogurt Desssing	2 tbsp	170
Chunky Blue Cheese & Olive Oil	2 tbsp	150
Classic Balsamic & Olive Oil	2 tbsp	150
Chunky Bluecheese Yogurt Dressing	2 tbsp	135
Organic Balsamic Vinaigrette	2 tbsp	135
Italian Vinaigrette	2 tbsp	120
Honey Mustard Yogurt Dressing	2 tbsp	115
Raspberry Merlot & Olive Oil	2 tbsp	50

Briannas® Dressing	Amount	Sodium (mg)
Rich Santa Fe Blend	2 tbsp	480
Blush Wine Vinaigrette	2 tbsp	420
Saucy Ginger Mandarin	2 tbsp	340
Asiago Caesar	2 tbsp	310
The New American Creamy Balsamic	2 tbsp	290
Classic Buttermilk Ranch	2 tbsp	280
Real French Vinaigrette	2 tbsp	260
True Blue Cheese	2 tbsp	250
Chipotle Cheddar	2 tbsp	240
Zesty French	2 tbsp	240
Rich Poppy Seed	2 tbsp	220
Dijon Honey Mustard	2 tbsp	170
Lively Lemon Tarragon	2 tbsp	150
Champagne Caper Vinaigrette	2 tbsp	105

Cardini's® Dressing	Amount	Sodium (mg)
Fat Free Caesar	2 tbsp	510
Roasted Asian Sesame	2 tbsp	370
Aged Parmesan Ranch	2 tbsp	300
Light Greek Vinaigrette	2 tbsp	280
Light Caesar	2 tbsp	260
Balsamic Vinaigrette	2 tbsp	250
Original Caesar	2 tbsp	240
Red Jalapeno Caesar	2 tbsp	240
Garlic Lemon Caesar	2 tbsp	230

Daily Adequate Intake is 1500 mg for adults

SODIUM

Continued

Balsamic Vinaigrette, Light	2 tbsp	220
Italian Dressing	2 tbsp	220
Honey Mustard	2 tbsp	180
Pear Vinaigrette	2 tbsp	150
Raspberry Pomegranate	2 tbsp	150

Cindys Kitchen® Dressing	Amount	Sodium (mg)
Real Blue Cheese	2 tbsp	250
Rosemary & Roasted Garlic Vinaigrette	2 tbsp	220
Avocado Vinaigrette	2 tbsp	210
Lemon & Shallot Vinaigrette	2 tbsp	190
Asiago Cracked Pepper Corn	2 tbsp	160
Balsamic Vinaigrette	2 tbsp	150
Fresh Buttermilk Ranch	2 tbsp	140
Roasted Garlic Caesar	2 tbsp	110
Honey Dijon Vinaigrette	2 tbsp	60
Pomegranate Vinaigrette, Low Sodium	2 tbsp	60

Drew's® Dressing	Amount	Sodium (mg)
Goodness	2 tbsp	290
Buttermilk Ranch	2 tbsp	250
Creamy Ranch	2 tbsp	240
Honey Dijon	2 tbsp	230
Lemon Goddess	2 tbsp	230
Asian Ginger	2 tbsp	210
Classic Italian	2 tbsp	210
Sesame Orange	2 tbsp	210
Shiitake Ginger	2 tbsp	210
Poppy Seed	2 tbsp	200
Romano Ceaser	2 tbsp	190
Roasted Red Pepper	2 tbsp	180
Classic Ceaser	2 tbsp	150
Rosemary Balsamic	2 tbsp	148
Thai Sesame Lime	2 tbsp	140
Aged Balsamic	2 tbsp	125
Roasted Garlic & Peppercorn	2 tbsp	95
Raspberry	2 tbsp	80
Greek Olive	2 tbsp	75
Smoked Tomato	2 tbsp	75

Daily Adequate Intake is 1500 mg for adults

SODIUM

Continued

Field Day® from Brystal Farms®	Amount	Sodium (mg)
Lemon Tahini	2 tbsp	420
Ranch	2 tbsp	230
Classic Italian	2 tbsp	210
Balsamic Vinaigrette	2 tbsp	125

Follow-Your-Heart® Dressing	Amount	Sodium (mg)
Vegan Lemon Herb	2 tbsp	290
Creamy Ranch	2 tbsp	240
Chipolte Lime Ranch	2 tbsp	230
Miso Ginger	2 tbsp	230
Vegan Caesar	2 tbsp	220
Low Fat Ranch	2 tbsp	220
Creamy Caesar	2 tbsp	210
Vegan Thousand Island	2 tbsp	210
Thick & Creamy Caesar	2 tbsp	190
Vegan Creamy Garlic	2 tbsp	180
High Omega Vegan Ranch	2 tbsp	150
High Omega Vegan Blue Cheese	2 tbsp	150
Vegan Honey Mustard	2 tbsp	125
Original Balsamic Vinaigrette	2 tbsp	95
Low Fat Balsamic Vinaigrette	2 tbsp	95

Girard's® Dressing	Amount	Sodium (mg)
Light Champagne	2 tbsp	470
Old Venice Italian	2 tbsp	470
Champagne	2 tbsp	450
Original French	2 tbsp	410
Romano Cheese Italian	2 tbsp	380
Blue Cheese Vinaigrette	2 tbsp	320
Caesar	2 tbsp	320
Chinese Chicken Salad	2 tbsp	320
Greek Feta Vinaigrette	2 tbsp	260
White Balsamic Vinaigrette	2 tbsp	250
Creamy Balsamic Vinaigrette	2 tbsp	220
Peach Mimosa Vinaigrette	2 tbsp	135
Apple Poppy Seed	2 tbsp	105
Raspberry	2 tbsp	70

Hidden Valley® Dressing	Amount	Sodium (mg)
Buttermilk Ranch Light	2 tbsp	310
Spicy Ranch	2 tbsp	310
Garden Vegetable Ranch	2 tbsp	270
Original Ranch	2 tbsp	260

Daily Adequate Intake is 1500 mg for adults

SODIUM

Continued

	Amount	Sodium (mg)
Original Ranch Light	2 tbsp	260
Old Fashioned Buttermilk Ranch	2 tbsp	240
Buttermilk	2 tbsp	230
Organic Original Ranch	2 tbsp	220
Cracked Peppercorn Ranch	2 tbsp	210
Bacon Ranch	2 tbsp	200
Coleslaw	2 tbsp	170

Hidden Valley® Farm House	Amount	Sodium (mg)
Creamy Balsamic with Herb	2 tbsp	290
Savory Bleu Cheese	2 tbsp	280
Southwest Chipotle	2 tbsp	280
Italian with Herb	2 tbsp	270
Original Italian with Herb	2 tbsp	270
Garden Tomato & Bacon	2 tbsp	260
Hickory Bacon & Onion	2 tbsp	260
Creamy Parmesan	2 tbsp	230
Homestyle Italian	2 tbsp	220
Original Caesar	2 tbsp	220
Roasted Onion Parmesan	2 tbsp	210
Pomegranate Vinaigrette	2 tbsp	100

Kens® Steak House	Amount	Sodium (mg)
Zesty Italian	2 tbsp	550
Italian with Olive Oil	2 tbsp	530
Italian Marinade	2 tbsp	460
Red Wine Vinegar Oil	2 tbsp	360
3 Cheese Italian	2 tbsp	350
Creamy Italian	2 tbsp	330
Italian & Aged Romano	2 tbsp	310
Thousand Island	2 tbsp	300
Chunky Blue Cheese	2 tbsp	290
Ranch	2 tbsp	290
Balsamic Vinaigrete	2 tbsp	280
Raspberry Fat Free	2 tbsp	280
Greek & Olive Oil	2 tbsp	270
Buttermilk Ranch	2 tbsp	260
Northern Italian Basil & Romano	2 tbsp	260
Pepper Corn Ranch	2 tbsp	260
Creamy Caesar	2 tbsp	250
Russian	2 tbsp	240
Balsamic & Honey	2 tbsp	160
Honey Mustard	2 tbsp	150
Sweet Vidalia Onion	2 tbsp	120

Daily Adequate Intake is 1500 mg for adults

SODIUM

Ken's® Lite Dressing	Amount	Sodium (mg)
Caesar	2 tbsp	550
Zesty italian	2 tbsp	440
Asian Sesame Ginger & Soy	2 tbsp	390
Chunky Bluecheese	2 tbsp	370
Creamy Caesar	2 tbsp	320
Balsamic Vinaigrete	2 tbsp	310
Ranch	2 tbsp	310
Thousand Island	2 tbsp	270
Northern Italian & Basil & Romano	2 tbsp	260
Poppy Seed	2 tbsp	150
Raspberry & Walnut Vinaigrette	2 tbsp	125
Sweet Vidalia Onion	2 tbsp	120

Kraft® Dressing	Amount	Sodium (mg)
Zesty Italian	2 tbsp	380
Sweet Honey Catalina	2 tbsp	380
Strawberry Balsamic	2 tbsp	360
Balsamic Vinaigrette	2 tbsp	350
Zesty Catalina	2 tbsp	340
Asian Toasted Sesame	2 tbsp	320
Chunky Blue Cheese	2 tbsp	320
Tomato Basil Balsamic	2 tbsp	320
Ranch	2 tbsp	300
Zesty Italian Anything	2 tbsp	300
Zesty Italian Dressing & Marinade	2 tbsp	300
Buttermilk Ranch	2 tbsp	290
Raspberry	2 tbsp	290
Coleslaw	2 tbsp	280
Creamy Poppyseed	2 tbsp	280
Classic Caesar	2 tbsp	270
Honey Mustard	2 tbsp	270
Ranch with Bacon	2 tbsp	270
Thousand Island	2 tbsp	270
Classic Ranch	2 tbsp	260
Green Goddnes	2 tbsp	260
Nesty Lime	2 tbsp	260
Peppercorn Ranch	2 tbsp	260
Roka Blue Cheese	2 tbsp	250
Cucumber Ranch	2 tbsp	240
Creamy French	2 tbsp	230
Creamy Italian	2 tbsp	220
Sweet Balsamic	2 tbsp	190
Sweet Balsamic Vinaigrette	2 tbsp	180

Daily Adequate Intake is 1500 mg for adults

SODIUM

Kraft® Fat Free Dressing	Amount	Sodium (mg)
Catalina Fat Free	2 tbsp	350
Classic Catalina Fat Free	2 tbsp	350
Zesty Italian Fat Free	2 tbsp	340
Ranch Fat Free	2 tbsp	330
Thousand Island Fat Free	2 tbsp	260

Kraft® Lite Dressing	Amount	Sodium (mg)
Ranch	2 tbsp	370
Classic Ranch	2 tbsp	350
Thousand Island	2 tbsp	340
Zesty Italian	2 tbsp	310
Raspberry	2 tbsp	240
Balsamic Vinaigrette	2 tbsp	210

Kroger® Dressing	Amount	Sodium (mg)
Roasted Red Pepper	2 tbsp	460
Zesty Italian Fat Free	2 tbsp	420
Balsamic & Basil Vinaigrette	2 tbsp	420
California French	2 tbsp	370
Chunky Blue Cheese	2 tbsp	360
Lite Creamy Caesar	2 tbsp	340
Creamy Buttermilk	2 tbsp	310
California & Honey French	2 tbsp	310
Greek	2 tbsp	290
Olive Oil & Vinegar	2 tbsp	290
Bacon & Honey French	2 tbsp	280
Russian	2 tbsp	260
Pepper Corn Ranch	2 tbsp	260
Lite Southwestern Ranch	2 tbsp	260
Three Cheese Ranch	2 tbsp	250
Poppy Seed	2 tbsp	240
Creamy Ranch	2 tbsp	240
Lite Raspberry Vinaigrette	2 tbsp	230
Honey Mustard	2 tbsp	220
Thousand Island	2 tbsp	200

Litehouse® Dressing	Amount	Sodium (mg)
Strawberry Balsamic	2 tbsp	360
Balsamic Vinaigrette	2 tbsp	350
Asian Toasted Sesame	2 tbsp	320
Tomato Basil Balsamic	2 tbsp	320
Barbecue Ranch	2 tbsp	290

Daily Adequate Intake is 1500 mg for adults

SODIUM

Continued

Sweet French	2 tbsp	280
Sesame Ginger	2 tbsp	270
Yogurt Bleu Cheese with Kefir	2 tbsp	270
Ceaser Dressing	2 tbsp	250
Tuscan House Italian	2 tbsp	250
Homestyle Ranch	2 tbsp	240
Original Thousand Island	2 tbsp	240
Pear Gorzonzola Dressing	2 tbsp	240
Creamy Cilantro	2 tbsp	230
Chunky Bleu Cheese	2 tbsp	220
Jalapeno Ranch	2 tbsp	220
Original Bleu Cheese	2 tbsp	220
Parmesan Caesar	2 tbsp	220
Yogurt Ranch with Kefir	2 tbsp	220
Ranch Dressing	2 tbsp	200
Organic Ranch	2 tbsp	190
Sweet Balsamic	2 tbsp	190
Ceaser-Caesar Dressing	2 tbsp	170
Honey Mustard	2 tbsp	140
Coleslaw Dressing	2 tbsp	130
Coleslaw with Pinapple	2 tbsp	110
Harvest Cranberry Greek	2 tbsp	110
Chunky Garlic Caesar	2 tbsp	85

Litehouse® Lite Dressing	Amount	Sodium (mg)
Zesty Italian	2 tbsp	310
Jalapeno Ranch Dressing	2 tbsp	270
Asian Toasted Sesame	2 tbsp	260
Bleu Cheese Dressing	2 tbsp	260
Coleslaw Dressing	2 tbsp	250
1000 Island Dressing	2 tbsp	240
Creamy Ranch Dressing	2 tbsp	240
Caesar Dressing	2 tbsp	220
Balsamic Vinaigrette	2 tbsp	210
Honey Dijon Vinaigrette	2 tbsp	150

Litehouse® Vinaigrette	Amount	Sodium (mg)
Zesty Italian Vinaigrette	2 tbsp	340
Bleu Cheese Vinaigrette	2 tbsp	280
Cherry Vinaigrette	2 tbsp	250
Greek Vinaigrette	2 tbsp	170
Balsamic Vinaigrette	2 tbsp	150
Fuji Apple Vinaigrette	2 tbsp	140
Red Wine Olive Oil Vinaigrette	2 tbsp	140
Organic Balsamic Vinaigrette	2 tbsp	135

Daily Adequate Intake is 1500 mg for adults

SODIUM

Continued

	Amount	Sodium (mg)
Pomegranate Blueberry Vinaigrette	2 tbsp	130
Harvest Cranberry Vinaigrette	2 tbsp	110
Huckleberry Vinaigrette	2 tbsp	105

Marie's Dressing	Amount	Sodium (mg)
Lite Chunky Blue Cheese	2 tbsp	290
Buttermilk Ranch	2 tbsp	260
Sesame Ginger	2 tbsp	250
Italian Vinaigrette	2 tbsp	240
Balsamic Vinaigrette	2 tbsp	210
Super Blue Cheese	2 tbsp	210
Yogurt Thousand Island	2 tbsp	200
Honey Dijon	2 tbsp	200
Honey Mustard	2 tbsp	200
Asiago Peppercorn	2 tbsp	200
Red Wine Vinaigrette	2 tbsp	200
Jalapeno Ranch	2 tbsp	200
Thousand Island	2 tbsp	190
Yogurt Blue Cheese	2 tbsp	190
Blue Cheese Vinaigrette	2 tbsp	190
Yogurt Ranch	2 tbsp	180
Greek Vinaigrette	2 tbsp	180
Yogurt Coleslaw	2 tbsp	180
Coleslaw	2 tbsp	170
Poppy Seed	2 tbsp	170
Chunky Blue Cheese	2 tbsp	160
Creamy Caesar	2 tbsp	160
Caesar	2 tbsp	150
Creamy Ranch	2 tbsp	150
Raspberry Vinaigrette	2 tbsp	100

Newman's® Own Dressing	Amount	Sodium (mg)
Lite Roasted Garlic Balsamic	2 tbsp	420
3 Cheese Balsamic	2 tbsp	380
Caesar	2 tbsp	380
Family Italian Recipe	2 tbsp	360
Lite Balsamic	2 tbsp	350
Creamy Ceasar	2 tbsp	340
Orange Ginger	2 tbsp	340
Parmesan & Roasted Garlic	2 tbsp	340
Low Fat Sesame Ginger	2 tbsp	330
Sesame Ginger	2 tbsp	330
Ranch	2 tbsp	310
Balsamic Vinaigrette	2 tbsp	290
Lite Honey Mustard	2 tbsp	280

Daily Adequate Intake is 1500 mg for adults

SODIUM

Continued

Greek Vinaigrette	2 tbsp	270
Lite Italian	2 tbsp	260
Poppy Seed	2 tbsp	220
Creamy Balsamic	2 tbsp	200
Honey French	2 tbsp	170
Olive Oil & Vinegar	2 tbsp	150
Lite Raspberry & Walnut	2 tbsp	120

Organic Ville®	Amount	Sodium (mg)
Miso Ginger	2 tbsp	270
French	2 tbsp	240
Herbs De Provence	2 tbsp	210
Non Dairy Ranch	2 tbsp	200
Non Dairy Thousand	2 tbsp	140
Non Dairy Coleslaw	2 tbsp	85

Sprouts®	Amount	Sodium (mg)
Chipote Ranch	2 tbsp	330
Sun-Dried Tomato	2 tbsp	310
Italian	2 tbsp	270
Ranch	2 tbsp	250
Balsamic	2 tbsp	240
Honey Dijon	2 tbsp	190
Caesar	2 tbsp	180
Rosemary Balsamic	2 tbsp	140
Roasted Garlic	2 tbsp	105
Wild Raspberry	2 tbsp	85
Raspberry	2 tbsp	80

Stater Brothers® Lite Dressing	Amount	Sodium (mg)
Lite Italian	2 tbsp	380
Lite Raspberry	2 tbsp	340
Lite Ranch	2 tbsp	270
Lite Caesar	2 tbsp	270
Lite Thousand Island	2 tbsp	250
Lite Balsamic Vinaigrette	2 tbsp	180

Stater Brothers® Brand Dressing	Amount	Sodium (mg)
Italian	2 tbsp	490
Catalina	2 tbsp	380
Fat Free Italian	2 tbsp	350
Caesar	2 tbsp	340
Roasted Red Pepper Italian Pamesan	2 tbsp	340
Thousand Island	2 tbsp	330

Daily Adequate Intake is 1500 mg for adults

SODIUM

Continued

Ranch	2 tbsp	280
Fat Free Ranch	2 tbsp	280
Bacon Ranch	2 tbsp	270

Target® Brand Dressing	Amount	Sodium (mg)
Caesar	2 tbsp	380
Zesty Italian	2 tbsp	350
Butter Milk Ranch	2 tbsp	340
Zesty Italian Reduced Fat	2 tbsp	340
Blue Cheese	2 tbsp	300
Balsamic Vinaigrette	2 tbsp	290
Greek	2 tbsp	280
Thousand Island	2 tbsp	270
Ranch	2 tbsp	260
Raspberry Reduced Fat	2 tbsp	240
Creamy French	2 tbsp	230

Vons® Safeway® Select Dressing	Amount	Sodium (mg)
Basil Sun-Dried Tomato	2 tbsp	460
Greek Feta	2 tbsp	350
Garlic Parmesan	2 tbsp	340
Olive Oil & Balsamic	2 tbsp	280
White Wine & Pear	2 tbsp	260
Sweet Citrus Herb	2 tbsp	250
Poppy Seed Carmelized Onion	2 tbsp	190
Classic Caesar	2 tbsp	160
Raspberry	2 tbsp	115
Red Wine & Rosemary & Thyme	2 tbsp	80

Walden Farm's® Dressing	Amount	Sodium (mg)
Asian	2 tbsp	290
Italian Sun Dried Tomato	2 tbsp	290
Bacon Ranch	2 tbsp	275
Honey Dijon Dressing	2 tbsp	270
Balsamic Vinaigrette	2 tbsp	260
Caesar Dressing	2 tbsp	260
Chipotle Ranch Dressing	2 tbsp	260
Sesame Ginger Dressing	2 tbsp	260
Zesty Italian	2 tbsp	260
Raspberry Vinaigrette	2 tbsp	250
Sweet Onion	2 tbsp	240
Buttermilk Ranch Dressing	2 tbsp	230
Ranch	2 tbsp	230
Creamy Italian	2 tbsp	225

Daily Adequate Intake is 1500 mg for adults

SODIUM

Italian	2 tbsp	225
Colesaw	2 tbsp	220
Creamy Bacon	2 tbsp	200
Russian	2 tbsp	190
Thousand Island Dressing	2 tbsp	190
French Dressing	2 tbsp	180

Whole Foods® 365® Dressing	Amount	Sodium (mg)
Ranch	2 tbsp	330
Herbes de Provence	2 tbsp	320
Italian	2 tbsp	290
Honey Musatrd	2 tbsp	280
Caesar	2 tbsp	280
Lemon Tahini	2 tbsp	240
Fig Balsamic	2 tbsp	230
Fat Free Balsamic	2 tbsp	230
Poppy Seed	2 tbsp	210
Lite Balsamic	2 tbsp	210
Balsamic	2 tbsp	210
Red Pepper & Feta	2 tbsp	120
Sundried Tomato	2 tbsp	115
Strawberry	2 tbsp	10

Wish Bone® Creamy Dressing	Amount	Sodium (mg)
Russian dressing	2 tbsp	340
Sweet & Spicy French	2 tbsp	330
Creamy Caesar	2 tbsp	290
Thousand Island	2 tbsp	290
Light Blue Cheese	2 tbsp	280
Light Ranch	2 tbsp	280
Light Thousand Island	2 tbsp	270
Chipotle Ranch	2 tbsp	260
Light Creamy Caesar	2 tbsp	250
Cheddar Bacon Ranch	2 tbsp	240
Chunky Blue Cheese	2 tbsp	240
Creamy Italian	2 tbsp	240
Light Parmesan Peppercorn Ranch	2 tbsp	240
Light Sweet & Spicy French	2 tbsp	240
Ranch Dressing	2 tbsp	230
Light Delux French	2 tbsp	220
Buffalo Blue Cheese	2 tbsp	210
Delux French	2 tbsp	170

Daily Adequate Intake is 1500 mg for adults

SODIUM

Wish Bone® Oil & Vinegar	Amount	Sodium (mg)
Fat Free Italian	2 tbsp	350
Fat Free Italian Dressing	2 tbsp	350
Light Italian dressing	2 tbsp	340
Robusto Italian	2 tbsp	340
Russian	2 tbsp	340
Romano Basil Vinaigrette	2 tbsp	330
Mediterranean Italian	2 tbsp	320
Sesame & Ginger	2 tbsp	300
Greek Vinaigrette	2 tbsp	290
Light Balsamic & Basil Vinaigrette	2 tbsp	290
Balsamic Italian Vinaigrette	2 tbsp	280
Balsamic Vinaigrette	2 tbsp	280
House Italian	2 tbsp	260
Light Raspberry Walnut	2 tbsp	260
Raspberrt Hazelnut Vinaigrette	2 tbsp	260
Olive Oil Vinaigrette	2 tbsp	250
Fat Free Red Wine Vinaigrette	2 tbsp	230
Red Wine Vinaigrette	2 tbsp	230
Superfruit Vinaigrette	2 tbsp	170

Sauces & Salsa	Amount	Sodium (mg)
Kikkoman Soy Sauce	1 tbsp	920
Kikkoman Teriyaki Marinade & Sauce	1 tbsp	610
Kikkoman Soy Sauce, less sodium	1 tbsp	575
Frank's Original Hot Sauce	1 tbsp	570
Kikkoman Original Teriyaki Sauce	1 tbsp	450
A-1 Steak Sauce	1 tbsp	280
Cholula Original Hot Sauce	1 tbsp	255
Louisiana Hot Sauce	1 tbsp	240
Heinz Chili Sauce	1 tbsp	230
Annie's Worchestersshire Sauce	1 tbsp	225
Lea Perrin's Worchestersshire Sauce	1 tbsp	195
Valentina Salsa Picante Hot Sauce	1 tbsp	192
Tobasco & Buffalo	1 tbsp	190
Heinz 57 Sauce	1 tbsp	150
Tobasco & Garlic	1 tbsp	150
Tobasco & Green Peppers	1 tbsp	150
Mrs Rentros Medium Salsa	1 tbsp	140
Pacer Original Picante Sauce	1 tbsp	125
Kraft Horseradish	1 tbsp	120
Tabasco Habanero	1 tbsp	120
Tobasco & Chipotle	1 tbsp	120
Buffalo Jalapeno Salsa	1 tbsp	115
La Victoria Red Taco Sauce	1 tbsp	110

Daily Adequate Intake is 1500 mg for adults

SODIUM

Tapato Salsa Picante Hot Sauce	1 tbsp	110
El Mexicano Salsa Verde Green Sauce	1 tbsp	100
Amys Salsa , medium	1 tbsp	95
Silver Star Flame Roasted Salsa	1 tbsp	75
Bristol's Own Salsa, mild	1 tbsp	68
Muir Glen Medium Salsa	1 tbsp	63
Robbie's Worchestersshire Sauce	1 tbsp	60
Tarter Sauce, Trader Joe's	1 tbsp	55
Tobasco Original Pepper Sauce	1 tbsp	35
Heinz No Salt Tomato Sauce	1 tbsp	5

SOUP

Albertson's® Chunky Brand	Amount	Sodium (mg)
Grilled Chicken	1 can	1880
Chicken, Broccoli, Cheese & Potato	1 can	1820
Clam Chowder	1 can	1780
Beef	1 can	1740
Sirlion Burger	1 can	1600
Chicken Noodle	1 can	1560
Chicken Corn Chowder	1 can	1520
Vegetable	1 can	1380
Creamy Chicken Dumplings	1 can	1280
Chicken Noodle, low sodium	1 can	820
Gumbo, low sodium	1 can	820

Albertson's® Traditional Brand	Amount	Sodium (mg)
Chicken Noodle	1 can	1380
Minestrone Penne	1 can	1380
Italian Style Wedding	1 can	1380
Lentil	1 can	1380
Clam Chowder	1 can	1320
Chicken & Wild Rice	1 can	1300

Amy's Organic Soup	Amount	Sodium (mg)
Cream of Tomato	1 can	1380
Hearty French Country Vegetable	1 can	1380
Hearty Rustic Italian	1 can	1380
Hearty Spanish Rice & Red Bean	1 can	1380
Mushroom Bisque with Porcini	1 can	1380
No Chicken Noodle	1 can	1380
Pasta & 3 Bean	1 can	1380
Chunky Tomato Bisque	1 can	1360
Chunky Vegetable	1 can	1360

Daily Adequate Intake is 1500 mg for adults

SODIUM

Continued

Fire Roasted Southwestern Vegetable	1 can	1360
Golden Lentil	1 can	1360
Hearty Minestrone with Vegetables	1 can	1360
Home Made Vegetable Soup & Chicken	1 can	1360
Lentil Vegetable	1 can	1360
Split Pea Soup	1 can	1340
Black Bean Vegetable Soup	1 can	1240
Cream of Mushroom	1 can	1180
Lentil Soup	1 can	1180
Butternut Squash	1 can	1160
Minestrone	1 can	1160
Thai Coconut	1 can	1160
Tuscan Bean & Rice	1 can	1160
Vegetable Barley	1 can	1160
Summer Corn & Vegetable	1 can	1120

Amy's Light in Sodium	Amount	Sodium (mg)
Chunky Tomato Bisque	1 can	680
Cream of Tomato	1 can	680
Lentil Vegetable	1 can	680
Split Pea	1 can	660
Butternut Squash	1 can	580
Lentil	1 can	580
Minestrone	1 can	580

Andersen's Soup	Amount	Sodium (mg)
Tomato Soup	1 can	1980
Split Pea Soup	1 can	1520
Split Pea with Bacon Soup	1 can	1500
Lentil Soup	1 can	1180

Bar Harbor® Soup	Amount	Sodium (mg)
Corn Chowder	1 can	1625
Clam Chowder	1 can	1375
Salmon Chowder	1 can	1350
Lobster Bisque	1 can	1080

Campbell's® Chunky Soup	Amount	Sodium (mg)
Beef with White Wild Rice	1 can	1780
Chicken Broccoli, Cheese & Potato	1 can	1780
Creamy Chicken & Dumplings	1 can	1780
Grilled Sirloin Steak & Vegetables	1 can	1780
New England Clam Chowder	1 can	1780
Old Fashioned Vegetable Beef	1 can	1780

Daily Adequate Intake is 1500 mg for adults

SODIUM

Steak "N" Potato Soup	1 can	1780
Baked Potato & Cheddar & Bacon Bits	1 can	1740
Beef with Country Vegetables	1 can	1720
Chicken Corn Chowder Soup	1 can	1720
Fajita Chicken with Rice & Beans	1 can	1700
Grilled Chicken Sausage Gumbo	1 can	1700
Grilled Chicken with Vegetables & Pasta	1 can	1700
Savory Chicken & White Wild Rice	1 can	1620
Potato Ham Chowder	1 can	1600
Classic Chicken Noodle Soup	1 can	1580
Hearty Beef Barley	1 can	1580
Roasted Beef with Mushrooms & Vegetables	1 can	1580
Savory Pot Roast	1 can	1580
Sirloin Burger & Country Vegetable	1 can	1580
Split Pea & Ham	1 can	1580
Hearty Bean & Ham	1 can	1560
Savory Vegetable	1 can	1540
Hearty Chicken with Vegetables	1 can	1420
Hearty Beef Noodle	1 can	1300
Hearty Italian Style Wedding	1 can	1300

Campbell's Chunky Healthy Request	Amount	Sodium (mg)
Beef with Country Vegetables	1 can	820
Chicken Corn Chowder Soup	1 can	820
Classic Chicken Noodle Soup	1 can	820
Grilled Chicken & Sausage Gumbo	1 can	820
Hearty Italian Style Wedding	1 can	820
Italian Style Wedding	1 can	820
New England Clam Chowder	1 can	820
Old Fashioned Vegetable Beef	1 can	820
Roasted Chicken & Country Vegetables	1 can	820
Savory Vegetable	1 can	820
Sirloin Burger & Country Vegetable	1 can	820

Campbell's® Home Style	Amount	Sodium (mg)
New England Clam Chowder	1 can	1780
Mexican Style Chcken Tortilla	1 can	1700
Chicken Noodle	1 can	1580
Chicken with White & Wild Rice	1 can	1580
Creamy Chicken & Herb Dumplings	1 can	1580
Harvest Tomato with Basil	1 can	1580
Italian Style Wedding	1 can	1580
Light Chicken Noodle	1 can	1580
Light Italian Style Wedding	1 can	1580
Vegetable Medley	1 can	1580

Daily Adequate Intake is 1500 mg for adults

SODIUM

Continued

Butternut Squash Bisque	1 can	1300
Creamy Gouda Bisque with Chicken	1 can	1300
Creole-Style Chicken,Red Beans & Rice	1 can	1300
Potato Broccoli & Cheese	1 can	1300
Southwest Style Potato	1 can	1300
Southwest Style White Chicken Chili	1 can	1300
Zesty Tomato Bisque	1 can	1300

Campbell's® Home Style Healthy Request	Amount	Sodium (mg)
Chicken with Whole Grain Pasta	1 can	820
Harvest Tomato with Basil	1 can	820
Italian Style Wedding, Micro Wavable	1 can	820
Mexican Style Chcken Tortilla	1 can	820
Savory Chicken & Brown Rice	1 can	820
Spicy Vegetable Chili	1 can	820

Campbell's® Kettle Style Soup	Amount	Sodium (mg)
Portobello Mushroom & Maderia Bisque	1 can	1540
Tuscan Style Chicken & White Beans	1 can	1520
Tomato with Sweet Basil	1 can	1500
Southwest Style Chicken Chili	1 can	1480
Burgurdy Beef Stew	1 can	1400

Campbell's® Microwavable Soup	Amount	Sodium (mg)
Homestyle Chicken Noodle	1 can	1780
Chunky Beef & Country Vegetables	1 can	1740
Chunky New England Clam Chowder	1 can	1740
Original Chicken Noodle	1 can	1740
Chunky Sirloin Burger & Country Vegetables	1 can	1600
Chunky Classic Chicken Noodle	1 can	1580
Chunky Grilled Chicken & Sausage Gumbo	1 can	1560
Creamy Tomato	1 can	960

Campbell's® 100% Natural	Amount	Sodium (mg)
New England Clam Chowder	1 can	1580
98 % Light New England Clam Chowder	1 can	1300
Butternut Squash Bisque	1 can	1300
Carmelized French Onion	1 can	1300
Chicken & Egg Noodle	1 can	1300
Chicken Tuscany	1 can	1300
Creamy Gouda Bisque with Chicken	1 can	1300
Creamy Potato & Roasted Garlic	1 can	1300
Creole-Style Chicken, Red Beans & Rice	1 can	1300

Daily Adequate Intake is 1500 mg for adults

SODIUM

Harvest Tomato with Basil	1 can	1300
Italian Style Wedding	1 can	1300
Mexican-Style Chicken Tortilla	1 can	1300
Nesty Tomato Bisque	1 can	1300
Potato Broccoli & Cheese	1 can	1300
Savory Chicken & Long Grain Rice	1 can	1300
Southwestern Style Vegetables	1 can	1300
Southwestern White Chicken Chili	1 can	1300

Campbell's® 100% Natural Healthy Request	Amount	Sodium (mg)
Chicken & Whole Grain Pasta	1 can	820
Harvest Tomato with Basil	1 can	820
Italian Style Wedding	1 can	820
Mexican Style Chicken Tortilla	1 can	820
Whole-Grain Pasta Fagioli	1 can	820

Campbell's® Soup at Hand	Amount	Sodium (mg)
Chicken with Mini Noodles Soup	1 container	980
Chicken & Stars Soup	1 container	960
Vegetable Beef, 70 Calories	1 container	930
Cream of Broccoli Soup	1 container	890
New England Clam Chowder	1 container	890
Creamy Chicken Soup	1 container	880
Creamy Tomato Parmesan Soup	1 container	780
Chicken with Mini Noodles, Less Sodium	1 container	730
CreamyTomato Soup	1 container	650
Vegetable with Mini Round Noodles	1 container	650
Classic Tomato Soup	1 container	645
Classic Tomato, 25% Less Sodium Soup	1 container	480

Campbell's® V8 Soup	Amount	Sodium (mg)
Garden Broccoli	1 can	960
Garden Vegetable	1 can	960
Golden ButterNut Squash	1 can	960
Potato Leek	1 can	960
South West Corn	1 can	960
Sweet Red Pepper	1 can	960
Tomato Herb	1 can	960

Daily Adequate Intake is 1500 mg for adults

SODIUM

Healthy Choice Micro Wavable	Amount	Sodium (mg)
Country Vegetable	1 can	960
Beef Pot Roast	1 can	940
Hearty Vegetable Barley	1 can	860
Chicken Tortilla	1 can	840
Butternut Squash	1 can	780
Cheese Tortellini	1 can	780
Chicken Noodles	1 can	780
Chicken with Rice	1 can	780
Mediterranean Style Chicken with Orzo	1 can	780
Thai Style Chicken Brown Rice	1 can	780
Tomato Basil	1 can	780

Healthy Valley Organic Soup	Amount	Sodium (mg)
Cream of Celery	1 can	1360
Cream of Chicken	1 can	1360
Cream of Mushroom	1 can	1360
Chicken Noodle	1 can	960
Chicken Rice	1 can	960
Less Sodium, 14 Garden Vegetable	1 can	960
Less Sodium, 5 Bean Vegetable	1 can	960
Less Sodium, Black Bean Vegetable	1 can	960
Less Sodium, Potato Leek	1 can	960
Less Sodium, Split Pea	1 can	960
Less Sodium, Split Pea & Carrots	1 can	960
Less Sodium, Vegetable	1 can	960
Less Sodium, Vegetable Barley	1 can	960
Less Sodium, Italian Minestrone	1 can	940
Less Sodium, Tomato Vegetable	1 can	940
Less Sodium, Corn & Vegetable	1 can	920
Less Sodium, Lentile & Carrots	1 can	900

Healthy Valley Organic Soup	Amount	Sodium (mg)
No Salt Added, Chicken Noodle	1 can	270
No Salt Added, Rice Primavera	1 can	270
No Salt Added, Split Pea	1 can	170
No Salt Added, Mushroom Barley	1 can	120
No Salt Added, Tomato	1 can	120
No Salt Added, Minestrone	1 can	100
No Salt Added, Vegetable	1 can	100
No Salt Added, Black Bean	1 can	60
No Salt Added, Lentile	1 can	60
No Salt Added, Potato Leek	1 can	60

Daily Adequate Intake is 1500 mg for adults

SODIUM

Imagine Natural Creation (17 oz)	Amount	Sodium (mg)
Tomato Bisque	1 container	1260
Loaded Baked Potato	1 container	1220
Savory Black Bean	1 container	1140
Chicken & Dumplings	1 container	1060
Chicken Corn Tortilla	1 container	960
Cicken Noodle	1 container	960

Imagine Natural Creation (32 oz)	Amount	Sodium (mg)
Creamy Tomato	1 container	2680
Creamy Sweet Potato	1 container	2400
Creamy Broccoli	1 container	2200
Creamy Butternut Squash	1 container	1760
Creamy Potato Leek	1 container	1760
Acorn Squash & Mango Soup	1 container	1720
Creamy Portobellow Mushroom	1 container	1680
Tuscan White Bean	1 container	1680
Creamy Tomato Basil	1 container	1640
Minestrone	1 container	1600
Creamy Corn & Lemon Grass	1 container	1560
Split Pea	1 container	1520
Southwestern Tortilla	1 container	1500
Homestyle Chicken Noodle	1 container	1460
Meatball with Orzo	1 container	1460
Chicken & Wild Rice	1 container	1420
Roasted Garlic Potato	1 container	1400
Creamy Chicken Soup	1 container	1360
Savory Lentil Apple	1 container	1360
Chicken Pot Pie Soup	1 container	1340
Fire Roasted Tomato Bisque	1 container	1340
Moroccan Chick Pea Bisque	1 container	1320
Corn Chipotle Bisque	1 container	1180

Imagine Natural Creation (32 oz) Light in Sodium	Amount	Sodium (mg)
Creamy Garden Tomato	1 container	1240
Cuban Black Bean Bisque	1 container	960
Creamy Butternut Squash	1 container	920
Creamy Harvest Corn	1 container	760
Creamy Sweet Potato	1 container	560

Daily Adequate Intake is 1500 mg for adults

SODIUM

Juanita's Mexican Gourmet Soup	Amount	Sodium (mg)
Beef & Vegetable	1 can	1380
Chicken Chipotle	1 can	1160
Chicken Tortilla	1 can	1140
Fiesta Chicken & Vegetable	1 can	1160
Zesty Vegetable & Pasta	1 can	1160

Muir Glen's Organic Soup	Amount	Sodium (mg)
Reduced Sodium Garden Vegetable	1 can	1920
Beef & Vegetable	1 can	1780
Tomato Basil	1 can	1760
Beef Barley	1 can	1700
Creamy Tomato Bisque	1 can	1680
Cajun Style Chicken Gumbo	1 can	1620
Chicken Noodle	1 can	1600
Reduced Sodium Chicken Noodle	1 can	1600
Chicken Tortilla	1 can	1590
Chicken & Wild Rice	1 can	1560
Classic Minestrone	1 can	1560
Garden Vegetable	1 can	1560
Homestyle Split Pea	1 can	1560
Savory Lentil	1 can	1560
South West Black Bean	1 can	1360

Pacific Natural Organic (17oz)	Amount	Sodium (mg)
Vegetable Lentil & Roasted Red Pepper	1 container	1520
Creamy Tomato	1 container	1500
Hearty Tomato Bisque	1 container	1500
Roasted Red Pepper & Tomato	1 container	1500
Rosmary Potato Chowder	1 container	1460
Curried Red Lentil Soup	1 container	1440
French Onion	1 container	1440
Chicken Noodle	1 container	1420
Minestrone with Chicken Meatballs	1 container	1400
Santa Fe Style Chicken	1 container	1400
Poblano Pepper & Corn Chowder	1 container	1380
Roasted Garlic Mushroom Lentil	1 container	1380
Chicken & Wild Rice	1 container	1320
Cashew Carrot Ginger	1 container	1300
Thai Sweet Potatos	1 container	1300
Chicken Spinach Penne	1 container	1220
Spicy Black Bean Soup	1 container	1200
Split Pea & Uncured Ham	1 container	1180
Butter Nut Squash Bisque	1 container	1160

Daily Adequate Intake is 1500 mg for adults

SODIUM

Continued

	Amount	Sodium (mg)
Chipotle Sweet Potatoes	1 container	1160
Chipotle Sweet Potatoes	1 container	1160
Creamy Butternut Squash	1 container	1100

Pacific Natural Organic (17 oz) Light in Sodium	Amount	Sodium (mg)
Creamy Tomato	1 container	760
Roasted Red Pepper & Tomato	1 container	740
Creamy Butternut Squash	1 container	560

Pacific Natural Organic (32 oz)	Amount	Sodium (mg)
Vegetable Lentil & Roasted R. Pepper	1 container	3040
Creamy Tomato	1 container	3000
Hearty Tomato Bisque	1 container	3000
Roasted Red Pepper & Tomato	1 container	3000
Rosmary Potato Chowder	1 container	2920
Curried Red Lentil Soup	1 container	2880
French Onion	1 container	2880
Minestrone with Chicken Meatballs	1 container	2880
Chicken Noodle	1 container	2840
Santa Fe Style Chicken	1 container	2800
Poblano Pepper & Corn Chowder	1 container	2760
Roasted Garlic Mushroom Lentil	1 container	2760
Chicken & Wild Rice	1 container	2640
Cashew Carrot Ginger	1 container	2600
Thai Sweet Potatos	1 container	2600
Chicken Spinach Penne	1 container	2440
Spicy Black Bean Soup	1 container	2360
Chipotle Sweet Potatoes	1 container	2320
Creamy Butter Nut Squash Bisque	1 container	2200
Creamy Butternut Squash	1 container	2200

Pacific Light in Sodium (32 oz)	Amount	Sodium (mg)
Creamy Tomato	1 container	1520
Roasted Red Pepper & Tomato	1 container	1480
Creamy Butternut Squash	1 container	1120

Progresso® High Fiber Soup	Amount	Sodium (mg)
Chicken Tuscany	1 can	1380
Creamy Tomato Basil	1 can	1380
Hearty Vegetable & Noodle	1 can	1380
Homestyle Minestrone	1 can	1380
Three Bean Chili with Beef	1 can	960

Daily Adequate Intake is 1500 mg for adults

SODIUM

Progresso® Light Soup	Amount	Sodium (mg)
Chicken & Dumplings	1 can	1380
Chicken Noodle	1 can	1380
New England Clam Chowder	1 can	1380
Chicken Vegetable Rotini	1 can	1320
Reduced Vegetable	1 can	980
Italian Style Meatball	1 can	960
Savory Vegetable Barley	1 can	960
Vegetable & Noodle	1 can	960
Beef Pot Roast	1 can	940
Homestyle Vegetable & Rice	1 can	940
Italian Style Vegetable	1 can	940
Vegetable	1 can	940
Zesty Southwestern Style Vegetable	1 can	940
Roasted Chicken & Vegetable	1 can	920
Zesty Santa Fee Style Chicken	1 can	920

Progresso® Reduced Sodium	Amount	Sodium (mg)
Beef & Vegetable	1 can	960
Italian Style Wedding	1 can	960
Tomato Parmesan	1 can	960
Chicken & Wild Rice	1 can	940
Chicken Noodle	1 can	940
Minestrone	1 can	940
Chicken Gumbo	1 can	900
Garden Vegetable	1 can	900

Progresso® Rich & Hearty Soups	Amount	Sodium (mg)
Chicken Corn Chowder with Bacon Flavor	1 can	1780
Creamy Roasted Chicken Wild Rice	1 can	1720
New England Clam Choder	1 can	1720
Loaded Potato with Bacon	1 can	1660
Hearty Roasted Chicken Pot Pie	1 can	1540
Roasted Chicken Pot Pies	1 can	1540
Beef Pot Roast & Country Vegetables	1 can	1380
Chicken Home Style Noodle	1 can	1380
Savory Beef Barley Vegetable	1 can	1380
Slow Cooked Vegetable Beef	1 can	1380
Steak & Homestyle Noodles	1 can	1380
Steak & Roasted Russet Potatoes	1 can	1380
Steak & Vegetables	1 can	1380
Steak Burger & County Vegetables	1 can	1380

Daily Adequate Intake is 1500 mg for adults

SODIUM

Progresso® Traditional Soup	Amount	Sodium (mg)
Chicken Cheese Enchilada	1 can	1780
New England Clam Chowder	1 can	1780
Potato Broccoli & Cheese Chowder	1 can	1720
New England Clam Chowder 99% fat free	1 can	1620
Southwestern Chicken Chowder	1 can	1480
Beef Barley 99% fat Free	1 can	1440
Beef & Vegetables	1 can	1380
Beef Barley	1 can	1380
Chickarima with Meat Balls	1 can	1380
Chicken & Orzo with Lemon	1 can	1380
Chicken Barley	1 can	1380
Chicken Noodle	1 can	1380
Hearty Chicken & Rotini	1 can	1380
Homestyle Chicken Vegetable, Pearl Pasta	1 can	1380
Italian Style Wedding	1 can	1380
Manhattan Clam Chowder	1 can	1380
Roasted Chicken Primavera	1 can	1380
Roasted Garlic Chicken	1 can	1380
Split Pea & Ham	1 can	1380
Turkey Noodle	1 can	1380
Chicken Noodle 99% fat Free	1 can	1340
Roasted Chicken Rotini	1 can	1340
Roasted Chicken with Garlic & Penne	1 can	1340
Chicken & Herb Dumplings	1 can	1300
Chicken & Sausage Gumbo	1 can	1300
Chicken & Wild Rice	1 can	1300
Chicken Rice & Vegetables	1 can	1280

Progresso® Vegetable Classic	Amount	Sodium (mg)
Creamy Mushroom	1 can	1780
Lentil	1 can	1620
Vegetable Italiano	1 can	1540
Hearty Penne in Chicken Broth	1 can	1420
Classic Hearty Tomato	1 can	1380
French Onion	1 can	1380
Garden Vegetable	1 can	1380
Green Split Pea with Bacon	1 can	1380
Hearty Black Bean	1 can	1380
Macaroni & Bean	1 can	1380
Minestrone	1 can	1380
Tomato Rotini	1 can	1380
Tomatao Basil	1 can	1360
Vegetarian Vegetable with Barley	1 can	1340
Vegetable	1 can	1320

Daily Adequate Intake is 1500 mg for adults

SODIUM

Continued

Minestrone, 99% fat Free	1 can	1200
Lentil, 99% fat Free	1 can	1000

Stater Brothers® Chunky Soup	Amount	Sodium (mg)
Grilled Chicken & Vegetable	1 can	1880
Hearty Beef & Vegetable	1 can	1780
Chicken Corn Chowder	1 can	1560
Hearty Vegetable	1 can	1380
Hearty Chicken Noodle	1 can	1380
Hearty Steak & Potato	1 can	1380
Hearty Chicken & Dumplings	1 can	1380
New England Clam Chowder	1 can	1340

Target's® Brand Soup	Amount	Sodium (mg)
Chicken & Dumplings	1 can	1780
Steak & Potato	1 can	1780
Chicken Corn Chowder	1 can	1740
Beef Dumplings	1 can	1600
Beef Barley	1 can	1580
Chunky Chicken Noodle	1 can	1580
Chicken Noodle	1 can	1380
Vegetable Minestrone	1 can	1300
Lentil	1 can	1200
New England Clam Chowder	1 can	1200
Home Style Vegetable	1 can	1120

The Original Soup-Man®	Amount	Sodium (mg)
Chicken Gumbo	1 container	2100
Crab & Corn Chowder	1 container	1960
Jambalaya	1 container	1960
Chicken Noodle	1 container	1560
Lentil	1 container	1300

Trader Joe's® Soup (32 oz)	Amount	Sodium (mg)
Creamy Tomato	1 container	3000
Tomato & Roasted Red Pepper	1 container	3000
Creamy Corn & Roasted Pepper	1 container	2360
Butternut Squash	1 container	2200
Latin Style Black Bean	1 container	2080
Sweet Potato Bisque	1 container	1640
Carrot Ginger	1 container	1280

Daily Adequate Intake is 1500 mg for adults

SODIUM

Vons® Safeway® Select Soup	Amount	Sodium (mg)
Creamy Parmesan Chicken noodle	1 container	1300
Garden Vegetables	1 container	1140
Thai Style Coconut Chicken	1 container	980
Sweet potato & Pumpkin	1 container	980
Italian Style White Bean	1 container	840

Vons® O® Organic Soup	Amount	Sodium (mg)
Southwestern Black Bean	1 container	1500
Lentil	1 container	1500
Chicken Noodle	1 container	1300
Tomato Basil	1 container	1260
Butternut Squash	1 container	900

Whole Foods® 365® Brands	Amount	Sodium (mg)
Beef & Barley	1 container	1500
Southwestern Black Bean	1 container	1500
Minestrone	1 container	1500
Lentil	1 container	1500
Chicken Tortilla	1 container	1380
Chicken & Wild Rice	1 container	1380
Thai Style Chicken Noodle	1 container	1380
Chicken Noodle	1 container	1300
Tomato & Basil	1 container	1260
Rustic Vegetable	1 container	960

Wolfgang Puck's Organic Soup	Amount	Sodium (mg)
Chicken & Egg Noodles	1 can	1840
Free Range Chicken Noodle	1 can	1720
Hearty Garden Vegetable	1 can	1700
Chicken with White & Wild Rice	1 can	1660
Thick Hearty Lentil & Vegetable	1 can	1640
Corn Chowder	1 can	1520
Vegetable Barley	1 can	1520
Black Bean	1 can	1500
Old Fashion Potato	1 can	1440
Thick Hearty Vegetable	1 can	1380
Chicken & Dumplings	1 can	1360
Classic Minestrone	1 can	1360
Tortilla	1 can	1360
Creamy Butternut Squash	1 can	1260
Tomato Basil Bisque	1 can	1180
Classic Tomato with Basil	1 can	960

Daily Adequate Intake is 1500 mg for adults

SODIUM

Turkey, Cooked	Amount	Sodium (mg)
Turkey bacon	3 oz	1942
Turkey sausage, reduced fat	3 oz	613
Liver	3 oz	83
Ground turkey, 93% lean	3 oz	77
Ground turkey, 85% lean	3 oz	69
Dark meat	3 oz	66
Ground turkey	3 oz	66
Light meat	3 oz	54
Ground turkey, fat free	3 oz	50
Breast meat	3 oz	44

Veal, Cooked	Amount	Sodium (mg)
Foreshank	3 oz	79
Loin	3 oz	79
Rib	3 oz	78
Ground	3 oz	71
Sirloin	3 oz	71
Breast	3 oz	58
Leg, top round	3 oz	57

VEGETABLES

Vegetables, Canned	Amount	Sodium (mg)
Sauerkraut	1 cup	1560
Tomato sauce	1 cup	1284
Asparagus	1 cup	695
Spinach	1 cup	689
Mushrooms	1 cup	663
Corn	1 cup	571
Stewed tomato	1 cup	564
Green peas	1 cup	495
Green beans	1 cup	376
Carrots	1 cup	353
Tomatoes	1 cup	343
Beets	1 cup	330
Tomato paste	1 cup	257
Spinach. Low sodium	1 cup	176
Sweet potato	1 cup	76
Tomato pure	1 cup	70
Pumpkin	1 cup	12
Green Beans, no salt added, drained	1 cup	3
Green Peas, no salt added, drained	1 cup	3

Daily Adequate Intake is 1500 mg for adults

SODIUM

Vegetables, Cooked	Amount	Sodium (mg)
Potatoes, mashed, whole milk & butter	1 cup	634
Hubbard squash, cubes	1 cup	500
Crookneck and Straightneck squash	1 cup	427
Beet greens	1 cup	347
Swiss chard	1 cup	313
Celery	1 cup	137
Beets	1 cup	131
Spinach	1 cup	126
Artichokes	1 cup	101
Carrots	1 cup	90
Sweet potato, mashed	1 cup	89
Broccoli	1 cup	64
Cabbage, Chinese Bok-Choy	1 cup	58
Dandelion greens	1 cup	46
Turnip greens	1 cup	42
Kohlrabi	1 cup	35
Rutabagas	1 cup	34
Brussels sprouts	1 cup	33
Collard greens	1 cup	30
Kale	1 cup	30
Spaghetti squash	1 cup	28
Asparagus	1 cup	25
Turnips	1 cup	25
Mustard greens	1 cup	22
Cauliflower	1 cup	19
Parsnips	1 cup	16
Cabbage	1 cup	12
Cabbage, Napa	1 cup	12
Yams, cubed	1 cup	11
Leaks	1 cup	10
Okra	1 cup	10
Acorn squash, cubes	1 cup	8
Butternut squash, cubes	1 cup	8
Onions	1 cup	6
Potatoes, flesh, baked	1 cup	6
Shiitake mushrooms	1 cup	6
Snow peas	1 cup	6
Zucchini,	1 cup	5
Split peas	1 cup	4
White mushrooms	1 cup	3
Pumpkin	1 cup	2
Scallop or Pattypan squash	1 cup	2
Summer squash	1 cup	2

Daily Adequate Intake is 1500 mg for adults

SODIUM

Continued

Winter squash	1 cup	2
Corn	1 cup	1
Eggplant	1 cup	1
Green beans	1 cup	1

Vegetables, Frozen	Amount	Sodium (mg)
Spinach	1 cup	184
Green peas	1 cup	115
Carrots	1 cup	86
Collard greens	1 cup	85
Cauliflower,	1 cup	32
Asparagus	1 cup	25
Turnip greens	1 cup	25
Brussels sprouts	1 cup	23
Broccoli	1 cup	20
Kale	1 cup	20
Okra	1 cup	6
Corn	1 cup	2
Rhubarb	1 cup	2
Green beans	1 cup	1

Vegetables, Raw	Amount	Sodium (mg)
Celery	1 cup	96
Swiss chard	1 cup	77
Carrots	1 cup	76
Spirulina, dried	1 tbsp	73
Cabbage, Chinese Bok-Choy	1 cup	46
Dandelion greens	1 cup	42
Cauliflower	1 cup	30
Broccoli	1 cup	29
Kale	1 cup	29
Spinach	1 cup	24
Savoy cabbage	1 cup	20
Cabbage, Red	1 cup	19
Cactus pads, nopales	1 cup	18
Green leaf lettuce	1 cup	16
Green onions & scallions	1 cup	16
Watercress	1 cup	14
Broccoli, Raab	1 cup	13
Cabbage	1 cup	13
Chicory greens	1 cup	13
Endive	1 cup	11
Radicchio	1 cup	9
Tomatoes	1 cup	9
Zucchini	1 cup	9

Daily Adequate Intake is 1500 mg for adults

SODIUM

Red leaf lettuce	1 cup	7
Tomatoes, cherry	1 cup	7
Iceburg lettuce	1 cup	6
Onions	1 cup	6
Red bell peppers	1 cup	6
Arugula	1 cup	5
Butternut squash	1 cup	5
Green bell peppers	1 cup	4
Romaine lettuce	1 cup	4
Snow peas	1 cup	4
White mushrooms	1 cup	4
Yellow bell peppers	1 large	4
Butterhead & boston lettuce	1 cup	3
Belgian endive	1 cup	2
Cucumbers	1 cup	2
Summer squash	1 cup	2
Tomatillos	1 cup	1
Shiitake mushrooms, dried	1 each	0

Daily Adequate Intake is 1500 mg for adults

Nutrient Data Collection Form

Food	Amount	Book Numbers	Multiply By	Estimated Nutrient Intake
Nutrient::	RDA:	Estimated:	% of RDA:	Total Estimated:

NOTES

SUGAR

The one environmental element on earth that has created a cluster of metabolic abnormalities and disturbances in humans is the dietary intake of sugar. Sugar is linked with the synthesis and storage of body fat, increased cholesterol levels, high blood pressure, impaired glucose metabolism, insulin resistance, and type-2 diabetes.

Dietary intake of sugar is a metabolic poison and should be minimized as much as possible. What Amount of sugar is needed by the body is easily derived from the metabolic break down of fruits, vegetables, and proteins.

SUGAR

Alcohol	Amount	Total Sugar (g)
White Wine	1 glass	1.4
Red Wine	1 glass	0.9
Beer, light, all types	1 bottle	0.3
Beer, regular, all types	1 bottle	0
Gin, Rum, Vodka, Whisky	1 shot	0

Beans, Canned	Amount	Total Sugar (g)
Baked beans, plain	1 cup	20.22
Kidney beans	1 cup	4.74
Pinto beans, mature	1 cup	2.45
Green beans	1 cup	2.00
Yellow beans	1 cup	1.47
Refried beans	1 cup	1.09
White beans, mature	1 cup	0.76
Navy beans	1 cup	0.73
Black-eyed peas	1 cup	x
Cranberry beans	1 cup	x
Fava beans	1 cup	x
Garbanzo beans	1 cup	x
Great Northern	1 cup	x
Lima beans	1 cup	x

Beans, Cooked	Amount	Total Sugar (g)
Natto	1 cup	8.6
Garbanzo beans	1 cup	7.9
Split peas	1 cup	5.7
Black-eyed peas	1 cup	5.6
Lima beans	1 cup	5.5
Soybeans, mature	1 cup	5.2
Lentils	1 cup	3.6
Mung beans, mature seeds	1 cup	3.5
Edamame	1 cup	3.4
Fava beans	1 cup	3.0
Green beans	1 cup	1.9
Yellow beans	1 cup	1.9
Navy beans	1 cup	0.7
White beans, mature	1 cup	0.6
Black Turtle beans, mature	1 cup	0.6
Pinto beans	1 cup	0.6
Kidney beans	1 cup	0.6
Adzuki	1 cup	x
Black beans	1 cup	x
Cranberry beans	1 cup	x

SUGAR

Great Northern	1 cup	x
Hyacinth beans	1 cup	x
Lupins, mature	1 cup	x
Moth beans	1 cup	x
Pigeon peas	1 cup	x
Soybeans, dry roasted	1 cup	x
Soybeans, green	1 cup	x
White beans, small	1 cup	x
Winged beans	1 cup	x
Yardlong beans, Chinese long beans	1 cup	x

Beef, Cooked	Amount	Total Sugar (g)
Beef ribs, trimmed to 1/8" fat	3 oz	0
Chuck roast, trimmed to 1/8" fat	3 oz	0
Filet Mignon, trimmed to 0" fat	3 oz	0
Ground beef, 75%	3 oz	0
Ground beef, 80%	3 oz	0
Ground beef, 85%	3 oz	0
Ground beef, 90%,	3 oz	0
Ground beef, 95%	3 oz	0
Porterhouse steak, trimmed to 0" fat	3 oz	0
Ribeye steak, trimmed to 0" fat	3 oz	0
Skirt Steak, trimmed to 0" fat	3 oz	0
T-Bone steak, trimmed 0" fat	3 oz	0
Top sirloin, trimmed to 1/8" fat	3 oz	0

Bread	Amount	Total Sugar (g)
Croissants, butter	1 medium	6.4
Bagel, wheat	4" bagel	6.0
Bagel, cinnamon & raisins	4" bagel	5.3
Bagel, plain	4" bagel	4.5
Potato bread	1 slice	4.0
Indian bread, Naan, whole wheat	1 piece	3.6
Mexican roll, bollilo	1 roll	3.5
Indian bread, Naan, plain	1 piece	3.2
Hamburger & Hotdog buns, plain	1 bun	2.7
Oatmeal bread	1 slice	2.2
English Muffin, plain	1 muffin	2.0
Bagel, oat bran	4" bagel	1.7
Multi-Grain, includes Whole-Grain	1 slice	1.7
Whole-Wheat	1 slice	1.6
Dinner Rolls, brown & serve	1 roll	1.6
Raisin bread	1 slice	1.5
Wheat	1 slice	1.4
Rye bread	1 slice	1.2

SUGAR

Continued

White	1 slice	1.1
Kaiser rolls	1 roll	1.0
Pita, white	6" pita	0.8
Egg bread	1 slice	0.7
French, and Sourdough	1 slice	0.6
Tortillas, flour	1 tortilla	0.6
Tortillas, corn	1 tortilla	0.2
Italian	1 slice	0.2
Pumpernickle	1 slice	0.2

CEREAL

Albertsons® Brand Cereal	Amount	Total Sugar (g)
Golden Wheat Puffs	1 cup	20
Raisin Bran Crunch Granola	1 cup	20
Good Day with Strawberry	1 cup	19
Cocoa Comets	1 cup	18
Raisin Bran	1 cup	17
Apple Crunchies	1 cup	16
Frosted Fruit O's	1 cup	15
Golden Corn Nuggets	1 cup	15
Frosted Flakes	1 cup	14
Honey Nut Toasted Oats	1 cup	12
Crunchy Oat Squares	1 cup	8
Honey Oats & Flakes	1 cup	8
Wheat Bran Flakes	1 cup	7
Multigrain	1 cup	6
Corn Flakes	1 cup	2
Crispy Rice	1 cup	2
Toasted Oats	1 cup	1

Arrowhead Mills®	Amount	Total Sugar (g)
Sweetened Shredded Wheat	1 cup	11
Sweetened Rice Flakes	1 cup	8
Maple Buckwheat Flakes	1 cup	5
Amaranth Flakes	1 cup	4
Oat Bran Flakes	1 cup	3
Spelt Flakes	1 cup	3
Kamut Flakes	1 cup	2
Shredded Wheat, Bite Size	1 cup	2
Sprouted Multigrain Flakes	1 cup	2

SUGAR

Continued

Barbara's	Amount	Total Sugar (g)
Shredded Oats Cinnamon Crunch	1 cup	15
Shredded Oats Vanilla Almond	1 cup	15
Shredded Minis Blueberry Burst	1 cup	14
Hole 'n Oats Honey Nut	1 cup	13
High Fiber Cranberry	1 cup	11
Shredded Oats Original	1 cup	10
Puffins Puffs Crunchy Cocoa	1 cup	9
Puffins Puffs Fruit Medley	1 cup	9
High Fiber Flax & Granola	1 cup	9
Puffins Cinnamon	1 cup	9
High Fiber Original	1 cup	8
Puffins Honey Rice	1 cup	8
Puffins Multigrain	1 cup	8
Puffins Peanut Butter	1 cup	8
Puffins Peanut Butter & Chocolate	1 cup	8
Puffins Original	1 cup	7
Shredded Spoonfuls Multigrain	1 cup	7
Corn Flakes	1 cup	4
Brown Rice Crisps	1 cup	1
Hole 'n Oats: Fruit Juice Sweetened	1 cup	1
Shredded Wheat	2 biscuits	0

Bear Naked®	Amount	Total Sugar (g)
Peak Protein, Original Granola	1 cup	24
Vanila Almond Crucnh Granola	1 cup	24
Fruit & Nut Ganola	1 cup	20
Banana Nut Granola	1 cup	16
Nut Cluster Crunch Cereal	1 cup	13

Cadia Organic	Amount	Total Sugar (g)
All Natural Raisin Bran	1 cup	18
Crunch	1 cup	12
Whole Grain Cadi-O's Toasted Oats	1 cup	11
Honey Kissed Cadi-O's	1 cup	9

Cascadian Farm®	Amount	Total Sugar (g)
Cinnamon Raisin Granola	1 cup	24
Maple Brown Sugar Granola	1 cup	21
Fruit & Nut Granola	1 cup	20
Oats & Honey Granola	1 cup	20
Dark Chocolate Almond Granola	1 cup	19
French Vanilla Almond Granola	1 cup	17
Raisin bran	1 cup	15

SUGAR

Hearty Morning	1 cup	12
Chocolate O's	1 cup	11
Fruit Ful O's	1 cup	11
Cinnamon Crunch	1 cup	8
Honey Nut O's	1 cup	7
Multi Gain Squares	1 cup	5
Purel O's	1 cup	1

Erewhon®	Amount	Total Sugar (g)
Cocoa Crispy Brown Rice	1 cup	11
Rice Twice, Gluten Free	1 cup	11
Raisin Bran	1 cup	10
Crispy Brown Rice, Strawberry Crisp	1 cup	8
Crispy Brown Rice, Mixed Berries	1 cup	6
Crispy Brown Rice, Gluten Free	1 cup	1
Crispy Brown Rice, No Salt Added	1 cup	1
Crispy Brown Rice, Original	1 cup	1
Corn Flakes, Gluten Free	1 cup	0

Ezekiel, 4:9	Amount	Total Sugar (g)
Cinnamon Flax	1 cup	16
Almond	1 cup	2
Golden Flax	1 cup	0
Original	1 cup	0

General Mills®	Amount	Total Sugar (g)
Oatmeal Crisp, Hearty Raisin	1 cup	19
Total Raisin Bran	1 cup	17
Raisin Nut Bran	1 cup	16
Oatmeal Crisp, Crunchy Almond	1 cup	15
Honey Nut Clusters	1 cup	14
Basic 4	1 cup	13
Cocoa Puffs	1 cup	13
Cookie Crisp	1 cup	13
Golden Grams	1 cup	13
Multi-Bran CHEX	1 cup	13
Reese's Puffs	1 cup	13
Total Cranberry Crunch	1 cup	13
Cinnamon Toast Crunch	1 cup	12
Honey Nut Chex	1 cup	12
Lucky Charms	1 cup	12
Chocolate Chex	1 cup	11
Cinnamon Chex	1 cup	10
Trix	1 cup	10

SUGAR

Dora The Explorer	1 cup	8
Total Whole Grain	1 cup	7
Wheat Chex	1 cup	7
Berry Berry Kix	1 cup	6
Wheaties	1 cup	5
Corn Chex	1 cup	3
Kix	1 cup	2
Rice Chex	1 cup	2

General Mills Cheerios®	Amount	Total Sugar (g)
Apple Cinnamon	1 cup	13
Frosted	1 cup	13
Banana Nut	1 cup	12
Chocolate	1 cup	12
Fruity	1 cup	12
Honey Nut	1 cup	12
Multi Grain Peanut Butter	1 cup	12
Yogurt Burst, Strawberry	1 cup	12
Crunch, Oat Clusters	1 cup	10
Berry Burst	1 cup	9
Cinnamon Burst	1 cup	9
Dulce de leche	1 cup	8
Multi Grain	1 cup	6
Original	1 cup	1

General Mills Fiber-One®	Amount	Total Sugar (g)
Raisin Bran Clusters	1 cup	14
Frosted Shredded Wheat	1 cup	12
Caramel Delight	1 cup	10
Honey Clusters	1 cup	6
Original Bran	1 cup	0

Glutino®	Amount	Total Sugar (g)
Frosted Corn & Rice Flakes	1 cup	10
Berry Sensible Beginning	1 cup	9
Corn Rice Flakes with Strawberries	1 cup	9
Apple & Cinnamon Rings	1 cup	8
Corn Rice Flakes	1 cup	8
Honey Nut Cereal	1 cup	8

Healthy Valley	Amount	Total Sugar (g)
Oat Bran Flakes & Raisins	1 cup	18
Oat Bran Almond Crunch	1 cup	18
Cranberry Crunch	1 cup	17

SUGAR

Continued

Low Fat Date & Almond Flavored Granola	1 cup	15
Low Fat Raisin Cinnamon Granola	1 cup	15
Oat Bran Flakes	1 cup	11
Heart Wise	1 cup	11
Fiber 7 Multigrain Flakes	1 cup	10
Multigrain Maple, Honey, Nut Squares	1 cup	10
Amaranth Flakes	1 cup	9
Golden Flax	1 cup	9
Multigrain Apple Cinnamon Squares	1 cup	4
Rice Crunch-EMS	1 cup	2
Corn Crunch-EMS	1 cup	2

Kashi®	Amount	Total Sugar (g)
Go Lean Crisp, Cinnamon Crumble	1 cup	13
Go Lean Crisp, Toasted Berry Crumble	1 cup	13
Go Lean Crunch	1 cup	13
Go Lean Crunch, Honey Almond Flax	1 cup	12
Heart to Heart, Oat Flakes & Blueberry Clusters	1 cup	12
Strawberry Fields	1 cup	11
Blackberry Hills	1 cup	10
Good Friends	1 cup	10
Berry Blossom	1 cup	9
Island Vanilla	27 biscuits	9
Cinnamon Harvest	28 biscuits	9
Go Lean	1 cup	9
Go Lean Vanilla Graham	1 cup	9
Heart to Heart, Nutty Chia Flax	1 cup	9
Berry Fruitful	29 biscuits	8
Honey Sunshine	1 cup	8
Indigo Morning	1 cup	8
Simply Maize	1 cup	8
Heart to Heart, Honey Toasted Oat	1 cup	7
Heart to Heart, Warm Cinnamon	1 cup	7
Autum Wheat	29 biscuits	7
7-Whole Grain Flakes	1 cup	6
7-Whole Grain Honey Puffs	1 cup	6
7-Whole Grain Nuggets	1 cup	6
7-Whole Grain Puffs	1 cup	0

Kellogg's®	Amount	Total Sugar (g)
All-Bran Bran Buds	1 cup	24
Cracklin' Oat Bran	1 cup	21
MUESLIX	1 cup	21
Honey Smacks	1 cup	20
Raisin Bran Crunch	1 cup	20

SUGAR

Raisin Bran	1 cup	18
Cocoa Krispies	1 cup	16
Frosted Rice Krispies	1 cup	16
Crunchy Nut Golden Honey Nut Flakes	1 cup	15
Frosted Flakes	1 cup	15
Krave Chocolate	1 cup	15
Smart Start, Strong Heart, Antioxidants	1 cup	14
Apple Jacks	1 cup	13
Crunchy Nut Roasted Nut & Honey O's	1 cup	13
Honey Crunch Corn Flakes	1 cup	13
Smorz	1 cup	13
CINNABON	1 cup	12
Fiberplus Berry Yogurt Crunch	1 cup	12
Froot Loops	1 cup	12
Rice Krispies Treats	1 cup	12
Frosted MINI-Wheats, Big-Bite	1 cup	11
Corn Pops	1 cup	10
All-Bran Original	1 cup	10
Fiberplus Cinnamon Oat Crunch	1 cup	9
All-Bran Complete Wheat Flakes	1 cup	7
Crispix	1 cup	4
Product 19	1 cup	4
Corn Flakes	1 cup	3
Rice Krispies	1 cup	3

Kellogg's Special-K®	Amount	Total Sugar (g)
Low Fat Granola	1 cup	18
Fruit & Yogurt	1 cup	14
Chocolately Delight	1 cup	12
Vanilla Almond	1 cup	12
Multigrain Oats & Honey	1 cup	12
Blueberry	1 cup	11
Cinnamon Pecan	1 cup	10
Red Berries	1 cup	9
Original	1 cup	4
Protein Plus	1 cup	3

Mom's Best®	Amount	Total Sugar (g)
Honey Ful Wheats	1 cup	20
Raisin Bran	1 cup	20
Crispy Coco Rice	1 cup	17
Honey Grahams	1 cup	13
Mallow Oats	1 cup	13
Toasted Cinnamon Squares	1 cup	13
Sweetened Wheat Fuls	1 cup	11

SUGAR

Honey Nut Toasty O's	1 cup	10
Oats & Honey Blend	1 cup	8
Toasted Wheat Fuls	1 cup	0

Nature's Path®	Amount	Total Sugar (g)
Acai Apple Granola	1 cup	17
Flax Plus Pumpkin Raisin Crunch	1 cup	17
Optimum Cranberry Ginger	1 cup	17
Pomegran Cherry Granola	1 cup	17
Pomegran Plus Granola	1 cup	17
Flax Plus Raisin Bran Flakes	1 cup	16
AGAVE Plus Granola	1 cup	13
Flax Plus Maple Pecan Crunch	1 cup	13
Flax Plus Pumpkin Flax Granola	1 cup	13
Flax Plus Redberry Crunch	1 cup	13
Flax Plus Vanilla Almond Granola	1 cup	13
Hemp Plus Granola	1 cup	13
Optimum Banana Almond	1 cup	12
Optimum Power Blueberry Cinnamon	1 cup	12
Peanut Butter Granola	1 cup	12
Smart Bran	1 cup	12
Crunchy Maple Sunrise	1 cup	11
Crunchy Vanilla Sunrise	1 cup	11
Heritage Crunch	1 cup	8
OATY BITES Whole Grain	1 cup	7
Whole O's	1 cup	6
Optimum Slim Low Fat Vanilla	1 cup	6
Flax Plus Multibran Flakes	1 cup	5
Heritage Flakes	1 cup	5
Heritage Heirloom	1 cup	5
Honeyed Corn Flakes	1 cup	5
Mesa Sunrise	1 cup	5
Millet Rice	1 cup	5
Multigrain Oat bran	1 cup	5

Peace All Natural	Amount	Total Sugar (g)
Walnut Spice Clusters & Flakes	1 cup	28
Cherry Almond Clusters & Flakes	1 cup	20
Golden Honey Granola	1 cup	17
Wild Berry Clusters & Flakes	1 cup	15
Maple Pecan	1 cup	11
Vanilla Almond Clusters & Flakes	1 cup	11
Mango Peach Passion Clusters & Flakes	1 cup	10

SUGAR

Continued

Post®	Amount	Total Sugar, g
Raisin Bran	1 cup	20
Golden Crisp	1 cup	19
Great Grains, Raisin, Date & Pecan	1 cup	18
Great Grains, Cranberry Almond Crunch	1 cup	16
Fruity Pebbles	1 cup	15
Cocoa Pebbles	1 cup	14
Blueberry Morning	1 cup	13
Honey Nut Shredded Wheat	1 cup	12
Shredded Wheat, Frosted, spoon-size	1 cup	12
Great Grains, Banana Nut Crunch	1 cup	11
Grape-Nuts Cereal	1 cup	10
Great Grains, Crunchy Pecan	1 cup	10
Bran Flakes	1 cup	7
Honeycomb Cereal	1 cup	7
Alpha-Bits	1 cup	6
Grape-Nuts Flakes	1 cup	6
Shredded Wheat, Original, spoon-size	1 cup	0.4
Shredded Wheat, Original, big-biscuit	2 biscuits	0.4
Shredded Wheat n' Bran	1 cup	0.4

Post® Honey Bunches of Oats®	Amount	Total Sugar (g)
Just Bunches, Cinnamonn	1 cup	20
Just Bunches, Honey Roasted	1 cup	20
Raisin Medley	1 cup	14
With Vanilla Bunches	1 cup	12
With Strawberries	1 cup	10
Honey Roasted	1 cup	8
Pecan Bunches	1 cup	8
With Almonds	1 cup	8
With Cinnamon Bunches	1 cup	8

Quaker®	Amount	Total Sugar (g)
Granola, Apple Cranberry Almond	1 cup	26
CAP'N Crunch	1 cup	16
Honey Graham OH'S	1 cup	16
CAP'N Crunch & Crunchberries	1 cup	15
CAP'N Crunch's OOPs! All Berries	1 cup	14
CAP'N Crunch's Peanut Butter Crunch	1 cup	12
LIFE Cereal, Cinnamon	1 cup	11
LIFE Cereal, Maple & Brown Sugar	1 cup	11
Oatmeal Squares	1 cup	9
Oatmeal Squares, Brown Sugar	1 cup	9
Oatmeal Squares, Cinnamon	1 cup	9

SUGAR

Continued

Oatmeal Squares, Golden Maple	1 cup	9
Oatmeal Squares, Honey Nut	1 cup	9
LIFE Cereal, Original	1 cup	8
Whole Hearts	1 cup	8
Corn Bran Crunch	1 cup	7
Toasted Multigrain Crisp	1 cup	7
Puffed Wheat	1 cup	0.21
Puffed Rice	1 cup	0

Trader Joe's® Brand Cereal	Amount	Total Sugar (g)
Organic Raisin Bran Clusters	1 cup	18
Raisin Bran Clusters	1 cup	18
Super Nutty Toffe Clusters	1 cup	15
Honey Nut O's*	1 cup	12
Frosted Flakes*	1 cup	12
Banana Nut Clusters	1 cup	12
Maple Pecan Clusters	1 cup	12
Very Berry Clusters	1 cup	12
Vanilla Almond Clusters	1 cup	11
Toasted Oatmeal Flakes	1 cup	9
Triple Berry O's*	1 cup	9
Bran Flakes*	1 cup	8
High Fiber Cereal	1 cup	8
Fruity O's	1 cup	8
Organic High Fiber O's	1 cup	7
MuitiGrain O's	1 cup	6
Puffed Wheat	1 cup	6
Crispy Rice	1 cup	3
Corn Flakes	1 cup	2
Joes O's	1 cup	1
Strawberry Yogurt Cereal*	1 cup	0
Raisin Bran	1 cup	0

Uncle Sam®	Amount	Total Sugar (g)
Wheat Berry Flakes, Flaxseed, & Strawberry	1 cup	9
Skinners Raisin Bran	1 cup	8
Wheat Berry Flakes, Flaxseed, Honey Almond	1 cup	7
Wheat Berry Flakes & Flaxseed, Original	1 cup	1

Vons® Safeway® Brand Cereal	Amount	Total Sugar (g)
Raisin Bran	1 cup	20
Crunchy Granola Raisin Bran	1 cup	20
Apple Orbits	1 cup	16
Honey Nut & Toasted Oats	1 cup	15

SUGAR

Continued

Cinnamon Live it Up	1 cup	11
Frosted Shredded Wheat, Bit Size	1 cup	11
Live It Up	1 cup	8
Oats & More with Honey	1 cup	8
Oats & More with Almond	1 cup	8
Bran Flakes	1 cup	7
Rice Pockets	1 cup	2
Toasted Oats	1 cup	2
Corn Flakes	1 cup	2
Cinnamon Crunch	1 cup	0

Vons® Eating Right® Cereal	Amount	Total Sugar (g)
Granola Cereal & Raisins	1 cup	23
Granola Cereal	1 cup	21
Cranberry Almond Multigrain	1 cup	12
Toasted Rice, Wheat Flakes & Strawberry	1 cup	9

Wall Mart® Brand Cereal	Amount	Total Sugar (g)
Extra Raisin Raisin Bran	1 cup	21
Crunchy Raisin Bran	1 cup	20
Raisin Bran	1 cup	18
Sugar Frosted Flakes	1 cup	17
Berry Crunch	1 cup	16
Apple Blast	1 cup	16
Honey Nut Spins	1 cup	15
Cinnamon Crunch	1 cup	13
Vanilla Almond Awake	1 cup	12
Crunchy Honey Oats with Almonds	1 cup	11
Fruit Spins	1 cup	11
Frosted Shredded Wheats	1 cup	11
Strawberry Awake	1 cup	10
Crunchy Honey Oats	1 cup	8
Toasted Wheat	1 cup	7
Bran Flakes	1 cup	7
Crunchy Nuggets	1 cup	6
Toasted Corn	1 cup	3
Toasted Rice	1 cup	2
Corn Flakes	1 cup	2
Crispy Rice	1 cup	2
Toasted Whole-Grain Oats	1 cup	1
Toasted Whole-Grain	1 cup	0
Honey Nut	1 cup	0

SUGAR

Whole Foods® 365® Brand Cereal	Amount	Total Sugar (g)
Raisin Bran	1 cup	15
Cocoa Rice Crisps	1 cup	12
Protein & Fiber	1 cup	12
Berry Flax Protein & Fiber Crunch	1 cup	10
High Fiber Morning O's	1 cup	9
Crunchy Cinnamon Squares	1 cup	8
Frosted Flakes	1 cup	8
Wheat Waffles	1 cup	7
Honey Flakes & Oat Clusters	1 cup	7
Whole Wheat Flakes	1 cup	7
Multi-Grain Morning O's	1 cup	6
Bran Flakes	1 cup	3
Brown Rice Crisp	1 cup	3
Corn Flakes	1 cup	2
Morning O's	1 cup	1
Wheat Squares	1 cup	0

Wild Harvest®	Amount	Total Sugar (g)
Crunchy Vanilla Almond Granola	1 cup	23
Blueberry Flax Granola	1 cup	21
Cherry Vanilla Granola	1 cup	18
Golden Honey & Flax Granola	1 cup	15
Wholesome Raisin Bran	1 cup	15
Cranberry Almond	1 cup	13
Mango Crisp	1 cup	13
Maple Pecan Flakes & Clusters	1 cup	12
Wild Berry Crisp	1 cup	11

Cereal, Cooked	Amount	Total Sugar (g)
Farina	1 cup	1.82
Oats, regular	1 cup	0.63
Malt-o-Meal plain	1 serving	0.35
White corn grits	1 cup	0.29
Yellow corn grits	1 cup	0.22
CREAM OF WHEAT, regular	1 cup	0.08

Cheese	Amount	Total Sugar (g)
Roquefort	1 oz	x
American, pasteurized process, imitation	1 oz	2.33
Cream cheese, fat free	1 oz	1.55
Feta	1 oz	1.16
Muenster, low fat	1 oz	0.98
Cream cheese	1 oz	0.91

SUGAR

Continued

Goat cheese, semisoft	1 oz	0.72
American, pasteurized process, fortified	1 oz	0.64
Gouda	1 oz	0.63
Goat cheese, hard type	1 oz	0.62
Fontina	1 oz	0.44
Mozzarella, non fat	1 oz	0.42
Swiss	1 oz	0.37
Swiss, low fat	1 oz	0.37
Muenster	1 oz	0.32
Mozzarella, whole milk	1 oz	0.29
Parmesan, grated	1 oz	0.26
Goat cheese, soft type	1 oz	0.25
Romano	1 oz	0.21
American, pasteurized process, low fat	1 oz	0.17
Mozzarella, part skim, low moisture	1 oz	0.17
Monterey, low fat	1 oz	0.16
Provolone	1 oz	0.16
Cheddar	1 oz	0.15
Cheddar, low fat	1 oz	0.15
Colby	1 oz	0.15
Provolone, reduced Fat	1 oz	0.15
Blue cheese	1 oz	0.14
Monterey	1 oz	0.14
Brie	1 oz	0.13
Gruyere	1 oz	0.10

Chicken, Cooked	Amount	Total Sugar (g)
All types	3 oz	0

CHILI

Chili, Amy's	Amount	Total Sugar (g)
Light in Sodium Medium Chili	1 can	10
Light in Sodium Spicy Chili	1 can	10
Medium Chili	1 can	10
Spicy Chili	1 can	10
Southwestern Black Bean Chili	1 can	10
Medium Chili with Vegetables	1 can	12
Black Bean Chili	1 can	6

Chili, Campbell's® Chunky	Amount	Total Sugar (g)
Chili with Beans Grilled Steak	1 can	18
Chili with Beans Roadhouse	1 can	16

SUGAR

Chili with Beans Firehouse	1 can	16
Beef Chili no Beans	1 can	14

Chili, Dennison®	Amount	Total Sugar (g)
Vegetarian Chili with Beans	1 can	12
Turkey Chili with Beans	1 can	6
Original Chili Con Carne with Beans	1 can	4
Hot Chili Con Carne with Beans	1 can	4
Chunky Chili Con Carne with Beans	1 can	4
Hot & Chunky Chili with Beans	1 can	2

Chili, Eden's	Amount	Total Sugar (g)
Kidney Bean & Kamut Chili	1 can	8
Pinto Bean & Spelt Chili	1 can	6
Great Northern Bean & Barley Chili	1 can	6
Black Bean & Quinoa Chili	1 can	6

Chili, Hardy Jack's	Amount	Total Sugar (g)
Chili no beans	1 can	6
Chili with beans	1 can	6

Chili, Healthy Valley	Amount	Total Sugar (g)
No salt added Tame Tomato Chili	1 can	22
Vegetarian Black Bean Mango Chili	1 can	18
Vegetarian Santa Fe White Bean Chili	1 can	18
Vegetarian Spicy Tomato Chili	1 can	18
Vegetarian 3 Bean Chipotle Chili	1 can	16
Vegetarian Black Bean Mole Chili	1 can	14

Chili, Hormel®	Amount	Total Sugar (g)
Cook-off Chipotle Chicken Chili	1 can	14
Cook-off Roasted Tomato Chili	1 can	14
Turkey Chili with Beans	1 can	12
Chili with Beans 99% fat free	1 can	12
Chili with Beans	1 can	10
Chunky Chili with Beans	1 can	10
Hot Chili with beans	1 can	10
Less Sodium Chili with Beans	1 can	10
Cook- off White Chicken Chili	1 can	10
Turkey Chili no Beans	1 can	8
Chili no Beans	1 can	6
Less Sodium Chili no Beans	1 can	6

SUGAR

Continued

Chili, Nalley's®	Amount	Total Sugar (g)
Thick Chili with beans	1 can	6
Original Chili with beans	1 can	6
Jalapeno Hot Chili with beans	1 can	4
Turkey Chili with beans	1 can	4

Chili, Stagg®	Amount	Total Sugar (g)
Vegetarian Garden Four Bean Chili	1 can	18
Dynamite Hot Chili with Beans	1 can	14
Classic Chili with Beans	1 can	14
Fiesta Grille Chili with Beans	1 can	14
Chunkero Chili with Beans	1 can	12
Country Brand Chili with Beans	1 can	12
Country Brand Chili Sweet Peppers	1 can	12
Silverado Beef Chili with Beans	1 can	12
Turkey Ranchero Chili with Beans	1 can	12
Steak House Chili no Beans	1 can	10
White Chicken Chili with Beans	1 can	10
Ranch House Chicken Chili & Beans	1 can	10
Laredo Chili, Beans & Jalapeno	1 can	6

Chili, Wolf Brand®	Amount	Total Sugar (g)
Spicy Chili with Beans	1 can	30
Homestyle Chili with Beans	1 can	22
Chili with Beans	1 can	6
Lean Beaf with Beans	1 can	6
Turkey Chili with Beans	1 can	6
Lean Beaf no Beans	1 can	6
Chili no Beans	1 can	4
Hot Chili no Beans	1 can	4
Turkey Chili no Beans	1 can	4

Cream	Amount	Total Sugar (g)
Sour Cream, cultured	1 tbsp	0.4
Whipped Topping, pressurized	1 tbsp	0.2
Half & Half	1 tbsp	0
Heavy Cream	1 tbsp	0
Light Coffe Cream	1 tbsp	0
Sour Cream, reduced fat	1 tbsp	0

SUGAR

Eggs	Amount	Total Sugar (g)
Egg whites, dried	1 ounce	1.5
Egg substitute, liquid, fat free	1/4 cup	1.2
Egg whole, scrambled	1 large	0.9
Egg whole, hard-boiled	1 large	0.6
Egg whites	1 large	0.2
Egg whole, poached	1 large	0.2
Egg whole, fried	1 large	0.2
Egg yolk	1 large	0.1
Egg whites, dried powder, stabilized	1 tbsp	0

FRUIT

Fruit, Canned	Amount	Total Sugar (g)
Plums	1 cup	58
Apricoits	1 cup	51
Peaches	1 cup	49
Pineapple	1 cup	43
Pears	1 cup	40
Applesauce, sweetened	1 cup	37
Applesauce, unsweetened	1 cup	23
Olives, green	5 large	0.07
Olives, black	5 large	0

Fruit, Canned	Amount	Fructose Sugar (g)
Pineapple, heavy syrup	1 cup	18.29
Applesauce, sweetened	1 cup	17.88
Pears	1 cup	15.69
Applesauce, unsweetened	1 cup	14.35
Peaches, drained	1 cup	7.66
Apricoits, heavy syrup	1 cup	x
Olives, black	5 large	x
Olives, green	5 large	x
Plums	1 cup	x

Fruit, Dried	Amount	Total Sugar (g)
Pears	1 cup	112
Currants	1 cup	97
Cranberries	1 cup	79
Figs	1 cup	71
Apricots	1 cup	69
Peaches	1 cup	67
Prunes, pitted	1 cup	66
Apples	1 cup	49

SUGAR

Fruit, Dried	Amount	Fructose Sugar (g)
Figs	1 cup	34.17
Prunes, pitted	1 cup	21.66
Peaches	1 cup	21.58
Apricots	1 cup	16.21
Apples	1 cup	x
Cranberries	1 cup	x
Currants	1 cup	x
Pears	1 cup	x

Fruit, Dried	Amount	Total Sugar (g)
Pears	1/4 cup	28
Currants	1/4 cup	24
Cranberries	1/4 cup	20
Figs	1/4 cup	18
Apricots	1/4 cup	17
Peaches	1/4 cup	17
Prunes, pitted	1/4 cup	17
Apples	1/4 cup	12

Fruit, Dried	Amount	Fructose Sugar (g)
Figs	1/4 cup	8.54
Prunes, pitted	1/4 cup	5.42
Peaches	1/4 cup	5.40
Apricots	1/4 cup	4.05
Apples	1/4 cup	x
Cranberries	1/4 cup	x
Currants	1/4 cup	x
Pears	1/4 cup	x

Fruit, Dried (in small portions)	Amount	Total Sugar (g)
Apricots	10 halves	19
Apples	5 rings	18
Peaches	3 halves	16
Pears	1 half	11
Apples	1 ring	4
Figs	1 fig	4
Prunes, pitted	1 prune	4

Fruit, Dried (in small portions)	Amount	Fructose Sugar (g)
Pears	1 half	11.00
Peaches	3 halves	5.26
Apricots	10 halves	4.36

SUGAR

Figs	1 fig	1.93
Prunes, pitted	1 prune	1.18
Apples	5 rings	x

Fruit, Frozen	Amount	Total Sugar (g)
Strawberries, sweetened, sliced	1 cup	61
Peaches, sliced	1 cup	55
Raspberries, unthawed	1 cup	54
Strawberries, sweetened, whole	1 cup	47
Blueberries	1 cup	45
Blackberries, unthawed	1 cup	16
Strawberries, unsweetened	1 cup	10

Fruit, Raw	Amount	Total Sugar (g)
Dates	1 cup	93
Raisins	1 cup	85
Prunes, uncooked	1 cup	66
Prunes, stewed	1 cup	62
Pomegrantes	1 cup	39
Grapes, red & green	1 cup	25
Mango	1 cup	23
Plantains	1 cup	22
Tangerine	1 cup	21
Sweet cherries, no pits	1 cup	20
Florida Oranges	1 cup	17
Pears	1 cup	16
Kiwi	1 cup	16
Pineapple	1 cup	16
Plums	1 cup	16
Grapefruit, pink & red, sections	1 cup	16
Apricots	1 cup	15
Blueberries	1 cup	14
Apples	1 cup	14
Navel oranges	1 cup	14
Honeydew	1 cup	14
Peachs	1 cup	13
Cataloupe	1 cup	13
Mulberries	1 cup	11
Papayas	1 cup	11
Nectarine	1 cup	11
Water mellon	1 cup	9
Strawberries	1 cup	8
Blackberries	1 cup	7
Avocado, Florida	1 cup	6

SUGAR

Raspberries	1 cup	5
Cranberries	1 cup	4
Jicama	1 cup	2
Avocado, California	1 cup	0.7

Fruit, Raw	Amount	Fructose Sugar (g)
Raisins	1 cup	43.04
Dates	1 cup	29.00
Prunes, uncooked	1 cup	21.68
Grapes, red & green	1 cup	12.28
Pears	1 cup	10.03
Sweet cherries, no pits	1 cup	8.27
Apples	1 cup	8.14
Kiwi, sliced	1 cup	7.83
Mango	1 cup	7.72
Blueberries	1 cup	7.36
Papayas	1 cup	5.41
Water mellon, diced	1 cup	5.11
Plums	1 cup	5.07
Honeydew	1 cup	5.03
Tangerine	1 cup	4.68
Grapefruit, pink & red, sections	1 cup	4.07
Strawberries	1 cup	4.05
Navel Oranges, sections	1 cup	3.71
Pineapple	1 cup	3.50
Blackberries	1 cup	3.46
Cantaloupe, cubes	1 cup	2.99
Raspberries	1 cup	2.89
Peachs	1 cup	2.60
Nectarine, slices	1 cup	1.86
Apricots	1 cup	1.55
Cranberries	1 cup	0.63
Avocado, Florida	1 cup	0.58
Avocado, California	1 cup	0.18
Florida Oranges, sections	1 cup	x
Jicama	1 cup	x
Plantains	1 cup	x
Prunes, stewed	1 cup	x

Fruit, Raw	Amount	Total Sugar (g)
Persimmons, small native	1 fruit	x
Pummelo	1 fruit	x
Mango	1 fruit	46
Pomegrantes	1 fruit	38

SUGAR

Cherimoya	1 fruit	30
Plantains	1 fruit	27
Raisins	1 small box	25
Dates	5 dates	22
Persimmons, Japanese	1 fruit	21
Apples, medium size	1 fruit	19
Prunes, uncooked	5 fruit	18
Pears	1 fruit	16
Banana, medium size	1 fruit	14
Florida Oranges	1 fruit	13
Peaches	1 fruit	13
Navel Oranges	1 fruit	12
Cherries	10 fruit	11
Nectarine	1 fruit	11
Papayas	1 fruit	11
Tangerine	1 fruit	9
Grapefruit, pink & red, sections	1/2 fruit	8
Grapes	10 grapes	8
Raisins	1 packet	8
Avocado, Florida	1 fruit	8
Grapes, red or green	10 fruit	8
Kiwi	1 fruit	7
Plums	1 fruit	7
Figs	1 fruit	7
Pineapple, slices	1/2" x 3"	5
Star fruit, Carambola	1 fruit	4
Pineapple guava, Feijoa	1 fruit	3
Chayote	1 fruit	3
Apricots	1 fruit	3
Strawberries	5 fruit	3
Kumquats	1 fruit	2
Avocado, California	1 fruit	0

Fruit, Raw	Amount	Fructose Sugar (g)
Raisins	1 small box	12.76
Apples, medium size	1 fruit	10.74
Pears	1 fruit	10.34
Dates	5 fruit	6.94
Prunes, uncooked	5 fruit	5.91
Papayas, small size	1 fruit	5.86
Banana, medium size	1 fruit	5.72
Cherries	10 fruit	4.40
Grapes	10 fruit	3.98
Kiwi	1 fruit	3.31
Navel Oranges	1 fruit	3.15

SUGAR

Peaches	1 fruit	2.30
Grapefruit, pink & red, sections	1/2 fruit	2.18
Tangerine	1 fruit	2.11
Plums	1 fruit	2.03
Figs, dried	1 fruit	1.93
Nectarine	1 fruit	1.86
Strawberries	5 fruit	1.46
Pineapple, slices	1/2" x 3"	1.06
Avocado, Florida	1 fruit	0.76
Apricots	1 fruit	0.33
Avocado, California	1 fruit	0.11
Florida Oranges	1 fruit	x
Kumquats	1 fruit	x
Plantains	1 fruit	x

Game Meat, Cooked	Amount	Total Sugar (g)
All types	3 oz	0

Grains, Cooked	Amount	Total Sugar (g)
Buckwheat	1 cup	1.5
Wild rice	1 cup	1.2
Egg & Spinach noodles	1 cup	1.1
Whole-Wheat spaghetti	1 cup	1.1
Macaroni	1 cup	0.8
Spaghetti	1 cup	0.8
Brown rice	1 cup	0.7
Egg noodles	1 cup	0.6
Pearled barley	1 cup	0.4
Bulgur	1 cup	0.2
Couscous	1 cup	0.2
Chow mein noodles	1 cup	0.1
White rice, long grain, regular	1 cup	0.1
Instant white rice	1 cup	0

Juice	Amount	Total Sugar (g)
Prune	1 cup	42
Grape	1 cup	36
Pomegranate	1 cup	32
Cranberry	1 cup	30
Apple & Grape blend	1 cup	27
Pineapple	1 cup	25
Apple	1 cup	24
Orange juice, canned, unsweetened	1 cup	22
Grapefruit, white, raw	1 cup	22

SUGAR

Continued

Orange, raw	1 cup	21
Blackberry	1 cup	19
Carrot	1 cup	9
Tomato	1 cup	9
Vegetable	1 cup	8
Lemon, raw	1 cup	6

Juice	Amount	Fructose Sugar (g)
Grape	1 cup	18.62
Apple & Grape blend	1 cup	16.15
Pomegranate	1 cup	15.86
Apple	1 cup	14.21
Cranberry	1 cup	12.57
Pineapple	1 cup	9.52
Orange	1 cup	6.05
Tomato	1 cup	3.74
Lemon, raw	1 cup	2.68
Carrot	1 cup	x
Grapefruit, white, raw	1 cup	x
Orange, raw	1 cup	x
Prune	1 cup	x
Vegetable	1 cup	x
Blackberry	1 cup	x

Lamb, Cooked	Amount	Total Sugar (g)
All types	3 oz	0

Milk	Amount	Total Sugar (g)
Canned, condensed, sweetened	1 cup	166
Canned, evaporated, non fat	1 cup	29
Canned, evaporated	1 cup	25
Human milk	1 cup	17
Low fat, 1%	1 cup	13
Non fat, fat free or skim liquid milk	1 cup	13
Reduced fat, 2%	1 cup	12
Whole milk, 3.25%	1 cup	12
Dry, instant, non fat	1/3 cup	12
Buttermilk, low fat	1 cup	12
Goat milk	1 cup	11
Soy milk, original, unfortified	1 cup	10
Coconut milk, canned	1 cup	x
Sheep milk	1 cup	x

SUGAR

Nuts & Seeds	Amount	Total Sugar (g)
Peanut butter, smooth style	1 oz	2.61
Pistachio	1 oz	2.17
Coconut, raw meat	1 oz	1.77
Cashews	1 oz	1.68
Peanuts	1 oz	1.45
Macadamia	1 oz	1.30
Hazelnuts	1 oz	1.23
Pecans	1 oz	1.13
Almonds	1 oz	1.10
Pine nuts	1 oz	1.02
English walnuts	1 oz	0.74
Sunflower seeds	1 oz	0.74
Brazil nuts	1 oz	0.66
Flaxseeds	1 oz	0.44
Pumpkin seeds	1 oz	0.40
Black walnuts	1 oz	0.31
Tahini, sesame butter	1 oz	0.14
Sesame seeds	1 oz	0.09
Chia seeds	1 oz	X

SALAD DRESSINGS

Annie's Organic Dressing	Amount	Total Sugar (g)
Thousand Island	2 tbsp	5
Papaya Poppy Seed	2 tbsp	4
Asian Sesame	2 tbsp	3
French Dressing	2 tbsp	3
Redwine & Olive Oil	2 tbsp	3
Sesame Ginger Vinaigrette	2 tbsp	3
Balsamic Vinaigrette	2 tbsp	2
Caesar Dressing	2 tbsp	2
Cowgirl Ranch Dressing	2 tbsp	2
Roasted Garlic Vinaigrette	2 tbsp	2
Buttermilk Dressing	2 tbsp	1
Green Garlic	2 tbsp	1
Green Goddess Dressing	2 tbsp	1
Pomegranate Vinaigrette	2 tbsp	1

Bernstein's Dressing	Amount	Total Sugar (g)
Herb Garden French	2 tbsp	6
Sweet Herb Italian	2 tbsp	5
Light Parmesan Garlic Ranch	2 tbsp	2
Light Roasted Garlic Balsamic	2 tbsp	2

SUGAR

Continued

Balsamic Italian	2 tbsp	1
Basil Parmesan	2 tbsp	1
Cheese & Garlic Italian	2 tbsp	1
Chunky Blue Cheese	2 tbsp	1
Fat Free Cheese & Garlic Italian	2 tbsp	1
Italian & Marinade	2 tbsp	1
Light Fantastic Cheese Fantastico	2 tbsp	1
Redwine & Garlic Italian	2 tbsp	1
Cheese Fantastico	2 tbsp	0
Creamy Caesar	2 tbsp	0
Restaurant Recipe Italian	2 tbsp	0

Best Food® Mayonnaise Dressing	Amount	Total Sugar (g)
Real Mayonnaise	2 tbsp	0
Light Mayonnaise	2 tbsp	0
Low Fat Mayonnaise	2 tbsp	0
Mayonnaise with Olive Oil	2 tbsp	0
Canola Cholesterol Free Mayonnaise	2 tbsp	0
Mayonesa Con Jugo De Lemon	2 tbsp	0

Bob's Big Boy® Dressing	Amount	Total Sugar (g)
Ranch	2 tbsp	1
Thousand Island	2 tbsp	1
Blue Cheese	2 tbsp	0
Roquefort	2 tbsp	0

Bolthouse Farms Dresssing	Amount	Total Sugar (g)
Honey Mustard Yogurt Dressing	2 tbsp	6
Zesty French Yogurt Dressing	2 tbsp	6
Classic Balsamic & Olive Oil	2 tbsp	5
Raspberry Merlot & Olive Oil	2 tbsp	5
Chunky Blue Cheese & Olive Oil	2 tbsp	3
Thousand Island Yogurt Dressing	2 tbsp	3
Asian Ginger & Olive Oil Vinaigrettes	2 tbsp	2
Caesar Parmigino Yogurt Dressing	2 tbsp	2
Classic Ranch Yogurt Dressing	2 tbsp	2
Salsa Ranch Yogurt Dressing	2 tbsp	2
Chunky Bluecheese Yogurt Dressing	2 tbsp	1

Brianna's Dressing	Amount	Total Sugar (g)
Blush Wine Vinaigrette	2 tbsp	14
Ginger Mandarin	2 tbsp	8
Lively Lemon Tarragon	2 tbsp	8

SUGAR

Dijon Honey Mustard	2 tbsp	7
Rich Poppyseed	2 tbsp	7
The New American	2 tbsp	5
Champagne Caper Vinaigrette	2 tbsp	4
Rich Santa Fe Blend	2 tbsp	4
True Blue Cheese	2 tbsp	4
Zesty French	2 tbsp	4
Chipotle Cheddar	2 tbsp	3
Classic Buttermilk Ranch	2 tbsp	2
Asiago Caesar	2 tbsp	1
Real French Vinaigrette	2 tbsp	0

Cardini's Dressings	Amount	Total Sugar (g)
Roasted Asian Sesame	2 tbsp	6
Asian Sesame	2 tbsp	6
Honey Mustard	2 tbsp	5
Pear Vinaigrette	2 tbsp	5
Balsamic Vinaigrette	2 tbsp	4
Raspberry Pomegranate	2 tbsp	4
Fat Free Caesar	2 tbsp	3
Aged Parmesan Ranch	2 tbsp	1
Light Caesar	2 tbsp	1
Italian	2 tbsp	0
Original Caesar	2 tbsp	0

Drew's® Dressing	Amount	Total Sugar (g)
Honey Dijon	2 tbsp	4
Poppy Seed	2 tbsp	4
Sesame Orange	2 tbsp	2
Buttermilk Ranch	2 tbsp	1
Classic Italian	2 tbsp	0
Greek Olive	2 tbsp	0
Lemon Goddess	2 tbsp	0
Roasted Garlic & Peppercorn	2 tbsp	0
Rosemary Balsamic	2 tbsp	0
Shiitake Ginger	2 tbsp	0
Smoked Tomato	2 tbsp	0
Thai Sesame Lime	2 tbsp	0

Girard's® Dressing	Amount	Total Sugar (g)
Spinach Salad Dressing	2 tbsp	12
Apple Poppy Seed	2 tbsp	8
Chinese Chicken Salad	2 tbsp	6
Creamy Balsamic Vinaigrette	2 tbsp	5

Continued

Peach Mimosa Vinaigrette	2 tbsp	5
White Balsamic Vinaigrette	2 tbsp	4
Light Caesar	2 tbsp	2
Blue Cheese Vinaigrette	2 tbsp	1
Caesar	2 tbsp	1
Champagne	2 tbsp	1
Greek Feta Vinaigrette	2 tbsp	1
Old Venice Italian	2 tbsp	1
Light Champagne	2 tbsp	1
Romano Cheese Italian	2 tbsp	1
Original French	2 tbsp	0

Hidden Valley® Creamy Dressing	Amount	Total Sugar (g)
Coleslaw	2 tbsp	4
Original Ranch Fat Free	2 tbsp	3
Buttermilk Ranch Light	2 tbsp	2
Original Ranch Light	2 tbsp	2
Classic Cheese Ranch	2 tbsp	1
Cracked Peppercorn Ranch	2 tbsp	1
Garden Vegetable Ranch	2 tbsp	1
Old Fashioned Buttermilk Ranch	2 tbsp	1
Original Ranch	2 tbsp	1
Spicy Ranch	2 tbsp	1
Bacon Ranch	2 tbsp	1

Hidden Valley® Farm House Dressing	Amount	Total Sugar (g)
Garden Tomato & Bacon	2 tbsp	5
Dijon Mustard Vinaigrette	2 tbsp	4
Savory Bleu Cheese	2 tbsp	3
Creamy Balsamic with Herb	2 tbsp	2
Hickory Bacon & Onion	2 tbsp	2
Homestyle Italian	2 tbsp	2
Original Italian with Herb	2 tbsp	2
Pomegranate Vinaigrette	2 tbsp	2
Creamy Parmesan	2 tbsp	1
Original Caesar	2 tbsp	1
Roasted Onion Parmesan	2 tbsp	1
Southwest Chipotle	2 tbsp	1

Ken's Steak House Dressing	Amount	Total Sugar (g)
Sweet Vidalia Onion	2 tbsp	10
Balsamic & Honey	2 tbsp	6
Honey Mustard	2 tbsp	6
Italian with Olive Oil	2 tbsp	4

SUGAR

Continued

Zesty Italian	2 tbsp	4
3 Cheese Italian	2 tbsp	3
Balsamic Vinaigrete	2 tbsp	3
Russian	2 tbsp	3
Thousand Island	2 tbsp	3
Creamy Italian	2 tbsp	2
Ranch Dressing	2 tbsp	2
Red Wine Vinegar Oil	2 tbsp	2
Buttermilk Ranch	2 tbsp	1
Caesar Dressing	2 tbsp	1
Chunky Blue Cheese	2 tbsp	1
Creamy Caesar	2 tbsp	1
Greek & Olive Oil	2 tbsp	1
Italian & Aged Romano	2 tbsp	1
Northern Italian Basil & Romano	2 tbsp	1
Peppercorn Ranch	2 tbsp	1
Italian Marinade	2 tbsp	0

Ken's® Lite Dressing	Amount	Total Sugar (g)
Sweet Vidalia Onion	2 tbsp	10
Asian Sesame Ginger & Soy	2 tbsp	7
Raspberry & Walnut Vinaigrette	2 tbsp	7
Thousand Island	2 tbsp	3
Caesar	2 tbsp	2
Ranch Dressing	2 tbsp	2
Blue Cheese Dressing	2 tbsp	1
Chunky Blue Cheese Dressing	2 tbsp	1
Creamy Caesar Dressing	2 tbsp	1
Zesty Italian	2 tbsp	1

Kraft® Dressing	Amount	Total Sugar (g)
Classic Catalina	2 tbsp	8
Coleslaw Dressing	2 tbsp	8
Creamy Poppyseed	2 tbsp	8
Sweet Balsamic Vinaigrette	2 tbsp	8
Sweet Honey Catalina	2 tbsp	8
Light Thousand Island	2 tbsp	7
Catalina Fat Free	2 tbsp	7
Creamy French	2 tbsp	6
Free Thousand Island	2 tbsp	5
Thousand Island	2 tbsp	4
Fat Free Ranch	2 tbsp	3
Buttermilk Ranch	2 tbsp	2
Cucumber Ranch	2 tbsp	2

SUGAR

Green Goddnes	2 tbsp	2
Light Zesty Italian	2 tbsp	2
Ranch with Backon	2 tbsp	2
Zesty Italian Anything	2 tbsp	2
Zesty Italian Dressing & Marinade	2 tbsp	2
Classic Caesar	2 tbsp	1
Creamy Italian	2 tbsp	1
Peppercorn Ranch	2 tbsp	1
Ranch	2 tbsp	1
Roka Blue Cheese	2 tbsp	1
Lite Ranch	2 tbsp	1

Litehouse® Dressing	Amount	Total Sugar (g)
Spinach Dressing	2 tbsp	9
Coleslaw Dressing	2 tbsp	8
Sesame Ginger	2 tbsp	8
Coleslaw with Pinapple	2 tbsp	7
Harvest Cranberry Greek	2 tbsp	6
Pear Gorzonzola	2 tbsp	6
Honey Mustard	2 tbsp	4
Barbecue Ranch	2 tbsp	3
Sweet French	2 tbsp	3
Buttermilk Ranch	2 tbsp	2
Jalapeno Ranch	2 tbsp	2
Organic Ranch	2 tbsp	2
Original Thousand Island	2 tbsp	2
Ranch Dressing	2 tbsp	2
Yogurt Ranch with Kefir	2 tbsp	2
Big Bleu Dressing	2 tbsp	1
Ceaser Dressing	2 tbsp	1
Ceaser-Caesar Dressing	2 tbsp	1
Chunky Bleu Cheese	2 tbsp	1
Creamy Cilantro	2 tbsp	1
Homestyle Ranch	2 tbsp	1
Original Bleu Cheese	2 tbsp	1
Parmesan Caesar	2 tbsp	1
Yogurt Bleu Cheese with Kefir	2 tbsp	1
Chunky Garlic Caesar	2 tbsp	0

Litehouse® Lite Dressing	Amount	Total Sugar (g)
Coleslaw Dressing	2 tbsp	8
Honey Dijon Vinaigrette	2 tbsp	8
1000 Island Dressing	2 tbsp	2
Jalapeno Ranch Dressing	2 tbsp	2
Ranch Dressing	2 tbsp	2

SUGAR

Continued

Bleu Cheese Dressing	2 tbsp	1
Caesar Dressing	2 tbsp	1
Creamy Ranch Dressing	2 tbsp	1

Litehouse® Vinaigrette Dressing	Amount	Total Sugar (g)
Cherry Vinaigrette	2 tbsp	9
Fuji Apple Vinaigrette	2 tbsp	6
Harvest Cranberry Vinaigrette	2 tbsp	6
Pomegranate Blueberry Vinaigrette	2 tbsp	5
Raspberry Walnut Vinaigrette	2 tbsp	5
Balsamic Vinaigrette	2 tbsp	4
Huckleberry Vinaigrette	2 tbsp	4
Bleu Cheese Vinaigrette	2 tbsp	3
Organic Balsamic Vinaigrette	2 tbsp	3
White Balsamic Vinaigrette	2 tbsp	3
Zesty Italian Vinaigrette	2 tbsp	3
Greek Vinaigrette	2 tbsp	1
Red Wine Olive Oil Vinaigrette	2 tbsp	1

Marie's Dressing	Amount	Total Sugar (g)
Spinach Salad Dressing	2 tbsp	10
Yogurt Coleslaw	2 tbsp	8
Coleslaw	2 tbsp	7
Poppy Seed	2 tbsp	7
Sesame Ginger	2 tbsp	6
Raspberry Vinaigrette	2 tbsp	6
Honey Dijon	2 tbsp	5
Honey Mustard	2 tbsp	5
Red Wine Vinaigrette	2 tbsp	5
Blue Cheese Vinaigrette	2 tbsp	4
Thousand Island	2 tbsp	3
Yogurt Thousand Island	2 tbsp	3
Balsamic Vinaigrette	2 tbsp	2
Italian Vinaigrette	2 tbsp	2
Yogurt Blue Cheese	2 tbsp	1
Lite Chunky Blue Cheese	2 tbsp	1
Buttermilk Ranch	2 tbsp	1
Yogurt Ranch	2 tbsp	1
Creamy Caesar	2 tbsp	1
Creamy Ranch	2 tbsp	1
Asiago Peppercorn	2 tbsp	1
Creamy Chipotle Ranch	2 tbsp	1
Lite Creamy Ranch	2 tbsp	1
Jalapeno Ranch	2 tbsp	1
Caesar	2 tbsp	0

SUGAR

Continued

Chunky Blue Cheese	2 tbsp	0
Super Blue Cheese	2 tbsp	0
Greek Vinaigrette	2 tbsp	0
Creamy Italian Garlic	2 tbsp	0

Newman's® Own Dressing	Amount	Total Sugar (g)
Orange Ginger	2 tbsp	8
Creamy Balsamic	2 tbsp	5
Honey French	2 tbsp	5
Poppy Seed	2 tbsp	5
3 Cheese Balsamic	2 tbsp	2
Balsamic Vinaigrette	2 tbsp	1
Caesar Dressing	2 tbsp	1
Greek Vinaigrette	2 tbsp	1
Olive Oil & Vinegar	2 tbsp	1
Parmesan & Roasted Garlic	2 tbsp	1
Ranch Dressing	2 tbsp	1
Creamy Ceasar	2 tbsp	0
Family Italian	2 tbsp	0

Newman's® Lite Dressing	Amount	Total Sugar (g)
Cranberry Walnut	2 tbsp	7
Honey Mustard	2 tbsp	5
Raspberry Walnut	2 tbsp	5
Roasted Garlic Balsamic	2 tbsp	3
Balsamic	2 tbsp	2
Caesar	2 tbsp	2
Italian	2 tbsp	0

Walden Farm's Dressing	Amount	Total Sugar (g)
Asian	2 tbsp	0
Bacon Ranch	2 tbsp	0
Balsamic Vinaigrette	2 tbsp	0
Bleu Cheese	2 tbsp	0
Buttermilk Ranch	2 tbsp	0
Caesar	2 tbsp	0
Chipotle Ranch	2 tbsp	0
Colesaw	2 tbsp	0
Creamy Bacon	2 tbsp	0
Creamy Italian	2 tbsp	0
French Dressing	2 tbsp	0
Honey Dijon Dressing	2 tbsp	0
Italian	2 tbsp	0
Italian Sun Dried Tomato	2 tbsp	0

SUGAR

Continued

Jersey Sweet Onion	2 tbsp	0
Ranch	2 tbsp	0
Raspberry Vinaigrette	2 tbsp	0
Russian	2 tbsp	0
Sesame Ginger	2 tbsp	0
Sweet Onion	2 tbsp	0
Thousand Island	2 tbsp	0
Zesty Italian	2 tbsp	0

Wish Bone® Creamy Dressing	Amount	Total Sugar (g)
Sweet & Spicy French	2 tbsp	7
Russian	2 tbsp	6
Delux French	2 tbsp	4
Light Delux French	2 tbsp	4
Light Sweet & Spicy French	2 tbsp	4
Thousand Island	2 tbsp	4
Fat Free Chunky Blue Cheese	2 tbsp	3
Light Thousand Island	2 tbsp	3
Creamy Italian Dressing	2 tbsp	2
Fat Free Ranch Dressing	2 tbsp	2
Light Ranch Dressing	2 tbsp	2
Chunky Blue Cheese	2 tbsp	1
Creamy Caesar	2 tbsp	1
Light Blue Cheese	2 tbsp	1
Light Creamy Caesar	2 tbsp	1
Ranch Dressing	2 tbsp	1
Light Parmesan Peppercorn Ranch	2 tbsp	0

Wish Bone® Oil & Vinegar Dressing	Amount	Total Sugar (g)
Fat Free Red Wine Vinaigrette	2 tbsp	6
Light Asian Sesame & Ginger	2 tbsp	5
Light Raspberry Walnut	2 tbsp	5
Raspberrt Hazelnut Vinaigrette	2 tbsp	5
Balsamic Italian Vinaigrette	2 tbsp	4
Italian	2 tbsp	4
Light Honey Dijon	2 tbsp	4
Red Wine Vinaigrette	2 tbsp	4
Superfruit Vinaigrette	2 tbsp	4
Balsamic Vinaigrette	2 tbsp	3
Bruschetta Italian	2 tbsp	3
Light Balsamic & Basil Vinaigrette	2 tbsp	3
Mediterranean Italian	2 tbsp	3
Olive Oil Vinaigrette	2 tbsp	3
Robusto Italian	2 tbsp	3
Fat Free Italian	2 tbsp	2

SUGAR

Fat Free Italian Dressing	2 tbsp	2
Greek Vinaigrette	2 tbsp	2
House Italian	2 tbsp	2
Light Italian dressing	2 tbsp	2
Romano Basil Vinaigrette	2 tbsp	1

Turkey, Cooked	Amount	Total Sugar (g)
All types	3 oz	0

VEGETABLES

Vegetables, Canned	Amount	Total Sugar (g)
Tomato paste	1 cup	32
Tomato pure	1 cup	12
Sweet potato	1 cup	11
Tomato sauce	1 cup	10
Beets	1 cup	9
Stewed tomatoes	1 cup	9
Pumpkin	1 cup	8
Yellow sweet corn	1 cup	7
Tomatoes	1 cup	6
Green peas	1 cup	5
Sauerkraut	1 cup	4
Mushrooms	1 cup	4
Carrots	1 cup	4
Asparagus	1 cup	3
Green beans	1 cup	1
Spinach	1 cup	1

Vegetables, Cooked	Amount	Total Sugar (g)
Cabbage, Napa	1 cup	x
Squash, Acorn	1 cup	x
Sweet potato, mashed	1 cup	18.7
Beets	1 cup	13.5
Rutabagas	1 cup	10.2
Squash, Hubbard	1 cup	10.0
Parsnips	1 cup	7.5
Squash, Winter, all varieties averaged	1 cup	6.8
Corn	1 cup	6.8
Snow peas	1 cup	6.4
Split peas	1 cup	5.7
Mushrooms, Shiitake	1 cup	5.6
Carrots	1 cup	5.4
Squash, Summer	1 cup	4.7

SUGAR

Turnips	1 cup	4.7
Kohlrabi	1 cup	4.6
Squash, Crookneck and Straightneck	1 cup	4.5
Onions	1 cup	4.5
Cabbage	1 cup	4.2
Butternut squash	1 cup	4.0
Squash, Spaghetti	1 cup	3.9
Okra	1 cup	3.8
White mushrooms	1 cup	3.7
Celery	1 cup	3.6
Eggplant	1 cup	3.2
Potatoes, mashed with Whole Milk & Butter	1 cup	3.1
Zucchini	1 cup	3.1
Brussels sprouts	1 cup	2.7
Squash, Scallop	1 cup	2.7
Cauliflower	1 cup	2.6
Pumpkin	1 cup	2.5
Asparagus	1 cup	2.3
Leaks	1 cup	2.2
Broccoli	1 cup	2.2
Potatoes, flesh, baked	1 cup	2.1
Green beans	1 cup	1.9
Swiss Chard	1 cup	1.9
Artichokes	1 cup	1.7
Kale	1 cup	1.6
Cabbage, Chinese Bok-Choy	1 cup	1.4
Beet greens	1 cup	0.9
Spinach	1 cup	0.8
Collard greens	1 cup	0.8
Turnip greens	1 cup	0.8
Yams, cubed	1 cup	0.7
Dandelion greens	1 cup	0.5
Mustard greens	1 cup	0.1

Vegetables, Frozen	Amount	Total Sugar (g)
Butternut squash	1 cup	x
Rhubarb, cooked with sugar	1 cup	68.9
Green peas	1 cup	7.4
Carrots	1 cup	6.0
Okra	1 cup	5.3
Spinach	1 cup	5.0
Brussels sprout	1 cup	3.2
Broccoli	1 cup	2.7
Cauliflower	1 cup	1.9
Kale	1 cup	1.7

SUGAR

Green beans	1 cup	1.7
Turnip greens	1 cup	1.2
Collard greens	1 cup	1.0
Spinach	1 cup	1.0
Asparagus	1 cup	0.6

Vegetables, Raw	Amount	Total Sugar (g)
Hubbard squash	1 cup	10.05
Onions	1 cup	6.78
Red bell peppers	1 cup	6.26
Carrots	1 cup	5.21
Tomatillos	1 cup	5.19
Tomatoes	1 cup	4.73
Crookneck and Straightneck squash	1 cup	4.46
Snow peas	1 cup	3.92
Spaghetti squash	1 cup	3.92
Tomatoes, cherry	1 cup	3.92
Green bell peppers	1 cup	3.58
Butternut squash	1 cup	3.08
Zucchini	1 cup	2.83
Scallop or Pattypan squash	1 cup	2.70
Cabbage, Red	1 cup	2.68
Summer squash	1 cup	2.49
Green onions & scallions	1 cup	2.33
Cabbage	1 cup	2.24
Celery	1 cup	2.20
Cauliflower	1 cup	1.91
Cucumbers	1 cup	1.74
Cabbage, Savoy	1 cup	1.59
Broccoli	1 cup	1.50
White mushrooms	1 cup	1.39
Iceburg lettuce	1 cup	1.08
Cactus pads, nopales	1 cup	0.99
Cabbage, Chinese Bok-Choy	1 cup	0.83
Romaine lettuce	1 cup	0.67
Butterhead & boston lettuce	1 cup	0.52
Green leaf lettuce	1 cup	0.44
Arugula	1 cup	0.40
Swiss chard	1 cup	0.40
Dandelion greens	1 cup	0.39
Radicchio	1 cup	0.24
Spirulina, dried	1 tbsp	0.22
Chicory greens	1 cup	0.20
Broccoli, Raab	1 cup	0.15
Endive	1 cup	0.13

SUGAR

Red leaf lettuce	1 cup	0.13
Spinach	1 cup	0.13
Shiitake mushrooms, dried	1 cup	0.08
Watercress	1 cup	0.07

Nutrient Data Collection Form

Food	Amount	Book Numbers	Multiply By	Estimated Nutrient Intake
Nutrient::	RDA:	Estimated:	% of RDA:	Total Estimated:

To download additional forms for free, go to www.TopNutrients4U.com

VITAMIN A

Vitamin A is a fat soluble vitamin needed in small amounts, but not daily.

It is required for fighting infections, bone growth, and proper vision. A deficiency is considered to be a nutritional disorder, caused by inadequate dietary intake and is aggravated by lack of dietary fat.

A deficiency most commonly affects the eyes with signs of night blindness or blurred vision in poor light. Because of the large amount of foods fortified with vitamin A and, the public's proneness for supplements, deficiency in America is unlikely, but toxicity is a genuine and real concern.

A wide range of toxicities has been identified in infants, preschool children, and the elders. The most serious effects documented from chronic toxicity are abnormal liver functions. In fact, chronic toxicity is really a reflection of how easily the human liver is inclined to accumulate vitamin A until concentrations become toxic.

Vitamin A is stored in the body to a much greater extent than other nutrients and 90% of this is stored in the liver. The liver extracts a portion of vitamin A from each meal and purposefully holds it in storage for future deficiencies. The body then metabolizes the last amount of the newly absorbed before it utilizes any liver reserves. This mechanism assures that the liver will accumulate vitamin A at each step of the food chain, if dietary intake is daily.

The amount of vitamin A that can be stored in the liver, before reaching toxic levels, directly correlates with the amount of dietary intake and duration of intake. Clinical symptoms appear to develop in a shorter period of time when higher levels are consumed.

Infants and young children seem to be more sensitive to increased intakes of vitamin A. In reported cases of vitamin A toxicity a fifty-seven year old women became critically ill after consuming 20 times the RDA for four years, whereas, a 15 year old boy became critically ill after only 1 month at the same intake. A 62 year old women became critically toxic from vitamin A after consuming 10 times the RDA for over ten years, whereas, a six year boy became critically ill after only 4 months at the same intake.

The liver possesses specialized sump cells known as Ito cells, whose sole purpose is for storage of vitamin A. When the cumulative intake of vitamin A exceeds the liver's limited capacity for storage the specialized cells will become engorged, saturated, and rupture. This leads to a condition known as hyper-vitaminosis A. An individual will now begin to experience tissue damage in multiple organs throughout the entire body with a broad spectrum of clinical abnormalities.

The daily amount needed to produce chronic toxicity is considerably lower than that required for acute toxicity. Long-term daily intakes that exceed biological needs but not large enough to induce acute toxicity or clinical signs will go unnoticed for years. Remember, the liver is a biochemical magnet for vitamin A and is stingy when it comes to letting go of any reserves.

If daily intake is constantly high, the liver will accumulate vitamin A and will continue to do so until a liver condition develops.

Blood levels of vitamin A may reflect dietary intake of vitamin A, but, it does not reflect liver concentrations of vitamin A, and are normally inadequate for estimating the body's vitamin A status. Because of the livers tremendous ability to clutch onto vitamin A, blood levels will indicate a problem only when liver concentrations are already dangerously too high or too low.

A more practical approach for preventive measures is to assess and monitor dietary intake. In documented cases of vitamin A toxicity, it was the physician's investigative efforts and analysis of the patient's diet that resulted in vitamin A toxicity as being the most plausible cause of the patient's symptoms.

In summary, there are no well-established therapeutic benefits to consuming intake of vitamin A above the RDA, and in fact, habitual ingestion of foods rich in vitamin A is associated with liver damage after an extended period of time, especially if intake overlaps with supplements.

Recommended daily intake is expressed in units of retinol activity equivalents (RAE) in microgram, mcg, quantities and includes the amount contributed from any carotenes. Never take a vitamin A supplement without consulting with your physician. For reported cases of vitamin A toxicity and clinical toxicity symptoms and signs see reference section.

VITAMIN A

Recommend Daily Intakes Levels for Vitamin A

Children	Vitamin A
1 to 3 year olds	300
4 to 8 year olds	400

Males	
9 to 13 year olds	600
19 to 30 years	900
31 to 50 years	900
51 to 70 years	900
Over 70	900

Females	
9 to 13 year olds	600
14 to 18 year olds	700
19 to 30 years	700
31 to 50 years	700
51 to 70 years	700
Over 70	700
Pregnancy	770
Lactation	1300

VITAMIN A

Alcohol	Amount	Vitamin A (mcg)
Beer, regular all types	1 bottle	0
Beer, light all types	1 bottle	0
Red Wine	1 glass	0
White Wine	1 glass	0
Gin, Rum, Vodka, Whisky	1 shot	0

Beans, Canned	Amount	Vitamin A (mcg)
Green beans	1 cup	28
Baked beans, plain	1 cup	13
Yellow beans	1 cup	8
Fava beans	1 cup	3
Black-eyed peas	1 cup	2
Garbanzo beans	1 cup	2
Cranberry beans	1 cup	0
Great Northern	1 cup	0
Kidney beans	1 cup	0
Lima beans	1 cup	0
Navy beans	1 cup	0
Pinto beans	1 cup	0
Refried beans	1 cup	0
White beans, mature	1 cup	0

Beans, Cooked	Amount	Vitamin A (mcg)
Green beans	1 cup	44
Yardlong beans, Chinese long beans	1 cup	24
Soybeans, green	1 cup	14
Yellow beans	1 cup	5
Black-eyed peas	1 cup	2
Fava beans	1 cup	2
Garbanzo beans, chickpeas	1 cup	2
Mothbeans	1 cup	2
Mung beans, mature seeds	1 cup	2
Adzuki	1 cup	0
Black beans	1 cup	0
Black Turtle beans, mature	1 cup	0
Cranberry beans	1 cup	0
Great Northern	1 cup	0
Hyacinth beans	1 cup	0
Kidney beans	1 cup	0
Lentils	1 cup	0
Lima beans	1 cup	0
Lupini beans	1 cup	0
Natto	1 cup	0

VITAMIN A

Continued

Navy beans	1 cup	0
Pigeon peas	1 cup	0
Pinto beans	1 cup	0
Soybeans, matured	1 cup	0
Soybeans, matured, dry roasted	1 cup	0
Split peas	1 cup	0
White beans, mature	1 cup	0
White beans, small	1 cup	0
Winged beans	1 cup	0
Edamame	1 cup	x

Beef, Cooked	Amount	Vitamin A (mcg)
Liver, pan-fried	3 oz	6582
Beef ribs, trim to 1/8" fat	3 oz	0
Brisket, lean, trim to 0" fat	3 oz	0
Chuck roast, trim to 1/8" fat	3 oz	0
Filet Mignon, trim to 0" fat	3 oz	0
Flank steak, lean, trim to 0" fat	3 oz	0
Ground beef, 75%, broiled	3 oz	0
Ground beef, 80%	3 oz	0
London Broil, top round	3 oz	0
Ground beef, 85%	3 oz	0
Ground beef, 90%	3 oz	0
Tri Tip steak, lean, trim to 0" fat	3 oz	0
Ground beef, 95%,	3 oz	0
Porterhouse steak, trim to 0" fat	3 oz	0
Ribeye steak, lean, trim 0" fat	3 oz	0
Skirt Steak, trim to 0" fat	3 oz	0
T-Bone steak, trim 0" fat	3 oz	0
Top sirloin, lean, trim to 1/8" fat	3 oz	0

Bread	Amount	Vitamin A (mcg)
Croissants, butter	1 each	117
Bagel, egg	4" bagel	35
Cornbread	1 piece	26
Egg bread	1 slice	25
Bagel, cinnamon & raisins	4" bagel	22
Potato bread	1 slice	8
Potato bread	1 slice	8
Indian bread, Naan, whole wheat	1 piece	2
Mexican roll, bollilo	1 roll	1
Bagel, oat bran	4" bagel	1
Oatmeal bread	1 slice	1
Bagel, plain	4" bagel	0
Bagel, wheat	4" bagel	0

RDA for adults is 700 mcg for females, and 900 mcg for males

Continued

Cracked Wheat	1 slice	0
Dinner Rolls, brown & serve	1 roll	0
English Muffin, plain	1 muffin	0
French, and Sourdough	1 slice	0
Hamburger & Hotdog buns, plain	1 bun	0
Italian	1 slice	0
Kaiser rolls	1 roll	0
Multi-Grain, includes Whole-Grain	1 slice	0
Pita, white	6" pita	0
Pumpernickle	1 slice	0
Raisen bread	1 slice	0
Reduced calorie wheat	1 slice	0
Rye bread	1 slice	0
Tortillas, corn	1 tortilla	0
Tortillas, flour	1 tortilla	0
White	1 slice	0
Whole-Wheat	1 slice	0
Indian bread, Naan, plain	1 piece	x

Butter	Amount	Vitamin A (mcg)
Regular dairy butter, salted	1 tbsp	97
Regular whipped butter, salted	1 tbsp	64

Cereal, General Mills®	Amount	Vitamin A (mcg)
Lucky Charms	1 cup	305
Cinnamon Chex	1 cup	300
Corn Chex	1 cup	286
Kix	1 cup	211
Wheaties	1 cup	199
Whole Grain Total	1 cup	199
Wheat Chex	1 cup	198
Golden Grams	1 cup	195
Honey Nut Chex	1 cup	193
Reese's Puffs	1 cup	191
Cocoa Puffs	1 cup	190
Cookie Crisp	1 cup	189
Dora The Explorer	1 cup	188
Multi-Bran CHEX	1 cup	179
Cinnamon Toast Crunch	1 cup	176
Rice Chex	1 cup	150
Total Raisin Bran	1 cup	149
Basic 4	1 cup	141
Trix	1 cup	140
Total Cranberry Crunch	1 cup	119
Berry Berry Kix	1 cup	109

RDA for adults is 700 mcg for females, and 900 mcg for males

VITAMIN A

Continued

	Amount	
Honey Nut Clusters	1 cup	0
Oatmeal Crisp, Crunchy Almond	1 cup	0
Oatmeal Crisp, Hearty Raisin	1 cup	0
Raisin Nut Bran	1 cup	0
Chocolate Chex	1 cup	x

Cereal, General Mills Cheerios®	Amount	Vitamin A (mcg)
Yogurt Burst, Strawberry	1 cup	300
Original	1 cup	277
Frosted	1 cup	207
Honey Nut	1 cup	200
Apple Cinnamon	1 cup	199
Oat Cluster Cheerios Crunch	1 cup	199
Berry Burst, Triple Berry	1 cup	198
Chocolate	1 cup	192
Fruity	1 cup	192
Banana Nut	1 cup	189
Multi Grain	1 cup	146
Cinnamon Burst	1 cup	x
Dulce De Leche Cheerios	1 cup	x
Honey Nut, Medley Crunch	1 cup	x

Cereal, General Mills Fiber One®	Amount	Vitamin A (mcg)
Caramel Delight	1 cup	149
Original Bran	1 cup	1
Frosted Shredded Wheat	1 cup	0
Honey Clusters	1 cup	0
Nutty Clusters & Almonds	1 cup	0
Raisin Bran Clusters	1 cup	0
80 Caloris, Chocolate Squares	1 cup	x
80 Caloris, Honey Squares	1 cup	x

Cereal, Kashi®	Amount	Vitamin A (mcg)
Heart to Heart, Honey Toasted Oat	1 cup	83
Heart to Heart, Oat Flakes & Blueberry Clusters	1 cup	63
Go Lean	1 cup	3
Good Friends	1 cup	3
Go Lean Crunch,	1 cup	1
Go Lean Crunch, Honey Almond Flax	1 cup	1
7-Whole Grain Flakes	1 cup	0
7-Whole Grain Honey Puffs	1 cup	0
7-Whole Grain Nuggets	1 cup	0
7-Whole Grain Puffs	1 cup	0
Autum Wheat	1 cup	0

RDA for adults is 700 mcg for females, and 900 mcg for males

VITAMIN A

Cinnamon Harvest	1 cup	0
Berry Blossom	1 cup	x
Go Lean Crisp, Toasted Berry Crumble	1 cup	x
Heart to Heart, Warm Cinnamon	1 cup	x
Honey Sunshine	1 cup	x
Island Vanilla	1 cup	x
Strawberry Fields	1 cup	x

Cereal, Kellogg's®	Amount	Vitamin A (mcg)
Frosted Rice Krispies	1 cup	506
Cocoa Krispies	1 cup	503
All-Bran Bran Buds	1 cup	450
Rice Krispies	1 cup	417
Smart Start, Strong Heart, Antioxidants	1 cup	372
All-Bran Original	1 cup	324
All-Bran Complete Wheat Flakes	1 cup	300
Cracklin' Oat Bran	1 cup	300
Raisin Bran	1 cup	261
Product 19	1 cup	224
Honey Smacks	1 cup	204
Rice Krispies Treats	1 cup	202
Honey Crunch Corn Flakes	1 cup	201
Frosted Flakes	1 cup	190
Raisin Bran Crunch	1 cup	162
Smorz	1 cup	150
Apple Jacks	1 cup	148
Froot Loops	1 cup	145
Crispix	1 cup	143
Corn Pops	1 cup	140
MUESLIX	1 cup	135
Corn Flakes	1 cup	127
Frosted MINI-Wheat's, Big-Bite	1 cup	0
CINNABON	1 cup	x
Crunchy Nut Golden Honey Nut Flakes	1 cup	x
Crunchy Nut Roasted Nut & Honey O's	1 cup	x
Fiberplus Berry Yogurt Crunch	1 cup	x
Fiberplus Cinnamon Oat Crunch	1 cup	x
Smart Start, Strong Heart, Toasted Oat	1 cup	x

Cereal, Kellogg's Special-K®	Amount	Vitamin A (mcg)
Chocolately Delight	1 cup	300
Cinnamon Pecan	1 cup	300
Fruit & Yogurt	1 cup	300
Vanilla Almond	1 cup	300
Blueberry	1 cup	298

VITAMIN A

Continued

Original	1 cup	225
Red Berries	1 cup	225
Low Fat Granola	1 cup	x
Multigrain Oats & Honey	1 cup	x
Protein Plus	1 cup	x

Cereal, Post®	Amount	Vitamin A, mcg
Grape-Nuts Cereal	1 cup	614
Bran Flakes	1 cup	300
Cocoa Pebbles	1 cup	300
Fruity Pebbles	1 cup	300
Golden Crisp	1 cup	300
Grape-Nuts Flakes	1 cup	300
Great Grains, Cranberry Almond Crunch	1 cup	299
Great Grains, Crunchy Pecan Cereal	1 cup	298
Great Grains, Raisin, Date & Pecan	1 cup	298
Raisin Bran	1 cup	224
Alpha-Bits	1 cup	222
Great Grains, Banana Nut Crunch	1 cup	222
Blueberry Morning	1 cup	176
Honeycomb Cereal	1 cup	145
Honey Nut Shredded Wheat	1 cup	0
Shredded Wheat n' Bran, spoon-size	1 cup	0
Shredded Wheat, Frosted, spoon-size	1 cup	0
Shredded Wheat, Original, big-biscuit	1 biscuit	0
Shredded Wheat, Original, spoon-size	1 cup	0

Post® Honey Bunches of Oats®	Amount	Vitamin A (mcg)
Just Bunches Honey Roasted	1 cup	336
Honey Roasted	1 cup	322
With Almonds	1 cup	290
Pecan Bunches	1 cup	289
With Vanilla Bunches	1 cup	221
With Cinnamon Bunches	1 cup	x
With Strawberries	1 cup	x

Cereal, Quaker®	Amount	Vitamin A (mcg)
Honey Graham OH'S	1 cup	230
Cinnamon Oatmeal Squares	1 cup	169
Oatmeal Squares	1 cup	167
Toasted Oatmeal Cereal, Honey Nut	1 cup	159
CAP'N Crunche's Peanut Butter Crunch	1 cup	8
CAP'N Crunch	1 cup	7
CAP'N Crunch with Crunch Berries	1 cup	7

RDA for adults is 700 mcg for females, and 900 mcg for males

VITAMIN A

Continued

Crunchy Bran	1 cup	3
Low Fat Granola with Raisins	1 cup	1
Oat Cinnamom LIFE	1 cup	1
Oat LIFE	1 cup	1
Ganola Oats, Wheat and Honey	1 cup	0
Ganola Oats, Wheat, Honey and Raisins	1 cup	0
Golden Maple Squares	1 cup	x
Granola Apple Cranberry Almond	1 cup	x
Maple Brown Sugar LIFE	1 cup	x
Toasted Oatmeal Cereal	1 cup	x

Cereal, Cooked	Amount	Vitamin A (mcg)
CREAM OF WHEAT, mix'n eat	1 packet	376
Oats, instant, fortified, plain	1 packet	329
White corn grits	1 cup	0
Yellow corn grits	1 cup	0
CREAM OF WHEAT, regular	1 cup	0
Farina	1 cup	0
Oats, regular, unenriched	1 cup	0

Cheese	Amount	Vitamin A (mcg)
Ricotta cheese, whole milk	1 cup	295
Ricotta cheese, part skim milk	1 cup	263
Cottage cheese, creamed, small curd	1 cup	83
Cottage cheese, lowfat, 2 %	1 cup	45
Cottage cheese, lowfat, 1 %	1 cup	25
Cottage cheese, nonfat	1 cup	3

Cheese	Amount	Vitamin A (mcg)
Goat cheese, hard type	1 oz	138
Goat cheese, semisoft	1 oz	115
Cream cheese	1 oz	104
American, pasteurized process, fortified	1 oz	90
Muenster	1 oz	84
Roquefort	1 oz	83
Goat cheese, soft type	1 oz	82
Gruyere	1 oz	77
Cheddar	1 oz	75
Colby	1 oz	75
Fontina	1 oz	74
Provolone	1 oz	67
Parmesan, grated	1 oz	65
Swiss	1 oz	62
Blue cheese	1 oz	56

RDA for adults is 700 mcg for females, and 900 mcg for males

VITAMIN A

Continued

Monterey	1 oz	56
Mozzarella, whole milk	1 oz	51
Muenster, low fat	1 oz	50
Brie	1 oz	49
Gouda	1 oz	47
Mozzarella, part skim milk, low moisture	1 oz	45
Monterey, low fat	1 oz	40
Provolone, reduced fat	1 oz	39
Mozzarella, nonfat	1 oz	36
Feta cheese	1 oz	35
Romano	1 oz	27
Cheddar, lowfat	1 oz	17
American, pasteurized process, low fat	1 oz	16
American, pasteurized process, imitation	1 oz	13
Swiss, low fat	1 oz	11
Cream cheese, fat free	1 oz	3

Cheese, Mexican	Amount	Vitamin A (mcg)
Queso fresco	1 oz	64
Mexican, blend	1 oz	49
Mexican, blend, reduced fat	1 oz	44
Queso anejo	1 oz	18
Queso chihuahua	1 oz	16
Queso asadero	1 oz	16

Chicken, Cooked	Amount	Vitamin A (mcg)
Chicken liver	3 oz	3384
Wing with skin, roasted	3 oz	40
Wing with skin, fried in flour	3 oz	32
Thigh with skin, fried with flour	3 oz	25
Breast with skin, roasted	3 oz	24
Drumstick with skin, fried in flour	3 oz	21
Cornish game hens, meat only	3 oz	17
Wing meat only, no skin, roasted	3 oz	15
Thigh with skin, roasted	3 oz	14
Breast with skin, fried with flour	3 oz	13
Drumstick with skin, roasted	3 oz	10
Thigh meat only, no skin, roasted	3 oz	7
Breast meat only, no skin, roasted	3 oz	5
Drumstick meat only, no skin, roasted	3 oz	5

RDA for adults is 700 mcg for females, and 900 mcg for males

VITAMIN A

Cream	Amount	Vitamin A (mcg)
Heavy Cream	1 tbsp	62
Light whipping cream	1 tbsp	42
Light Coffe Cream	1 tbsp	27
Sour Cream, cultured	1 tbsp	21
Half & Half	1 tbsp	15
Sour Cream, reduced fat	1 tbsp	15
Whipped Topping, pressurized	1 tbsp	6

Eggs	Amount	Vitamin A (mcg)
Egg whole, fried	1 large	101
Egg whole, scrambled	1 large	98
Egg whole, poached	1 large	80
Egg whole, hard-boiled	1 large	74
Egg yolk	1 large	65
Egg substitute, liquid, fat free	1/4 cup	7
Egg whites, raw	1 large	0
Egg whites, dried	1 ounce	0
Egg whites, dried powder, stabilized	1 tbsp	0

Fish, Canned	Amount	Vitamin A (mcg)
Atlantic Sardines, in oil	3 oz	27
Light tuna, in oil	3 oz	20
Light tuna, in water	3 oz	14
White (albacore) tuna, in water	3 oz	5
White (albacore) tuna, in oil	3 oz	4

Fish, Cooked	Amount	Vitamin A (mcg)
Bluefin tuna	3 oz	643
Atlantic herring, pickeled	3 oz	219
King mackerel	3 oz	214
Rainbow trout, farmed	3 oz	85
Sockeye salmon	3 oz	59
Sea bass	3 oz	54
Coho salmon, farmed	3 oz	50
Atlantic mackerel	3 oz	46
Coho salmon, wild	3 oz	43
Grouper	3 oz	42
Alaskan halibut	3 oz	41
Swordfish	3 oz	37
Pink salmon	3 oz	36
Whiting	3 oz	32
Florida pompano	3 oz	31

RDA for adults is 700 mcg for females, and 900 mcg for males

VITAMIN A

Continued

Freshwater bass	3 oz	30
Snapper	3 oz	30
Keta (chum) salmon	3 oz	29
Spanish mackerel	3 oz	28
Striped bass	3 oz	26
Yellowtail	3 oz	26
Chinook salmon, smoked	3 oz	22
Northern pike	3 oz	20
Walleye pike	3 oz	20
Orange roughy	3 oz	20
Pacific & Jack mackerel	3 oz	20
Atlantic croaker	3 oz	20
Atlantic & Pacific halibut	3 oz	20
Yellowfin tuna	3 oz	19
Haddock	3 oz	18
Greenland halibut	3 oz	15
Walleye pollock	3 oz	14
Cat fish, wild	3 oz	13
Rainbow trout, wild	3 oz	13
Atlantic perch	3 oz	13
Atlantic cod	3 oz	12
Atlantic salmon, wild	3 oz	11
Atlantic pollock	3 oz	10
Flounder & Sole	3 oz	10
Carp	3 oz	8
Pacific cod	3 oz	2
Cat fish, farmed	3 oz	1
Cat fish, breaded & fried	3 oz	0
Tilapia	3 oz	0
Chinook salmon	3 oz	x
Skipjack (aku) tuna	3 oz	x
Atlantic salmon, farmed	3 oz	x

Fish, Shellfish, Cooked	Amount	Vitamin A (mcg)
Clams, canned	3 oz	127
Clams, breaded & fried	3 oz	77
Oysters, breaded & fried	3 oz	76
Shrimp	3 oz	76
Octopus	3 oz	76
Blue crab cakes	3 oz	48
Shrimp, breaded & fried	3 oz	48
Queen crab	3 oz	44
Scallops, breaded & fried	3 oz	19
Eastern oysters, farmed	3 oz	16
Eastern oysters, wild	3 oz	17

VITAMIN A

Continued

Crayfish	3 oz	13
Squid, fried	3 oz	9
Alaskan king crab	3 oz	8
Abalone	3 oz	2
Northern lobster	3 oz	1
Blue crab	3 oz	1
Blue crab, canned	3 oz	1
Alaskan king crab, imitation	3 oz	0
Shrimp, canned	3 oz	0

Fruit, Canned	Amount	Vitamin A (mcg)
Apricots	1 cup	160
Peaches	1 cup	45
Plums	1 cup	34
Olives, black	5 large	4
Pineapple	1 cup	3
Olives, green	5 large	3
Applesauce, unsweetened	1 cup	2
Applesauce, sweetened	1 cup	0
Pears	1 cup	0

Fruit, Dried	Amount	Vitamin A (mcg)
Apricots	1 cup	234
Peaches	1 cup	173
Prunes	1 cup	68
Currants	1 cup	6
Figs	1 cup	0
Pears	1 cup	0
Apples	1 cup	0
Cranberries	1 cup	0

Fruit, Frozen	Amount	Vitamin A (mcg)
Peaches	1 cup	35
Blackberries, unthawed	1 cup	9
Raspberries	1 cup	8
Blueberries	1 cup	5
Strawberries	1 cup	3

Fruit, Raw	Amount	Vitamin A (mcg)
Elderberries	1 cup	442
Cantaloupe, cubes	1 cup	270
Apricots	1 cup	158
Grapefruit, pink or red	1 cup	133
Mango	1 cup	89

RDA for adults is 700 mcg for females, and 900 mcg for males

VITAMIN A

Plantains	1 cup	83
Papaya	1 cup	68
Prunes, uncooked	1 cup	68
Tangerine	1 cup	66
Water mellon	1 cup	43
Stewed prunes	1 cup	42
Plums	1 cup	28
Peachs	1 cup	27
Nectarine	1 cup	24
Oranges, all commerical grades	1 cup	20
Avocado, California	1 cup	16
Avocado, Florida	1 cup	16
Blackberries	1 cup	16
Black currants	1 cup	13
Kiwi	1 cup	7
Cheeries, sweet, no pits	1 cup	5
Grapes, red & green	1 cup	5
Honeydew	1 cup	5
Pineapple	1 cup	5
Apples	1 cup	4
Blueberries	1 cup	4
Cranberries	1 cup	3
Pears	1 cup	2
Raspberries	1 cup	2
Strawberries	1 cup	2
Jicama, raw	1 cup	1
Mulberries	1 cup	1
Dates	1 cup	0
Figs	1 cup	0
Pomegranates	1 cup	0
Raisins	1 cup	0

Fruit, Raw	Amount	Vitamin A (mcg)
Cantaloupe	1/2 fruit	466
Mango	1 fruit	181
Persimmons, Japanese	1 fruit	136
Plantains	1 fruit	100
Papayas	1 fruit	74
Grapefruit, pink or red	1/2 fruit	71
Apricots	1 fruit	34
Tangerine	1 fruit	30
Nectarine	1 fruit	22
Avocado, Florida	1 fruit	21
Prunes, uncooked	5 fruit	19
Peaches	1 fruit	16

RDA for adults is 700 mcg for females, and 900 mcg for males

VITAMIN A

Oranges	1 fruit	14
Plums	1 fruit	11
Avocado, California	1 fruit	10
Apples	1 fruit	4
Banana	1 fruit	4
Star fruit, Carambola	1 fruit	3
Kiwi	1 fruit	3
Kumquats	1 fruit	3
Cherries	10 cherries	2
Pears	1 fruit	2
Pineapple	1/2" x 3" slice	1
Strawberries	5 fruit	1
Pineapple guava, Feijoa	1 fruit	0
Chayote	1 fruit	0
Cherimoya	1 fruit	0
Dates	5 dates	0
Figs, dried	1 fig	0
Pummelo	1 fruit	0
Raisins	1 small box	0
Raisins	1 packet	0
Raspberries	10 fruit	0
Persimmons, small native	1 fruit	x

Game Meat, Cooked	Amount	Vitamin A (mcg)
Duck	3 oz	20
Bison, ground	3 oz	0
Caribou	3 oz	0
Deer	3 oz	0
Deer, ground	3 oz	0
Elk	3 oz	0
Elk, ground	3 oz	0
Rabbit	3 oz	0
Squirrel	3 oz	0
Wild boar	3 oz	0
Antelope	3 oz	x
Buffalo, steak, free range	3 oz	x

Grains, Cooked	Amount	Vitamin A (mcg)
Egg & Spinach noodles	1 cup	16
Spaghetti, spinach	1 cup	11
Egg noodles	1 cup	10
Pearled barley	1 cup	0
Quinoa	1 cup	0
Spelt	1 cup	0
Kamut	1 cup	0

VITAMIN A

Millet	1 cup	0
Wild rice	1cup	0
Bulgur	1 cup	0
Macaroni, Whole-Wheat	1 cup	0
Spaghetti, Whole-Wheat	1 cup	0
Brown rice	1 cup	0
Buckwheat	1 cup	0
Couscous	1 cup	0
Macaroni	1 cup	0
Oat bran	1 cup	0
Oats, regular, unenriched	1 cup	0
Rice noodles	1 cup	0
Soba noodles	1 cup	0
Spaghetti	1 cup	0
White rice, regular long grain	1 cup	0

Herbs & Spices	Amount	Vitamin A (mcg)
Paprika	1 tsp	57
Chili powder	1 tsp	40
Cilantro	1/4 cup	13
Dill weed, dried	1 tsp	3
Spearmint	1 tsp	3
Tarragon, dried, ground	1 tsp	3
Thyme, dried, ground	1 tsp	3
Bay leaf, crumbled	1 tsp	2
Chervil, dried	1 tsp	2
Chives, raw, chopped	1 tsp	2
Coriander, dried, leaves	1 tsp	2
Oregano, dried, ground	1 tsp	2
Rosemary, dried	1 tsp	2
Sage, ground	1 tsp	2
Thyme, dried, leaves	1 tsp	2
All-spice, ground	1 tsp	1
Basil, dried & ground	1 tsp	1
Capers, canned	1 tsp	1
Curry powder	1 tsp	1
Pepper, black, ground	1 tsp	1
Anise seed	1 tsp	0
Caraway seeds	1 tsp	0
Celery seeds	1 tsp	0
Cinnamon powder	1 tsp	0
Cloves, ground	1 tsp	0
Garlic powder	1 tsp	0
Ginger, ground	1 tsp	0
Nutmeg, ground	1 tsp	0

RDA for adults is 700 mcg for females, and 900 mcg for males

VITAMIN A

Continued

Onion powder	1 tsp	0
Parsley, dried	1 tsp	0
Saffron	1 tsp	0
Turmeric, ground	1 tsp	0

Juice	Amount	Vitamin A (mcg)
Carrot	1 cup	2256
Vegetable	1 cup	189
Grapefruit, raw	1 cup	133
Tomato	1 cup	56
Orange, raw	1 cup	25
Cranberry, cocktail	1 cup	0
Grape	1 cup	0
Lemon, raw	1 cup	0
Pineapple	1 cup	0
Prune	1 cup	0
Apple	1 cup	0
Pomegranate	1 cup	0

Lamb, Cooked	Amount	Vitamin A (mcg)
All types	3 oz	0

Milk	Amount	Vitamin A (mcg)
Canned, evaporated, nonfat	1 cup	302
Canned, condensed, sweetened	1 cup	226
Dry, instant, nonfat	1/3 cup	163
Human milk	1 cup	150
Nonfat, Fat Free or Skim Milk	1 cup	149
Lowfat milk, 1%	1 cup	142
Goat milk	1 cup	139
Reduced fat, 2%	1 cup	134
Whole, 3.25% Fat	1 cup	112
Sheep milk	1 cup	108
Buttermilk, cultured, lowfat	1 cup	34
Coconut milk, canned	1 cup	0
Soy milk, original, unfortified	1 cup	0

Nuts & Seeds	Amount	Vitamin A (mcg)
Pistachio	1 oz	6
Black walnuts	1 oz	1
Chia seeds	1 oz	1
Pecans	1 oz	1
Sunflower seeds	1 oz	1
Tahini	1 oz	1

RDA for adults is 700 mcg for females, and 900 mcg for males

VITAMIN A

Continued

Almonds	1 oz	0
Brazilnuts	1 oz	0
Cashews	1 oz	0
Coconut, raw meat	1 oz	0
English walnuts	1 oz	0
Flaxseed	1 oz	0
Hazelnuts	1 oz	0
Macadamia	1 oz	0
Peanut butter, smooth style	1 oz	0
Peanuts	1 oz	0
Pine nuts	1 oz	0
Pumpkin seeds	1 oz	0
Sesame seeds	1 oz	0

Oils	Amount	Vitamin A (mcg)
Cod liver fish oil	1 tbsp	4080
Avocado oil	1 tbsp	0
Canola oil	1 tbsp	0
Coconut oil	1 tbsp	0
Corn oil	1 tbsp	0
Cottonseed oil	1 tbsp	0
Flaxseed oil	1 tbsp	0
Grapeseed oil	1 tbsp	0
Menhaden fish oil	1 tbsp	0
Olive oil	1 tbsp	0
Palm kernal vegetable oil	1 tbsp	0
Peanut oil	1 tbsp	0
Safflower, high linoleic acid, oil	1 tbsp	0
Safflower, high oleic acid, oil	1 tbsp	0
Salmon fish oil	1 tbsp	0
Salmon oil	1 tbsp	0
Sesame oil	1 tbsp	0
Soybean lecithin oil	1 tbsp	0
Soybean oil	1 tbsp	0
Soybean, partially hydrogenated oil	1 tbsp	0
Sunflower, high linoleic acid	1 tbsp	0
Sunflower, high oleic acid	1 tbsp	0
Walnut oil	1 tbsp	0
Wheat Gem oil	1 tbsp	0

Pork, Cooked	Amount	Vitamin A (mcg)
Braunschweiger sausage	3 oz	3587
Liverwurst spread	1/4 cup	2250
Sausage	3 oz	10

RDA for adults is 700 mcg for females, and 900 mcg for males

VITAMIN A

Continued

Bacon	3 oz	9
Italian sausage	3 oz	8
Back ribs	3 oz	5
Spareribs	3 oz	3
Center loin chops	3 oz	2
Bratwurst	3 oz	2
Sirloin pork chops	3 oz	2
Center loin pork chop	3 oz	2
Polish sausage	3 oz	0
Canadian-style bacon	3 oz	0
Cured ham	3 oz	0
Tenderloin	3 oz	0

Turkey, Cooked	Amount	Vitamin A (mcg)
Turkey liver	3 oz	9138
Ground turkey, 93% lean	3 oz	26
Ground turkey, 85% lean	3 oz	25
Ground turkey	3 oz	20
Ground turkey, fat free	3 oz	7
Dark meat	3 oz	4
Light meat	3 oz	3
Turkey sausage, reduced fat	3 oz	2
Turkey bacon	3 oz	0
Breast meat	3 oz	0

Veal, Cooked	Amount	Vitamin A (mcg)
Breast	3 oz	x
Foreshank	3 oz	x
Ground	3 oz	0
Leg, top round	3 oz	0
Loin	3 oz	0
Rib	3 oz	0
Sirloin	3 oz	0

Vegetables, Canned	Amount	Vitamin A (mcg)
Pumpkin	1 cup	1906
Spinach	1 cup	1049
Sweet potato	1 cup	898
Carrots	1 cup	815
Tomato paste	1 cup	199
Asparagus	1 cup	99
Green peas	1 cup	75
Tomato sauce	1 cup	54
Green beans	1 cup	28

RDA for adults is 700 mcg for females, and 900 mcg for males

VITAMIN A

Stewed tomatoes	1 cup	23
Corn	1 cup	8
Beets	1 cup	2
Sauerkraut	1 cup	1
Mushrooms	1 cup	0

Vegetables, Cooked	Amount	Vitamin A (mcg)
Sweet potato, mashed	1 cup	2581
Carrots	1 cup	1329
Butternut squash	1 cup	1144
Sweet potato, baked	1 medium	1096
Spinach	1 cup	943
Kale	1 cup	885
Collard greens	1 cup	771
Hubbard squash	1 cup	687
Pumpkin	1 cup	612
Beet greens	1 cup	552
Turnip greens	1 cup	549
Swiss chard	1 cup	536
Winter squash, all varieties averaged	1 cup	535
Mustard greens	1 cup	442
Bok-Choy	1 cup	360
Dandelion greens	1 cup	359
Raab broccoli	1 cup	193
Broccoli	1 cup	120
Crookneck and Straightneck squash	1 cup	101
Zucchini	1 cup	101
Asparagus	1 cup	90
Snow peas	1 cup	83
Broccilini	1 cup	72
Brussels sprouts	1 cup	61
Green beans	1 cup	44
Acorn squash	1 cup	43
Leaks	1 cup	43
Celery	1 cup	39
Cactus pad, nopales	1 cup	33
Okra	1 cup	22
Summer squash, all varieties averaged	1 cup	20
Corn	1 cup	19
Potatoes, mashed with whole milk	1 cup	15
Napa cabbage	1 cup	14
Spaghetti squash	1 cup	9
Yams, cubed	1 cup	8
Scallop or Pattypan squash	1 cup	7
Cabbage	1 cup	6

RDA for adults is 700 mcg for females, and 900 mcg for males

VITAMIN A

Beets	1 cup	3
Kohlrabi	1 cup	3
Artichokes	1 cup	2
Eggplant	1 cup	2
Cauliflower	1 cup	1
Split peas	1 cup	1
Onions	1 cup	0
Parsnips	1 cup	0
Potatoes, flesh, baked	1 cup	0
Rutabagas	1 cup	0
Shitake mushrooms	1 cup	0
Turnips	1 cup	0
White mushrooms	1 cup	0

Vegetables, Frozen	Amount	Vitamin A (mcg)
Carrots	1 cup	1235
Spinach	1 cup	1146
Collard greens	1 cup	978
Kale	1 cup	956
Turnip greens	1 cup	882
Butternut squash	1 cup	401
Green peas	1 cup	168
Broccoli	1 cup	94
Asparagus	1 cup	72
Brussels sprouts	1 cup	71
Green beans	1 cup	38
Okra	1 cup	28
Corn	1 cup	16
Rhubarb	1 cup	10
Cauliflower	1 cup	0

Vegetables, Raw	Amount	Vitamin A (mcg)
Enoki mushrooms	1 cup	x
Carrots	1 cup	918
Butternut squash	1 cup	745
Mustard spinach	1 cup	742
Kale	1 cup	515
Dandelion greens	1 cup	279
Romaine lettuce	1 cup	244
Red bell peppers	1 cup	234
Green leaf lettuce	1 cup	207
Bok-Choy	1 cup	156
Spinach	1 cup	141
Swiss chard	1 cup	110

RDA for adults is 700 mcg for females, and 900 mcg for males

VITAMIN A

Continued

Red leaf lettuce	1 cup	105
Butterhead or boston lettuce	1 cup	91
Chicory greens	1 cup	83
Tomatoes	1 cup	76
Tomatoes, cherry	1 cup	63
Endive	1 cup	54
Watercress	1 cup	54
Snow peas	1 cup	53
Raab Broccoli	1 cup	52
Green onions & scallions	1 cup	50
Red cabbage	1 cup	39
Savoy cabbage	1 cup	35
Broccoli	1 cup	27
Green bell peppers	1 cup	27
Celery	1 cup	26
Arugula	1 cup	24
Nopales	1 cup	20
Yellow bell peppers	1 large	19
Iceburg lettuce	1 cup	14
Summer squash	1 cup	11
Zucchini	1 cup	11
Tomatillos	1 cup	8
Cucumbers	1 cup	5
Cabbage	1 cup	4
Oyster mushrooms	1 cup	2
Spirulina, dried	1 tbsp	2
Belgian endive	1 cup	1
Cauliflower	1 cup	0
Crimini mushrooms	1 cup	0
Onions	1 cup	0
Portabella mushrooms	1 cup	0
Radicchio	1 cup	0
Shiitake mushrooms, dried	1 each	0
White Mushrooms	1 cup	0

Yogurt	Amount	Vitamin A (mcg)
Plain yogurt, whole milk	8 oz	61
Plain yogurt, low fat	8 oz	32
Plain yogurt, skim milk	8 oz	5
Plain greek yogurt, non fat	8 oz	2

RDA for adults is 700 mcg for females, and 900 mcg for males

Nutrient Data Collection Form

Food	Amount	Book Numbers	Multiply By	Estimated Nutrient Intake
Nutrient::	RDA:	Estimated:	% of RDA:	Total Estimated:

NOTES

VITAMIN B1

Vitamin B1 known as thiamine is the first discovered of the eight known B-complex vitamins. It is water-soluble and needed daily in milligrams (mg) quantities. Several enzymes needed for carbohydrate metabolism are thiamine dependent. Because of this, excessive intake of carbohydrates with a low intake of thiamine may lead to a thiamine deficiency.

Clinically a deficiency is characterized by neurological and cardiovascular diseases, and is associated with lactic acidosis and high levels of C-reactive proteins. The early deficiency signs are reduced stamina, irritability, inability to focus, and painful leg cramps. Other signs such as numbness and tingling of the feet with a stiffness of the ankles known as dry beriberi may or may not be present at that time. In advanced stages the signs are shortness of breath, rapid heart rate, swollen legs and ankles, enlarged heart, and fatigue known as wet or cardiac beriberi. If not corrected, this could bring on the onset of an insidious crippling health condition with permanent brain damage known as Wernicke Koraskoff Syndrome.

This is most common in alcoholics because of their extremely imbalanced diet. Alcoholics alternate between periodic binges and marginal diets during periods of abstinence. During binges alcohol inhibits the body's ability to activate, transport, absorb, and store thiamine. During abstinence, an alcoholic's anorexia type behavior renders the diet inadequate to replenish the thiamine lost from alcohol consumption.

Deficiency is also found in critically ill children, breast-fed infants from thiamine deficient mothers, and infants fed formulas lacking adequate thiamine known as infantile beriberi. The beginning stages of deficiency are over looked because the earliest symptoms such as fatigue, headaches, and mood swings are non-specific or too generalized and mimic symptoms of more common ailments. Since deficiencies are suspected in only alcoholics, it is likely that a deficiency can exist but goes unsuspected in non-alcoholics.

VITAMIN B1

Studies report low blood thiamine concentrations upon admission
to hospitals for 7% of school children, 28% of infants admitted
to intensive care units, 21% of adults, and 80% of alcoholics. To
summarize the above, the medical profession has identified several
diseases resulting directly from a vitamin B1 deficiency. The more
severe diseased states are uncommon, but less severe thiamine
deficiencies do occur and the longer the deficiency exist the sicker the
person becomes.

Recommend Daily Intakes Levels for Vitamin B1

Children	Vitamin B1, mg
1 to 3 year olds	.5
4 to 8 year olds	.6
Males	
9 to 13 year olds	.9
14 to 18 year olds	1.2
19 to 30 years	1.2
31 to 50 years	1.2
51 to 70 years	1.2
Over 70	1.2
Females	
9 to 13 year olds	.9
14 to 18 year olds	1.0
19 to 30 years	1.1
31 to 50 years	1.1
51 to 70 years	1.1
Over 70	1.1
Pregnancy	1.4
Lactation	1.4

VITAMIN B1

Alcohol	Amount	Vitamin B1 (mg)
Beer, light, all types	1 bottle	0.018
Beer, regular, all types	1 bottle	0.018
Red Wine	3.5 fl oz	0.007
White Wine	3.5 fl oz	0.007
Gin, Rum, Vodka, Whisky	1 shot	0.003

Beans, Canned	Amount	Vitamin B1 (mg)
Great Northern	1 cup	0.375
Navy beans	1 cup	0.369
Kidney beans	1 cup	0.271
White beans, mature	1 cup	0.252
Baked beans, plain	1 cup	0.244
Black-eyed peas	1 cup	0.182
Lima beans	1 cup	0.133
Pinto beans	1 cup	0.125
Cranberry beans	1 cup	0.101
Refried beans	1 cup	0.083
Garbanzo beans	1 cup	0.077
Fava beans	1 cup	0.051
Green beans	1 cup	0.024
Yellow beans	1 cup	0.023

Beans, Cooked	Amount	Vitamin B1 (mg)
Hyacinth beans	1 cup	0.524
Winged beans	1 cup	0.507
Soybeans, green	1 cup	0.468
Navy beans	1 cup	0.431
White beans, small	1 cup	0.422
Black beans	1 cup	0.420
Black Turtle beans, mature	1 cup	0.416
Soybeans, matured, dry roasted	1 cup	0.397
Cranberry beans	1 cup	0.372
Split peas	1 cup	0.372
Black-eyed peas	1 cup	0.345
Lentils	1 cup	0.335
Mung beans, mature seeds	1 cup	0.331
Pinto beans	1 cup	0.330
Edamame	1 cup	0.310
Lima beans	1 cup	0.303
Kidney beans	1 cup	0.283
Great Northern	1 cup	0.280
Natto	1 cup	0.280
Mungo beans, mature seeds	1 cup	0.270

RDA is 1.2 mg for adults

VITAMIN B1

Soybeans, matured	1 cup	0.267
Adzuki	1 cup	0.264
Pigeon peas	1 cup	0.245
Lupini beans	1 cup	0.222
Mothbeans	1 cup	0.219
White beans, mature	1 cup	0.211
Garbanzo beans, chickpeas	1 cup	0.190
Fava beans	1 cup	0.165
Green beans	1 cup	0.092
Yellow beans	1 cup	0.092
Yardlong beans, Chinese long beans	1 cup	0.088

Beef, Cooked	Amount	Vitamin B1 (mg)
Tri Tip steak, lean, trim to 0" fat	3 oz	0.111
Filet Mignon, trim to 0" fat	3 oz	0.053
Porterhouse steak, trim	3 oz	0.100
T-Bone steak, trim to 0" fat	3 oz	0.100
Skirt Steak, trim to 0" fat	3 oz	0.076
Brisket, lean, trim to 0" fat	3 oz	0.065
Top Sirloin, lean, trim to 1/8" fat	3 oz	0.062
London Broil, top round	3 oz	0.060
Beef ribs, trim to 1/8" fat	3 oz	0.060
Chuck roast, trim to 1/8" fat	3 oz	0.060
Ribeye steak, lean, trim 0" fat	3 oz	0.059
Flank steak, lean, trim to 0" fat	3 oz	0.057
Ground beef, 75%	3 oz	0.042
Ground beef, 80%	3 oz	0.041
Ground beef, 85%	3 oz	0.039
Ground beef, 90%	3 oz	0.037
Ground beef, 95%	3 oz	0.036

Beef, Cooked	Amount	Vitamin B1 (mg)
Tri Tip steak, lean, trim to 0" fat	1 cooked lb	0.581
T-bone steak, trim to 0" fat	1 cooked lb	0.458
Porterhouse steak, trim to 0" fat	1 cooked lb	0.449
Skirt steak, trim to 0" fat	1 cooked lb	0.408
Flank steak, lean, trim to 0" fat	1 cooked lb	0.345
Beef ribs, trim to 1/8" fat	1 cooked lb	0.318
Chuck roast, trim to 1/8" fat	1 cooked lb	0.318
Brisket, lean, trim to 0" fat	1 cooked lb	0.304
Flank steak, lean, trim to 0" fat	1 steak	0.291
Top Sirloin, trim to 1/8" fat	1 cooked lb	0.223
Ribeye steak, boneless, trim to 0" fat	1 steak	0.146
Ribeye filet, lean, trim to 0" fat	1 filet	0.119

RDA is 1.2 mg for adults

Continued

Top Sirloin, choice filet, trim to 0" fat	1 filet	0.088
Filet Mignon, tenderloin, trim to 0" fat	1 steak	0.073

Beef, Cooked	Amount	Vitamin B1 (mg)
Ground beef, 80%	1/4 lb patty	0.037
Ground beef, 90%	1/4 lb patty	0.036
Ground beef, 85%	1/4 lb patty	0.035
Ground beef, 75%	1/4 lb patty	0.034
Ground beef, 95%	1/4 lb patty	0.034

Bread	Amount	Vitamin B1 (mg)
Indian bread, Naan, plain	1 piece	0.702
Mexican roll, bollilo	1 roll	0.666
Bagel plain	4" bagel	0.535
Bagel, egg	4" bagel	0.477
Bagel, wheat	4" bagel	0.395
Pita, white	6" pita	0.359
Bagel, oat bran	4" bagel	0.348
Bagel, cinnamon & raisins	4" bagel	0.342
English Muffin, plain	1 muffin	0.272
Kaiser rolls	1 roll	0.272
Croissants, butter	1 each	0.221
White	1 slice	0.205
Indian bread, Naan, whole wheat	1 piece	0.187
Egg bread	1 slice	0.175
Hamburger & Hotdog buns, plain	1 bun	0.172
Tortillas, flour	1 tortilla	0.172
Dinner Rolls, brown & serve	1 roll	0.147
Cornbread	1 piece	0.146
Rye bread	1 slice	0.139
French or Sourdough	1 slice	0.108
Oatmeal bread	1 slice	0.108
Pumpernickle	1 slice	0.105
Whole-Wheat	1 slice	0.099
Reduced calorie wheat	1 slice	0.097
Italian	1 slice	0.095
Reduced calorie white	1 slice	0.094
Wheat	1 slice	0.093
Cracked Wheat	1 slice	0.090
Raisin bread	1 slice	0.088
Reduced calorie rye	1 slice	0.084
Multi-Grain, includes Whole-Grain	1 slice	0.073
Potato bread	1 slice	0.060
Tortillas, corn	1 tortilla	0.024

RDA is 1.2 mg for adults

VITAMIN B1

Butter	Amount	Vitamin B1 (mg)
Regular dairy butter, salted	1 tbsp	0.001
Regular dairy whipped butter, salted	1 tbsp	0

Cereal, General Mills	Amount	Vitamin B1 (mg)
Total Whole Grain	1 cup	2.000
Total Raisin Bran	1 cup	1.484
Total Cranberry Crunch	1 cup	1.200
Wheaties	1 cup	1.008
Corn Chex	1 cup	0.744
Multi-Bran CHEX	1 cup	0.689
Lucky Charms	1 cup	0.625
Chocolate Chex	1 cup	0.555
Raisin Nut Bran	1 cup	0.523
Cinnamon Chex	1 cup	0.516
Cocoa Puffs	1 cup	0.504
Dora The Explorer	1 cup	0.504
Reese's Puffs	1 cup	0.503
Wheat Chex	1 cup	0.501
Honey Nut Chex	1 cup	0.500
Golden Grams	1 cup	0.496
Cookie Crisp	1 cup	0.485
Kix	1 cup	0.469
Cinnamon Toast Crunch	1 cup	0.455
Honey Nut Clusters	1 cup	0.399
Basic 4	1 cup	0.385
Rice Chex	1 cup	0.378
Trix	1 cup	0.352
Berry Berry Kix	1 cup	0.290
Oatmeal Crisp, Crunchy Almond	1 cup	0.110
Oatmeal Crisp, Hearty Raisins	1 cup	0.062

Cereal, General Mills Cheerios®	Amount	Vitamin B1 (mg)
Multi Grain	1 cup	1.500
Yogurt Burst, Strawberry	1 cup	1.066
Original	1 cup	0.580
Chocolate	1 cup	0.504
Crunch, Oat Clusters	1 cup	0.504
Apple Cinnamon	1 cup	0.500
Berry Burst	1 cup	0.500
Frosted	1 cup	0.500
Fruity	1 cup	0.500
Honey Nut	1 cup	0.500
Banana Nut	1 cup	0.485

RDA is 1.2 mg for adults

VITAMIN B1

Cereal, General Mills Fiber One®	Amount	Vitamin B1 (mg)
Original	1 cup	0.800
Caramel Delight	1 cup	0.400
Raisin Bran Clusters	1 cup	0.385
Honey Clusters	1 cup	0.364
Frosted Shredded Wheat	1 cup	0.360

Cereak, Kashi®	Amount	Vitamin B1 (mg)
Go Lean	1 cup	0.265
Autum Wheat	1 cup	0.197
Island Vanilla	1 cup	0.187
Heart to Heart, Honey Toasted Oat	1 cup	0.176
Good Friends	1 cup	0.106
Berry Blossom	1 cup	0.096
Honey Sunshine	1 cup	0.092
Go Lean Crunch, Honey Almond Flax	1 cup	0.085
Heart to Heart, Warm Cinnamon	1 cup	0.079
Heart to Heart, Wild Blueberry	1 cup	0.077
Go Lean Crisp, Toasted Berry Crumble	1 cup	0.075
Go Lean Crunch,	1 cup	0.032
7-Whole Grain Honey Puffs	1 cup	0.030
7-Whole Grain Puffs	1 cup	0.023

Cereal, Kellogg's®	Amount	Vitamin B1 (mg)
ALL-BRAN Complete Wheat Flakes	1 cup	1.999
Product 19	1 cup	1.500
Smart Start, Strong Heart Antioxidants	1 cup	1.500
All-Bran Original	1 cup	1.407
All-Bran Bran Buds	1 cup	1.126
Frosted Flakes	1 cup	0.799
Fiberplus Cinnamon Oat Crunch	1 cup	0.700
MUESLIX	1 cup	0.657
Crispix	1 cup	0.525
Fiberplus Berry Yogurt Crunch	1 cup	0.525
Rice Krispies Treats	1 cup	0.520
Rice Krispies	1 cup	0.513
Cracklin' Oat Bran	1 cup	0.503
Cocoa Krispies	1 cup	0.500
Crunchy Nut, Golden Honey Nut Flakes	1 cup	0.500
Crunchy Nut, Roasted Nut & Honey O's	1 cup	0.500
Frosted Rice Krispies	1 cup	0.500
Honey Crunch Corn Flakes	1 cup	0.500
Krave Chocolate	1 cup	0.500
Honey Smacks	1 cup	0.500

RDA is 1.2 mg for adults

VITAMIN B1

Raisin Bran	1 cup	0.444
CINNABON	1 cup	0.438
Froot Loops	1 cup	0.387
Raisin Bran Crunch	1 cup	0.376
Apple Jacks	1 cup	0.375
Corn Flakes	1 cup	0.375
Corn Pops	1 cup	0.375
Smorz	1 cup	0.375
Frosted MINI-Wheat's, Big-Bite	5 biscuits	0.269

Cereal, Kellogg's Special-K®	Amount	Vitamin B1 (mg)
Low Fat Granola	1 cup	1.050
Multigrain Oats & Honey	1 cup	0.788
Vanilla Almond	1 cup	0.724
Chocolately Delight	1 cup	0.711
Blueberry	1 cup	0.700
Cinnamon Pecan	1 cup	0.700
Fruit & Yogurt	1 cup	0.700
Protein Plus	1 cup	0.696
Original	1 cup	0.524
Red Berries	1 cup	0.524

Cereal, Post®	Amount	Vitamin B1, mg
Grape-Nuts Cereal	1 cup	1.162
Bran Flakes	1 cup	0.520
Great Grains, Raisins, Date & Pecan	1 cup	0.513
Great Grains, Cranberry Almond Crunch	1 cup	0.512
Fruity Pebbles	1 cup	0.504
Golden Crisp	1 cup	0.504
Cocoa Pebbles	1 cup	0.503
Grape-Nuts Flakes	1 cup	0.503
Great Grains, Crunchy Pecan	1 cup	0.485
Alpha-Bits	1 cup	0.390
Shredded Wheat, Frosted, spoon-size	1 cup	0.374
Honey Nut Shredded Wheat	1 cup	0.372
Great Grains, Banana Nut Crunch	1 cup	0.354
Raisin Bran	1 cup	0.354
Blueberry Morning	1 cup	0.308
Honeycomb Cereal	1 cup	0.256
Shredded Wheat, Original, spoon-size	1 cup	0.142
Shredded Wheat n' Bran, spoon-size	1 cup	0.094
Shredded Wheat, Original, big-biscuit	1 biscuit	0.064

RDA is 1.2 mg for adults

VITAMIN B1

Post® Honey Bunches of Oats®	Amount	Vitamin B1 (mg)
Just Bunches, Honey Roasted	1 cup	0.596
With Cinnamon Bunches	1 cup	0.520
With Almonds	1 cup	0.512
Pecan Bunches	1 cup	0.503
With Strawberries	1 cup	0.496
Honey Roasted	1 cup	0.489
With Vanilla Bunches	1 cup	0.392

Cereal, Quaker®	Amount	Vitamin B1 (mg)
Toasted Oarmeal Cereal	1 cup	0.782
Toasted Oarmeal Cereal, Honey Nut	1 cup	0.688
Honey Graham OH'S	1 cup	0.660
Oat Cinnamon LIFE	1 cup	0.588
CAP'N Crunch	1 cup	0.581
CAP'N Crunch with Crunch Berries	1 cup	0.574
Maple Brown Sugar LIFE	1 cup	0.574
CAP'N Crunch's Peanut Butter Crunch	1 cup	0.551
Oat LIFE	1 cup	0.546
Cinnamon Oatmeal Squares	1 cup	0.421
Ganola Oats, Wheat and Honey	1 cup	0.419
Ganola Oats, Wheat, Honey and Raisins	1 cup	0.387
Oatmeal Squares	1 cup	0.382
Golden Maple Squares	1 cup	0.382
Granola Apple Cranberry Almond	1 cup	0.337
Low Fat Granolia with Raisins	1 cup	0.304
Crunchy Bran	1 cup	0.182

Cereal, Cooked	Amount	Vitamin B1 (mg)
Oats, instant, fortified, plain	1 packet	0.460
Farina	1 cup	0.301
Yellow corn grits	1 cup	0.249
White corn grits	1 cup	0.208
Oats, regular, unenriched	1 cup	0.178
CREAM OF WHEAT, regular	1 cup	0.138

Cheese	Amount	Vitamin B1 (mg)
Cottage cheese, low fat, 2 %	1 cup	0.093
Cottage cheese, creamed, small curd	1 cup	0.061
Ricotta, part skim milk	1 cup	0.052
Cottage cheese, low fat, 1 %	1 cup	0.047
Cottage cheese, non fat, uncreamed	1 cup	0.033
Ricotta, whole milk	1 cup	0.032

RDA is 1.2 mg for adults

VITAMIN B1

Cheese	Amount	Vitamin B1 (mg)
Feta	1 oz	0.044
Goat cheese, hard type	1 oz	0.040
Mozzarella, part skim milk, low moisture	1 oz	0.029
Brie	1 oz	0.020
Goat cheese, semisoft type	1 oz	0.020
Goat cheese, soft type	1 oz	0.020
Swiss	1 oz	0.018
Gruyere	1 oz	0.017
Cream cheese, fat free	1 oz	0.011
Roqufort	1 oz	0.011
Romano	1 oz	0.010
Gouda	1 oz	0.009
Mozzarella, whole milk	1 oz	0.009
American, pasteurized process, low fat	1 oz	0.008
Blue cheese	1 oz	0.008
Cheddar	1 oz	0.008
Parmesan, grated	1 oz	0.008
Cream cheese	1 oz	0.006
Fontina	1 oz	0.006
Monterey, low fat	1 oz	0.006
Mozzarella, non fat	1 oz	0.006
Swiss, low fat	1 oz	0.006
Provolone	1 oz	0.005
Provolone, reduced fat	1 oz	0.005
American, pasteurized process, fortified	1 oz	0.004
Colby	1 oz	0.004
Monterey	1 oz	0.004
Muenster	1 oz	0.004
Cheddar, low fat,	1 oz	0.003
Muenster, low fat	1 oz	0.003
American, pasteurized process, imitation	1 oz	0

Cheese, Mexican	Amount	Vitamin B1 (mg)
Queso blanco	1 oz	0.014
Queso fresco	1 oz	0.012
Queso seco	1 oz	0.011
Mexican, blend, reduced fat	1 oz	0.009
Mexican, blend	1 oz	0.006
Queso anejo	1 oz	0.006
Queso asadero	1 oz	0.006
Queso chihuahua	1 oz	0.005

RDA is 1.2 mg for adults

VITAMIN B1

Chicken, Cooked	Amount	Vitamin B1 (mg)
Thigh, with skin, fried	1 thigh	0.102
Breast, skin, fried with flour	1/2 breast	0.080
Drumstick, no skin, roasted	1 drumstick	0.078
Breast, no skin, roasted	1/2 breast	0.060
Drumstick, with skin, fried	1 drumstick	0.040
Thigh, no skin, roasted	1 thigh	0.038

Chicken, Cooked	Amount	Vitamin B1 (mg)
Thigh meat only, no skin, roasted	3 oz	0.081
Thigh with skin, fried with flour	3 oz	0.080
Drumstick meat only, roasted	3 oz	0.079
Drumstick with skin, roasted	3 oz	0.075
Thigh with skin, roasted	3 oz	0.074
Breast with skin, roasted	3 oz	0.070
Drumstick with skin, fried in flour	3 oz	0.069
Cornish game hens, meat only	3 oz	0.064
Breast with skin, fried with flour	3 oz	0.060
Breast meat only, no skin, roasted	3 oz	0.056
Wing with skin, fried in flour	3 oz	0.049
Wing meat only, no skin, roasted	3 oz	0.040
Wing with skin, roasted	3 oz	0.036

Cream	Amount	Vitamin B1 (mg)
Half & Half	1 tbsp	0.005
Light Coffe Cream	1 tbsp	0.005
Sour Cream, reduced fat	1 tbsp	0.005
Sour Cream, cultured	1 tbsp	0.004
Heavy Cream	1 tbsp	0.003
Whipped Topping, pressurized	1 tbsp	0.001

Eggs	Amount	Vitamin B1 (mg)
Egg substitute, liquid, fat free	1/4 cup	0.072
Egg whole, hard-boiled	1 large	0.033
Egg yolk	1 large	0.029
Egg whole, scrambled	1 large	0.024
Egg whole, fried	1 large	0.020
Egg whole, poached	1 large	0.016
Egg whites, dried powder, stabilized	1 tbsp	0.003
Egg whites	1 large	0.001
Egg whites, dried	1 ounce	0.001

RDA is 1.2 mg for adults

VITAMIN B1

Fish, Canned	Amount	Vitamin B1 (mg)
Atlantic Sardines, in oil	3 oz	0.068
Light tuna, in oil	3 oz	0.032
Light tuna, in water	3 oz	0.026
White (albacore) tuna, in oil	3 oz	0.014
White (albacore) tuna, in water	3 oz	0.007

Fish, Cooked	Amount	Vitamin B1 (mg)
Florida pompano	3 oz	0.578
Atlantic salmon, farmed	3 oz	0.289
Walleye pike	3 oz	0.265
Bluefin tuna	3 oz	0.236
Atlantic salmon, wild	3 oz	0.234
Cat fish, wild	3 oz	0.193
Sockeye salmon	3 oz	0.183
Yellowtail	3 oz	0.149
Atlantic mackerel	3 oz	0.135
Rainbow trout, wild	3 oz	0.129
Rainbow trout, farmed	3 oz	0.122
Carp	3 oz	0.119
Pacific mackerel	3 oz	0.115
Yellowfin tuna	3 oz	0.114
Sea bass	3 oz	0.110
Spanish mackerel	3 oz	0.110
King mackerel	3 oz	0.098
Striped bass	3 oz	0.098
Coho salmon, farmed	3 oz	0.085
Tilapia	3 oz	0.079
Keta (chum) salmon	3 oz	0.078
Pink salmon	3 oz	0.077
Atlantic croaker	3 oz	0.076
Swordfish	3 oz	0.076
Atlantic cod	3 oz	0.075
Freshwater bass	3 oz	0.074
Alaskan halibut	3 oz	0.071
Grouper	3 oz	0.069
Coho salmon, wild	3 oz	0.064
Cat fish, breaded & fried	3 oz	0.062
Greenland halibut	3 oz	0.062
Whiting	3 oz	0.058
Northern pike	3 oz	0.057
Atlantic & Pacific halibut	3 oz	0.049
Atlantic pollock	3 oz	0.046
Walleye pollock	3 oz	0.046
Snapper	3 oz	0.045

RDA is 1.2 mg for adults

VITAMIN B1

Continued

Atlantic perch	3 oz	0.039
Orange roughy	3 oz	0.038
Chinook salmon	3 oz	0.037
Pacific cod	3 oz	0.032
Skipjack (aku) tuna	3 oz	0.032
Atlantic herring, pickeled	3 oz	0.031
Flounder	3 oz	0.022
Cat fish, farmed	3 oz	0.020
Chinock salmon, smoked	3 oz	0.020
Haddock	3 oz	0.020

Fish, Shellfish, Cooked	Amount	Vitamin B1 (mg)
Abalone	3 oz	0.187
Oysters, breaded & fried	3 oz	0.128
Shrimp, breaded & fried	3 oz	0.110
Eastern oysters, farmed	3 oz	0.110
Clams, breaded & fried	3 oz	0.085
Queen crab	3 oz	0.082
Crab cakes	3 oz	0.076
Squid, fried	3 oz	0.048
Octopus	3 oz	0.048
Alaskan king crab	3 oz	0.045
Crayfish	3 oz	0.042
Scallops, breaded & fried	3 oz	0.036
Shrimp	3 oz	0.027
Alaskan king crab, imitation	3 oz	0.026
Eastern oysters, wild	3 oz	0.021
Clams, canned	3 oz	0.020
Blue crab, canned	3 oz	0.020
Northern lobster	3 oz	0.020
Blue crab	3 oz	0.020
Shrimp, canned	3 oz	0.006

Fruit, Canned	Amount	Vitamin B1 (mg)
Pineapple	1 cup	0.229
Applesauce, unsweetened	1 cup	0.063
Apricots	1 cup	0.052
Applesauce, sweetened	1 cup	0.043
Plums	1 cup	0.041
Peaches	1 cup	0.029
Pears	1 cup	0.027
Olives, black	5 large	0.003
Olives, green	5 large	0.001

RDA is 1.2 mg for adults

VITAMIN B1

Fruit, Dried	Amount	Vitamin B1 (mg)
Currants	1 cup	0.230
Figs	1 cup	0.127
Apricots	1 cup	0.019
Pears	1 cup	0.014
Cranberries	1 cup	0.008
Peaches	1 cup	0.003
Apples	1 cup	0

Fruit, Frozen	Amount	Vitamin B1 (mg)
Raspberries	1 cup	0.048
Blueberries	1 cup	0.046
Blackberries, unthawed	1 cup	0.044
Strawberries	1 cup	0.041
Peaches	1 cup	0.030

Fruit, Raw	Amount	Vitamin B1 (mg)
Avocado, California	1 cup	0.172
Oranges	1 cup	0.157
Raisins	1 cup	0.154
Pineapple	1 cup	0.130
Tangerines, sections	1 cup	0.113
Grapes, red & green	1 cup	0.110
Elderberries	1 cup	0.102
Grapefruit, pink or red, sections	1 cup	0.099
Prunes, uncooked	1 cup	0.089
Plantains	1 cup	0.077
Dates	1 cup	0.076
Cataloupe	1 cup	0.066
Honeydew	1 cup	0.065
Stewed prunes	1 cup	0.060
Black currants	1 cup	0.056
Blueberries	1 cup	0.054
Apricots	1 cup	0.050
Water mellon	1 cup	0.050
Kiwi	1 cup	0.049
Nectarine	1 cup	0.049
Mango	1 cup	0.046
Plums	1 cup	0.046
Cherries, without pits	1 cup	0.042
Mulberries	1 cup	0.041
Strawberries, sliced	1 cup	0.040
Raspberries	1 cup	0.039
Peachs	1 cup	0.037

RDA is 1.2 mg for adults

VITAMIN B1

Papayas	1 cup	0.033
Blackberries	1 cup	0.029
Jicama	1 cup	0.024
Apples	1 cup	0.021
Pears	1 cup	0.019
Cranberries	1 cup	0.012

Fruit, Raw	Amount	Vitamin B1 (mg)
Cherimoya	1 fruit	0.237
Pummelo	1 fruit	0.207
Pomegranates	1 fruit	0.187
Oranges	1 fruit	0.114
Avocado, California	1 fruit	0.105
Mango	1 fruit	0.094
Plantains	1 fruit	0.093
Grapefruit, pink or red	1/2 fruit	0.053
Chayote	1 fruit	0.051
Tangerine	1 fruit	0.051
Persimmons, Japanese	1 fruit	0.050
Raisins	1 small box	0.046
Nectarine	1 fruit	0.044
Pineapple	1/2" x 3" slice	0.039
Banana	1 fruit	0.037
Papayas, small size	1 fruit	0.036
Peaches	1 fruit	0.031
Avocado, Florida	1 fruit	0.030
Prunes, uncooked	5 fruit	0.024
Apples	1 fruit	0.023
Cherries	10 fruit	0.022
Kiwi	1 fruit	0.019
Dates	5 fruit	0.018
Pears	1 fruit	0.018
Plums	1 fruit	0.018
Raisins	1 packet	0.015
Strawberries	5 fruit	0.014
Apricots	1 fruit	0.010
Figs, dried	1 fruit	0.007
Kumquats	1 fruit	0.007
Olives, green	5 large	0.003
Olives, black	5 large	0.001
Persimmons, small native	1 fruit	x

RDA is 1.2 mg for adults

VITAMIN B1

Game Meat, Cooked	Amount	Vitamin B1 (mg)
Deer, ground	3 oz	0.428
Wild boar	3 oz	0.264
Antelope	3 oz	0.221
Duck	3 oz	0.221
Caribou	3 oz	0.212
Deer	3 oz	0.153
Buffalo, steak, free range	3 oz	0.144
Bison, ground	3 oz	0.110
Elk, ground	3 oz	0.106
Squirrel	3 oz	0.051
Rabbit	3 oz	0.017
Elk, roasted	3 oz	x

Grains, Cooked	Amount	Vitamin B1 (mg)
Egg noodles	1 cup	0.462
Egg & Spinach noodles	1 cup	0.392
Macaroni	1 cup	0.384
Spaghetti	1 cup	0.384
Oat bran	1 cup	0.350
White rice, regular long grain	1 cup	0.258
Kamut	1 cup	0.206
Spelt	1 cup	0.200
Quinoa	1 cup	0.200
Brown rice	1 cup	0.187
Millet	1 cup	0.184
Whole-Wheat spaghetti	1 cup	0.151
Barley, pearled	1 cup	0.130
Instant white rice	1 cup	0.124
Soba noodles	1 cup	0.107
Bulgur	1 cup	0.104
Couscous	1 cup	0.099
Wild rice	1cup	0.085
Buckwheat	1 cup	0.067
Amaranth	1 cup	0.037
Rice noodles	1 cup	0.032

Herbs & Spices	Amount	Vitamin B1 (mg)
Garlic powder	1 tsp	0.013
Onion powder	1 tsp	0.011
Caraway seeds	1 tsp	0.008
Coriander, dried	1 tsp	0.008
Paprika	1 tsp	0.008
Anise seed	1 tsp	0.007

RDA is 1.2 mg for adults

VITAMIN B1

Celery seeds	1 tsp	0.007
Chili powder	1 tsp	0.007
Thyme, dried, ground	1 tsp	0.007
Rosemary, dried	1 tsp	0.006
Sage, ground	1 tsp	0.005
Coriander, seeds	1 tsp	0.004
Curry powder	1 tsp	0.004
Dill weed, dried	1 tsp	0.004
Tarragon, dried, ground	1 tsp	0.004
Cloves, ground	1 tsp	0.003
Oregano, dried	1 tsp	0.003
Parsley, dried	1 tsp	0.003
Turmeric, ground	1 tsp	0.003
All-spice, ground	1 tsp	0.002
Chervil, dried	1 tsp	0.002
Pepper, black, ground	1 tsp	0.002
Basil, dried & ground	1 tsp	0.001
Chives, raw, chopped	1 tsp	0.001
Cinnamon powder	1 tsp	0.001
Ginger, ground	1 tsp	0.001
Basil, fresh, chopped	1 tsp	0
Bay leaf, crumbled	1 tsp	0
Capers, canned	1 tsp	0
Rosemary, fresh	1 tsp	0
Thyme, fresh	1 tsp	0

Juice	Amount	Vitamin B1 (mg)
Orange juice, raw	1 cup	0.223
Carrot	1 cup	0.217
Pineapple	1 cup	0.145
Tomato	1 cup	0.114
Vegetable	1 cup	0.104
Grapefruit juice, raw	1 cup	0.099
Lemon juice, raw	1 cup	0.059
Apple	1 cup	0.052
Grape	1 cup	0.043
Prune	1 cup	0.041
Pomegranate	1 cup	0.037
Cranberry, cocktail	1 cup	0

Lamb, Cooked	Amount	Vitamin B1 (mg)
Cubed, for stew or kabob	3 oz	0.094
Chops, loin, lean, trim to 1/4" fat	3 oz	0.085
Ground	3 oz	0.085
Leg, whole, trim to 1/4" fat	3 oz	0.085

RDA is 1.2 mg for adults

VITAMIN B1

Rib, lean, trim to 1/4" fat	3 oz	0.085
Foreshank, trim to 1/8" fat	3 oz	0.042

Milk	Amount	Vitamin B1 (mg)
Dry, instant, non fat	1 cup	0.281
Canned, condensed, sweetened	1 cup	0.275
Sheep milk	1 cup	0.159
Soy milk, original, unfortified	1 cup	0.146
Canned, evaporated	1 cup	0.118
Goat milk	1 cup	0.117
Canned, evaporated, non fat	1 cup	0.115
Whole milk, 3.25%	1 cup	0.112
Non fat, fat free or skim liquid milk	1 cup	0.110
Reduced fat, 2%	1 cup	0.095
Buttermilk, low fat	1 cup	0.083
Coconut milk, canned	1 cup	0.050
Low fat, 1%	1 cup	0.049
Human milk	1 cup	0.034

Nuts & Seeds	Amount	Vitamin B1 (mg)
Flaxseeds	1 oz	0.466
Sunflower seeds	1 oz	0.420
Tahini	1 oz	0.346
Macadamia	1 oz	0.339
Pistachio nuts	1 oz	0.247
Sesame seeds	1 oz	0.224
Pecans	1 oz	0.187
Hazelnuts	1 oz	0.182
Peanuts	1 oz	0.181
Chia seeds	1 oz	0.176
Brazil nuts	1 oz	0.175
Trail mix, regular, salted	1 oz	0.131
Trail mix, tropical	1 oz	0.128
Cashews	1 oz	0.120
Trail mix, regular with chocolate chips	1 oz	0.117
Pine nuts	1 oz	0.103
English walnuts	1 oz	0.097
Pumpkin seeds	1 oz	0.077
Almonds	1 oz	0.060
Mixed nuts, roasted with peanuts, no salt	1 oz	0.057
Peanut butter, smooth style	1 oz	0.021
Coconut, raw meat	1 oz	0.019
Black walnuts	1 oz	0.016

　　RDA is 1.2 mg for adults

VITAMIN B1

Nuts & Seeds	Amount	Vitamin B1 (mg)
Flaxseeds	1/4 cup	0.690
Hazelnuts, chopped	1/4 cup	0.690
Sunflower seeds	1/4 cup	0.518
Macadamia	1/4 cup	0.400
Sesame seeds	1/4 cup	0.285
Pistachio	1/4 cup	0.268
Peanuts	1/4 cup	0.234
Brazilnuts	1/4 cup	0.205
Tahini	1 tbsp	0.183
Trail mix, regular, salted	1/4 cup	0.173
Flaxseeds	1 tbsp	0.169
Pecans, halves	1/4 cup	0.163
Trail mix, tropical	1/4 cup	0.158
Trail mix, regular with chocolate chips	1/4 cup	0.151
Pine nuts	1/4 cup	0.123
Pumpkin seeds	1/4 cup	0.088
English walnuts, halves	1/4 cup	0.085
Almonds	1/4 cup	0.075
Sesame seeds	1 tbsp	0.071
Mixed nuts, roasted with peanuts, no salt	1/4 cup	0.068
Peanut butter, smooth	1/4 cup	0.047
Black walnuts	1/4 cup	0.018
Coconut meat, shredded	1/4 cup	0.013
Peanut butter, smooth	1 tbsp	0.012
Cashews	1/4 cup	x
Chia seeds	1/4 cup	x

Pork, Cooked	Amount	Vitamin B1 (mg)
Tenderloin	3 oz	0.802
Canadian-style bacon	3 oz	0.700
Cured ham, lean	3 oz	0.578
Sirloin pork chops	3 oz	0.555
Italian sausage	3 oz	0.530
Cured ham	3 oz	0.511
Chops, broiled	3 oz	0.509
Center loin pork chops	3 oz	0.509
Chops, lean, pan-fried	3 oz	0.482
Chops, pan-fried	3 oz	0.456
Polish sausage	3 oz	0.427
Backribs	3 oz	0.391
Bratwurst	3 oz	0.390
Canadian-style bacon	2 slices	0.383
Spareribs	3 oz	0.347
Bacon	3 oz	0.343

RDA is 1.2 mg for adults

VITAMIN B1

Continued

Sausage	3 oz	0.250
Braunschweiger	3 oz	0.212
Liverwurst spread	1/4 cup	0.150
Sausage	1 patty	0.079
Bacon	3 slices	0.077
Sausage	2 links	0.076

Turkey, Cooked	Amount	Vitamin B1 (mg)
Ground turkey, 93% lean	3 oz	0.068
Ground turkey	3 oz	0.065
Ground turkey, 85% lean	3 oz	0.057
Ground turkey, fat free	3 oz	0.057
Turkey sausage, reduced fat	3 oz	0.056
Dark meat	3 oz	0.051
Turkey bacon	3 oz	0.051
Breast meat	3 oz	0.037
Light meat	3 oz	0.030

Veal, Cooked	Amount	Vitamin B1 (mg)
Ground	3 oz	0.060
Breast	3 oz	0.051
Leg, top round	3 oz	0.051
Sirloin	3 oz	0.051
Foreshank	3 oz	0.042
Loin	3 oz	0.042
Rib	3 oz	0.042

Vegetables, Canned	Amount	Vitamin B1 (mg)
Green peas	1 cup	0.221
Tomato Paste	1 cup	0.157
Asparagus	1 cup	0.148
Mushrooms	1 cup	0.133
Stewed tomatoes	1 cup	0.117
Tomatoes	1 cup	0.108
Yellow sweet corn	1 cup	0.086
Tomato pure	1 cup	0.063
Pumpkin	1 cup	0.059
Tomato sauce	1 cup	0.059
Sweet potato	1 cup	0.049
Spinach	1 cup	0.034
Sauerkraut	1 cup	0.030
Carrots	1 cup	0.026
Green beans	1 cup	0.020
Beets	1 cup	0.017

RDA is 1.2 mg for adults

VITAMIN B1

Vegetables, Cooked	Amount	Vitamin B1 (mg)
Split peas	1 cup	0.372
Okra	1 cup	0.211
Snow peas	1 cup	0.205
Potatoes, mashed with whole milk	1 cup	0.187
Sweet potato, mashed	1 cup	0.184
Spinach	1 cup	0.171
Beet greens	1 cup	0.168
Brussels sprouts	1 cup	0.167
Butternut squash	1 cup	0.148
Rutabagas	1 cup	0.139
Yellow sweet corn	1 cup	0.139
Dandelion greens	1 cup	0.137
Parsnips	1 cup	0.129
Yams, cubed	1 cup	0.129
Potatoes, flesh, baked	1 cup	0.128
Asparagus	1 cup	0.117
White mushrooms	1 cup	0.114
Carrots	1 cup	0.103
Broccoli	1 cup	0.098
Cabage	1 cup	0.092
Green beans	1 cup	0.092
Onions	1 cup	0.088
Artichokes	1 cup	0.084
Summer squash	1 cup	0.079
Collard greens	1 cup	0.076
Pumpkin	1 cup	0.076
Eggplant	1 cup	0.075
Kale	1 cup	0.069
Kohlrabi	1 cup	0.066
Celery	1 cup	0.065
Turnip greens	1 cup	0.065
Acorn squash	1 cup	0.063
Zucchini	1 cup	0.063
Swiss chard	1 cup	0.060
Mustard greens	1 cup	0.057
Shitake mushrooms	1 cup	0.054
Bok-Choy	1 cup	0.052
Cauliflower	1 cup	0.052
Beets	1 cup	0.046
Turnips	1 cup	0.042
Winter squash	1 cup	0.033
Leeks	1 cup	0.027
Napa cabbage	1 cup	0.005

RDA is 1.2 mg for adults

VITAMIN B1

Vegetables, Frozen	Amount	Vitamin B1 (mg)
Green peas	1 cup	0.453
Brussels sprouts	1 cup	0.160
Spinach	1 cup	0.148
Okra	1 cup	0.134
Butternut squash	1 cup	0.120
Asparagus	1 cup	0.117
Broccoli	1 cup	0.101
Turnip greens	1 cup	0.089
Collard greens	1 cup	0.080
Cauliflower	1 cup	0.067
Kale	1 cup	0.056
Yellow sweet corn	1 cup	0.049
Green beans	1 cup	0.047
Carrots	1 cup	0.044
Rhubarb	1 cup	0.043

Vegetables, Raw	Amount	Vitamin B1 (mg)
Spirulina, dried	1 tbsp	0.167
Butternut squash	1 cup	0.140
Dandelion greens	1 cup	0.104
Shiitake mushrooms, dried	1 each	0.100
Snow peas	1 cup	0.094
Green bell peppers	1 cup	0.085
Red bell peppers	1 cup	0.080
Kale	1 cup	0.074
Onions	1 cup	0.074
Carrots	1 cup	0.073
Tomatoes	1 cup	0.067
Raab broccoli	1 cup	0.065
Broccoli	1 cup	0.062
Tomatillos	1 cup	0.058
White mushrooms	1 cup	0.057
Belgian endive	1 cup	0.056
Green onions & scallions	1 cup	0.055
Tomatoes, cherry	1 cup	0.055
Summer squash	1 cup	0.054
Yellow bell peppers	1 large	0.052
Zucchini	1 cup	0.051
Cauliflower	1 cup	0.050
Savoy cabbage	1 cup	0.049
Red cabbage	1 cup	0.045
Cabbage	1 cup	0.043
Endive	1 cup	0.040
Romaine lettuce	1 cup	0.040

RDA is 1.2 mg for adults

VITAMIN B1

Continued

Green leaf lettuce	1 cup	0.039
Butterhead or boston lettuce	1 cup	0.031
Watercress	1 cup	0.031
Bok-Choy	1 cup	0.028
Cucumber	1 cup	0.028
Celery	1 cup	0.025
Iceburg lettuce	1 cup	0.023
Spinach	1 cup	0.023
Red leaf lettuce	1 cup	0.018
Chicory greens	1 cup	0.017
Swiss chard	1 cup	0.014
Prickley pear cactus pads	1 cup	0.010
Arugula	1 cup	0.009
Radicchio	1 cup	0.006

Yogurt	Amount	Vitamin B1 (mg)
Plain yogurt, skim milk	8 oz	0.109
Plain yogurt, low fat milk	8 oz	0.100
Plain yogurt, whole milk	8 oz	0.066
Plain Greek Yogurt, nonfat	6 oz	0.039

Nutrient Data Collection Form

Food	Amount	Book Numbers	Multiply By	Estimated Nutrient Intake
Nutrient::	RDA:	Estimated:	% of RDA:	Total Estimated:

To download additional forms for free, go to www.TopNutrients4U.com

Vitamin B3 known as niacin is the third member of the B-complex vitamins. It is water soluble and needed daily in milligrams (mg). Vitamin B3 generates energy from metabolism of carbohydrates and other macronutrients.

Deficiencies affect the skin, digestion, and nervous systems. Deficiency symptoms are dark and scaly pigmented rashes in skin areas exposed to sun light. Your digestive system will be upset and this will result in vomiting and diarrhea. Neurological symptoms are headaches, fatigue, depression, and possible memory loss. All this describes the signs of a disease known as pellagra. It is a disease of adults and usually occurs after 20 years of age. Historically pellagra occurs in populations that eat large amounts of foods low in both niacin and the amino acid tryptophane.

Science has shown that a portion of dietary tryptophane is converted into niacin within the body. To take into account the combined effects of both niacin and tryptophane's contribution to the niacin pool, a new unit of measurement was created known as niacin equivalents (NE). The established RDA is in mg of niacin equivalents (NE), except for infants younger than six months which are expressed as preformed niacin. For all the food groups we could find the tryptophane values we have calculated the units in niacin equivalents (NE) in mg. For the foods we could not find the tryptophane values we have left the units in niacin mg.

VITAMIN B3

The recommended daily allowance, RDA, in niacin equivalents.

Recommend Daily Intakes Levels for Vitamin B3

Children	Vitamin B3, mg
1 to 3 year olds	6
4 to 8 year olds	8

Males	
9 to 13 year olds	12
14 to 18 year olds	16
19 to 30 years	16
31 to 50 years	16
51 to 70 years	16
Over 70	16

Females	
9 to 13 year olds	12
14 to 18 year olds	14
19 to 30 years	14
31 to 50 years	14
51 to 70 years	14
Over 70	14
Pregnancy	18
Lactation	17
Lactation	1.6

VITAMIN B3

Alcohol	Amount	Niacin (mg)
Regular Beer	1 bottle	1.8
Light Beer	1 bottle	1.4
Red Wine	1 glass	0.3
White Wine	1 glass	0.2
Gin, Rum, Vodka, Whisky	1 shot	0.005

Beans, Canned	Amount	Niacin Equivalents (mg)
Baked beans, plain	1 cup	3
Black-eyed peas	1 cup	3
Cranberry beans	1 cup	4
Fava beans	1 cup	5
Garbanzo beans	1 cup	2
Great Northern beans	1 cup	5
Green beans	1 cup	5
Kidney beans	1 cup	4
Lima beans	1 cup	3
Navy beans	1 cup	5
Pinto beans	1 cup	3
Refried beans	1 cup	4
White beans, mature	1 cup	4
Yellow beans	1 cup	0.6

Beans, Cooked	Amount	Niacin Equivalents (mg)
Adzuki	1 cup	x
Soybeans, matured, dry roasted	1 cup	9.898
Winged beans	1 cup	8.111
Soybeans, matured	1 cup	7.619
Soybeans, green	1 cup	6.750
Natto	1 cup	6.500
Mungo beans, mature seeds	1 cup	5.033
Split peas	1 cup	4.777
Lentils	1 cup	4.766
Edamame	1 cup	4.668
Lupini beans	1 cup	4.288
Navy beans	1 cup	4.214
Cranberry beans	1 cup	4.179
Great Northern	1 cup	4.122
Kidney beans	1 cup	4.056
Black Turtle beans, mature	1 cup	3.958
Black beans	1 cup	3.886
Mung beans	1 cup	3.733
Mung beans, mature seeds	1 cup	3.732
White beans, mature	1 cup	3.684

RDA is 12 to 18 mg for adults

VITAMIN B3

Lima beans	1 cup	3.674
White beans, small	1 cup	3.653
Pinto beans	1 cup	3.627
Black-eyed peas	1 cup	3.546
Fava beans	1 cup	3.242
Garbanzo beans, chickpeas	1 cup	3.180
Pigeon peas	1 cup	3.162
Hyacinth beans	1 cup	2.997
Mothbeans	1 cup	2.648
Green beans	1 cup	1.185
Yellow beans	1 cup	1.184
Yardlong beans, Chinese long beans	1 cup	1.155

Beef, Cooked	Amount	Niacin Equivalents (mg)
Flank steak, lean, trim to 0" fat	3 oz	9
Filet Mignon, trim to 0" fat	3 oz	9
Top Sirloin, lean, trim to 1/8" fat	3 oz	9
Tri Tip steak, lean, trim to 0" fat	3 oz	8
Rib eye steak, lean, trim 0" fat	3 oz	7
London Broil, top round, trim to 0" fat	3 oz	7
T-Bone steak, trim 0" fat	3 oz	7
Ground beef, 95%	3 oz	7
Porterhouse steak, trim to 0" fat	3 oz	7
Brisket, lean, trim to 0" fat	3 oz	7
Skirt Steak, trim to 0" fat	3 oz	7
Ground beef, 90%	3 oz	7
Beef ribs, trim to 1/8" fat	3 oz	7
Ground beef, 85%	3 oz	6
Chuck roast, trim to 1/8" fat	3 oz	6
Ground beef, 80%	3 oz	6
Ground beef, 75%,	3 oz	6

Beef, Cooked	Amount	Niacin Equivalents (mg)
Flank steak, lean, trim to 0" fat	1 cooked lb	50
Top Sirloin, trim to 1/8" fat	1 cooked lb	46
Tri Tip steak, lean, trim to 0" fat	1 cooked lb	45
Flank steak, lean, trim to 0" fat	1 steak	42
T-bone steak, trim to 0" fat	1 cooked lb	39
Porterhouse steak, trim to 0" fat	1 cooked lb	39
Brisket, lean, trim to 0" fat	1 cooked lb	39
Skirt steak, trim to 0" fat	1 cooked lb	38
Beef ribs, trim to 1/8" fat	1 cooked lb	35
Chuck roast, trim to 1/8" fat	1 cooked lb	33
Ribeye steak, boneless, trim to 0" fat	1 steak	18

　　　　　　RDA is 12 to 18 mg for adults

VITAMIN B3

Continued

Top Sirloin, choice filet, trim to 0" fat	1 filet	15
Ribeye filet, lean, trim to 0" fat	1 filet	14
Filet Mignon, tenderloin, trim to 0" fat	1 steak	13

Beef, Cooked	Amount	Niacin Equivalents (mg)
Ground beef, 95%	1/4 lb patty	7
Ground beef, 90%	1/4 lb patty	7
Ground beef, 85%	1/4 lb patty	6
Ground beef, 80%	1/4 lb patty	5
Ground beef, 75%	1/4 lb patty	5

Bread	Amount	Niacin Equivalents (mg)
Bagel, oat bran	4" bagel	5.524
Bagel, plain	4" bagel	5.371
Bagel, egg	4" bagel	4.914
Bagel, cinnamon & raisins	4" bagel	4.424
Pita, white	6 1/2 " pita	3.829
Kaiser rolls	1 roll	3.533
English Muffin, plain	1 muffin	3.353
Egg bread	1 slice	2.689
Cornbread, drymix	1 piece	2.017
Dinner rolls, brown & serve	1 roll	1.886
Whole-Wheat	1 slice	1.753
Rye bread	1 slice	1.735
Tortillas, flour	1 tortilla	1.696
French, or Sourdough	1 slice	1.690
Multi-Grain, and Whole-Grain	1 slice	1.584
Pumpernickle	1 slice	1.506
Cracked Wheat	1 slice	1.385
Oatmeal bread	1 slice	1.364
Raisin bread	1 slice	1.268
Italian	1 slice	1.226
Tortillas, corn	1 tortilla	0.572
Hamburger & hotdog buns, plain	1 bun	x
Wheat	1 slice	x
White	1 slice	x
Bagel, wheat	4" bagel	x

Cereal, General Mills®	Amount	Niacin (mg)
Total Whole Grain	1 cup	26.680
Total Raisin Bran	1 cup	19.981
Total Cranberry Crunch	1 cup	16.000
Wheaties	1 cup	13.320
Cinnamon Toast Crunch	1 cup	9.848

RDA is 12 to 18 mg for adults

VITAMIN B3

Multi-Bran CHEX	1 cup	9.337
Lucky Charms	1 cup	9.108
Chocolate Chex	1 cup	7.125
Cinnamon Chex	1 cup	6.680
Honey Nut Chex	1 cup	6.667
Raisin Nut Bran	1 cup	6.664
Cocoa Puffs	1 cup	6.660
Dora The Explorer	1 cup	6.660
Cookie Crisp	1 cup	6.656
Golden Grams	1 cup	6.655
Reese's Puffs	1 cup	6.651
Wheat Chex	1 cup	6.643
Kix	1 cup	5.820
Honey Nut Clusters	1 cup	5.016
Basic 4	1 cup	5.005
Rice Chex	1 cup	4.995
Trix	1 cup	4.992
Corn Chex	1 cup	4.991
Oatmeal Crisp, Hearty Raisin	1 cup	4.030
Berry Berry Kix	1 cup	4.013
Oatmeal Crisp, Crunchy Almond	1 cup	3.685

Cereal, General Mills Cheerios®	Amount	Niacin (mg)
Multi Grain	1 cup	20.000
Banana Nut	1 cup	6.683
Apple Cinnamon	1 cup	6.667
Berry Burst	1 cup	6.667
Frosted	1 cup	6.667
Fruity	1 cup	6.667
Honey Nut	1 cup	6.667
Chocolate	1 cup	6.660
CRUNCH, Oat Clusters	1 cup	6.660
Original	1 cup	5.348

Cereal, General Mills Fiber One®	Amount	Niacin (mg)
Original Bran	1 cup	10.000
Frosted Shredded Wheat	1 cup	7.980
Raisin Bran Clusters	1 cup	5.005
Caramel Delight	1 cup	5.000
Honey Clusters	1 cup	4.992

Cereal, Kashi®	Amount	Niacin (mg)
Autum Wheat	1 cup	2.808
Island Vanilla	1 cup	2.640

RDA is 12 to 18 mg for adults

VITAMIN B3

Continued

Good Friends	1 cup	2.120
Berry Blossom	1 cup	0.960
Go Lean Crunch, Honey Almond Flax	1 cup	0.870
Honey Sunshine	1 cup	0.840
7-Whole Grain Honey Puffs	1 cup	0.780
Heart to Heart, Wild Blueberry	1 cup	0.660
Heart to Heart, Honey Toasted Oat	1 cup	0.638
7-Whole Grain Puffs	1 cup	0.608
Heart to Heart, Warm Cinnamon	1 cup	0.396
Go Lean	1 cup	0.208
Go Lean Crisp, Toasted Berry Crumble	1 cup	0.204
Go Lean Crunch	1 cup	0.159

Cereal, Kellogg's®	Amount	Niacin (mg)
All-Bran Complete Wheat Flakes	1 cup	26.680
Product 19	1 cup	20.010
Smart Start, Strong Heart, Antioxidants	1 cup	20.000
All-Bran Bran Buds	1 cup	15.045
Frosted Flakes	1 cup	11.620
Fiberplus Cinnamon Oat Crunch	1 cup	9.344
All-Bran Original	1 cup	9.176
MUESLIX	1 cup	8.209
Raisin Bran	1 cup	8.142
Fiberplus Berry Yogurt Crunch	1 cup	6.996
Crispix	1 cup	6.989
Rice Krispies Treats	1 cup	6.800
Frosted Rice Krispies	1 cup	6.680
Cracklin' Oat Bran	1 cup	6.664
Crunchy Nut Roasted Nut & Honey O's	1 cup	6.660
Honey Smacks	1 cup	6.660
Cocoa Krispies	1 cup	6.655
Crunchy Nut Golden Honey Nut Flakes	1 cup	6.655
Krave Chocolate	1 cup	6.655
Honey Crunch Corn Flakes	1 cup	6.640
CINNABON	1 cup	5.520
Rice Krispies	1 cup	5.210
Apple Jacks	1 cup	5.012
Corn Flakes	1 cup	5.012
Corn Pops	1 cup	5.010
Smorz	1 cup	5.010
Froot Loops	1 cup	4.988
Raisin Bran Crunch	1 cup	4.982
Frosted MINI-Wheats, Big-Bite	5 biscuits	3.563

VITAMIN B3

Cereal, Kellogg's Special-K®	Amount	Niacin (mg)
Low Fat Granola	1 cup	14.040
Multigrain Oats & Honey	1 cup	10.494
Vanilla Almond	1 cup	9.720
Chocolately Delight	1 cup	9.465
Fruit & Yogurt	1 cup	9.344
Blueberry	1 cup	9.320
Protein Plus	1 cup	9.280
Original	1 cup	7.006
Red Berries	1 cup	7.006
Cinnamon Pecan	1 cup	5.320

Cereal, Post®	Amount	Niacin, mg
Grape-Nuts Cereal	1 cup	16.936
Bran Flakes	1 cup	6.680
Great Grains, Raisin, Date & Pecan	1 cup	6.673
Fruity Pebbles	1 cup	6.660
Golden Crisp	1 cup	6.660
Great Grains, Cranberry Almond Crunch	1 cup	6.656
Great Grains, Crunchy Pecan	1 cup	6.656
Cocoa Pebbles	1 cup	6.651
Grape-Nuts Flakes	1 cup	6.651
Great Grains, Banana Nut Crunch	1 cup	5.015
Raisin Bran	1 cup	5.015
Alpha-Bits	1 cup	5.010
Shredded Wheat, Frosted, spoon-size	1 cup	5.002
Honey Nut Shredded Wheat	1 cup	4.997
Blueberry Morning	1 cup	4.004
Honeycomb Cereal	1 cup	3.328
Shredded Wheat, Original, spoon-size	1 cup	2.764
Shredded Wheat n' Bran, spoon-size	1 cup	2.450
Shredded Wheat, Original, big-biscuit	1 biscuit	1.312

Post® Honey Bunches of Oats®	Amount	Niacin, mg
Just Bunches Honey Roasted	1 cup	7.487
Honey Roasted	1 cup	7.120
With Cinnamon Bunches	1 cup	6.680
With Almonds	1 cup	6.656
With Strawberries	1 cup	6.655
Pecan Bunches	1 cup	6.651
With Vanilla Bunches	1 cup	4.984

RDA is 12 to 18 mg for adults

VITAMIN B3

Cereal, Quaker	Amount	Niacin (mg)
Toasted Oatmeal Cereal	1 cup	9.510
Toasted Oatmeal Cereal, Honey Nut	1 cup	8.987
Honey Gram OH'S	1 cup	8.795
Oat Cinnamon LIFE	1 cup	7.823
CAP'N Crunch	1 cup	7.727
Maple Brown Sugar LIFE	1 cup	7.625
CAP'N Crunch with Crunch Berries	1 cup	7.617
Crunchy Bran	1 cup	7.340
CAP'N Crunch's Peanut Butter Crunch	1 cup	7.330
Cinnamon Oatmeal Squares	1 cup	5.610
Golden Maple Squares	1 cup	5.513
Oatmeal Squares	1 cup	5.508
Oat LIFE	1 cup	3.696
Ganola Oats, Wheat and Honey	1 cup	2.354
Ganola Oats, Wheat, Honey and Raisins	1 cup	2.168
Low Fat Granolia with Raisins	1 cup	1.958
Granola Apple Cranberry Almond	1 cup	1.891

Cereal, Cooked	Amount	Niacin (mg)
Malt-o-Meal plain	1 serving	7.574
Oats, instant, fortified, plain	1 cup	7.078
Cream of Wheat, mix'n eat	1 packet	4.970
Farina	1 cup	3.568
White corn grits	1 cup	2.053
Yellow corn grits	1 cup	1.775
WHEATENA	1 cup	1.336
Cream of Wheat, regular	1 cup	1.305
Oats, regular, unenriched	1 cup	0.526

Cheese	Amount	Niacin Equivalents (mg)
Cottage cheese, lowfat, 2 %	1 cup	6.127
Cottage cheese, creamed, small curd	1 cup	5.739
Ricotta, part skim milk	1 cup	5.708
Cottage cheese, lowfat, 1 %	1 cup	5.489
Ricotta, whole milk	1 cup	5.389
Cottage cheese, nonfat, uncreamed	1 cup	3.525

Cheese	Amount	Niacin (mg)
Mozzarella, nonfat	1 oz	0.034
Muenster, low fat	1 oz	0.028
Monterey, low fat	1 oz	0.025
Swiss, low fat	1 oz	0.025
American, pasteurized process, low fat	1 oz	0.022
American, pasteurized process, imitation	1 oz	0.017

Cheese	Amount	Niacin Equivalents (mg)
Mozzarella, part skim milk, low moisture	1 oz	2.879
Parmesan, grated	1 oz	2.482
Mozzarella, whole milk	1 oz	2.462
Goat cheese, hard type	1 oz	2.197
Romano	1 oz	2.055
Gruyere	1 oz	2.013
Swiss	1 oz	1.926
Blue cheese	1 oz	1.755
Fontina	1 oz	1.743
Gouda	1 oz	1.685
Provolone	1 oz	1.677
Provolone, reduced fat	1 oz	1.661
Roquefort	1 oz	1.641
Brie	1 oz	1.625
Muenster	1 oz	1.579
Cheddar	1 oz	1.540
Monterey	1 oz	1.509
Colby	1 oz	1.459
Goat cheese, semisoft	1 oz	1.392
Cheddar, lowfat	1 oz	1.364
Feta cheese	1 oz	1.231
American, pasteurized process, fortified	1 oz	1.122
Goat cheese, soft type	1 oz	1.039
Cream cheese, fat free	1 oz	0.932
Cream cheese	1 oz	0.374
American, pasteurized process, imitation	1 oz	x
American, pasteurized process, low fat	1 oz	x
Monterey, low fat	1 oz	x
Mozzarella, nonfat	1 oz	x
Muenster, low fat	1 oz	x
Swiss, low fat	1 oz	x

RDA is 12 to 18 mg for adults

VITAMIN B3

Cheese, Mexican	Amount	Niacin Equivalents (mg)
Mexican, blend	1 oz	1.715
Queso asadero	1 oz	1.317
Queso anejo	1 oz	1.025
Queso chihuahua	1 oz	0.976
Queso seco	1 oz	x
Mexican, blend, reduced fat	1 oz	x
Queso blanco	1 oz	x
Queso fresco	1 oz	x

Chicken, Cooked	Amount	Niacin Equivalents (mg)
Breast with skin, fried with flour	1/2 breast	19.410
Breast with skin, roasted	1/2 breast	18.000
Breast meat only, no skin, roasted	1/2 breast	16.970
Thigh with skin, fried in flour	1 thigh	7.423
Drumstick, with skin, fried	1 drumstick	5.458
Drumstick, no skin, roasted	1 drumstick	x
Thigh meat only, no skin, roasted	1 thigh	x

Chicken, Cooked	Amount	Niacin Equivalents (mg)
Breast with skin, fried with flour	3 oz	17.678
Breast meat only, no skin, roasted	3 oz	16.788
Breast with skin, roasted	3 oz	15.620
Wing meat only, no skin, roasted	3 oz	11.265
Thigh with skin, fried with flour	3 oz	10.187
Wing with skin, roasted	3 oz	9.717
Wing with skin, fried in flour	3 oz	9.675
Drumstick with skin, fried in flour	3 oz	9.481
Cornish game hens, meat only	3 oz	9.182
Thigh meat only, no skin, roasted	3 oz	9.090
Drumstick meat only, no skin, roasted	3 oz	8.452
Thigh with skin, roasted	3 oz	8.254
Drumstick with skin, roasted	3 oz	7.992

Cream	Amount	Niacin Equivalents (mg)
Half & Half	1 tbsp	0.112
Sour cream, reduced fat	1 tbsp	0.110
Light Coffe Creamer	1 tbsp	0.109
Sour cream cultured	1 tbsp	0.079
Heavy whipping cream	1 tbsp	0.072
Whipped topping, pressurized	1 tbsp	0.018

RDA is 12 to 18 mg for adults

VITAMIN B3

Eggs	Amount	Niacin Equivalents (mg)
Egg whites, dried	1 ounce	4.961
Egg substitute, liquid, fat free	1/4 cup	1.717
Egg whites, dried powder, stabilized	1 tbsp	1.534
Egg whole, scrambled	1 large	1.426
Egg whole, fried	1 large	1.421
Egg whole, poached	1 large	1.415
Egg whole, hard boiled	1 large	1.298
Egg whites	1 large	0.715
Egg yolk, raw	1 large	0.504

Fish, Canned	Amount	Niacin Equivalents (mg)
Light tuna, in oil	3 oz	15.162
White (albacore) tuna, in oil	3 oz	14.143
Light tuna, in water	3 oz	11.582
White (albacore) tuna, in water	3 oz	8.679

Fish, Cooked	Amount	Niacin Equivalents (mg)
Yellowfin tuna	3 oz	23.193
Skipjack, (aku), tuna	3 oz	20.426
Bluefin tuna	3 oz	13.709
Pacific and Jack mackerel	3 oz	13.150
King mackerel	3 oz	13.010
Sockeye salmon	3 oz	12.810
Chinook salmon	3 oz	12.620
Atlantic salmon, wild	3 oz	12.598
Yellowtail	3 oz	12.110
Pink salmon	3 oz	11.900
Swordfish	3 oz	11.616
Keta (chum) salmon	3 oz	11.347
Atlantic & Pacific halibut	3 oz	10.740
Coho salmon, wild	3 oz	10.491
Atlantic salmon, farmed	3 oz	10.354
Coho, farmed	3 oz	10.134
Alaskan halibut	3 oz	10.060
Atlantic mackerel	3 oz	9.605
Rainbow trout, farmed	3 oz	9.599
Rainbow trout, wild	3 oz	8.537
Spanish mackerel	3 oz	7.983
Tilapia	3 oz	7.783
Atlantic pollock	3 oz	7.336
Haddock	3 oz	7.184
Walleye pollock	3 oz	7.090
Florida pompano	3 oz	6.980

RDA is 12 to 18 mg for adults

VITAMIN B3

Chinock salmon, smoked	3 oz	6.912
Pacific rockfish	3 oz	6.662
Atlantic croaker	3 oz	6.605
Northern pike	3 oz	6.297
Walleye pike	3 oz	6.281
Striped bass	3 oz	5.791
Atlantic cod	3 oz	5.769
Carp	3 oz	5.418
Sea bass	3 oz	5.365
Pollock	3 oz	5.257
Whiting	3 oz	5.153
Cat fish, farmed	3 oz	5.132
Freshwater bass	3 oz	5.127
Atlantic herring, pickeled	3 oz	5.057
Cat fish, wild	3 oz	4.960
Orange roughy	3 oz	4.814
Cat fish, breaded & fried	3 oz	4.774
Greenland halibut	3 oz	4.551
Snapper	3 oz	4.461
Pacific cod	3 oz	4.409
Grouper	3 oz	4.257
Atlantic perch	3 oz	4.249
Flounder and Sole	3 oz	3.869

Fish, Shellfish, Cooked	Amount	Niacin Equivalents (mg)
Octopus	3 oz	7.946
Queen crab	3 oz	7.119
Shrimp, breaded & fried	3 oz	6.842
Blue crab cakes	3 oz	6.448
Shrimp	3 oz	5.959
Blue crab	3 oz	5.535
Blue crab, canned	3 oz	5.535
Clams, canned	3 oz	5.291
Crayfish	3 oz	5.255
Squid, fried	3 oz	5.079
Northern lobster	3 oz	5.073
Alaskan king crab	3 oz	4.956
Abalone	3 oz	4.782
Scallops, breaded & fried	3 oz	4.246
Clams, breaded & fried	3 oz	4.137
Shrimp, canned	3 oz	3.107
Eastern oysters, breaded & fried	3 oz	2.885
Eastern oysters, wild	3 oz	2.677
Eastern oysters, farmed	3 oz	2.623
Alaskan king crab, imitation	3 oz	1.594

RDA is 12 to 18 mg for adults

VITAMIN B3

Fruit, Canned	Amount	Niacin (mg)
Peaches	1 cup	1.609
Apricoits	1 cup	0.970
Plums	1 cup	0.751
Pineapple	1 cup	0.729
Pears	1 cup	0.644
Applesauce, unsweetened	1 cup	0.205
Applesauce, sweetened	1 cup	0.184
Olives, green	5 large	0.032
Olives, black	5 large	0.008

Fruit, Dried	Amount	Niacin (mg)
Peaches	1 cup	7.000
Apricots	1 cup	3.366
Pears	1 cup	2.470
Currants	1 cup	2.326
Cranberries	1 cup	1.200
Figs	1 cup	0.922
Apples	1 cup	0.797

Fruit, Frozen	Amount	Niacin (mg)
Blackberries	1 cup	1.823
Peaches	1 cup	1.633
Strawberries, sweetened	1 cup	0.747
Strawberries, unsweetened	1 cup	0.688
Blueberries	1 cup	0.582
Raspberries	1 cup	0.575

Fruit, Raw	Amount	Niacin (mg)
Stewed prunes	1 cup	1.793
Blackberries	1 cup	0.930
Raspberries	1 cup	0.736
Pomegranates	1 cup	0.656
Black currants	1 cup	0.336

Fruit, Raw	Amount	Niacin Equivalents (mg)
Avocado, California	1 cup	5.364
Prunes, uncooked	1 cup	4.008
Avocado, Florida	1 cup	2.614
Raisins	1 cup	2.311
Dates	1 cup	2.173
Nectarine	1 cup	1.726
Peachs	1 cup	1.655

RDA is 12 to 18 mg for adults

VITAMIN B3

Continued

Mango	1 cup	1.454
Apricots	1 cup	1.407
Plantains	1 cup	1.382
Cantaloupe	1 cup	1.224
Kiwi	1 cup	1.064
Elderberries	1 cup	1.042
Pineapple	1 cup	0.958
Plums	1 cup	0.938
Strawberries, sliced	1 cup	0.858
Honeydew	1 cup	0.844
Tangerines, sections	1 cup	0.800
Oranges	1 cup	0.775
Grapefruit, pink or red, sections	1 cup	0.769
Papayas	1 cup	0.718
Blueberries	1 cup	0.686
Jicama	1 cup	0.607
Grapes, red & green	1 cup	0.584
Cherries, without pits	1 cup	0.470
Water mellon	1 cup	0.454
Pears	1 cup	0.303
Cranberries	1 cup	0.151
Apples	1 cup	0.131
Black currants	1 cup	x
Blackberries	1 cup	x
Pomegranates	1 cup	x
Raspberries	1 cup	x
Stewed prunes	1 cup	x
Mulberries	1 cup	x

Fruit, Raw	Amount	Niacin Equivalents (mg)
Avocado, Florida	1 fruit	3.460
Avocado, California	1 fruit	3.167
Plantains	1 fruit	1.678
Nectarine	1 fruit	1.630
Prunes, uncooked	5 prunes	1.094
Banana	1 fruit	0.968
Peaches	1 fruit	0.957
Raisins	1 small box	0.696
Oranges	1 fruit	0.569
Dates	5 dates	0.519
Kiwi	1 fruit	0.442
Grapefruit, pink or red	1/2 fruit	0.418
Plums	1 fruit	0.375
Tangerine	1 fruit	0.364
Strawberries	5 fruit	0.315

Continued

Apricots	1 fruit	0.293
Pineapple	1/2" x 3" slice	0.282
Pears	1 fruit	0.282
Cherries	10 fruit	0.243
Raisins	1 packet	0.224
Apples	1 fruit	0.153
Figs, dried	1 fruit	0.085
Kumquats	1 fruit	x
Pomegranates	1 fruit	x

Game Meat, Cooked	Amount	Niacin (mg)
Deer, ground	3 oz	7.868
Buffalo, steak, free range	3 oz	5.967
Deer	3 oz	5.704
Rabbit	3 oz	5.440
Caribou	3 oz	4.922
Bison, ground	3 oz	4.735
Elk, ground	3 oz	4.522
Duck	3 oz	4.335
Squirrel	3 oz	3.944
Wild boar	3 oz	3.578
Antelope	3 oz	x
Elk, roasted	3 oz	x

Grains, Cooked	Amount	Niacin Equivalents (mg)
Kamut	1 cup	6.358
Egg noodles	1 cup	4.473
Macaroni	1 cup	4.298
Spaghetti	1 cup	4.248
Pearled barley	1 cup	4.239
White rice, regular, long-grain	1 cup	4.149
Egg & Spinach noodles	1 cup	4.141
Brown rice	1 cup	4.047
Spinach spaghetti	1 cup	3.492
Wild rice	1 cup	3.444
Millet	1 cup	3.414
Bulgur	1 cup	3.270
Buckwheat	1 cup	2.946
Couscous	1 cup	2.826
Macaroni, Whole-Wheat	1 cup	2.607
Spaghetti, Whole-Wheat	1 cup	2.607
Oat bran	1 cup	2.398
Quinoa	1 cup	2.362
Oats, regular, unenriched	1 cup	2.093
Soba noodles	1 cup	1.948

RDA is 12 to 18 mg for adults

VITAMIN B3

Rice noodles	1 cup	0.444
Amaranth	1 cup	x
Spelt	1 cup	x

Herbs & Spices	Amount	Niacin (mg)
Chili powder	1 tsp	0.313
Paprika	1 tsp	0.231
Ginger, ground	1 tsp	0.173
Tarragon, dried, ground	1 tsp	0.143
Tumeric, ground	1 tsp	0.113
Oregano, dried	1 tsp	0.084
Caraway seeds	1 tsp	0.076
Curry powder	1 tsp	0.069
Thyme, dried, ground	1 tsp	0.069
Basil, dried & ground	1 tsp	0.069
Anise seed	1 tsp	0.064
Coriander, dried	1 tsp	0.064
Celery seeds	1 tsp	0.061
All-spice, ground	1 tsp	0.054
Basil, fresh	1/4 cup	0.054
Parsley, dried	1 tsp	0.050
Thyme, dried, leaves	1 tsp	0.049
Sage, ground	1 tsp	0.040
Coriander, seed	1 tsp	0.038
Cinnamon powder	1 tsp	0.035
Cloves, dried, ground	1 tsp	0.033
Chervil, dried	1 tsp	0.032
Dill weed, dried	1 tsp	0.028
Pepper, black, ground	1 tsp	0.026
Garlic powder	1 tsp	0.025
Capers, canned	1 tsp	0.018
Dill weed, fresh	5 sprigs	0.016
Thyme, fresh	1 tsp	0.015
Bay leaf, crumbled	1 tsp	0.012
Rosemary, dried	1 tsp	0.012
Safron	1 tsp	0.010
Onion powder	1 tsp	0.008
Rosemary, fresh	1 tsp	0.006
Chives, raw, chopped	1 tsp	0.006

Juice	Amount	Niacin (mg)
Prune	1 cup	2.010
Vegetable, cocktail	1 cup	1.757
Tomato	1 cup	1.635
Orange, raw	1 cup	0.992

RDA is 12 to 18 mg for adults

VITAMIN B3

Continued

Carrot	1 cup	0.911
Pomegranate	1 cup	0.580
Pineapple	1 cup	0.498
Grapefruit, raw	1 cup	0.494
Grape	1 cup	0.336
Lemon, raw	1 cup	0.222
Apple	1 cup	0.181
Cranberry, cocktail	1 cup	0.104

Lamb, Cooked	Amount	Niacin Equivalents (mg)
Cubed, for stew or kabob	3 oz	10.268
Chops, loin, lean, trim to 1/4" fat	3 oz	10.201
Rib, lean, trim to 1/4" fat	3 oz	10.151
Leg, whole, trim to 1/4" fat	3 oz	9.835
Ground	3 oz	9.795
Foreshank, trim to 1/8" fat	3 oz	9.341

Milk	Amount	Niacin Equivalents (mg)
Canned, condensed, sweetened	1 cup	6.359
Dry, instant, nonfat	1 cup	6.222
Canned, evaporated, nonfat	1 cup	5.011
Sheep milk	1 cup	4.455
Soy milk, original & vanila	1 cup	2.780
Goat milk	1 cup	2.459
Coconut milk, canned	1 cup	2.340
Nonfat, fat free or skim liquid milk	1 cup	1.980
Lowfat, 1%	1 cup	1.977
Reduced fat, 2%	1 cup	1.924
Buttermilk, lowfat	1 cup	1.858
Whole milk, 3.25%	1 cup	1.850
Human milk	1 cup	1.135

Nuts & Seeds	Amount	Niacin Equivalents (mg)
Peanut butter, smooth style	1 oz	4.866
Peanuts	1 oz	4.604
Chia seeds	1 oz	4.569
Pumpkin seeds	1 oz	4.130
Sunflower seeds	1 oz	4.013
Tahini	1 oz	3.295
Sesame seeds	1 oz	3.113
Mixed nuts, roasted with peanuts, no salt	1 oz	2.582
Flaxseed	1 oz	2.273
Trail mix, regular, salted	1 oz	2.119
Trail mix, regular with chocolate chips	1 oz	2.015

RDA is 12 to 18 mg for adults

VITAMIN B3

Almonds	1 oz	1.976
Pine nuts	1 oz	1.744
Pistachio nuts	1 oz	1.652
Cashew	1 oz	1.651
Black walnuts	1 oz	1.633
Hazelnuts	1 oz	1.426
English walnuts	1 oz	1.119
Macadamia	1 oz	1.017
Trail mix, tropical	1 oz	0.770
Pecans	1 oz	0.764
Brazilnuts	1 oz	0.750
Coconut, meat	1 oz	0.336

Nuts & Seeds	Amount	Niacin Equivalents (mg)
Peanut butter, smooth style	1/4 cup	11.078
Peanuts	1/4 cup	5.921
Sunflower seeds	1/4 cup	4.950
Pumpkin seeds	1/4 cup	4.708
Sesame seeds	1/4 cup	3.958
Flaxseeds	1/4 cup	3.377
Mixed nuts, roasted with peanuts, no salt	1/4 cup	3.100
Trail mix, regular, salted	1/4 cup	2.800
Peanut butter, smooth style	1 tbsp	2.744
Trail mix, regular with chocolate chips	1/4 cup	2.591
Almonds	1/4 cup	2.493
Pine nuts	1/4 cup	2.081
Black walnuts	1/4 cup	1.797
Pistachio	1/4 cup	1.783
Tahini	1 tbsp	1.751
Hazelnuts, chopped	1/4 cup	1.435
Macadamia	1/4 cup	1.195
Sesame seeds	1 tbsp	0.989
English walnuts, halves	1/4 cup	0.981
Trail mix, tropical	1/4 cup	0.952
Brazilnuts	1/4 cup	0.881
Flaxseeds	1 tbsp	0.834
Pecans, halves	1/4 cup	0.672
Coconut meat, shredded	1/4 cup	0.241

Pork, Cooked	Amount	Niacin Equivalents (mg)
Bacon	3 oz	13.884
Chops, lean, pan-fried	3 oz	13.200
Chops, pan-fried	3 oz	12.474
Sirloin pork chops	3 oz	12.122
Chops, broiled	3 oz	10.758

RDA is 12 to 18 mg for adults

VITAMIN B3

Center loin pork chops	3 oz	10.758
Backribs	3 oz	10.374
Tenderloin	3 oz	10.175
Spareribs	3 oz	9.887
Canadian-style bacon	3 oz	9.278
Braunschweiger	3 oz	9.163
Bratwurst	3 oz	8.992
Cured ham, lean	3 oz	8.517
Sausage	3 oz	7.519
Cured ham	3 oz	7.258
Italian sausage	3 oz	5.823
Polish sausage	3 oz	4.878
Liverwurst spread	1/4 cup	3.748

Turkey, Cooked	Amount	Niacin Equivalents (mg)
Light meat	3 oz	14.538
Ground turkey, fat free	3 oz	13.767
Ground turkey	3 oz	11.831
Breast meat	3 oz	11.219
Dark meat	3 oz	9.865
Ground turkey, 85% lean	3 oz	9.837
Ground turkey, 93% lean	3 oz	9.827
Turkey sausage, reduced fat	3 oz	4.549
Turkey bacon	3 oz	x

Vegetables, Canned	Amount	Niacin Equivalents (mg)
Tomato paste	1 cup	9.409
Tomato puree	1 cup	4.131
Asparagus	1 cup	3.159
Yellow sweet corn	1 cup	3.051
Mushrooms	1 cup	3.035
Tomato sauce	1 cup	2.789
Green peas	1 cup	2.580
Spinach	1 cup	2.180
Stewed tomatos	1 cup	2.121
Tomatoes, red, ripe	1 cup	2.025
Pumpkin	1 cup	1.432
Sweet potato	1 cup	1.182
Carrots	1 cup	1.006
Sauerkraut	1 cup	0.653
Beets	1 cup	0.586
Green beans	1 cup	0.577

RDA is 12 to 18 mg for adults

VITAMIN B3

Vegetables, Cooked	Amount	Niacin Equivalents (mg)
White mushrooms	1 cup	7.575
Split peas	1 cup	4.777
Potatoes, mashed with whole milk	1 cup	3.364
Sweet potato, mashed	1 cup	3.298
Yellow sweet corn	1 cup	3.075
Asparagus	1 cup	2.735
Potatoes, flesh, baked	1 cup	2.485
Raab broccoli	1 cup	2.446
Butternut squash	1 cup	2.436
Acorn squash	1 cup	2.356
Shiitake mushrooms	1 cup	2.275
Spinach	1 cup	2.082
Okra	1 cup	1.827
Broccoli	1 cup	1.746
Snow peas	1 cup	1.712
Beet greens	1 cup	1.686
Brussels sprouts	1 cup	1.680
Rutabagas	1 cup	1.616
Winter squash	1 cup	1.465
Pumpkin	1 cup	1.379
Carrots	1 cup	1.273
Collard greens	1 cup	1.234
Mustard greens	1 cup	1.189
Green beans	1 cup	1.185
Swiss chard	1 cup	1.163
Bok-Choy	1 cup	1.161
Summer squash	1 cup	1.156
Kale	1 cup	1.150
Beets	1 cup	1.130
Zucchini	1 cup	1.101
Turnip greens	1 cup	1.075
Onions	1 cup	1.046
Cauliflower	1 cup	1.008
Kohlrabi	1 cup	0.944
Nopales	1 cup	0.791
Celery	1 cup	0.746
Eggplant	1 cup	0.727
Turnips	1 cup	0.649
Cabbage	1 cup	0.639
Leeks	1 cup	0.308
Artichokes	1 cup	X
Broccolini	1 cup	X
Dandelion Greens	1 cup	X
Parsnips	1 cup	X

RDA is 12 to 18 mg for adults

VITAMIN B3

Vegetables, Frozen	Amount	Niacin Equivalents (mg)
Spinach	1 cup	4.034
Green peas	1 cup	3.301
Yellow sweet corn	1 cup	3.013
Asparagus	1 cup	2.734
Turnip greens	1 cup	2.351
Collard greens	1 cup	2.163
Brussels sprouts	1 cup	1.865
Broccoli	1 cup	1.826
Butternut squash	1 cup	1.797
Kale	1 cup	1.640
Okra	1 cup	1.566
Cauliflower	1 cup	1.191
Green beans	1 cup	0.883
Carrots	1 cup	0.786
Rhubarb	1 cup	x

Vegetables, Raw	Amount	Niacin Equivalents (mg)
Oyster mushrooms	1 cup	4.862
Portabella mushrooms	1 cup	4.365
Crimini mushrooms	1 cup	3.403
White mushrooms	1 cup	2.925
Yellow bell peppers	1 large	2.055
Butternut squash	1 cup	2.013
Spirulina, dried	1 tbsp	1.980
Red bell peppers	1 cup	1.759
Carrots	1 cup	1.298
Tomatoes	1 cup	1.252
Kale	1 cup	1.120
Broccoli	1 cup	1.045
Snow peas	1 cup	1.021
Mustard spinach	1 cup	1.017
Green bell peppers	1 cup	1.015
Cauliflower	1 cup	0.892
Green onions & scallions	1 cup	0.858
Raab broccoli	1 cup	0.771
Shiitake mushrooms	1 each	0.770
Summer squash	1 cup	0.750
Zucchini	1 cup	0.693
Celery	1 cup	0.567
Prickley pear cactus pads, nopales	1 cup	0.553
Onions	1 cup	0.553
Shiitake mushrooms, dried	1 each	0.525

RDA is 12 to 18 mg for adults

Continued

Bok-Choy	1 cup	0.517
Savoy cabbage	1 cup	0.443
Red cabbage	1 cup	0.426
Spinach	1 cup	0.417
Belgian endive	1 cup	0.377
Butterhead & boston lettuce	1 cup	0.313
Cabbage	1 cup	0.297
Chicory greens	1 cup	0.295
Green leaf lettuce	1 cup	0.293
Romaine lettuce	1 cup	0.275
Radicchio	1 cup	0.269
Swiss chard	1 cup	0.244
Watercress	1 cup	0.235
Endive	1 cup	0.233
Red leaf lettuce	1 cup	0.190
Cucumber	1 cup	0.185
Iceburg lettuce	1 cup	0.151
Arugula	1 cup	x
Dandelion greens	1 cup	x
Tomatillos	1 cup	x

Yogurt	Amount	Niacin (mg)
Plain yogurt, skim milk	8 oz	0.281
Plain yogurt, low fat milk	8 oz	0.259
Plain yogurt, whole milk	8 oz	0.170

Nutrient Data Collection Form

Food	Amount	Book Numbers	Multiply By	Estimated Nutrient Intake
Nutrient::	RDA:	Estimated:	% of RDA:	Total Estimated:

To download additional forms for free, go to www.TopNutrients4U.com

VITAMIN B6

Vitamin B6 known as pyridoxine is the sixth member of the B-complex vitamins. It is water soluble and needed daily in milligrams (mg) quantities. It is the generic name for six organic compounds involved with enzymatic reactions of the immunity and nervous systems, hence deficiencies will affect the skin, mucous membranes, and nerve tissues.

Classical deficiency symptoms include depression, confusion, irritability, anemia, adolescent acne, sores or cracks at corners of the mouth, swollen red tongue, and oral ulcers may develop. Studies in infants indicate that B-6 deficiency upsets the cerebral metabolism and causes convulsions in infants that feed from milk formulas deficient in B-6. Studies associate low plasma concentrations of B-6 with cardiovascular disease, DNA damage, degeneration of pancreatic beta-cells, increased plasma concentrations of C-reactive proteins, and decreased plasma concentrations of omega-3 and omega-6 polyunsaturated fatty acids.

Vitamin B-6 is required for the formation of mood-enhancing neurotransmitters such as serotonin which may explain the depression symptoms. Vitamin B-6 is needed for the routine conversion of dietary tryptophane to vitamin B-3, thus a deficiency in B-6 will lead to a deficiency in B-3, which might explain pellagra-like skin lesions and dermatitis seen in deficiencies of both vitamins.

Scientist has identified as many as 103 enzymatic reactions requiring vitamin B-6, of which the above are only a few. Infants, elderly, alcoholics, and women taking contraceptive drugs are at high risk of a deficiency.

The recommended daily allowance, RDA, for B6 is in milligrams, mg.

Recommend Daily Intakes Levels for Vitamin B6

Children	Vitamin B6, mg
1 to 3 year olds	.5
4 to 8 year olds	.6

Males	
9 to 13 year olds	1.0
14 to 18 year olds	1.3
19 to 30 years	1.3
31 to 50 years	1.3
51 to 70 years	1.7
Over 70	1.7

Females	
9 to 13 year olds	1.0
14 to 18 year olds	1.2
19 to 30 years	1.3
31 to 50 years	1.3
51 to 70 years	1.5
Over 70	1.5
Pregnancy	1.9
Lactation	2.0

VITAMIN B6

Alcohol	Amount	Vitamin B6 (mg)
Regular Beer	1 bottle	0.164
Light Beer	1 bottle	0.120
Red Wine	1 glass	0.084
White Wine	1 glass	0.074
Gin, Rum, Vodka, Whisky	1 shot	0

Beans, Canned	Amount	Vitamin B6 (mg)
Garbanzo beans, chickpeas	1 cup	1.135
Great Northern	1 cup	0.278
Navy beans	1 cup	0.270
Refried beans	1 cup	0.262
Lima beans	1 cup	0.219
Baked beans, plain	1 cup	0.213
Kidney beans	1 cup	0.205
White beans, mature	1 cup	0.196
Pinto beans	1 cup	0.178
Cranberry beans	1 cup	0.143
Fava beans	1 cup	0.115
Black-eyed peas	1 cup	0.108
Yellow beans	1 cup	0.057
Green beans	1 cup	0.046

Beans, Cooked	Amount	Vitamin B6 (mg)
Soybeans, matured	1 cup	0.402
Pinto beans	1 cup	0.392
Lentils	1 cup	0.352
Lima beans	1 cup	0.303
Navy beans	1 cup	0.251
Garbanzo beans, chickpeas	1 cup	0.228
Natto	1 cup	0.228
White beans, small	1 cup	0.227
Adzuki	1 cup	0.221
Kidney beans	1 cup	0.212
Soybeans, matured, dry roasted	1 cup	0.209
Great Northern	1 cup	0.207
Soybeans, green	1 cup	0.180
Black-eyed peas	1 cup	0.171
White beans, mature	1 cup	0.166
Mothbeans	1 cup	0.165
Edamame	1 cup	0.155
Cranberry beans	1 cup	0.143
Black Turtle beans, mature	1 cup	0.142
Mung beans, mature seeds	1 cup	0.135

VITAMIN B6

Fava beans	1 cup	0.122
Black beans	1 cup	0.119
Split peas	1 cup	0.094
Pigeon peas	1 cup	0.084
Winged beans	1 cup	0.081
Hyacinth beans	1 cup	0.072
Green beans	1 cup	0.070
Yellow beans	1 cup	0.070
Yardlong beans, Chinese long beans	1 cup	0.025
Lupini beans	1 cup	0.015

Beef, Cooked	Amount	Vitamin B6 (mg)
Top Sirloin, lean, trim to 1/8" fat	3 oz	0.537
Flank steak, lean, trim to 0" fat	3 oz	0.509
Filet Mignon, trim to 0" fat	3 oz	0.490
Tri Tip steak, lean, trim to 0" fat	3 oz	0.387
Ground beef, 95%	3 oz	0.350
Ground beef, 90%	3 oz	0.337
Ground beef, 85%	3 oz	0.325
Ribeye steak, lean, trim 0" fat	3 oz	0.315
Ground beef, 80%	3 oz	0.312
Porterhouse steak, trim to 0" fat	3 oz	0.310
T-Bone steak, trim 0" fat	3 oz	0.307
Ground beef, 75%, broiled	3 oz	0.298
Skirt Steak, trim to 0" fat	3 oz	0.273
Brisket, lean, trim to 0" fat	3 oz	0.270
London Broil, top round, trim to 0" fat	3 oz	0.238
Chuck roast, trim to 1/8" fat	3 oz	0.221
Beef ribs, trim to 1/8" fat	3 oz	0.196

Beef, Cooked	Amount	Vitamin B6 (mg)
Flank steak, lean, trim to 0" fat	1 steak	2.719
Top Sirloin, trim to 1/8" fat	1 lb cooked	2.561
Flank steak, lean, trim to 0" fat	1 lb cooked	2.294
Tri Tip steak, lean, trim to 0" fat	1 lb cooked	2.009
Porterhouse steak, trim to 0" fat	1 lb cooked	1.656
T-bone steak, trim to 0" fat	1 lb cooked	1.637
Skirt steak, trim to 0" fat	1 lb cooked	1.456
Brisket, lean, trim to 0" fat	1 lb cooked	1.444
Chuck roast, trim to 1/8" fat	1 lb cooked	1.180
Beef ribs, trim to 1/8" fat	1 lb cooked	1.044
Filet Mignon, tenderloin, trim to 0" fat	1 steak	0.804
Ribeye steak, boneless, trim to 0" fat	1 steak	0.784
Top Sirloin, choice filet, trim to 0" fat	1 filet	0.756
Ribeye filet, lean, trim to 0" fat	1 filet	0.614

RDA is 1.3 to 1.7 mg for adults

VITAMIN B6

Beef, Ground, Cooked	Amount	Vitamin B6 (mg)
Ground beef, 95%	1/4 lb patty	0.338
Ground beef, 90%	1/4 lb patty	0.326
Ground beef, 85%	1/4 lb patty	0.294
Ground beef, 80%	1/4 lb patty	0.283
Ground beef, 75%	1/4 lb patty	0.246

Bread	Amount	Vitamin B6 (mg)
Bagel, wheat	4" bagel	0.144
Indian bread, Naan, whole wheat	1 piece	0.136
Mexican roll, bollilo	1 roll	0.103
Indian bread, Naan, plain	1 piece	0.086
Bagel, egg	4" bagel	0.077
Cracked Wheat	1 slice	0.076
Potato bread	1 slice	0.074
Potato bread	1 slice	0.074
Multi-Grain, and Whole-Grain	1 slice	0.068
Cornbread	1 piece	0.062
Bagel plain	4" bagel	0.059
Tortillas, corn	1 tortilla	0.057
Bagel, cinnamon & raisins	4" bagel	0.055
Bagel, oat-bran	4" bagel	0.045
Pumpernickle	1 slice	0.040
English Muffin, plain	1 muffin	0.035
Croissants, butter	1 medium	0.033
Hamburger & Hotdog buns, plain	1 bun	0.031
Italian	1 slice	0.031
Wheat	1 slice	0.030
Reduced calorie wheat	1 slice	0.029
Dinner Rolls, brown & serve	1 roll	0.027
Egg bread	1 slice	0.026
French or Sourdough	1 slice	0.025
Rye bread	1 slice	0.024
White	1 slice	0.021
Kaiser rolls	1 roll	0.020
Pita, white	6" pita	0.020
Biscuit, buttermilk, refrigerated dough	2 1/2"	0.018
Oatmeal bread	1 slice	0.018
Raisen bread	1 slice	0.018
Reduced calorie rye	1 slice	0.018
Tortillas, flour	1 tortilla	0.016
Reduced calorie white	1 slice	0.010
Whole-Wheat	1 slice	0.010

RDA is 1.3 to 1.7 mg for adults

VITAMIN B6

Butter	Amount	Vitamin B6 (mg)
Regular dairy butter, salted	1 tbsp	0
Regular dairy whipped butter, salted	1 tbsp	0

CEREAL

Cereal, General Mills®	Amount	Vitamin B6 (mg)
Total Whole Grain	1 cup	2.667
Total Raisin Bran	1 cup	2.000
Total Cranberry Crunch	1 cup	1.600
Wheaties	1 cup	1.333
Lucky Charms	1 cup	1.084
Multi-Bran Chex	1 cup	0.800
Chocolate Chex	1 cup	0.711
Cocoa Puffs	1 cup	0.667
Cookie Crisp	1 cup	0.667
Dora The Explorer	1 cup	0.667
Golden Grams	1 cup	0.667
Honey Nut Chex	1 cup	0.667
Reese's Puffs	1 cup	0.667
Wheat Chex	1 cup	0.667
Raisin Nut Bran	1 cup	0.666
Cinnamon Chex	1 cup	0.664
Corn Chex	1 cup	0.600
Cinnamon Toast Crunch	1 cup	0.587
Kix	1 cup	0.552
Basic 4	1 cup	0.500
Honey Nut Clusters	1 cup	0.500
Rice Chex	1 cup	0.500
Trix	1 cup	0.500
Berry Berry Kix	1 cup	0.400
Oatmeal Crisp, Hearty Raisin	1 cup	0.397
Oatmeal Crisp, Crunchy Almond	1 cup	0.367

Cereal, General Mills Cheerios®	Amount	Vitamin B6 (mg)
Yogurt Burst	1 cup	0.800
Apple Cinnamon	1 cup	0.667
Banana Nut	1 cup	0.667
Berry Burst	1 cup	0.667
Chocolate	1 cup	0.667
Crunch, Oat Clusters	1 cup	0.667
Frosted	1 cup	0.667
Fruity	1 cup	0.667

RDA is 1.3 to 1.7 mg for adults

Continued

Honey Nut	1 cup	0.667
Original	1 cup	0.533
Multi Grain	1 cup	.5

Cereal, General Mills Fiber One®	Amount	Vitamin B6 (mg)
Original Bran	1 cup	1
Frosted Shredded Wheat	1 cup	0.600
Caramel Delight	1 cup	0.500
Honey Clusters	1 cup	0.500
Raisin Bran Clusters	1 cup	0.500

Cereal, Kashi®	Amount	Vitamin B6 (mg)
Heart to Heart, Honey Toasted Oat	1 cup	2.684
Heart to Heart, Warm Cinnamon	1 cup	2.631
Heart to Heart, Wild Blueberry	1 cup	2.013
Go Lean	1 cup	0.280
Island Vanilla	1 cup	0.165
Autum Wheat	1 cup	0.154
Good Friends	1 cup	0.143
Go Lean Crunch, Honey Almond Flax	1 cup	0.080
7-Whole Grain Honey Puffs	1 cup	0.071
7-Whole Grain Puffs	1 cup	0.063
Berry Blossom	1 cup	0.028
Go Lean Crunch	1 cup	0.016
Honey Sunshine	1 cup	0.016
Go Lean Crisp, Toasted Berry Crumble	1 cup	0.007

Cereal, Kellogg's®	Amount	Vitamin B6 (mg)
All-Bran Original	1 cup	7.440
All-Bran Bran Buds	1 cup	6.009
MUESLIX	1 cup	3.037
All-Bran Complete Wheat Flakes	1 cup	2.668
Product 19	1 cup	2.001
Smart Start, Strong Heart, Antioxidants	1 cup	2.000
Frosted Flakes	1 cup	1.502
Raisin Bran	1 cup	1.087
Fiberplus Cinnamon Oat Crunch	1 cup	0.939
Crispix	1 cup	0.699
Fiberplus Berry Yogurt Crunch	1 cup	0.689
Crunchy Nut, Roasted Nut & Honey O's	1 cup	0.684
Rice Krispies	1 cup	0.682
Honey Crunch Corn Flakes	1 cup	0.680
Rice Krispies Treats	1 cup	0.680
Frosted Rice Krispies	1 cup	0.668

RDA is 1.3 to 1.7 mg for adults

VITAMIN B6

Cracklin' Oat Bran	1 cup	0.666
Honey Smacks	1 cup	0.666
Cocoa Krispies	1 cup	0.665
Crunchy Nut, Golden Honey Nut Flakes	1 cup	0.665
Krave Chocolate	1 cup	0.665
CINNABON	1 cup	0.549
Smorz	1 cup	0.510
Apple Jacks	1 cup	0.501
Corn Flakes	1 cup	0.501
Corn Pops	1 cup	0.501
Froot Loops	1 cup	0.499
Raisin Bran Crunch	1 cup	0.498
Frosted MINI-Wheat's, Big-Bite	1 cup	0.356

Cereal, Kellogg's Special-K®	Amount	Vitamin B6 (mg)
Original	1 cup	2.015
Low Fat Granolia	1 cup	1.352
Multigrain Oats & Honey	1 cup	1.045
Chocolately Delight	1 cup	0.988
Vanilla Almond	1 cup	0.952
Fruit & Yogurt	1 cup	0.939
Blueberry	1 cup	0.920
Cinnamon Pecan	1 cup	0.920
Protein Plus	1 cup	0.889
Red Berries	1 cup	0.713

Cereal, Post®	Amount	Vitamin B6, mg
Grape-Nuts Cereal	1 cup	2.784
Great Grains, Crunchy Pecan	1 cup	0.693
Fruity Pebbles	1 cup	0.684
Golden Crisp	1 cup	0.684
Bran Fl;akes	1 cup	0.680
Great Grains, Raisin, Date & Pecan	1 cup	0.660
Cocoa Pebbles	1 cup	0.657
Grape-Nuts Flakes	1 cup	0.657
Great Grains, Cranberry Almond Crunch	1 cup	0.640
Alpha-Bits	1 cup	0.510
Shredded Wheat, Frosted, spoon-size	1 cup	0.499
Honey Nut Shredded Wheat	1 cup	0.496
Great Grains, Banana Nut Crunch	1 cup	0.472
Raisin Bran	1 cup	0.472
Blueberry Morning	1 cup	0.396
Honeycomb Cereal	1 cup	0.341
Shredded Wheat, Original, big-biscuit	1 biscuit	0.289

RDA is 1.3 to 1.7 mg for adults

VITAMIN B6

Continued

Shredded Wheat, Original, spoon-size	1 cup	0.069
Shredded Wheat n' Bran, spoon-size	1 cup	0.033

Post® Honey Bunches of Oats®	Amount	Vitamin B6 (mg)
Honey Roasted	1 cup	1.056
Just Bunches Honey Roasted	1 cup	0.766
With Strawberries	1 cup	0.703
With Almonds	1 cup	0.683
With Cinnamon Bunches	1 cup	0.680
Pecan Bunches	1 cup	0.657
With Vanilla Bunches	1 cup	0.504

Cereal, Quaker®	Amount	Vitamin B6 (mg)
Toasted Oatmeal Cereal	1 cup	0.933
Toasted Oatmeal Cereal, Honey Nut	1 cup	0.882
Honey Graham OH'S	1 cup	0.879
LIFE Cereal, Cinnamon	1 cup	0.782
CAP'N Crunch	1 cup	0.770
LIFE Cereal, Maple Brown Sugar	1 cup	0.766
CAP'N Crunch with Crunch Berries	1 cup	0.759
CAP'N Crunch's Peanut Butter Crunch	1 cup	0.734
Crunchy Bran	1 cup	0.734
Oatmeal Squares, Cinnamon	1 cup	0.561
Oatmeal Squares, Golden Maple	1 cup	0.552
Oatmeal Squares	1 cup	0.551
LIFE Cereal, Original	1 cup	0.371
Granola Apple Cranberry Almond	1 cup	0.189

Cereal, Cooked	Amount	Vitamin B6 (mg)
Malt-o-Meal, plain	1 serving	0.520
Farina	1 cup	0.229
White corn grits	1 cup	0.111
Yellow corn grits	1 cup	0.085
CREAM OF WHEAT, regular	1 cup	0.033
Oats, regular, unenriched	1 cup	0.012

Cheese	Amount	Vitamin B6 (mg)
Cottage cheese, lowfat 1 %	1 cup	0.154
Ricotta, whole milk	1 cup	0.106
Cottage cheese, creamed, small curd	1 cup	0.104
Cottage cheese, lowfat 2 %	1 cup	0.050
Ricotta, part skim milk	1 cup	0.049
Cottage cheese, nonfat, uncreamed	1 cup	0.023

RDA is 1.3 to 1.7 mg for adults

VITAMIN B6

Cheese	Amount	Vitamin B6 (mg)
Feta cheese	1 oz	0.120
Goat cheese, soft type	1 oz	0.071
Brie	1 oz	0.067
Blue cheese	1 oz	0.047
Roquefort	1 oz	0.035
Fontina	1 oz	0.024
Romano	1 oz	0.024
Swiss	1 oz	0.024
Goat cheese, hard type	1 oz	0.023
Gouda	1 oz	0.023
Gruyere	1 oz	0.023
Mozzarella, non fat	1 oz	0.023
American, pasteurized process, low fat	1 oz	0.022
Colby	1 oz	0.022
Monterey	1 oz	0.022
Monterey, low fat	1 oz	0.022
Mozzarella, part skim milk, low moisture	1 oz	0.022
Swiss, low fat	1 oz	0.022
Cheddar	1 oz	0.021
Provolone	1 oz	0.021
Provolone, reduced fat	1 oz	0.020
Goat cheese, semisoft	1 oz	0.017
Muenster, low fat	1 oz	0.017
Muenster	1 oz	0.016
American, pasteurized process, fortified	1 oz	0.015
Cream cheese, fat free	1 oz	0.014
Parmesan, grated	1 oz	0.014
Cheddar, low fat	1 oz	0.013
Cream cheese	1 oz	0.010
Mozzarella, whole milk	1 oz	0.010
American, pasteurized process, imitation	1 oz	0.008
Cheez Whiz, pasteurized process	1 oz	x
Velveeta, pasteurized process	1 oz	x

Cheese, Mexican	Amount	Vitamin B6 (mg)
Queso seco	1 oz	0.026
Mexican, blend, reduced fat	1 oz	0.024
Queso blanco	1 oz	0.024
Queso fresco	1 oz	0.022
Mexican, blend	1 oz	0.017
Queso chihuahua	1 oz	0.016
Queso asadero	1 oz	0.015
Queso anejo	1 oz	0.013

RDA is 1.3 to 1.7 mg for adults

VITAMIN B6

Chicken, Cooked	Amount	Vitamin B6 (mg)
Breast, no skin, roasted	1/2 breast	0.568
Breast, no skin, roasted	1/2 breast	0.516
Thigh, with skin, fried	1 thigh	0.224
Thigh, no skin, roasted	1 thigh	0.182
Drumstick, no skin, roasted	1 drumstick	0.172
Drumstick, with skin, fried	1 drumstick	0.172

Chicken, Cooked	Amount	Vitamin B6 (mg)
Breast meat only, no skin, roasted	3 oz	0.510
Wing meat only, no skin, roasted	3 oz	0.502
Breast with skin, fried with flour	3 oz	0.493
Breast with skin, roasted	3 oz	0.476
Thigh meat only, no skin, roasted	3 oz	0.389
Wing with skin, roasted	3 oz	0.357
Thigh with skin, roasted	3 oz	0.348
Wing with skin, fried in flour	3 oz	0.348
Drumstick meat only, no skin, roasted	3 oz	0.342
Drumstick with skin, roasted	3 oz	0.321
Cornish game hens, meat only	3 oz	0.304
Drumstick with skin, fried in flour	3 oz	0.298
Thigh with skin, fried with flour	3 oz	0.280

Cream	Amount	Vitamin B6 (mg)
Sour cream cultured	1 tbsp	0.007
Half & Half	1 tbsp	0.006
Light Coffe cream	1 tbsp	0.005
Heavy Whipping	1 tbsp	0.004
Sour cream reduced fat	1 tbsp	0.002
Whipped topping, pressurized	1 tbsp	0.001

Eggs	Amount	Vitamin B6 (mg)
Egg whole, fried	1 large	0.085
Egg whole, scrambled	1 large	0.082
Egg substitute, liquid, fat free	1/4 cup	0.080
Egg whole, poached	1 large	0.072
Egg whole, hard-boiled	1 large	0.061
Egg yolk	1 large	0.058
Egg whites, dried	1 ounce	0.010
Egg whites	1 large	0.002
Egg whites, dried powder, stabilized	1 tbsp	0.002

RDA is 1.3 to 1.7 mg for adults

VITAMIN B6

Fish, Canned	Amount	Vitamin B6 (mg)
White (albacore) tuna, in oil	3 oz	0.366
Light tuna, in water	3 oz	0.271
White (albacore) tuna, in water	3 oz	0.184
Atlantic Sardines, in oil	3 oz	0.142
Light tuna, in oil	3 oz	0.094

Fish, Cooked	Amount	Vitamin B6 (mg)
Atlantic salmon, farmed	3 oz	1.254
Yellowfin tuna, fresh	3 oz	0.882
Skipjack (aku) tuna	3 oz	0.834
Atlantic salmon, wild	3 oz	0.802
Pink salmon	3 oz	0.592
Sockeye salmon	3 oz	0.589
Atlantic & Pacific halibut	3 oz	0.537
Swordfish	3 oz	0.523
Coho salmon, farmed	3 oz	0.483
Coho salmon, wild	3 oz	0.483
Bluefin tuna	3 oz	0.446
King mackerel	3 oz	0.434
Greenland halibut	3 oz	0.412
Chinook salmon	3 oz	0.393
Keta (chum) salmon	3 oz	0.393
Atlantic mackerel	3 oz	0.391
Sea bass	3 oz	0.391
Snapper	3 oz	0.391
Spanish mackerel	3 oz	0.391
Rainbow trout, farmed	3 oz	0.328
Pacific mackerel	3 oz	0.324
Grouper	3 oz	0.298
Rainbow trout, wild	3 oz	0.294
Striped bass	3 oz	0.294
Atlantic pollock	3 oz	0.281
Pollock	3 oz	0.280
Walleye pollock	3 oz	0.280
Haddock	3 oz	0.278
Atlantic cod	3 oz	0.241
Chinock salmon, smoked	3 oz	0.236
Alaskan halibut	3 oz	0.226
Atlantic croaker	3 oz	0.221
Pacific rockfish	3 oz	0.205
Florida pompano	3 oz	0.196
Carp	3 oz	0.186
Cat fish, breaded & fried	3 oz	0.161

RDA is 1.3 to 1.7 mg for adults

Continued

Yellowtail	3 oz	0.157
Whiting	3 oz	0.153
Cat fish, farmed	3 oz	0.150
Atlantic herring, pickeled	3 oz	0.145
Freshwater bass	3 oz	0.117
Walleye pike	3 oz	0.117
Pacific cod	3 oz	0.116
Northern pike	3 oz	0.115
Tilapia	3 oz	0.105
Flounder & Sole	3 oz	0.098
Cat fish, wild	3 oz	0.090
Atlantic perch	3 oz	0.071
Perch	3 oz	0.071
Orange roughy	3 oz	0.057

Fish, Shellfish, Cooked	Amount	Vitamin B6 (mg)
Octopus	3 oz	0.551
Shrimp	3 oz	0.206
Alaskan king crab	3 oz	0.153
Queen crab	3 oz	0.147
Crab cakes	3 oz	0.145
Blue crab	3 oz	0.133
Blue crab, canned	3 oz	0.133
Abalone	3 oz	0.128
Scallops, breaded & fried	3 oz	0.119
Alaskan king crab, imitation	3 oz	0.110
Northern lobster	3 oz	0.101
Shrimp, breaded & fried	3 oz	0.083
Crayfish	3 oz	0.065
Eastern oysters, farmed	3 oz	0.065
Oysters, breaded & fried	3 oz	0.054
Clams, breaded & fried	3 oz	0.051
Squid, fried	3 oz	0.049
Eastern oysters, wild	3 oz	0.038
Clams, canned	3 oz	0.014
Shrimp, canned	3 oz	0.008

Fruit, Canned	Amount	Vitamin B6 (mg)
Pineapple	1 cup	0.188
Apricots	1 cup	0.139
Plums	1 cup	0.070
Applesauce, sweetened	1 cup	0.069
Applesauce, unsweetened	1 cup	0.066
Peaches	1 cup	0.050

RDA is 1.3 to 1.7 mg for adults

VITAMIN B6

Pears	1 cup	0.037
Olives, green	5 large	0.004
Olives, black	5 large	0.002

Fruit, Dried	Amount	Vitamin B6 (mg)
Currants	1 cup	0.426
Apricots	1 cup	0.186
Figs	1 cup	0.158
Pears	1 cup	0.130
Apples	1 cup	0.107
Peaches	1 cup	0.107
Cranberries	1 cup	0.046

Fruit, Frozen	Amount	Vitamin B6 (mg)
Blueberries	1 cup	0.136
Blackberries, unthawed	1 cup	0.092
Raspberries	1 cup	0.085
Strawberries	1 cup	0.076
Peaches	1 cup	0.045

Fruit, Raw	Amount	Vitamin B6 (mg)
Avocado, California	1 cup	0.660
Stewed prunes	1 cup	0.541
Plantains	1 cup	0.443
Prunes, uncooked	1 cup	0.357
Elderberries	1 cup	0.334
Raisins	1 cup	0.252
Dates	1 cup	0.243
Mango	1 cup	0.196
Pineapple	1 cup	0.185
Tangerine	1 cup	0.152
Honeydew	1 cup	0.150
Grapes, red & green	1 cup	0.138
Grapefruit, pink & red, sections	1 cup	0.122
Cantaloupe	1 cup	0.115
Kiwi	1 cup	0.113
Oranges	1 cup	0.108
Apricots	1 cup	0.089
Strawberries	1 cup	0.078
Blueberries	1 cup	0.075
Cherries, without pits	1 cup	0.075
Black currants	1 cup	0.074
Mulberries	1 cup	0.070
Raspberries	1 cup	0.068

RDA is 1.3 to 1.7 mg for adults

VITAMIN B6

Water mellon	1 cup	0.068
Cranberries	1 cup	0.057
Papayas	1 cup	0.055
Apples	1 cup	0.051
Plums	1 cup	0.048
Pears	1 cup	0.045
Blackberries	1 cup	0.043
Jicama	1 cup	0.042
Peachs	1 cup	0.038
Nectarine	1 cup	0.036

Fruit, Raw	Amount	Vitamin B6 (mg)
Cherimoya	1 fruit	0.604
Plantains	1 fruit	0.535
Banana	1 fruit	0.433
Avocado, California	1 fruit	0.405
Mango	1 fruit	0.400
Pummelo	1 fruit	0.219
Persimmons, Japanese	1 fruit	0.168
Chayote	1 fruit	0.154
Avocado, Florida	1 fruit	0.110
Prunes, uncooked	5 fruit	0.097
Oranges	1 fruit	0.079
Raisins	1 small box	0.075
Tangerine	1 fruit	0.069
Grapefruit, pink & red	1/2 fruit	0.065
Papayas	1 fruit	0.060
Dates	5 fruit	0.059
Apples	1 fruit	0.057
Pineapple	1/2" x 3" slice	0.056
Kiwi	1 fruit	0.043
Pears	1 fruit	0.041
Cherries	10 fruit	0.040
Nectarine	1 fruit	0.032
Peaches	1 fruit	0.032
Pineapple guava, Feijoa	1 fruit	0.028
Strawberries	5 fruit	0.028
Raisins	1 packet	0.024
Apricots	1 fruit	0.019
Plums	1 fruit	0.019
Star fruit, Carambola	1 fruit	0.015
Figs, dried	1 fruit	0.009
Kumquats	1 fruit	0.007
Olives	5 large	0.002
Persimmons, small native	1 fruit	x

RDA is 1.3 to 1.7 mg for adults

VITAMIN B6

Game Meat, Cooked	Amount	Vitamin B6 (mg)
Buffalo, steak, free range	3 oz	0.675
Deer, ground	3 oz	0.398
Elk, ground	3 oz	0.357
Wild boar	3 oz	0.355
Bison, ground	3 oz	0.319
Squirrel	3 oz	0.314
Rabbit	3 oz	0.289
Caribou	3 oz	0.272
Duck	3 oz	0.212
Antelope	3 oz	x
Elk, roasted	3 oz	x

Grains, Cooked	Amount	Vitamin B6 (mg)
White rice, long-grain, enriched	1 cup	0.303
Brown rice	1 cup	0.283
Amaranth	1 cup	0.278
Wild rice	1cup	0.221
Quinoa	1 cup	0.200
Millet	1 cup	0.188
Egg & Spinach noodles	1 cup	0.182
Pearled barley	1 cup	0.181
Spelt	1 cup	0.155
Bulgur	1 cup	0.151
White rice, long-grain, regular	1 cup	0.147
Kamut	1 cup	0.143
Buckwheat	1 cup	0.129
Whole Wheat Spaghetti	1 cup	0.111
Instant white rice	1 cup	0.083
Couscous	1 cup	0.080
Egg noodles	1 cup	0.074
Macaroni	1 cup	0.069
Spaghetti	1 cup	0.069
Oat bran	1 cup	0.055
Chow mein noodles	1 cup	0.050
Soba noodles	1 cup	0.046
Rice noodles	1 cup	0.011

Herbs & Spices	Amount	Vitamin B6 (mg)
Chili powder	1 tsp	0.057
Garlic powder	1 tsp	0.051
Paprika	1 tsp	0.049
Turmeric, ground	1 tsp	0.040
Tarragon, dried, ground	1 tsp	0.039

RDA is 1.3 to 1.7 mg for adults

VITAMIN B6

Continued

	Amount	Vitamin B6 (mg)
Pepper, black, ground	1 tsp	0.032
Curry powder	1 tsp	0.023
Rosemary, dried	1 tsp	0.021
Basil, dried & ground	1 tsp	0.019
Oregano, dried	1 tsp	0.019
Sage, ground	1 tsp	0.019
Celery seeds	1 tsp	0.018
Dill weed, dried	1 tsp	0.017
Onion powder	1 tsp	0.017
Anise seed	1 tsp	0.014
Parsley, dried	1 tsp	0.014
Ginger, ground	1 tsp	0.011
Bay leaf, crumbled	1 tsp	0.010
Caraway seeds	1 tsp	0.008
Cloves, dried, ground	1 tsp	0.008
Thyme, dried	1 tsp	0.008
Saffron	1 tsp	0.007
Chervil, dried	1 tsp	0.006
All-spice, ground	1 tsp	0.004
Cinnamon powder	1 tsp	0.004
Coriander, dried	1 tsp	0.004
Thyme, fresh	1 tsp	0.003
Dill weed, fresh	5 sprigs	0.002
Rosemary, fresh	1 tsp	0.002
Chives, raw	1 tsp	0.001

Juice	Amount	Vitamin B6 (mg)
Prune	1 cup	0.558
Carrot	1 cup	0.512
Vegetable	1 cup	0.339
Tomato	1 cup	0.270
Pineapple	1 cup	0.250
Lemon juice, raw	1 cup	0.112
Grapefruit juice, raw	1 cup	0.109
Pomegranate	1 cup	0.100
Orange juice, raw	1 cup	0.099
Grape	1 cup	0.081
Apple	1 cup	0.045
Cranberry	1 cup	0

RDA is 1.3 to 1.7 mg for adults

VITAMIN B6

Lamb, Cooked	Amount	Vitamin B6 (mg)
Leg, whole, trim to 1/4" fat	3 oz	0.128
Rib, lean, trim to 1/4" fat	3 oz	0.128
Cubed, for stew or kabob	3 oz	0.119
Ground	3 oz	0.119
Chops, loin, lean, trim to 1/4" fat	3 oz	0.110
Foreshank, trim to 1/8" fat	3 oz	0.085

Milk	Amount	Vitamin B6 (mg)
Soy milk, original, unfortified	1 cup	0.187
Canned, condensed, sweetened	1 cup	0.156
Sheep milk	1 cup	0.147
Canned, evaporated, non fat	1 cup	0.141
Canned, evaporated	1 cup	0.126
Goat milk	1 cup	0.112
Reduced fat, 2%	1 cup	0.093
Nonfat, fat free or skim	1 cup	0.091
Lowfat, 1%	1 cup	0.090
Whole milk, 3.25%	1 cup	0.088
Buttermilk, low fat	1 cup	0.083
Dry, instant, non fat	1/3 cup	0.079
Coconut milk, canned	1 cup	0.063
Human milk	1 cup	0.027

Nuts & Seeds	Amount	Vitamin B6 (mg)
Pistachio	1 oz	0.482
Sunflower seeds	1 oz	0.381
Sesame seeds	1 oz	0.224
Black walnuts	1 oz	0.165
Hazelnuts	1 oz	0.160
Peanut butter, smooth style	1 oz	0.154
English walnuts	1 oz	0.152
Flaxseeds	1 oz	0.134
Cashews	1 oz	0.118
Peanuts	1 oz	0.099
Trail mix, tropical	1 oz	0.093
Mixed nuts, roasted with peanuts, no salt	1 oz	0.084
Trail mix, regular, salted	1 oz	0.084
Macadamia	1 oz	0.078
Trail mix, regular with chocolate chips	1 oz	0.073
Pecans	1 oz	0.060
Almonds	1 oz	0.041
Pumpkin seeds	1 oz	0.041

RDA is 1.3 to 1.7 mg for adults

VITAMIN B6

Continued

Brazilnuts	1 oz	0.029
Pine nuts	1 oz	0.027
Coconut, raw meat	1 oz	0.015
Chia seeds	1 oz	x

Nuts & Seeds	Amount	Vitamin B6 (mg)
Pistachio	1/4 cup	0.523
Sunflower seeds	1/4 cup	0.471
Peanut butter, smooth	1/4 cup	0.350
Sesame seeds	1/4 cup	0.284
Flaxseeds	1/4 cup	0.199
Black walnuts	1/4 cup	0.182
Hazelnuts, chopped	1/4 cup	0.162
English walnuts	1/4 cup	0.134
Peanuts	1/4 cup	0.127
Trail mix, tropical	1/4 cup	0.114
Trail mix, regular, salted	1/4 cup	0.112
Mixed nuts, roasted with peanuts, no salt	1/4 cup	0.101
Trail mix, regular with chocolate chips	1/4 cup	0.095
Macadamia	1/4 cup	0.092
Peanut butter, smooth	1 tbsp	0.087
Sesame seeds	1 tbsp	0.071
Pecans, halves	1/4 cup	0.052
Almonds	1/4 cup	0.051
Flaxseeds	1 tbsp	0.049
Pumpkin seeds	1/4 cup	0.046
Brazilnuts	1/4 cup	0.034
Pine nuts	1/4 cup	0.032
Tahini	1 tbsp	0.022
Coconut meat, shredded	1/4 cup	0.011
Cashews	1/4 cup	x
Chia seeds	1/4 cup	x

Pork, Cooked	Amount	Vitamin B6 (mg)
Chops, broiled	3 oz	0.569
Chops, lean, pan-fried	3 oz	0.478
Chops, pan-fried	3 oz	0.446
Cured ham, lean	3 oz	0.399
Canadian-style bacon	3 oz	0.382
Backribs	3 oz	0.351
Cured ham	3 oz	0.323
Spareribs	3 oz	0.298
Italian sausage	3 oz	0.280
Bratwurst	3 oz	0.278
Sausage	3 oz	0.278

RDA is 1.3 to 1.7 mg for adults

VITAMIN B6

Polish sausage	3 oz	0.162
Sausage	1 patty	0.088
Sausage	2 links	0.085
Bacon	3 slices	0.066

Turkey, Cooked	Amount	Vitamin B6 (mg)
Ground turkey, fat free	3 oz	0.772
Light meat	3 oz	0.686
Ground turkey	3 oz	0.538
Breast meat	3 oz	0.476
Ground turkey, 93% lean	3 oz	0.400
Dark meat	3 oz	0.372
Ground turkey, 85% lean	3 oz	0.326
Turkey bacon	3 oz	0.272
Turkey sausage, reduced fat	3 oz	0.199

Veal, Cooked	Amount	Vitamin B6 (mg)
Ground	3 oz	0.331
Leg, top round	3 oz	0.306
Loin	3 oz	0.289
Sirloin	3 oz	0.272
Breast	3 oz	0.246
Foreshank	3 oz	0.225
Rib	3 oz	0.212

Vegetables, Canned	Amount	Vitamin B6 (mg)
Tomato paste	1 cup	0.566
Tomato pure	1 cup	0.315
Sauerkraut	1 cup	0.307
Tomatoes	1 cup	0.266
Asparagus	1 cup	0.266
Tomato sauce	1 cup	0.238
Spinach	1 cup	0.214
Carrots	1 cup	0.164
Pumpkin	1 cup	0.157
Sweet potato	1 cup	0.122
Yellow corn	1 cup	0.116
Beets	1 cup	0.097
Mushrooms	1 cup	0.095
Green peas	1 cup	0.095
Stewed tomatos	1 cup	0.043
Green beans	1 cup	0.039

RDA is 1.3 to 1.7 mg for adults

VITAMIN B6

Vegetables, Cooked	Amount	Vitamin B6 (mg)
Sweet potato, mashed	1 cup	0.541
Potatoes, mashed with whole milk	1 cup	0.487
Spinach	1 cup	0.436
Acorn squash	1 cup	0.398
Potatoes, flesh, baked	1 cup	0.367
Hubbard squash	1 cup	0.353
Winter squash, all varieties averaged	1 cup	0.330
Broccoli	1 cup	0.312
Yams, cubes	1 cup	0.310
Okra	1 cup	0.299
Bok-Choy	1 cup	0.282
Brussels sprouts	1 cup	0.278
Onions	1 cup	0.271
Turnip greens	1 cup	0.259
Butternut squash	1 cup	0.254
Kohlrabi	1 cup	0.254
Collard greens	1 cup	0.243
Carrots	1 cup	0.239
Shitake mushrooms	1 cup	0.231
Snow peas	1 cup	0.230
Cauliflower	1 cup	0.215
Yellow corn	1 cup	0.207
Beet greens	1 cup	0.190
Kale	1 cup	0.179
Rutabagas	1 cup	0.173
Cabbage	1 cup	0.168
Dandelion greens	1 cup	0.168
Scallop or Pattypan squash	1 cup	0.153
Spaghetti squash	1 cup	0.153
Swiss chard	1 cup	0.149
White mushrooms	1 cup	0.148
Parsnips	1 cup	0.145
Zucchini	1 cup	0.144
Crookneck and Straightneck squash	1 cup	0.140
Mustard greens	1 cup	0.137
Artichokes	1 cup	0.136
Celery	1 cup	0.129
Leeks	1 cup	0.118
Summer squash, all varieties averaged	1 cup	0.117
Beets	1 cup	0.114
Pumpkin	1 cup	0.108
Turnips	1 cup	0.105
Split peas	1 cup	0.094
Eggplant	1 cup	0.085

RDA is 1.3 to 1.7 mg for adults

VITAMIN B6

Continued

Green beans	1 cup	0.070
Napa cabbage	1 cup	0.040
Asparagus	1 cup	0.036

Vegetables, Frozen	Amount	Vitamin B6 (mg)
Brussels sprouts	1 cup	0.448
Spinach	1 cup	0.258
Broccoli	1 cup	0.239
Green peas	1 cup	0.181
Butternut squash	1 cup	0.166
Yellow corn	1 cup	0.162
Asparagus	1 cup	0.142
Carrots	1 cup	0.123
Turnip greens	1 cup	0.110
Okra	1 cup	0.068
Rhubarb	1 cup	0.048

Vegetables, Raw	Amount	Vitamin B6 (mg)
Red bell peppers	1 cup	0.434
Green bell peppers	1 cup	0.334
Yellow bell peppers	1 large	0.312
Summer squash	1 cup	0.246
Mustard spinach	1 cup	0.229
Butternut squash	1 cup	0.216
Onions	1 cup	0.192
Cauliflower	1 cup	0.184
Zucchini	1 cup	0.184
Kale	1 cup	0.182
Snow peas	1 cup	0.157
Broccoli	1 cup	0.154
Carrots	1 cup	0.152
Red cabbage	1 cup	0.146
Tomatoes	1 cup	0.144
Dandelion greens	1 cup	0.138
Bok-Choy	1 cup	0.136
Savoy cabbage	1 cup	0.133
Tomatoes, cherry	1 cup	0.119
Celery	1 cup	0.089
Cabbage	1 cup	0.087
Tomatillos	1 cup	0.074
White mushrooms	1 cup	0.073
Raab broccoli	1 cup	0.068
Green onions & scallions	1 cup	0.061
Prickley pear cactus pads	1 cup	0.060

RDA is 1.3 to 1.7 mg for adults

VITAMIN B6

Continued

Spinach	1 cup	0.059
Green leaf lettuce	1 cup	0.050
Butterhead & boston lettuce	1 cup	0.045
Watercress	1 cup	0.044
Cucumbers	1 cup	0.042
Romaine lettuce	1 cup	0.041
Belgian endive	1 cup	0.038
Swiss chard	1 cup	0.036
Shiitake mushrooms, dried	1 cup	0.035
Chicory greens	1 cup	0.030
Red leaf lettuce	1 cup	0.028
Spirulina, dried	1 tbsp	0.025
Iceberg lettuce	1 cup	0.023
Radicchio	1 cup	0.023
Arugula	1 cup	0.015

Yogurt	Amount	Vitamin B6 (mg)
Plain yogurt, skim milk	8 oz	0.120
Plain yogurt, low fat milk	8 oz	0.111
Plain Greek yogurt, nonfat	8 oz	0.107
Plain yogurt, whole milk	8 oz	0.073

Nutrient Data Collection Form

Food	Amount	Book Numbers	Multiply By	Estimated Nutrient Intake
Nutrient::	RDA:	Estimated:	% of RDA:	Total Estimated:

VITAMIN B12

Vitamin B12 known as cobalamine is the last of the water soluble B-complex vitamins. It is the only B-vitamin we cannot get from plants. Vitamin B12 is an essential nutrient that must be supplied by dietary meat or dairy products. It is needed for development and maintenance of red blood cells, DNA synthesis, and the entire nervous system.

The earliest deficiency symptoms may be mouth and tongue sores that clear up after a month and a feeling of being weak and tired. As deficiency continues pale skin, sore swollen red tongue and/or bleeding gums may appear. Long-term deficiencies results in neurological destruction of nerve endings and bone-disorders with symptoms including depression, poor memory, loss of balance, impaired urination like incontinence, and numbness and tingling of hands, feet, and toes.

The classical vitamin B12 deficiency most commonly discussed is in association with a condition known as pernicious anemia, which is a decrease in normal red blood cells that occurs when your intestines cannot properly absorb vitamin B12.

Vitamin B-12 is stored in the liver, and body reserves last for years, but after depletion blood levels may appear within normal ranges. For this reason a slow deterioration of nerve cells could be taking place without any symptoms.

VITAMIN B12

The recommended daily allowance, RDA, are in micrograms, mcg.

Recommend Daily Intakes Levels for Vitamin B12

Children	B12, mcg
1 to 3 year olds	.9
4 to 8 year olds	1.2

Males	
9 to 13 year olds	1.8
14 to 18 year olds	2.4
19 to 30 years	2.4
31 to 50 years	2.4
51 to 70 years	2.4
Over 70	2.4

Females	
9 to 13 year olds	1.8
14 to 18 year olds	2.4
19 to 30 years	2.4
31 to 50 years	2.4
51 to 70 years	2.4
Over 70	2.4
Pregnancy	2.6
Lactation	2.8

VITAMIN B12

Alcohol	Amount	Vitamin B12 (mcg)
White Wine	1 glass	0
Red Wine	1 glass	0
Light Beer	1 bottle	0
Regular Beer	1 bottle	0
Gin, Rum, Vodka, or Whisky	1 shot	0

Beans, Canned	Amount	Vitamin B12 (mcg)
Baked beans, plain	1 cup	0
Black-eyed peas	1 cup	0
Cranberry beans	1 cup	0
Fava beans	1 cup	0
Garbanzo beans	1 cup	0
Great Northern	1 cup	0
Green beans	1 cup	0
Lima beans, large	1 cup	0
Navy beans	1 cup	0
Pinto beans	1 cup	0
Red kidney beans	1 cup	0
Refried beans	1 cup	0
White beans	1 cup	0
Yellow beans	1 cup	0

Beans, Cooked	Amount	Vitamin B12 (mcg)
Adzuki	1 cup	0
Black beans	1 cup	0
Black Turtle beans, mature	1 cup	0
Black-eyed peas	1 cup	0
Cranberry beans	1 cup	0
Edamame	1 cup	0
Fava beans	1 cup	0
Garbanzo beans, chickpeas	1 cup	0
Great Northern	1 cup	0
Green beans	1 cup	0
Hyacinath beans	1 cup	0
Kidney beans	1 cup	0
Lentils	1 cup	0
Lima beans	1 cup	0
Lupini beans	1 cup	0
Mothbeans	1 cup	0
Mung beans, mature seeds	1 cup	0
Natto	1 cup	0
Navy beans	1 cup	0
Pigeon peas	1 cup	0

RDA is 2.4 mcg for adults

VITAMIN B12

Pinto beans	1 cup	0
Soybeans, green	1 cup	0
Soybeans, matured	1 cup	0
Soybeans, matured, dry roasted	1 cup	0
Split peas	1 cup	0
White beans, mature	1 cup	0
White beans, small	1 cup	0
Winged beans	1 cup	0
Yardlong beans, Chinese long beans	1 cup	0
Yellow beans	1 cup	0

Beef, Cooked	Amount	Vitamin B12 (mcg)
Flat Iron Steak	3 oz	4.39
Filet Mignon, trim to 0" fat	3 oz	3.48
Skirt Steak, trim to 0" fat	3 oz	3.16
Ribeye steak, lean, trim 0" fat	3 oz	2.65
Tri Tip steak, lean, trim to 0" fat	3 oz	2.45
Ground beef, 75%	3 oz	2.39
Ground beef, 80%	3 oz	2.32
London Broil, top round, trim to 0" fat	3 oz	2.30
Ground beef, 85%	3 oz	2.24
Beef ribs, trim to 1/8" fat	3 oz	2.18
Ground beef, 90%	3 oz	2.18
Ground beef, 95%	3 oz	2.10
Brisket, lean, trim to 0" fat	3 oz	2.06
Chuck roast, trim to 1/8" fat	3 oz	1.93
T-Bone steak, trim 0" fat	3 oz	1.86
Porterhouse steak, trim to 0" fat	3 oz	1.85
Top Sirloin, lean, trim to 1/8" fat	3 oz	1.43
Flank steak, lean, trim to 0" fat	3 oz	1.36

Beef, Cooked	Amount	Vitamin B12 (mcg)
Skirt steak, trim to 0" fat	1 lb	16.87
Tri Tip steak, lean, trim to 0" fat	1 lb	13.06
Beef ribs, trim to 1/8" fat	1 lb	11.62
Brisket, lean, trim to 0" fat	1 lb	10.99
Chuck roast, trim to 1/8" fat	1 lb	10.31
T-bone steak, trim to 0" fat	1 lb	9.93
Porterhouse steak, trim to 0" fat	1 lb	9.89
Flank steak, lean, trim to 0" fat	1 lb	7.26
Top Sirloin, trim to 1/8" fat	1 lb	7.22
Ribeye steak, boneless, trim to 0" fat	1 steak	6.58
Flank steak, lean, trim to 0" fat	1 steak	6.13
Filet Mignon, tenderloin, trim to 0" fat	1 steak	4.80

RDA is 2.4 mcg for adults

Top Sirloin, choice filet, trim to 0" fat	1 filet	4.71
Ribeye filet, lean, trim to 0" fat	1 filet	4.40

Beef, Ground, Cooked	Amount	Vitamin B12 (mcg)
Ground beef, 80%	1/4 lb patty	2.10
Ground beef, 90%	1/4 lb patty	2.10
Ground beef, 85%	1/4 lb patty	2.03
Ground beef, 95%	1/4 lb patty	2.03
Ground beef, 75%	1/4 lb patty	1.97

Bread	Amount	Vitamin B12 (mcg)
All types	1 serving	0

Butter	Amount	Vitamin B12 (mcg)
Regular dairy butter, salted	1 tbsp	0.02
Regular dairy whipped butter, salted	1 tbsp	0.01

Cereal, General Mills®	Amount	Vitamin B12 (mcg)
Total Whole Grain	1 cup	8.00
Total Raisin Bran	1 cup	5.99
Total Cranberry Crunch	1 cup	4.80
Wheaties	1 cup	4.00
Lucky Charms	1 cup	2.45
Corn Chex	1 cup	2.39
Chocolate Chex	1 cup	2.13
Raisin Nut Bran	1 cup	2.03
Cocoa Puffs	1 cup	2.02
Dora The Explorer	1 cup	2.02
Cookie Crisp	1 cup	2.01
Reese's Puffs	1 cup	2.01
Wheat Chex	1 cup	2.01
Cinnamon Chex	1 cup	2.00
Honey Nut Chex	1 cup	2.00
Golden Grams	1 cup	1.98
Cinnamon Toast Crunch	1 cup	1.78
Rice Chex	1 cup	1.51
Trix	1 cup	1.50
Basic 4	1 cup	1.48
Honey Nut Clusters	1 cup	1.48
Kix	1 cup	1.37
Multi-Bran Chex	1 cup	1.30
Berry Berry Kix	1 cup	1.19
Oatmeal Crisp, Crunchy Almond	1 cup	0
Oatmeal Crisp, Hearty Raisin	1 cup	0

RDA is 2.4 mcg for adults

VITAMIN B12

Cereal, General Mills Cheerios®	Amount	Vitamin B12 (mcg)
Multi Grain	1 cup	6.20
Yogurt Burst	1 cup	4.00
Banana Nut	1 cup	2.02
Chocolate	1 cup	2.02
Crunch & Oat Clusters	1 cup	2.02
Apple Cinnamon	1 cup	2.00
Berry Burst	1 cup	2.00
Frosted	1 cup	2.00
Fruity	1 cup	2.00
Original	1 cup	1.86
Honey Nut	1 cup	1.60

Cereal, General Mills Fiber One®	Amount	Vitamin B12 (mcg)
Original Bran	1 cup	3.02
Honey Clusters	1 cup	1.51
Caramel Delight	1 cup	1.50
Frosted Shredded Wheat	1 cup	1.50
Raisin Bran Clusters	1 cup	1.49

Cereal, Kashi®	Amount	Vitamin B12 (mcg)
Heart to Heart, Honey Toasted Oat	1 cup	8.01
Heart to Heart, Warm Cinnamon	1 cup	7.79
Heart to Heart, Wild Blueberry	1 cup	6.05
Kashi U	1 cup	6.05
7-Whole Grain Honey Puffs	1 cup	0
7-Whole Grain Puffs	1 cup	0
Berry Blossom	1 cup	0
Go Lean	1 cup	0
Go Lean Crunch,	1 cup	0
Go Lean Crunch, Honey Almond Flax	1 cup	0
Good Friends	1 cup	0
Good Friends, Cinna-Raisin Crunch	1 cup	0
Honey Sunshine	1 cup	0
Autum Wheat	1 cup	0

Cereal, Kellogg's®	Amount	Vitamin B12 (mcg)
All-Bran Bran Buds	1 cup	18.02
All-Bran Original	1 cup	11.66
MUESLIX	1 cup	9.03
All-Bran Complete Wheat Flakes	1 cup	8.00
Product 19	1 cup	6.00
Smart Start, Strong Heart, Antioxidants	1 cup	6.00
Frosted Flakes	1 cup	3.40

RDA is 2.4 mcg for adults

VITAMIN B12

Continued

Fiberplus Cinnamon Oat Crunch	1 cup	2.82
Raisin Bran	1 cup	2.54
Fiberplus Berry Yogurt Crunch	1 cup	2.12
Rice Krispies	1 cup	2.10
Cracklin' Oat Bran	1 cup	2.03
Crunchy Nut Roasted Nut & Honey O's	1 cup	2.02
Honey Smacks	1 cup	2.02
Frosted Rice Krispies	1 cup	2.00
Honey Crunch Corn Flakes	1 cup	2.00
Cocoa Krispies	1 cup	1.98
Crunchy Nut Golden Honey Nut Flakes	1 cup	1.98
Krave Chocolate	1 cup	1.98
Crispix	1 cup	1.80
CINNABON	1 cup	1.62
Apple Jacks	1 cup	1.51
Corn Flakes	1 cup	1.51
Froot Loops	1 cup	1.51
Corn Pops	1 cup	1.50
Smorz	1 cup	1.50
Raisin Bran Crunch	1 cup	1.48
Rice Krispies Treats	1 cup	1.40
Frosted MINI-Wheat's, Big-Bite	1 cup	1.08

Cereal, Kellogg's Special-K®	Amount	Vitamin B12 (mcg)
Original	1 cup	6.01
Low fat Granolia	1 cup	4.16
Multigrain Oats & Honey	1 cup	3.14
Chocolately Delight	1 cup	2.89
Vanilla Almond	1 cup	2.84
Fruit & Yogurt	1 cup	2.82
Blueberry	1 cup	2.80
Cinnamon Pecan	1 cup	2.80
Protein Plus	1 cup	2.78
Red Berries	1 cup	2.11

Cereal, Post®	Amount	Vitamin B12, mcg
Grape-Nuts Cereal	1 cup	7.3
Bran Flakes	1 cup	2.0
Cocoa Pebbles	1 cup	2.0
Fruity Pebbles	1 cup	2.0
Golden Crisp	1 cup	2.0
Grape-Nuts Flakes	1 cup	2.0
Great Grains, Crunchy Pecan	1 cup	2.0
Great Grains, Raisins, Date & Pecan	1 cup	2.0
Great Grains, Cranberry Almond Crunch	1 cup	2.0

RDA is 2.4 mcg for adults

VITAMIN B12

Alpha-Bits	1 cup	1.5
Great Grains, Banana Nut Crunch	1 cup	1.5
Honey Nut Shredded Wheat	1 cup	1.5
Raisin Bran	1 cup	1.5
Shredded Wheat, Frosted, spoon-size	1 cup	1.5
Blueberry Morning	1 cup	1.2
Honeycomb Cereal	1 cup	1.0
Shredded Wheat, Original, big-biscuit	1 biscuit	1
Shredded Wheat n' Bran, spoon-size	1 cup	0
Shredded Wheat, Original, spoon-size	1 cup	0

Post® Honey Bunches of Oats®	Amount	Vitamin B12, mcg
Honey Roasted	1 cup	3.87
Just Bunches Honey Roasted	1 cup	2.21
Pecan Bunches	1 cup	2.01
With Almonds	1 cup	2.01
With Cinnamon Bunches	1 cup	2.00
With Strawberries	1 cup	1.98
With Vanilla Bunches	1 cup	1.51

Cereal, Quaker®	Amount	Vitamin B12 (mcg)
Ganola Oats, Wheat and Honey	1 cup	0.17
Low Fat Granola with Raisins	1 cup	0.05
CAP'N Crunch	1 cup	0
CAP'N Crunch with Crunch Berries	1 cup	0
CAP'N Crunch's Peanut Butter	1 cup	0
Cinnamon Oatmeal Squares	1 cup	0
Crunchy Bran	1 cup	0
Honey Graham OH'S	1 cup	0
Oat Cinnamon Life	1 cup	0
Oatmeal Squares	1 cup	0
Shreaded Wheat, plain	1 cup	0

Cheese	Amount	Vitamin B12 (mcg)
Cottage cheese, lowfat, 1%	1 cup	1.42
Cottage cheese, lowfat, 2%	1 cup	1.02
Cottage cheese, creamed, small curd	1 cup	0.97
Ricotta, whole milk	1 cup	0.84
Ricotta, part skim milk	1 cup	0.71
Cottage cheese, nonfat, uncreamed	1 cup	0.67

RDA is 2.4 mcg for adults

VITAMIN B12

Cheese	Amount	Vitamin B12 (mcg)
Swiss	1 oz	0.95
Mozzarella, part skim milk, low moisture	1 oz	0.65
Mozzarella, whole milk	1 oz	0.65
Parmesan, grated	1 oz	0.64
Feta	1 oz	0.48
Fotina	1 oz	0.48
Brie cheese	1 oz	0.47
Swiss, low fat	1 oz	0.47
Gruyere	1 oz	0.45
Gouda	1 oz	0.44
American, pasteurized process, fortified	1 oz	0.43
Muenster	1 oz	0.42
Muenster, low fat	1 oz	0.41
Provolone	1 oz	0.41
Provolone, reduced fat	1 oz	0.41
Blue cheese	1 oz	0.35
Romano	1 oz	0.32
Cream cheese, fat free	1 oz	0.27
Mozzarella, nonfat	1 oz	0.26
Cheddar	1 oz	0.24
Monterey	1 oz	0.24
Colby	1 oz	0.23
Monterey, low fat	1 oz	0.23
American, pasteurized process, low fat	1 oz	0.22
American, pasteurized process, imitation	1 oz	0.20
Roquefort	1 oz	0.18
Cheddar, lowfat	1 oz	0.14
Cream cheese	1 oz	0.07
Goat cheese, semisoft	1 oz	0.06
Goat cheese, soft type	1 oz	0.05
Goat cheese, hard type	1 oz	0.03
Cheez Whiz, pasteurized process	1 oz	x
Velveeta, pasteurized process	1 oz	x

Cheese, Mexican	Amount	Vitamin B12 (mcg)
Queso fresco	1 oz	0.48
Mexican, blend, reduced fat	1 oz	0.47
Queso anejo	1 oz	0.39
Mexican, blend	1 oz	0.35
Queso chihuahua	1 oz	0.29
Queso asadero	1 oz	0.28

RDA is 2.4 mcg for adults

VITAMIN B12

Chicken, Cooked	Amount	Vitamin B12 (mcg)
Breast, no skin	1/2 breast	0.3
Breast, skin, fried with flour	1/2 breast	0.3
Drumstick, with skin, fried	1 drumstick	0.2
Thigh, no skin	1 thigh	0.2
Thigh,with skin, fried	1 thigh	0.2
Drumstick, no skin	1 drumstick	0.1

Chicken, Cooked	Amount	Vitamin B12 (mcg)
Thigh with skin, roasted	3 oz	0.36
Drumstick with skin, roasted	3 oz	0.35
Thigh meat only, no skin, roasted	3 oz	0.34
Drumstick meat only, no skin, roasted	3 oz	0.33
Breast with skin, fried with flour	3 oz	0.29
Breast with skin, roasted	3 oz	0.29
Wing meat only, no skin, roasted	3 oz	0.29
Breast meat only, no skin, roasted	3 oz	0.27
Drumstick with skin, fried in flour	3 oz	0.27
Cornish game hens, meat only	3 oz	0.26
Thigh with skin, fried with flour	3 oz	0.26
Wing with skin, roasted	3 oz	0.25
Wing with skin, fried in flour	3 oz	0.24

Eggs	Amount	Vitamin B12 (mcg)
Egg whole, hard-boiled	1 large	0.6
Egg whole, scrambled	1 large	0.5
Egg whole, fried	1 large	0.4
Egg whole, poached	1 large	0.4
Egg yolk	1 large	0.3
Egg substitute, liquid, fat free	1/4 cup	0.2
Egg whites, dried	1 ounce	0.05
Egg whites, dried powder, stabilized	1 tbsp	0.04
Egg whites	1 large	0

Fish, Canned	Amount	Vitamin B12 (mcg)
Atlantic Sardines, in oil	3 oz	7.60
Light tuna, in water	3 oz	2.17
Light tuna, in oil	3 oz	1.90
White (albacore) tuna , in oil	3 oz	1.87
White (albacore) tuna , in water	3 oz	1.00

RDA is 2.4 mcg for adults

VITAMIN B12

Fish, Cooked	Amount	Vitamin B12 (mcg)
Atlantic mackerel	3 oz	16.15
King mackerel	3 oz	15.30
Bluefin tuna	3 oz	9.25
Spanish mackerel	3 oz	5.95
Rainbow trout, wild	3 oz	5.36
Sockeye salmon	3 oz	4.80
Coho salmon, wild	3 oz	4.25
Pink salmon	3 oz	4.02
Atlantic herring, pickeled	3 oz	3.60
Pacific mackerel	3 oz	3.60
Rainbow trout, farmed	3 oz	3.49
Atlantic pollock	3 oz	3.13
Walleye pollock	3 oz	3.11
Keta (chum) salmon	3 oz	2.94
Chinook salmon, smoked	3 oz	2.77
Coho salmon, farmed	3 oz	2.69
Atlantic salmon, wild	3 oz	2.59
Catfish, wild	3 oz	2.46
Chinook salmon	3 oz	2.44
Atlantic salmon, farmed	3 oz	2.38
Catfish, farmed	3 oz	2.36
Alaskan halibut	3 oz	2.17
Yellowfin tuna	3 oz	2.00
Freshwater bass	3 oz	1.96
Pacific cod	3 oz	1.96
Walleye pike	3 oz	1.96
Northern pike	3 oz	1.95
Skipjack (aku) tuna	3 oz	1.86
Haddock	3 oz	1.81
Atlantic croaker	3 oz	1.78
Catfish, breaded & fried	3 oz	1.60
Tilapia	3 oz	1.58
Atlantic perch	3 oz	1.46
Swordfish	3 oz	1.40
Carp	3 oz	1.25
Flounder	3 oz	1.10
Halibut	3 oz	1.10
Atlantic & Pacific halibut	3 oz	1.08
Yellowtail	3 oz	1.06
Florida pompano	3 oz	1.02
Atlantic cod	3 oz	0.89
Greenland halibut	3 oz	0.82
Grouper	3 oz	0.59
Orange roughy	3 oz	0.40

RDA is 2.4 mcg for adults

VITAMIN B12

Fish, Shellfish, Cooked	Amount	Vitamin B12 (mcg)
Clams, breaded & fried	3 oz	34.23
Octopus	3 oz	30.60
Eastern oysters, farmed	3 oz	20.66
Clams, canned	3 oz	15.84
Oysters, breaded & fried	3 oz	13.29
Eastern oysters, wild	3 oz	10.97
Alaskan king crab	3 oz	9.78
Queen crab	3 oz	8.82
Blue crab cakes	3 oz	5.05
Blue crab	3 oz	2.83
Crab, blue, canned	3 oz	2.83
Crayfish	3 oz	1.83
Shrimp, breaded & fried	3 oz	1.59
Shrimp	3 oz	1.41
Northern lobster	3 oz	1.22
Scallops, breaded & fried	3 oz	1.12
Squid, fried	3 oz	1.05
Shrimp, canned	3 oz	0.63
Abalone	3 oz	0.59
Alaskan king crab, imitation	3 oz	0.48

Fruit	Amount	Vitamin B12 (mcg)
All types	1 cup	0

Game Meat, Cooked	Amount	Vitamin B12 (mcg)
Antelope	3 oz	x
Elk, roasted	3 oz	x
Caribou	3 oz	5.64
Rabbit	3 oz	5.53
Squirrel	3 oz	5.53
Elk, ground	3 oz	2.18
Deer, ground	3 oz	1.97
Bison, ground	3 oz	1.94
Buffalo, steak, free range	3 oz	1.42
Wild boar	3 oz	0.60
Duck	3 oz	0.34

Grains, Cooked	Amount	Vitamin B12 (mcg)
All types	1 cup	0

Herbs & Spices	Amount	Vitamin B12 (mcg)
All types	1 tsp	0

RDA is 2.4 mcg for adults

VITAMIN B12

Juice	Amount	Vitamin B12 (mcg)
All types	1 cup	0

Lamb, Cooked	Amount	Vitamin B12 (mcg)
Cubed, for stew or kabob	3 oz	2.58
Rib, lean, trim to 1/4" fat	3 oz	2.24
Ground	3 oz	2.22
Leg, whole, trim to 1/4 " fat	3 oz	2.20
Chops, loin, lean, trim to 1/4" fat	3 oz	2.10
Foreshank, trim to 1/8" fat	3 oz	1.94

Milk	Amount	Vitamin B12 (mcg)
Sheep milk	1 cup	1.7
Canned, condensed, sweet	1 cup	1.3
Reduced fat, 2%	1 cup	1.3
Non fat, fat free or skim milk	1 cup	1.2
Low fat 1%	1 cup	1.1
Whole milk , 3.25%	1 cup	1.1
Dry, instant, non fat	1/3 cup	0.9
Canned, evaporated, non fat	1 cup	0.6
Buttermilk, low fat	1 cup	0.5
Canned, evaporated	1 cup	0.4
Goat milk	1 cup	0.2
Human milk	1 cup	0.1
Coconut milk, canned	1 cup	0
Soy milk, original & vanila, unfortified	1 cup	0

Nuts & Seeds	Amount	Vitamin B12 (mcg)
All types	1 oz	0

Pork, Cooked	Amount	Vitamin B12 (mcg)
Braunschweiger	3 oz	17.08
Liverwurst spread	1/4 cup	7.40
Italian sausage	3 oz	1.10
Spareribs	3 oz	0.92
Polish sausage	3 oz	0.83
Chops, lean pan-fried	3 oz	0.68
Chops, pan-fried	3 oz	0.67
Canadian-style bacon	3 oz	0.66
Sirloin pork chops	3 oz	0.64
Backribs	3 oz	0.63
Bratwurst	3 oz	0.62
Cured ham, lean	3 oz	0.60

VITAMIN B12

Continued

Cured ham	3 oz	0.54
Center loin pork chops	3 oz	0.50
Chops, broiled	3 oz	0.50
Tenderloin	3 oz	0.48
Canadian-style bacon	2 slices	0.4
Sausage	1 patty	0.3
Sausage	2 links	0.3
Bacon	3 slices	0.2

Turkey, Cooked	Amount	Vitamin B12 (mcg)
Ground turkey, 93% lean	3 oz	1.53
Dark meat	3 oz	1.40
Ground turkey, 85% lean	3 oz	1.19
Ground turkey	3 oz	1.14
Ground turkey, fat free	3 oz	0.57
Breast meat	3 oz	0.33
Light meat	3 oz	0.31
Turkey bacon	3 oz	0.31
Turkey sausage, reduced fat	3 oz	0.24

Veal, Cooked	Amount	Vitamin B12 (mcg)
Foreshank	3 oz	1.37
Breast	3 oz	1.26
Rib	3 oz	1.24
Sirloin	3 oz	1.21
Ground	3 oz	1.08
Loin	3 oz	1.05
Leg, top round	3 oz	0.99

VEGETABLES	Amount	Vitamin B12 (mcg)
All types	1 cup	0

Yogurt	Amount	Vitamin B12 (mcg)
Greek, plain, non fat	8 oz	1.7

RDA is 2.4 mcg for adults

Nutrient Data Collection Form

Food	Amount	Book Numbers	Multiply By	Estimated Nutrient Intake
Nutrient::	RDA:	Estimated:	% of RDA:	Total Estimated:

To download additional forms for free, go to www.TopNutrients4U.com

NOTES

VITAMIN C

Vitamin C known as <u>ascorbic acid</u> is a water soluble vitamin needed daily in milligrams. It is needed for repair and maintenance of bones and teeth, and for the growth, development, and protection of blood vessels, joints, ligaments, and tendons. Vitamin C is most commonly known for its antioxidant capabilities since it is known to protect artery walls against oxidative damage. Vitamin-C is nature's water soluble anti-oxidant. However, it is a mischaracterization to think of vitamin-C solely as an antioxidant since it has so many different functions. Deficiency is associated with scurvy, cancer, heart disease, and high blood pressure. Deficiency symptoms include anemia, bleeding gums with loose teeth, joint pains and swelling, slow wound healing, and frequent infections

The recommended daily allowance, RDA, for vitamin C are in milligrams, mg.

Recommend Daily Intake Levels for Vitamin C

Children	Vitamin C, mg
1 to 3 year olds	15
4 to 8 year olds	25
Males	
9 to 13 year olds	45
14 to 18 year olds	75
19 to 30 years	90
31 to 50 years	90
51 to 70 years	90
Over 70	90
Females	
9 to 13 year olds	45
14 to 18 year olds	65
19 to 30 years	75
31 to 50 years	75
51 to 70 years	75
Over 70	75
Pregnancy	85
Lactation	120

VITAMIN C

Alcohol	Amount	Vitamin C (mg)
White Wine	1 glass	0
Red Wine	1 glass	0
Light Beer	1 bottle	0
Regular Beer	1 bottle	0
Gin, Rum, Vodka, or Whisky	1 shot	0

Beans, Canned	Amount	Vitamin C (mg)
Refried beans	1 cup	14
Yellow beans	1 cup	7
Black-eyed peas	1 cup	7
Fava beans	1 cup	5
Green beans	1 cup	4
Great Northern	1 cup	3
Cranberry beans	1 cup	2
Kidney beans	1 cup	2
Navy beans	1 cup	2
Pinto beans	1 cup	2
Garbanzo beans	1 cup	0
Baked beans, plain	1 cup	0
Lima beans	1 cup	0
White beans, mature	1 cup	0

Beans, Cooked	Amount	Vitamin C (mg)
Soybeans, green	1 cup	31.0
Natto	1 cup	22.0
Yardlong beans, Chinese long beans	1 cup	16.8
Green beans	1 cup	12.1
Yellow beans	1 cup	12.1
Edamame	1 cup	9.5
Soybeans, matured, dry roasted	1 cup	4.3
Lentils	1 cup	3.0
Soybeans, matured	1 cup	2.9
Great Northern	1 cup	2.3
Garbanzo beans, chickpeas	1 cup	2.1
Kidney beans	1 cup	2.1
Mung beans, mature seeds	1 cup	2.0
Lupini beans	1 cup	1.8
Mothbeans	1 cup	1.8
Mungo beans, mature seeds	1 cup	1.8
Navy beans	1 cup	1.6
Pinto beans	1 cup	1.4
Split peas	1 cup	0.8
Black-eyed peas	1 cup	0.7

VITAMIN C

Fava beans	1 cup	0.5
Adzuki	1 cup	0
Black beans	1 cup	0
Cranberry beans	1 cup	0
Hyacinth beans	1 cup	0
Lima beans	1 cup	0
Black Turtle beans, mature	1 cup	0
Pigeon peas	1 cup	0
White beans, mature	1 cup	0
White beans, small	1 cup	0
Winged beans	1 cup	0

Beaf, Cooked	Amount	Vitamin C (mg)
All types	3 oz	0

Bread	Amount	Vitamin C (mg)
English Muffin, plain	1 muffin	1.0
Bagel, plain	4" bagel	0.9
Bagel, cinnamon & raisins	4" bagel	0.6
Bagel, egg	4" bagel	0.5
Mexican roll, bollilo	1 roll	0.2
Bagel, oat bran	4" bagel	0.2
Cornbread, dry mix	1 piece	0.1
French, sourdough	1 slice	0.1
Reduced calorie rye	1 slice	0.1
Reduced calorie wheat	1 slice	0.1
Rye bread	1 slice	0.1
Wheat	1 slice	0.1
Dinner Rolls, brown & serve	1 roll	0.1
Croissants, butter	1 each	0.1
Indian bread, Naan, whole wheat	1 piece	0
Bagel, wheat	4" bagel	0
Cracked Wheat	1 slice	0
Potato bread	1 slice	0
Egg bread	1 slice	0
Multi-Grain, and Whole-Grain	1 slice	0
Oatmeal bread	1 slice	0
Pita, white	6" pita	0
Pumpernickle	1 slice	0
Raisen bread, enriched	1 slice	0
Reduced calorie white	1 slice	0
White	1 slice	0
Whole-Wheat	1 slice	0
Italian	1 slice	0
Hamburger & Hotdog buns, plain	1 bun	0

RDA is 60 mg

VITAMIN C

Kaiser rolls	1 roll	0
Tortillas, flour	1 tortilla	0
Tortillas, corn	1 tortilla	0
Indian bread, Naan, plain	1 piece	x

Cereal, General Mills®	Amount	Vitamin C (mg)
Total Whole Grain	1 cup	80.0
Lucky Charms	1 cup	9.6
Corn Chex	1 cup	9.0
Chocolate Chex	1 cup	8.5
Cinnamon Chex	1 cup	8.0
Cocoa Puffs	1 cup	8.0
Cookie Crisp	1 cup	8.0
Dora The Explorer	1 cup	8.0
Golden Grams	1 cup	8.0
Honey Nut Chex	1 cup	8.0
Multi-Bran CHEX	1 cup	8.0
Reese's Puffs	1 cup	8.0
Wheat Chex	1 cup	8.0
Wheaties	1 cup	8.0
Cinnamon Toast Crunch	1 cup	7.1
Kix	1 cup	6.1
Honey Nut Clusters	1 cup	6.0
Rice Chex	1 cup	6.0
Trix	1 cup	6.0
Berry Berry Kix	1 cup	4.8
Basic 4	1 cup	0
Oatmeal Crisp, Crunchy Almond	1 cup	0
Oatmeal Crisp, Hearty Raisin	1 cup	0
Raisin Nut Bran	1 cup	0
Total Cranberry Crunch	1 cup	0
Total Raisin Bran	1 cup	0

Cereal, General Mills® Cheerios	Amount	Vitamin C (mg)
Banana Nut	1 cup	20
Chocolate	1 cup	20
Fruity	1 cup	20
Multi Grain	1 cup	16
Apple Cinnamon	1 cup	8
Berry Burst	1 cup	8
Frosted	1 cup	8
Crunch & Oat Clusters	1 cup	8
Honey Nut	1 cup	8
Yogurt Burst, Strawberry	1 cup	8
Original	1 cup	7

VITAMIN C

Cereal, General Mills Fiber One	Amount	Vitamin C (mg)
Original Bran	1 cup	12
Caramel Delight	1 cup	6
Honey Clusters	1 cup	0
Raisin Bran Clusters	1 cup	0
Frosted Shredded Wheat	1 cup	0

Cereal, Kashi®	Amount	Vitamin C (mg)
Heart to Heart, Honey Toasted Oat	1 cup	40.0
Heart to Heart, Warm Cinnamon	1 cup	39.2
Heart to Heart, Oat Flakes & Blueberry Clusters	1 cup	30.2
Strawberry Fields	1 cup	10.4
Berry Blossom	1 cup	2.4
Indigo Morning	1 cup	1.4
7-Whole Grain Flakes	1 cup	0
7-Whole Grain Honey Puffs	1 cup	0
7-Whole Grain Nuggets	1 cup	0
7-Whole Grain Puffs	1 cup	0
Autum Wheat	29 biscuits	0
Berry Fruitful	29 biscuits	0
Cinnamon Harvest	28 biscuits	0
Go Lean	1 cup	0
Go Lean Crisp, Cinnamon Crumble	1 cup	0
Go Lean Crisp, Toasted Berry Crumble	1 cup	0
Go Lean Crunch,	1 cup	0
Go Lean Crunch, Honey Almond Flax	1 cup	0
Good Friends	1 cup	0
Honey Sunshine	1 cup	0
Island Vanilla	27 biscuits	0
Simply Maize	1 cup	x

Cereal, Kellogg's®	Amount	Vitamin C (mg)
All-Bran Complete Wheat Flakes	1 cup	80
Product 19	1 cup	60
Cocoa Krispies	1 cup	20
Cracklin' Oat Bran	1 cup	20
Fiberplus Cinnamon Oat Crunch	1 cup	20
Frosted Rice Krispies	1 cup	20
Krave Chocolate	1 cup	20
CINNABON	1 cup	19
All-Bran Bran Buds	1 cup	18
Rice Krispies	1 cup	18
Froot Loops	1 cup	15
Apple Jacks	1 cup	15

RDA is 60 mg

VITAMIN C

Continued

Fiberplus Berry Yogurt Crunch	1 cup	15
Smart Start, Strong Heart Antioxidants	1 cup	15
Smorz	1 cup	15
All-Bran Original	1 cup	12
Frosted Flakes	1 cup	10
Crunchy Nut Golden Honey Nut Flakes	1 cup	8.3
Honey Smacks	1 cup	8.0
Honey Crunch Corn Flakes	1 cup	8.0
Rice Krispies Treats	1 cup	8.0
Crunchy Nut Roasted Nut & Honey O's	1 cup	7.9
Corn Flakes	1 cup	6.2
Corn Pops	1 cup	6.1
Crispix	1 cup	6.1
Raisin Bran Crunch	1 cup	1.6
MUESLIX	1 cup	0.3
Frosted MINI-Wheat's, Big-Bite	1 cup	0
Raisin Bran	1 cup	0

Cereal, Kellogg's Special-K®	Amount	Vitamin C (mg)
Multigrain Oats & Honey	1 cup	31
Vanilla Almond	1 cup	28
Fruit & Yogurt	1 cup	28
Chocolately Delight	1 cup	28
Blueberry	1 cup	28
Cinnamon Pecan	1 cup	28
Protein Plus	1 cup	28
Red Berries	1 cup	21
Original	1 cup	21
Low Fat Granola	1 cup	1

Cereal, Post®	Amount	Vitamin C, mg
Great Grains, Cranberry Almond Crunch	1 cup	16.0
Fruity Pebbles	1 cup	8.0
Alpha-Bits	1 cup	4.0
Shredded Wheat, Original, big-biscuit	1 biscuit	2.5
Raisin Bran	1 cup	0.5
Blueberry Morning	1 cup	0.4
Great Grains, Raisin, Date & Pecan	1 cup	0.4
Great Grains, Banana Nut Crunch	1 cup	0.1
Great Grains, Crunchy Pecan	1 cup	0.1
Bran Flakes	1 cup	0
Cocoa Pebbles	1 cup	0
Golden Crisp	1 cup	0
Grape-Nuts Cereal	1 cup	0
Grape-Nuts Flakes	1 cup	0

RDA is 60 mg

VITAMIN C

Honey Nut Shredded Wheat	1 cup	0
Honeycomb Cereal	1 cup	0
Shredded Wheat n' Bran, spoon-size	1 cup	0
Shredded Wheat, Frosted, spoon-size	1 cup	0
Shredded Wheat, Original, spoon-size	1 cup	0

Post® Honey Bunches of Oats®	Amount	Vitamin C (mg)
With Strawberries	1 cup	6.4
Pecan Bunches	1 cup	2.0
With Cinnamon Bunches	1 cup	0.2
Honey Roasted	1 cup	0
Just Bunches Honey Roasted	1 cup	0
With Almonds	1 cup	0
With Vanilla Bunches	1 cup	0

Cereal, Quaker®	Amount	Vitamin C (mg)
Oatmeal Squares, Golden Maple	1 cup	17.5
Honey Graham OH'S	1 cup	10.5
Oatmeal Squares, Cinnamon	1 cup	6.7
Oatmeal Squares	1 cup	6.4
Toasted Multigrain Crisp	1 cup	5.3
Granola Apple Cranberry Almond	1 cup	3.0
CAP'N Crunch's OOPs! All Berries	1 cup	0.1
CAP'N Crunch	1 cup	0
CAP'N Crunch with Crunch Berries	1 cup	0
CAP'N Crunch's Peanut Butter Crunch	1 cup	0
Crunchy Bran	1 cup	0
LIFE Cereal, Cinnamon	1 cup	0
LIFE Cereal, Maple & Brown Sugar	1 cup	0
LIFE Cereal, Original	1 cup	0
Puffed Rice	1 cup	0
Puffed Wheat	1 cup	0

Cereal, Cooked	Amount	Vitamin C (mg)
Malt-o-Meal, plain	1 serving	0.3
Farina	1 cup	0
CREAM OF WHEAT, regular	1 cup	0
Oats, regular, unenriched	1 cup	0
WHEATENA	1 cup	0
White corn grits	1 cup	0
Yellow corn grits	1 cup	0

RDA is 60 mg

VITAMIN C

Cheese	Amount	Vitamin C (mg)
All types	1 oz	0

Chicken, cooked	Amount	Vitamin C (mg)
All types	3 oz	0

Cream	Amount	Vitamin C (mg)
Half & Half	1 tbsp	0.1
Heavy cream	1 tbsp	0.1
Light Coffe cream	1 tbsp	0.1
Sour cream, cultured	1 tbsp	0.1
Sour cream, reduced fat	1 tbsp	0.1
Whipped topping, pressurized	1 tbsp	0.1

Eggs, Cooked	Amount	Vitamin C (mg)
All types	1 large	0

FISH	Amount	Vitamin C (mg)
All types	3 oz	0

Fruit, Canned	Amount	Vitamin C (mg)
Pineapple	1 cup	19
Apricots	1 cup	8
Peaches	1 cup	7
Applesauce, sweetened	1 cup	4
Pears	1 cup	3
Applesauce, unsweetened	1 cup	2
Plums	1 cup	1
Olives, black	5 large	0.2
Olives, green	5 large	0

Fruit, Dried	Amount	Vitamin C (mg)
Pears	1 cup	13
Peaches	1 cup	8
Currants	1 cup	7
Apples	1 cup	3
Figs	1 cup	2
Apricots	1 cup	1
Cranberries	1 cup	0.2

RDA is 60 mg

VITAMIN C

Fruit, Frozen	Amount	Vitamin C (mg)
Peaches	1 cup	236
Strawberries	1 cup	106
Raspberries	1 cup	41
Blackberries, unthawed	1 cup	5
Blueberries	1 cup	2

Fruit, Raw	Amount	Vitamin C (mg)
Black currants	1 cup	203
Kiwi	1 cup	167
Strawberries	1 cup	98
Navel oranges	1 cup	98
Papayas	1 cup	88
Valencias Oranges	1 cup	87
Florida Oranges	1 cup	83
Pineapple	1 cup	79
Grapefruit, pink & red, sections	1 cup	72
Mango	1 cup	60
Cantaloupe	1 cup	59
Elderberries	1 cup	52
Tangerine	1 cup	52
Mulberries	1 cup	51
Avocado, Florida	1 cup	40
Raspberries	1 cup	32
Honeydew	1 cup	31
Blackberries	1 cup	30
Plantains	1 cup	27
Jicama	1 cup	26
Avocado, California	1 cup	20
Pomegranates	1 cup	18
Grapes, red or green	1 cup	17
Apricots	1 cup	17
Plums	1 cup	16
Blueberries	1 cup	14
Cranberries	1 cup	13
Water Mellon	1 cup	12
Cherries	1 cup	11
Peaches	1 cup	10
Nectarine	1 cup	8
Stewed prunes	1 cup	7
Pears	1 cup	7
Apples	1 cup	6
Raisins	1 cup	3
Prunes, uncooked	1 cup	1
Dates	1 cup	1

RDA is 60 mg

VITAMIN C

Fruit, Raw	Amount	Vitamin C (mg)
Pummelo	1 fruit	371
Mango	1 fruit	122
Papayas	1 fruit	96
Navel Oranges	1 fruit	83
Kiwi	1 fruit	64
Florida Oranges	1 fruit	63
Valencias Oranges	1 fruit	59
Avocado, Florida	1 fruit	53
Grapefruit, pink & red, sections	1/2 fruit	38
Strawberries	5 fruit	35
Plantains	1 fruit	33
Star fruit, Carambola	1 fruit	31
Cherimoya	1 fruit	30
Pomegranates	1 fruit	29
Pineapple	1/2" x 3" slice"	24
Tangerine	1 fruit	24
Persimmons, small native	1 fruit	17
Chayote	1 fruit	16
Pineapple guava, Feijoa	1 fruit	14
Persimmons, Japanese	1 fruit	13
Avocado, California	1 fruit	12
Banana	1 fruit	10
Peaches	1 fruit	9
Kumquats	1 fruit	8
Nectarine	1 fruit	7
Apples	1 fruit	6
Plums	1 fruit	6
Pears	1 fruit	6
Cherries, no pits	10 fruit	6
Apricots	1 fruit	4
Raisins	1 small box	1
Prunes, uncooked	5 prunes	0
Raisins	1 packet	0
Olives, black	5 large	0
Dates	5 dates	0
Figs, dried	1 fig	0
Olives, green	5 large	0

Game Meat, Cooked	Amount	Vitamin C (mg)
All types	3 oz	0

Grains, Cooked	Amount	Vitamin C (mg)
All grains	1 cup	0

VITAMIN C

Herbs & Spices	Amount	Vitamin C (mg)
Coriander, dried	1 tsp	3.4
Tarragon, dried, ground	1 tsp	0.8
All-spice, ground	1 tsp	0.7
Rosemary, dried	1 tsp	0.7
Chives, raw, chopped	1 tsp	0.6
Parsley, dried	1 tsp	0.6
Saffron	1 tsp	0.6
Thyme, dried	1 tsp	0.6
Thyme, fresh	1 tsp	0.6
Turmeric, ground	1 tsp	0.6
Dill weed, dried	1 tsp	0.5
Onion powder	1 tsp	0.5
Anise seed	1 tsp	0.4
Caraway seeds	1 tsp	0.4
Coriander, seeds	1 tsp	0.4
Bay leaf, crumbled	1 tsp	0.3
Celery seeds	1 tsp	0.3
Chili powder	1 tsp	0.3
Curry powder	1 tsp	0.2
Sage, ground	1 tsp	0.2
Cinnamon powder	1 tsp	0.1
Ginger, ground	1 tsp	0.1
Basil, dried & ground	1 tsp	0
Cloves, dried, ground	1 tsp	0
Garlic powder	1 tsp	0
Oregano, dried	1 tsp	0
Paprika	1 tsp	0
Pepper, black, ground	1 tsp	0

Juice	Amount	Vitamin C (mg)
Orange juice, raw	1 cup	124
Cranberry	1 cup	107
Grapefruit juice, raw	1 cup	94
Lemon juice, raw	1 cup	94
Vegetable	1 cup	67
Tomato	1 cup	44
Pineapple	1 cup	25
Carrot	1 cup	20
Prune	1 cup	11
Apple	1 cup	2
Grape	1 cup	0.3
Pomegranate	1 cup	0.2

RDA is 60 mg

VITAMIN C

Lamb, Cooked	Amount	Vitamin C (mg)
All types	3 oz	0

Milk	Amount	Vitamin C (mg)
Human milk	1 cup	12
Sheep milk	1 cup	10
Canned, condensed, sweetened	1 cup	8
Canned, evaporated	1 cup	5
Goat milk	1 cup	3
Canned, evaporated, non fat	1 cup	3
Buttermilk, low fat	1 cup	2
Coconut milk, canned	1 cup	2
Dry, instant, non fat	1/3 cup	1
Reduced fat , 2%	1 cup	0.50
Lowfat, 1%	1 cup	0
Nonfat, fat free or skim	1 cup	0
Soy milk, original, unfortified	1 cup	0
Whole milk, 3.25%	1 cup	0

Nuts & Seeds	Amount	Vitamin C (mg)
Hazelnuts	1 oz	1.8
Pistachio	1 oz	1.6
Coconut, raw meat	1 oz	0.9
Black walnuts	1 oz	0.5
Chia seeds	1 oz	0.5
Pumpkin seeds	1 oz	0.5
English walnuts	1 oz	0.4
Sunflower seeds	1 oz	0.4
Macadamia	1 oz	0.3
Pecans	1 oz	0.3
Brazilnuts	1 oz	0.2
Flaxseeds	1 oz	0.2
Pine nuts	1 oz	0.2
Cashews	1 oz	0.1
Almonds	1 oz	0
Peanut butter, smooth style	1 oz	0
Peanuts	1 oz	0
Sesame seeds	1 oz	0
Tahini	1 oz	0

Nuts & Seeds	Amount	Vitamin C (mg)
Hazelnuts	1/4 cup	1.80
Pistachio	1/4 cup	1.70
Coconut, raw meat	1/4 cup	0.90

RDA is 60 mg

VITAMIN C

Continued

Pumpkin seeds	1/4 cup	0.60
Black walnuts	1/4 cup	0.50
Sunflower seeds	1/4 cup	0.50
Macadamia	1/4 cup	0.40
English walnuts	1/4 cup	0.30
Flaxseeds	1/4 cup	0.30
Pecans	1/4 cup	0.30
Pine nuts	1/4 cup	0.30
Brazilnuts	1/4 cup	0.20
Flaxseeds	1 tbsp	0.10
Almonds	1/4 cup	0
Peanut butter, smooth style	1/4 cup	0
Peanuts	1/4 cup	0
Sesame seeds	1/4 cup	0
Tahini	1/4 cup	0
Cashews	1/4 cup	x
Chia seeds	1/4 cup	x

Pork, Cooked	Amount	Vitamin C (mg)
Polish sausage	3 oz	0.9
Sausage	3 oz	0.6
Sausage	1 patty	0.2
Sausage	2 links	0.2
Italian sausage	3 oz	0.1
Spareribs	3 oz	0
Chops, lean pan-fried	3 oz	0
Chops, pan-fried	3 oz	0
Canadian-style bacon	3 oz	0
Backribs	3 oz	0
Bratwurst	3 oz	0
Cured ham, lean	3 oz	0
Cured ham	3 oz	0
Chops, broiled	3 oz	0
Canadian-style bacon	2 slices	0
Bacon	3 slices	0

Turkey, Cooked	Amount	Vitamin C (mg)
All types	3 oz	0

Vegetables, Canned	Amount	Vitamin C (mg)
Asparagus	1 cup	45
Sauerkraut	1 cup	35
Spinach	1 cup	31
Tomatoes	1 cup	22

RDA is 60 mg

VITAMIN C

Sweet potato	1 cup	21
Stewed tomatoes	1 cup	20
Corn	1 cup	17
Grean peas	1 cup	16
Pumpkin	1 cup	10
Beets	1 cup	7
Green beans	1 cup	6
Carrots	1 cup	4
Mushrooms	1 cup	0

Vegetables, Cooked	Amount	Vitamin C (mg)
Mustard Spinach	1 cup	117
Broccoli	1 cup	101
Brussels sprouts	1 cup	97
Kohlrabi	1 cup	89
Snow Peas	1 cup	77
Lambsquarters	1 cup	67
Cabbage	1 cup	56
Cauliflower	1 cup	55
Cabbage, Red	1 cup	52
Cabbage, Chinese, Bok-Choy	1 cup	44
Sweet potato, mashed	1 cup	42
Turnip greens	1 cup	40
Beet greens	1 cup	36
Mustard greens	1 cup	35
Collard greens	1 cup	35
Kale	1 cup	33
Rutabagas	1 cup	32
Swiss chard	1 cup	32
Butternut squash	1 cup	31
Raab broccoli	1 cup	31
Okra	1 cup	26
Broccolini	1 cup	25
Cabbage, Savoy	1 cup	25
Zucchini	1 cup	23
Acorn squash	1 cup	22
Crookneck and Straightneck squash	1 cup	21
Parsnips	1 cup	20
Hubbard squash	1 cup	20
Winter squash, all varieties, averaged	1 cup	20
Scallop or Pattypan squash	1 cup	19
Dandelion greens	1 cup	19
Turnips	1 cup	18
Spinach	1 cup	18
Potatoes, flesh, baked	1 cup	16

RDA is 60 mg

VITAMIN C

Continued

	Amount	Vitamin C (mg)
Yams, cubes	1 cup	16
Asparagus	1 cup	14
Potatoes, mashed with whole milk	1 cup	13
Artichokes	1 cup	12
Green beans	1 cup	12
Onions	1 cup	12
Pumpkin	1 cup	12
Summer squash	1 cup	10
Celery	1 cup	9
Yellow corn	1 cup	8
Prickley pear cactus pads (nopales)	1 cup	8
White mushrooms	1 cup	6
Beets	1 cup	6
Carrots	1 cup	6
Spaghetti squash	1 cup	5
Leeks	1 cup	4
Cabbage, Napa	1 cup	4
Eggplant	1 cup	1
Split peas	1 cup	1
Shitake mushrooms	1 cup	0

Vegetables, Frozen	Amount	Vitamin C (mg)
Broccoli	1 cup	74
Brussels sprouts	1 cup	71
Collard greens	1 cup	45
Asparagus	1 cup	44
Turnip greens	1 cup	36
Kale	1 cup	33
Okra	1 cup	18
Green peas	1 cup	16
Butternut squash	1 cup	8
Rhubarb	1 cup	8
Yellow corn	1 cup	6
Green beans	1 cup	6
Spinach	1 cup	4
Carrots	1 cup	3

Vegetables, Raw	Amount	Vitamin C (mg)
Yellow bell peppers	1 large	341
Mustard spinach	1 cup	195
Red bell peppers	1 cup	190
Green bell peppers	1 cup	120
Kale	1 cup	80
Broccoli	1 cup	79
Snow peas	1 cup	59

RDA is 60 mg

VITAMIN C

Continued

Cauliflower	1 cup	48
Red cabbage	1 cup	40
Bok-Choy	1 cup	32
Butternut squash	1 cup	29
Cabbage	1 cup	26
Tomatoes	1 cup	25
Savoy Cabbage	1 cup	22
Zucchini	1 cup	20
Tomatoes	1 cup	20
Dandelion greens	1 cup	19
Summer squash	1 cup	19
Green onions & scallions	1 cup	19
Tomatillos	1 cup	15
Watercress	1 cup	15
Onions	1 cup	12
Swiss chard	1 cup	11
Spinach	1 cup	8
Broccoli, raab	1 cup	8
Prickley pear cactus pads	1 cup	8
Chicory greens	1 cup	7
Carrots	1 cup	7
Green leaf lettuce	1 cup	5
Celery	1 cup	4
Endive	1 cup	3
Radicchio	1 cup	3
Arugula	1 cup	3
Cucumbers	1 cup	3
Belgian endive	1 cup	3
Romaine lettuce	1 cup	2
Butterhead & boston lettuce	1 cup	2
Iceburg lettuce	1 cup	2
White mushrooms	1 cup	2
Red leaf lettuce	1 cup	1
Spirulina, dried	1 tbsp	0.7
Shiitake mushrooms, dried	1 each	0.1

RDA is 60 mg

Nutrient Data Collection Form

Food	Amount	Book Numbers	Multiply By	Estimated Nutrient Intake
Nutrient::	RDA:	Estimated:	% of RDA:	Total Estimated:

To download additional forms for free, go to www.TopNutrients4U.com

VITAMIN D

Vitamin-D & Bone Disease

Vitamin-D is a fat soluble vitamin your body synthesizes when your skin is exposed to sunlight. It is commonly known because of its requirement for the absorption of calcium. By controlling calcium absorption, vitamin-D fulfills its primary function which is to maintain a constant supply of calcium circulating within the blood. It is estimated that only 15% of calcium intake can be absorbed without vitamin-D. Even if your diet is rich in calcium, the body cannot absorb an adequate amount without vitamin-D, and most of the calcium will pass through the body unused. Since calcium absorption is a requirement for the formation and maintenance of bones throughout life, vitamin-D may play a more important role than calcium.

Well-accepted studies have shown prevention of bone fractures when vitamin-D was taken with calcium. Calcium intake by itself did not reduce the risk of bone fractures, and long-term studies do not support benefits of a high intake of calcium in preventing the risk of bone fractures.

A severe vitamin-D deficiency will cause dangerously low levels of calcium circulating in the blood, known as hypocalcemia. When clinical symptoms appear, it will require emergency care.

Overall vitamin-D metabolism is regulated by blood levels of both phosphorus and the parathyroid hormones, and both are regulated by dietary intake of phosphorus.

In one experiment of healthy men, a high phosphorus intake reduced blood concentrations of vitamin-D. When dietary phosphorus was restricted for ten days, blood levels of vitamin-D increased immediately and within a week stabilized at almost twice the value than when phosphorus intake was normal. In a second experiment, a phosphorus restriction from 1500 mg to 500 mg increased concentrations of vitamin D by 80%.

In a third experiment, 7 healthy adult males participated in a dietary phosphorus restriction under strictly controlled and normal metabolic conditions. Blood levels of phosphorus and vitamin-D were measured hourly over a 24 hour period before and after the experiment. Results showed a phosphorus restriction from 2300mg /

day to 625 mg / day after 8 days increased blood levels of vitamin-D by 53%. Clearly, one must first manage dietary intake of phosphorus before considering the management of vitamin D.

It is difficult to meet your vitamin D needs from diet alone. Most foods that humans normally eat contain very little or no vitamin D. You could spend your whole life eating food that contains very little vitamin D, and as long as you had exposure to sunlight you could be healthy. You cannot say that about any other vitamin.

Vitamin D is unlike anything else with respect to classical nutrition which requires humans to eat food. Vitamin D does not require humans to eat food; it requires humans to have some exposure to sunlight since sunlight is a fundamental requirement for human survival.

Given concern about skin cancer, many are cautious regarding sun exposure. Exposure of arms and legs (with no sunscreen) for only 30 minutes twice a week between 10 AM and 3 PM could be adequate to prevent a vitamin D deficiency in a large percent of the population.

In a geriatric nursing home study, sun exposure three times a week for twelve weeks was as effective at increasing serum concentrations of vitamin D as was 400 IU / day of vitamin D supplements.

A vitamin D deficiency in the general public can become alarmingly high during the winter and spring depending on geography. People living at higher latitudes or in northern states are at increased risk of a deficiency and may require vitamin D supplemental support for a period of time simply because of where they live.

During childhood, deficiency may cause soft bones, growth retardation, and skeletal deformities; later in life it has been associated with hip fractures, muscle weakness, and depression. A prolonged deficiency leads to a bone softening disease known as osteomalacia, common in the elderly who are too often confined indoors. Chronic deficiency is associated with increased incidences of osteoporosis, schizophrenia, depression, and congestive heart failure.

Concerning toxicity, excessive amounts of vitamin D supplements can poison the body by causing dangerously high levels of calcium known as hypercalcemia. Hypercalcemia is a common metabolic emergency which occurs when serum calcium levels exceed a safe range and has been found in cases of vitamin D toxicity. Most cases of toxicity involved oral intake amounts much higher than the recommended daily amount.

In summary, optimum bone health in humans is dependent on exposure to sunlight and so is the metabolism of vitamin D and calcium, and the safest way to manage your vitamin D metabolism is to first manage dietary intake of phosphorus.

The recommended adequate intake for vitamin D is expressed as micrograms (mcg) of cholecalciferol (D3) and assumes an absence of adequate exposure to sunlight. Never take a vitamin D supplement without consulting with a physician.

Recommend Adequate Intakes Levels for Vitamin D

Children	D3, mcg
1 to 3 year olds	10
4 to 8 year olds	10
Mails	
9 to 13 year olds	15
14 to 18 year olds	15
19 to 30 years	15
31 to 50 years	15
51 to 70 years	15
Over 70	20
Female	
9 to 13 year olds	15
14 to 18 year olds	15
19 to 30 years	15
31 to 50 years	15
51 to 70 years	15
Over 70	20
Pregnancy & Lactation	15

REPORTED CASES of VITAMIN D DEFICIENCY

A 10-day-old boy born in September is admitted to an emergency ward for uncontrollable seizures. Upon admission his left sided arm and leg are twitching, and lip smacking with right-sided head turning. Episodes lasted approximately 30 seconds and were occurring up to 7 times an hour. Laboratory test revealed calcium and vitamin D levels below acceptable ranges with elevated parathyroid hormone levels. An investigation noted, the baby had been breast feed, the mother had a diet low in calcium, she reported not taking any prenatal vitamins, and always wearing sunscreen when outdoors. Laboratory test of the mother revealed although her calcium levels were within an acceptable range her vitamin D and parathyroid hormones levels were abnormal confirming a vitamin D deficiency in both the mother and child.

The baby was managed with intravenous calcium gluconate infusion and oral intake of calcium and vitamin D. The seizures resolved within 48 hours and the infant was discharged home with oral calcium and vitamin D. Two weeks after discharge the infant was seizure free with normal laboratory test. Attending physicians conclude a vitamin D deficiency in infants and mothers is a re-emerging public health issue and sunscreen with a sun protection of 8 reduces the skins production of vitamin D by 98%.

A 67 year-old man with no past medial history was found in a coma during winter and admitted to the intensive care unit. Physical exam showed constricted pupils, irregular heartbeat, and spastic lower extremities. Laboratory data included low calcium and phosphorus levels, high thyroid stimulus hormone levels with normal renal and liver functions. He was diagnosed with stroke, atrial fibrillation, and hypocalcemia. He was given intravenous calcium gluconate 1000 mg (elementary calcium 90 mg) and regained consciousness in 7 days. Further work-up for hypocalcemia revealed low vitamin D levels and parathyroid hormone levels were 891.6 pg/ml with normal being below 72 pg/ml. On day 9 he was started on 50,000 IU of vitamin D daily for two weeks in conjunction with oral 500 mg of elemental calcium plus vitamin D three times daily. It took 28 days for all laboratory test to return to normal. This patient who was critically ill had hypocalcemia, hyperparathyroidism, and a vitamin D deficiency. Attending physicains reported the patients positive response to treatment with vitamin D supported a vitamin D deficiency as the most plausible cause for hypocalcemia.

VITAMIN D REFERENCES

1984 Phosphate deprivation increases serum 1,25-(OH)2-vitamin D concentrations in healthy men. *William J. Maierhofer, Richard W. Gray, Jacob Lemann Jr. Kidney International. 1984, Vol. 25, 571-575.*

1986 Oral intake of phosphorus can determine the serum concentration of 1,25-dihydroxyvitamin D by determining its production rate in humans. *A.A. Portale, B.P. Halloran, M.M. Murphy, R.C. Morris. Journal of Clinical Investigation. 1986, Vol. 77, No. 1, 7-12.*

1989 Physiologic regulation of the serum concentration of 1,25-dihydroxyvitamin D by phosphorus in normal men. *Portale AA, Halloran BP, Morris RC Jr. Journal Clinical Investigation. May 1989, Vol. 83, No.5, 1494-1499.*

2004 Nutritional rickets among children in the United States: review of cases reported between 1986 and 2003. *Pamala Weisburg, Kelly S. Scanlon, Ruowei Li, Mary Cogswell. American Journal Clinical Nutrition. December 2004, Vol. 80, No. 6, 1697s-1705s.*

2007 Vitamin D deficiency. *Michael F. Hollock, M.D. Ph.D., New England Journal of Medicine. July 2007, Vol. 357: 266-281.*

2007 Hypovitaminosis D in British adults and age 45 years: nationwide cohort study of dietary and lifestyle predictors. *Elina Hypponen., Chris Power. American Journal Clinical Nutrition. March 2007, Vol. 85, No. 3, 860-868.*

2009 Prevalence and associations of 25-hydroxyvitamin D deficiency in U.S. children: NHANES 2001-2004. *Juhi Kumar, M.D., MPH, Paul*

Munter, PhD, Frederick J. Kaskel, M.D., PhD., Susan M. Hailpern PhD, MS., Michael L. Melamed, M.D., MHS. *Pediatrics September 1, 2009, Vol. 24, No. 3, e362-e370.*

2009 **Vitamin D deficiency as an ignored cause of hypocalcemia in acute illness: Report of 2 Cases and Review of Literature.** *Hiroshi Noto, Howard J. Heller. The Open Endocronolgy Journal. 2009, Vol. 3,1-4.*

2013 **Effect of calcium plus vitamin D supplementation during pregnancy in Brazilian adolescent mothers: a randomized placebo-controlled trial.** *Maria Eduarda L. Diogenes, Flavia F. Bezerra, Elaine P. Rezende, Marcia Fernanda Taveria, Isabel Pinhal, Carmen M. Donangelo. American Journal of Clinical Nutrition. July 2013, Vol. 98, No. 1*

VITAMIN D

Alcohol	Amount	Vitamin D3 (mcg)
White Wine	1 glass	0
Red Wine	1 glass	0
Light Beer	1 bottle	0
Regular Beer	1 bottle	0
Gin, Rum, Vodka, or Whisky	1 shot	0

Beans, Canned	Amount	Vitamin D3 (mcg)
Baked beans	1 cup	0
Black-eyed peas	1 cup	0
Cranberry beans	1 cup	0
Fava beans	1 cup	0
Garbanzo beans	1 cup	0
Great Northern	1 cup	0
Green beans	1 cup	0
Lima beans, large	1 cup	0
Navy beans	1 cup	0
Pinto beans	1 cup	0
Red kidney beans	1 cup	0
Refried beans	1 cup	0
White beans	1 cup	0
Yellow beans	1 cup	0

Beans, Cooked	Amount	Vitamin D3 (mcg)
Adzuki	1 cup	0
Black beans	1 cup	0
Black Turtle beans, mature	1 cup	0
Black-eyed peas	1 cup	0
Cranberry beans	1 cup	0
Edamame	1 cup	0
Fava beans	1 cup	0
Garbanzo beans, chickpeas	1 cup	0
Great Northern	1 cup	0
Green beans	1 cup	0
Hyacinath beans	1 cup	0
Kidney beans	1 cup	0
Lentils	1 cup	0
Lima beans	1 cup	0
Lupini beans	1 cup	0
Mothbeans	1 cup	0
Mung beans, mature seeds	1 cup	0
Natto	1 cup	0
Navy beans	1 cup	0
Pigeon peas	1 cup	0

Adequate Intakes 5 to 15 mcg for adults

VITAMIN D

Continued

Pinto beans	1 cup	0
Soybeans, green	1 cup	0
Soybeans, matured	1 cup	0
Soybeans, matured, dry roasted	1 cup	0
Split peas	1 cup	0
White beans, mature	1 cup	0
White beans, small	1 cup	0
Winged beans	1 cup	0
Yardlong beans, Chinese long beans	1 cup	0
Yellow beans	1 cup	0

Beef, Cooked	Amount	Vitamin D3 (mcg)
Chuck roast, trimmed to 1/8" fat	3 oz	0.3
London Broil, top round	3 oz	0.3
Ground beef, 75%	3 oz	0.2
Ground beef, 80%	3 oz	0.2
Filet Mignon, trimmed to 0" fat	3 oz	0.1
Ground beef, 85%	3 oz	0.2
Ground beef, 90%	3 oz	0.2
Ground beef, 95%	3 oz	0.2
Top sirloin, lean, trimmed to 1/8" fat	3 oz	0.2
Ribeye steak, lean, trimmed 0" fat	3 oz	0.1

Beef, Cooked	Amount	Vitamin D3 (mcg)
Chuck roast, trimmed to 1/8" fat	1 lb cooked	1.8
Top Sirloin, trimmed to 1/8" fat	1 lb cooked	0.9
Ribeye steak, boneless, trimmed to 0" fat	1 steak	0.2
Filet Mignon, tenderloin, trimmed to 0" fat	1 steak	0.1
Ribeye filet, lean, trimmed to 0" fat	1 filet	0.1
Top Sirloin, choice filet, trimmed to 0" fat	1 filet	0.1
Beef ribs, trimmed to 1/8" fat	1 lb cooked	x
Brisket, lean, trimmed to 0" fat	1 lb cooked	x
Flank steak, lean, trimmed to 0" fat	1 lb cooked	x
Flank steak, lean, trimmed to 0" fat	1 steak	x
Porterhouse steak, trimmed to 0" fat	1 lb cooked	x
Skirt steak, trimmed to 0" fat	1 lb cooked	x
T-bone steak, trimmed to 0" fat	1 lb cooked	x
Tri Tip steak, lean, trimmed to 0" fat	1 lb cooked	x

Adequate Intakes 5 to 15 mcg for adults

VITAMIN D

Beef, Ground, Cooked	Amount	Vitamin D3 (mcg)
Ground beef, 80%	1/4 lb patty	0.2
Ground beef, 85%	1/4 lb patty	0.2
Ground beef, 90%	1/4 lb patty	0.2
Ground beef, 95%	1/4 lb patty	0.2
Ground beef, 75%	1/4 lb patty	0.1

Bread	Amount	Vitamin D3 (mcg)
All types	1 serving	0

Butter	Amount	Vitamin D3 (mcg)
Regular dairy butter, salted	1 tbsp	0.2
Regular dairy whipped butter, salted	1 tbsp	0.1

Cereal, General Mills®	Amount	Vitamin D3 (mcg)
Total Whole Grain	1 cup	3.3
Total Raisin Bran	1 cup	2.5
Total Cranberry Crunch	1 cup	2.0
Corn Chex	1 cup	1.5
Chocolate Chex	1 cup	1.4
Lucky Charms	1 cup	1.4
Cinnamon Chex	1 cup	1.3
Cocoa Puffs	1 cup	1.3
Cookie Crisp	1 cup	1.3
Dora The Explorer	1 cup	1.3
Golden Grams	1 cup	1.3
Honey Nut Chex	1 cup	1.3
Multi-Bran CHEX	1 cup	1.3
Reese's Puffs	1 cup	1.3
Wheat Chex	1 cup	1.3
Wheaties	1 cup	1.3
Cinnamon Toast Crunch	1 cup	1.2
Basic 4	1 cup	1.0
Rice Chex	1 cup	1.0
Trix	1 cup	1.0
Berry Berry Kix	1 cup	0.8
Kix	1 cup	0.8
Honey Nut Clusters	1 cup	0
Oatmeal Crisp, Crunchy Almond	1 cup	0
Oatmeal Crisp, Hearty Raisin	1 cup	0
Raisin Nut Bran	1 cup	0

Adequate Intakes 5 to 15 mcg for adults

VITAMIN D

Cereal, General Mills Cheerios®	Amount	Vitamin D3 (mcg)
Apple Cinnamon	1 cup	1.3
Banana Nut	1 cup	1.3
Berry Burst	1 cup	1.3
Chocolate	1 cup	1.3
Crunch & Oat Clusters	1 cup	1.3
Frosted	1 cup	1.3
Fruity	1 cup	1.3
Honey Nut	1 cup	1.3
Yogurt Burst, strawberry	1 cup	1.3
Multi Grain	1 cup	1
Original	1 cup	1

Cereal, General Mills Fiber One®	Amount	Vitamin D3 (mcg)
Honey Clusters	1 cup	1.5
Raisin Bran Clusters	1 cup	1.5
Caramel Delight	1 cup	1
Bran Cereal	1 cup	0
Frosted Shreaded Wheat	1 cup	0

Cereal, Kashi®	Amount	Vitamin D3 (mcg)
7-Whole Grain Puffs	1 cup	0
Berry Blossom	1 cup	0
Go Lean	1 cup	0
Go Lean Crunch	1 cup	0
Go Lean Crunch, Honey Almond Flax	1 cup	0
Golden Goodness	1 cup	0
Good Friends	1 cup	0
Heart to Heart, Honey Toasted Oat	1 cup	0
Heart to Heart, Warm Cinnamon	1 cup	0
Heart to Heart, Wild Blueberry	1 cup	0

Cereal, Kellogg's®	Amount	Vitamin D3 (mcg)
All-Bran Bran Buds	1 cup	3.0
All-Bran Original	1 cup	2.7
Raisin Bran	1 cup	2.3
Cocoa Krispies	1 cup	2.0
Frosted Flakes	1 cup	2.0
Frosted Rice Krispies	1 cup	2.0
Rice Krispies	1 cup	1.8
All-Bran Complete Wheat Flakes	1 cup	1.4
Crunchy Nut, Golden Honey Nut Flakes	1 cup	1.4
Honey Crunch Corn Flakes	1 cup	1.4
Krave Chocolate	1 cup	1.4

Adequate Intakes 5 to 15 mcg for adults

Continued

Rice Krispies Treats	1 cup	1.4
Cracklin' Oat Bran	1 cup	1.3
Crunchy Nut, Roasted Nut & Honey O's	1 cup	1.3
Fiberplus Cinnamon Oat Crunch	1 cup	1.3
Honey Smacks	1 cup	1.3
CINNABON	1 cup	1.2
Apple Jacks	1 cup	1.0
Corn Flakes	1 cup	1.0
Corn Pops	1 cup	1.0
Crispix	1 cup	1.0
Fiberplus Berry Yogurt Crunch	1 cup	1.0
Froot Loops	1 cup	1.0
Product 19	1 cup	1.0
Raisin Bran Crunch	1 cup	1.0
Smart Start Strong Heart Antioxidants	1 cup	1.0
Smorz	1 cup	1.0
MUESLIX	1 cup	0.6
Frosted MINI-Wheats, Big-Bite	1 cup	0.0

Cereal, Kellogg's Special-K®	Amount	Vitamin D3 (mcg)
Low Fat Granolia	1 cup	1.5
Multigrain Oats & Honey	1 cup	1.5
Fruit & Yogurt	1 cup	1.4
Blueberry	1 cup	1.3
Chocolately Delight	1 cup	1.3
Cinnamon Pecan	1 cup	1.3
Vanilla Almond	1 cup	1.3
Original	1 cup	0
Protein plus	1 cup	0
Red Berries	1 cup	0

Cereal, Post®	Amount	Vitamin D3, mcg
Cocoa Pebbles	1 cup	2.7
Fruity Pebbles	1 cup	2.7
Golden Crisp	1 cup	2.7
Alpha-Bits	1 cup	2.0
Grape Nuts Cereal	1 cup	2.0
Honeycomb Cereal	1 cup	1.7
Bran Flakes	1 cup	1.3
Grape Nuts Flakes	1 cup	1.3
Great Grains, Cranberry Almond Crunch	1 cup	1.3
Great Grains, Crunch Pecan	1 cup	1.3

VITAMIN D

Continued

Great Grains, Raisins, Dates & Pecans	1 cup	1.3
Great Grains, Banana Nut Crunch	1 cup	1.0
Raisin Bran	1 cup	1.0
Blueberry Morning	1 cup	0.8
Honey Nut Shreaded Wheat	1 cup	0
Shredded Wheat n' Bran, spoon-size	1 cup	0
Shredded Wheat, Frosted, spoon-size	1 cup	0
Shredded Wheat, Original, big-biscuit	1 biscuit	0
Shredded Wheat, Original, spoon-size	1 cup	0

Post® Honey Bunches of Oats®	Amount	Vitamin D3, mcg
Honey Roasted	1 cup	1.8
Just Bunches Honey Roasted	1 cup	1.5
Pecan Bunches	1 cup	1.3
With Almonds	1 cup	1.3
With Cinnamon Bunches	1 cup	1.3
With Strawberries	1 cup	1.3
With Vanilla Bunches	1 cup	1.0

Cereal, Quaker®	Amount	Vitamin D3 (mcg)
CAP'N Crunch	1 cup	0
CAP'N Crunch & Crunchberries	1 cup	0
CAP'N Crunch's OOPs! All Berries	1 cup	0
CAP'N Crunch's Peanut Butter Crunch	1 cup	0
Corn Bran Crunch	1 cup	0
Honey Graham OH'S	1 cup	0
LIFE Cereal, Cinnamon	1 cup	0
LIFE Cereal, Maple & Brown Sugar	1 cup	0
LIFE Cereal, Original	1 cup	0
Oatmeal Squares	1 cup	0
Oatmeal Squares, Cinnamon	1 cup	0
Oatmeal Squares, Golden Maple	1 cup	0
Puffed Rice	1 cup	0
Puffed Wheat	1 cup	0
Toasted Multigrain Crisp	1 cup	0
Granola, Apple, Cranberry, & Almond	1 cup	x

Cereal, Cooked	Amount	Vitamin D3 (mcg)
All cereals	1 cup	0

Adequate Intakes 5 to 15 mcg for adults

VITAMIN D

Cheese	Amount	Vitamin D3 (mcg)
Ricotta, whole milk	1 cup	0.5
Ricotta, part skim milk	1 cup	0.2
Cottage cheese, creamed, small curd	1 cup	0.2
Cottage cheese, low fat, 1 %	1 cup	0
Cottage cheese, lowf at, 2 %	1 cup	0
Cottage cheese, non fat, uncreamed	1 cup	0

Cheese	Amount	Vitamin D3 (mcg)
American, pasteurized process, fortified	1 oz	2.1
Cheddar	1 oz	0.2
Colby	1 oz	0.2
Cream cheese	1 oz	0.2
Fontina	1 oz	0.2
Goat cheese, hard type	1 oz	0.2
Gruyere	1 oz	0.2
Monterey	1 oz	0.2
Muenster	1 oz	0.2
Blue cheese	1 oz	0.1
Brie	1 oz	0.1
Feta	1 oz	0.1
Goat cheese, semisoft type	1 oz	0.1
Goat cheese, soft type	1 oz	0.1
Gouda	1 oz	0.1
Monterey, low fat	1 oz	0.1
Mozzarella, part skim milk, low moisture	1 oz	0.1
Mozzarella, whole milk	1 oz	0.1
Muenster, low fat	1 oz	0.1
Parmesan, grated	1 oz	0.1
Provolone	1 oz	0.1
Provolone, reduced fat	1 oz	0.1
Romano	1 oz	0.1
Swiss	1 oz	0.1
American, pasteurized process, imitation	1 oz	0
American, pasteurized process, low fat	1 oz	0
Cheddar, lowfat	1 oz	0
Cream cheese, fat free	1 oz	0
Mozzarella, nonfat	1 oz	0
Swiss, low fat	1 oz	0
Cheez Whiz, pasteurized process	1 oz	x
Velveeta, pasteurized process	1 oz	x

VITAMIN D

Cheese, Mexican	Amount	Vitamin D3 (mcg)
Queso fresco	1 oz	0.8
Queso seco	1 oz	0.5
Queso blanco	1 oz	0.2
Mexican, blend	1 oz	0.1
Queso anejo	1 oz	0.1
Queso asadero	1 oz	0.1
Queso chihuahua	1 oz	0.1
Mexican, blend, reduced fat	1 oz	0.1

Chicken, Cooked	Amount	Vitamin D3 (mcg)
Breast, with skin, fried in batter	1/2 breast	0.1
Breast, no skin, roasted	1/2 breast	0.1
Thigh, no skin, roasted	1 thigh	0.1

Chicken, Cooked	Amount	Vitamin D3 (mcg)
Breast with skin, fried with flour	3 oz	x
Drumstick with skin, fried in flour	3 oz	x
Thigh with skin, fried with flour	3 oz	x
Wing with skin, fried in flour	3 oz	x
Thigh meat only, no skin, roasted	3 oz	0.2
Thigh with skin, roasted	3 oz	0.2
Cornish game hens, meat only	3 oz	0.1
Breast meat only, no skin, roasted	3 oz	0.1
Breast with skin, roasted	3 oz	0.1
Drumstick with skin, roasted	3 oz	0.1
Wing meat only, no skin, roasted	3 oz	0.1
Wing with skin, roasted	3 oz	0.1
Drumstick meat only, no skin, roasted	3 oz	0
Chicken liver	3 oz	0

Cream	Amount	Vitamin D3 (mcg)
Heavy Whipping Cream	1 tbsp	0.1
Light Coffe Cream	1 tbsp	0.1
Light Whipping Cream	1 tbsp	0.1
Half & Half	1 tbsp	0
Sour Cream, cultured	1 tbsp	0
Sour Cream, reduced fat, cultured	1 tbsp	0
Whipped topping, pressurized	1 tbsp	0

Adequate Intakes 5 to 15 mcg for adults

VITAMIN D

Eggs	Amount	Vitamin D3 (mcg)
Egg whole, hard-boiled	1 large	1.1
Egg whole, scrambled	1 large	1.1
Egg whole, poached	1 large	1.0
Egg whole, fried	1 large	1.0
Egg substitute, liquid, fat free	1/4 cup	1.0
Egg yolk	1 large	0.9
Egg whites, raw	1 large	0
Egg whites, dried	1 ounce	0
Egg whites, dried powder, stabilized	1 tbsp	0

Fish, Canned	Amount	Vitamin D3 (mcg)
Light tuna, in oil	3 oz	5.7
Atlantic Sardines, in oil	3 oz	4.1
White (albacore) tuna, in water	3 oz	1.7
Light tuna, in water	3 oz	1.0
White (albacore) tuna, in oil	3 oz	x

Fish, Cooked	Amount	Vitamin D3 (mcg)
Alaskan halibut	3 oz	x
Atlantic croaker	3 oz	x
Atlantic mackerel	3 oz	x
Atlantic pollock	3 oz	x
Atlantic salmon, farmed	3 oz	x
Atlantic salmon, wild	3 oz	x
Bluefin tuna	3 oz	x
Carp	3 oz	x
Catfish, breaded & fried	3 oz	x
Catfish, wild	3 oz	x
Chinook salmon	3 oz	x
Coho salmon, farmed	3 oz	x
Florida pompano	3 oz	x
Freshwater bass	3 oz	x
Greenland halibut	3 oz	x
Grouper	3 oz	x
Keta (chum) salmon	3 oz	x
King mackerel	3 oz	x
Northern pike	3 oz	x
Orange roughy	3 oz	x
Rainbow trout, wild	3 oz	x
Sea bass	3 oz	x
Skipjack (aku) tuna	3 oz	x
Spanish mackerel	3 oz	x

VITAMIN D

Striped bass	3 oz	X
Walleye pike	3 oz	X
Yellowtail	3 oz	X

Fish, Cooked	Amount	Vitamin D3 (mcg)
Rainbow trout, farmed	3 oz	16.2
Chinook salmon, smoked	3 oz	14.5
Swordfish	3 oz	14.1
Sockeye salmon	3 oz	11.1
Pink salmon	3 oz	11.0
Pacific mackerel	3 oz	9.7
Coho salmon, wild	3 oz	9.6
Atlantic & Pacific halibut	3 oz	4.9
Pacific rockfish	3 oz	3.9
Tilapia	3 oz	3.1
Flounder and Sole	3 oz	3.0
Atlantic herring, pickeled	3 oz	2.4
Yellowfin tuna	3 oz	1.7
Whiting	3 oz	1.5
Atlantic perch	3 oz	1.2
Walleye pollock	3 oz	1.1
Haddock	3 oz	0.5
Pacific cod	3 oz	0.5
Catfish, farmed	3 oz	0.3

Fish, Shellfish, Cooked	Amount	Vitamin D3 (mcg)
Abalone	3 oz	X
Clams, breaded & fried	3 oz	X
Eastern oysters, farmed	3 oz	X
Eastern oysters, wild	3 oz	X
Queen crab	3 oz	X
Shrimp, breaded & fried	3 oz	0.1
Shrimp	3 oz	0.1
Clams, canned	3 oz	0.1
Northern lobster	3 oz	0
Alaskan king crab, imitation	3 oz	0
Blue crab	3 oz	0
Blue crab, canned	3 oz	0
Crayfish	3 oz	0
Octopus	3 oz	0
Shrimp, canned	3 oz	0

Fruit	Amount	Vitamin D3 (mcg)
All types	1 cup	0

Adequate Intakes 5 to 15 mcg for adults

VITAMIN D

Game Meat, Cooked	Amount	Vitamin D3 (mcg)
Antelope	3 oz	x
Bison, ground	3 oz	x
Buffalo, steak, free range	3 oz	x
Elk, ground	3 oz	x
Elk, roasted	3 oz	x
Duck	3 oz	0.1
Caribou	3 oz	0
Deer, ground	3 oz	0
Rabbit	3 oz	0
Squirrel	3 oz	0
Wild boar	3 oz	0

Grains, Cooked	Amount	Vitamin D3 (mcg)
All types	1 cup	0

Juice, unfortified	Amount	Vitamin D3 (mcg)
All types	1 cup	0

Lamb, Cooked	Amount	Vitamin D3 (mcg)
Cubed, for stew or kabob	3 oz	x
Foreshank, trimmed to 1/8" fat	3 oz	x
Chops, loin, lean, trimmed to 1/4" fat	3 oz	0.1
Ground	3 oz	0.1
Leg, whole, trimmed to 1/4" fat	3 oz	0.1
Rib, lean, trimmed to 1/4" fat	3 oz	0.1

Milk	Amount	Vitamin D3 (mcg)
Sheep milk	1 cup	x
Canned, evaporated, nonfat	1 cup	5.1
Canned, evaporated	1 cup	5.0
Goat milk	1 cup	3.2
Whole milk, 3.25%	1 cup	3.2
Lowfat, 1%	1 cup	2.9
Reduced fat, 2%	1 cup	2.9
Non fat, fat free or skim milk	1 cup	2.9
Dry, instant, non fat	1/3 cup	2.5
Canned, condensed, sweetened	1 cup	0.6
Human milk	1 cup	0.2
Coconut milk, Canned	1 cup	0
Buttermilk, low fat	1 cup	0
Soy milk, original & vanila, unfortified	1 cup	0

VITAMIN D

Nuts & Seeds	Amount	Vitamin D3 (mcg)
All nuts and seeds	1 oz	0

Oil	Amount	Vitamin D3 (mcg)
Cod liver oil	1 tbsp	34

Pork, Cooked	Amount	Vitamin D3 (mcg)
Spareribs	3 oz	2.2
Backribs	3 oz	1.0
Braunschweiger	3 oz	1.0
Canadian-style bacon	3 oz	0.9
Bratwurst	3 oz	0.9
Italian sausage	3 oz	0.8
Cured ham, lean	3 oz	0.8
Center loin pork chops	3 oz	0.7
Chops, broiled	3 oz	0.7
Sirloin pork chops	3 oz	0.6
Sausage	3 oz	0.6
Cured ham	3 oz	0.6
Chops, pan-fried	3 oz	0.5
Canadian-style bacon	2 slices	0.5
Chops, lean, pan-fried	3 oz	0.4
Ground pork	3 oz	0.4
Tenderloin	3 oz	0.3
Bacon, pan-fried	3 slices	0.2
Sausage	1 patty	0.2
Sausage	2 links	0.2
Polish sausage	3 oz	x
Liverwurst spread	1/4 cup	x

Salad Dressing	Amount	Vitamin D3 (mcg)
All types	1 tbsp	0

Turkey, Cooked	Amount	Vitamin D3 (mcg)
Dark meat	3 oz	0.3
Light meat	3 oz	0.3
Turkey sausage, reduced fat	3 oz	0.3
Turkey bacon	3 oz	0.3
Breast meat only	3 oz	0.2
Ground turkey	3 oz	0.2
Ground turkey, 93% lean	3 oz	0.2
Ground turkey, 85% lean	3 oz	0.2
Ground turkey, fat free	3 oz	0.2

Adequate Intakes 5 to 15 mcg for adults

VITAMIN D

Veal, Cooked	Amount	Vitamin D3 (mcg)
Ground	3 oz	0
Leg, top round	3 oz	0
Loin	3 oz	0
Sirloin	3 oz	0
Breast	3 oz	x
Foreshank	3 oz	x
Rib	3 oz	x

Vegetables	Amount	Vitamin D3 (mcg)
All vegetables	1 cup	0

Yogurt	Amount	Vitamin D3 (mcg)
Plain yogurt, whole milk	8 oz	0.2
Plain yogurt, low fat	8 oz	0
Plain yogurt, skim milk	8 oz	0
Plain greek yogurt, non fat	8 oz	0

Nutrient Data Collection Form

Food	Amount	Book Numbers	Multiply By	Estimated Nutrient Intake
Nutrient::	RDA:	Estimated:	% of RDA:	Total Estimated:

To download additional forms for free, go to www.TopNutrients4U.com

VITAMIN E

Vitamin E known as d-alpha-tocopherol is a fat soluble vitamin who functions to protect membrane cells against free radical damage. Vitamin-E is nature's fat soluble anti-oxidant. Free radicals are regular by-products your body produces during normal metabolism, and become damaging only in the absence of antioxidants.

Since vitamin E is fat soluble the amount required is largely dependent upon the amount of polyunsaturated fats in the diet. Adequate dietary intake of vitamin E may be difficult to achieve on diets which focus exclusively on non-fat food choices. Persons who cannot absorb dietary fat due to an inability to secrete bile acids or disorders of fat metabolism are at high risk of a deficiency.

Deficiency is usually characterized with some form of nerve degeneration in hands and feet. General deficiency signs include muscle weakness, leg cramps, tingling in arms, legs, hands, and feet, and cognitive decline.

The recommended daily allowance, RDA, for vitamin E activity is expressed in milligrams (mg) of d-alpha-tocopherol.

Recommend Daily Intakes Levels of Vitamin E

Children	Vitamin E, mg
1 to 3 year olds	6
4 to 8 year olds	7

Males	
9 to 13 year olds	11
14 to 18 year olds	15
19 to 30 years	15
31 to 50 years	15
51 to 70 years	15
Over 70	15

Females	
9 to 13 year olds	11
14 to 18 year olds	15
19 to 30 years	15
31 to 50 years	15
51 to 70 years	15
Over 70	15
Pregnancy	15
Lactation	19

VITAMIN E

Alcohol	Amount	Vitamin E (mg)
Red Wine	1 glass	0
White Wine	1 glass	0
Light Beer	1 bottle	0
Regular Beer	1 bottle	0
Gin, Rum, Vodka, Whisky	1 shot	0

Beans, Canned	Amount	Vitamin E (mg)
White beans, mature	1 cup	2.07
Navy beans	1 cup	2.04
Pinto beans	1 cup	1.37
Yellow beans	1 cup	0.44
Baked beans, plain	1 cup	0.38
Refried beans	1 cup	0.12
Green beans	1 cup	0.05
Kidney beans, mature	1 cup	0.05
Blackeyed peas	1 cup	x
Cranberry beans	1 cup	x
Fava beans	1 cup	x
Garbanzo	1 cup	x
Great Northern	1 cup	x
Lima beans, mature	1 cup	x

Beans, Cooked	Amount	Vitamin E (mg)
White beans, mature	1 cup	1.68
Black Turtle beans, mature	1 cup	1.61
Pinto beans	1 cup	1.61
Edamame	1 cup	1.05
Soybeans, mature	1 cup	0.60
Garbanzo beans	1 cup	0.57
Green beans	1 cup	0.56
Yellow beans	1 cup	0.56
Black-eyed peas	1 cup	0.48
Lima beans	1 cup	0.34
Mung beans, mature seeds	1 cup	0.30
Lentils	1 cup	0.22
Split peas	1 cup	0.06
Kidney beans	1 cup	0.05
Fava beans	1 cup	0.03
Natto	1 cup	0.02
Navy beans	1 cup	0.02
Adzuki	1 cup	x
Black beans	1 cup	x
Cranberry beans	1 cup	x

RDA is 15 mg for adults

Continued

Great Northern	1 cup	x
Hyacinath beans	1 cup	x
Lupini beans	1 cup	x
Mothbeans	1 cup	x
Pigeon peas	1 cup	x
Soybeans, green	1 cup	x
Soybeans, mature, dry roasted	1 cup	x
White beans, small	1 cup	x
Winged beans	1 cup	x
Yardlong beans, Chinese long beans	1 cup	x

Beef, Cooked	Amount	Vitamin E (mg)
Ground beef, 75%	3 oz	0.40
Ground beef, 80%	3 oz	0.40
Ground beef, 85%	3 oz	0.38
Brisket, lean, trimmed to 0" fat	3 oz	0.37
London Broil, top round, trim to 0" fat	3 oz	0.37
Filet Mignon, trimmed to 0" fat	3 oz	0.12
Ground beef, 90%	3 oz	0.35
Flank steak, lean, trimmed to 0" fat	3 oz	0.32
Top Sirloin, lean, trimmed to 1/8" fat	3 oz	0.32
Ground beef, 95%	3 oz	0.31
T-bone steak, trimmed 0" fat	3 oz	0.20
Chuck roast, trimmed to 1/8" fat	3 oz	0.18
Tri Tip steak, lean, trimmed to 0" fat	3 oz	0.15
Porterhouse steak, trimmed to 0" fat	3 oz	0.15
Skirt steak, trimmed to 0" fat	3 oz	0.08

Beef, Cooked	Amount	Vitamin E (mg)
Top Sirloin, trimmed to 1/8" fat	1 lb cooked	2.00
Brisket, lean, trimmed to 0" fat	1 lb cooked	1.95
Flank steak, lean, trimmed to 0" fat	1 lb cooked	1.73
Flank steak, lean, trimmed to 0" fat	1 steak	1.46
Chuck roast, trimmed to 1/8" fat	1 lb cooked	0.95
Porterhouse steak, trimmed to 0" fat	1 lb cooked	0.82
T-bone steak, trimmed to 0" fat	1 lb cooked	0.82
Tri Tip steak, lean, trimmed to 0" fat	1 lb cooked	0.77
Skirt steak, trimmed to 0" fat	1 lb cooked	0.45
Filet Mignon, tenderloin, trimmed to 0" fat	1 steak	0.16
Beef ribs, trimmed to 1/8" fat	1 lb cooked	x
Ribeye filet, lean, trimmed to 0" fat	1 filet	x
Ribeye steak, boneless, trimmed to 0" fat	1 steak	x
Top Sirloin, choice filet, trimmed to 0" fat	1 filet	x

VITAMIN E

Beef, Ground, Cooked	Amount	Vitamin E (mg)
Ground beef, 85%	1/4 lb patty	0.38
Ground beef, 80%	1/4 lb patty	0.36
Ground beef, 90%	1/4 lb patty	0.34
Ground beef, 75%	1/4 lb patty	0.33
Ground beef, 95%	1/4 lb patty	0.30

Bread	Amount	Vitamin E (mg)
Indian bread, Naan, whole wheat	1 piece	1.40
Indian bread, Naan, plain	1 piece	0.71
Croissants, butter	1 medium	0.48
Bagel, oat bran	4" bagel	0.35
Bagel, wheat	4" bagel	0.31
Bagel, cinnamon & raisins	4" bagel	0.28
Kaiser rolls	1 roll	0.24
English Muffin, plain	1 muffin	0.18
Pita, white	6" pita	0.18
Potato bread	1 slice	0.15
Whole-Wheat	1 slice	0.15
Oatmeal bread	1 slice	0.13
Pumpernickle	1 slice	0.13
Rye bread	1 slice	0.11
Egg bread	1 slice	0.10
Multi-Grain, and Whole-Grain	1 slice	0.10
Bagel plain	4" bagel	0.09
Dinner Rolls, brown & serve	1 roll	0.08
Raisen bread	1 slice	0.07
Tortillas, corn	1 tortilla	0.07
Italian	1 slice	0.06
Tortillas, flour	1 tortilla	0.06
White bread	1 slice	0.06
French or Sourdough	1 slice	0.05
Wheat bread	1 slice	0.05
Reduced calorie white	1 slice	0.04
Hamburger & Hotdog buns, plain	1 bun	0.03
Mexican roll, bollilo	1 roll	0

Butter	Amount	Vitamin E (mg)
Regular dairy butter, salted	1 tbsp	0.33
Regular dairy whipped butter, salted	1 tbsp	0.22

VITAMIN E

Cereal, General Mills®	Amount	Vitamin E (mg)
Total Whole Grain	1 cup	18.00
Total Raisin Bran	1 cup	13.50
Total Cranberry Crunch	1 cup	10.80
Reese's Puffs	1 cup	9.14
Oatmeal Crisp, Crunchy Almond	1 cup	1.17
Raisin Nut Bran	1 cup	1.01
Cinnamon Toast Crunch	1 cup	0.83
Cinnamon Chex	1 cup	0.60
Basic 4	1 cup	0.57
Wheat Chex	1 cup	0.43
Multi-Bran Chex	1 cup	0.34
Dora The Explorer	1 cup	0.33
Rice Chex	1 cup	0.30
Golden Grams	1 cup	0.26
Cocoa Puffs	1 cup	0.25
Honey Nut Chex	1 cup	0.24
Wheaties	1 cup	0.23
Honey Nut Clusters	1 cup	0.22
Oatmeal Crisp, Hearty Raisin	1 cup	0.22
Cookie Crisp	1 cup	0.20
Trix	1 cup	0.18
Lucky Charms	1 cup	0.16
Berry Berry Kix	1 cup	0.14
Corn Chex	1 cup	0.09
Kix	1 cup	0.07
Chocolate Chex	1 cup	x

Cereal, General Mills Cheerios®	Amount	Vitamin E (mg)
Multi Grain	1 cup	4.72
Apple Cinnamon	1 cup	1.90
Berry Burst	1 cup	0.80
Honey Nut	1 cup	0.36
Original	1 cup	0.19
Fruity	1 cup	0.18
Frosted	1 cup	0.16
Yogurt Burst Strawberry	1 cup	0.13

Cereal, General Mills Fiber One®	Amount	Vitamin E (mg)
Caramel Delight	1 cup	0.58
Original Bran	1 cup	0.36
Honey Clusters	1 cup	0.17
Raisin Bran Clusters	1 cup	0
80 Calorie Chocolate Squares	1 cup	x

RDA is 15 mg for adults

VITAMIN E

Continued

| 80 Calorie Honey Squares | 1 cup | x |
| Frosted Shredded Wheat | 1 cup | x |

Cereal, Kashi®	Amount	Vitamin E (mg)
Heart to Heart, Warm Cinnamon	1 cup	25.9
Heart to Heart, Wild Blueberry	1 cup	20.3
Heart to Heart, Honey Toasted Oat	1 cup	18.0
Honey Sunshine	1 cup	17.7
Berry Blossom	1 cup	11.5
Kashi U	1 cup	9.95
Go Lean Crisp Toasted Berry Crumble	1 cup	2.28
Go Lean Crunch, Honey Almond Flax	1 cup	1.98
Go Lean Crunch,	1 cup	1.42
Autum Wheat	1 cup	0.52
Good Friends	1 cup	0.45
Go Lean	1 cup	0.32
7 whole Grain Honey Puffs	1 cup	0.25
7 whole Grain Puffs	1 cup	0.17

Cereal, Kellogg's®	Amount	Vitamin E (mg)
Fiberplus Cinnamon Oat Crunch	1 cup	18.05
All-Bran Complete Wheat Flakes	1 cup	17.92
Fiberplus Berry Yogurt Crunch	1 cup	13.59
Product 19	1 cup	13.50
Smart Start, Strong Heart, Antioxidants	1 cup	13.50
Rice Krispies	1 cup	7.73
MUESLIX	1 cup	5.91
Frosted Rice Krispies	1 cup	4.50
Cocoa Krispies	1 cup	4.38
All-Bran Original	1 cup	0.77
Raisin Bran	1 cup	0.39
Frosted MINI-Wheat's, Big-Bite	1 cup	0.28
Honey Crunch Corn Flakes	1 cup	0.23
Raisin Bran Crunch	1 cup	0.19
Rice Krispies Treats	1 cup	0.16
Honey Smacks	1 cup	0.15
Smorz	1 cup	0.14
Corn Pops	1 cup	0.04
Crispix	1 cup	0.04
Froot Loops	1 cup	0.04
Apple Jacks	1 cup	0.03
Corn Flakes	1 cup	0.03
Frosted Flakes	1 cup	0.03
All-Bran Bran Buds	1 cup	0
CINNABON	1 cup	0

RDA is 15 mg for adults

VITAMIN E

Continued

Cracklin' Oat Bran	1 cup	0
Crunchy Nut Roasted Nut & Honey O's	1 cup	0
Crunchy Nut Golden Honey Nut Flakes	1 cup	x
Krave Chocolate	1 cup	x

Cereal, Kelloggs Special-K®	Amount	Vitamin E (mg)
Low Fat Granola	1 cup	9.45
Original	1 cup	4.74
Red Berries	1 cup	4.74
Vanilla Almond	1 cup	0.54
Chocolately Delight	1 cup	0.22
Cinnamon Pecan	1 cup	0.18
Blueberry	1 cup	0
Fruit & Yogurt	1 cup	0
Multigrain Oats & Honey	1 cup	0
Protein Plus	1 cup	x

Cereal, Post®	Amount	Vitamin E, mg
Great Grains, Cranberry Almond Crunch	1 cup	3.60
Grape-Nuts Cereal	1 cup	0.71
Honey Nut Shredded Wheat	1 cup	0.71
Blueberry Morning	1 cup	0.69
Great Grains, Banana Nut Crunch	1 cup	0.69
Great Grains, Crunchy Pecan	1 cup	0.51
Shredded Wheat n' Bran, spoon-size	1 cup	0.51
Great Grains, Raisin, Date & Pecan	1 cup	0.42
Raisin Bran	1 cup	0.32
Shredded Wheat, Original, spoon-size	1 cup	0.32
Grape-Nuts Flakes	1 cup	0.31
Bran Flakes	1 cup	0.30
Shredded Wheat, frosted, spoon-size	1 cup	0.17
Golden Crisp	1 cup	0.12
Alpha-Bits	1 cup	0.09
Cocoa Pebbles	1 cup	0.05
Fruity Pebbles	1 cup	0.05
Honeycomb Cereal	1 cup	0.04
Shredded Wheat, Original, big-biscuit	1 biscuit	0

Post® Honey Bunches of Oats®	Amount	Vitamin E (mg)
Just Bunches Honey Roasted	1 cup	1.56
With Almonds	1 cup	0.79
With Vanilla Bunches	1 cup	0.52
Honey Roasted	1 cup	0.49
Pecan Bunches	1 cup	0.19

RDA is 15 mg for adults

VITAMIN E

Continued

With Cinnamon Bunches	1 cup	x
With Strawberries	1 cup	x

Cereal, Quaker®	Amount	Vitamin E (mg)
Oatmeal Squares, Cinnamon	1 cup	1.73
Oatmeal Squares	1 cup	1.67
Granola, Apple, Cranberry, & Almond	1 cup	1.60
Oatmeal Squares, Golden Maple	1 cup	1.27
Toasted Multigrain Crisp	1 cup	1.00
Puffed Wheat	1 cup	0.30
LIFE Cereal, Original	1 cup	0.26
CAP'N Crunch's Peanut Butter Crunch	1 cup	0.24
Corn Bran Crunch	1 cup	0.24
LIFE Cereal, Maple & Brown Sugar	1 cup	0.24
LIFE Cereal, Cinnamon	1 cup	0.23
CAP'N Crunch	1 cup	0.22
CAP'N Crunch & Crunchberries	1 cup	0.22
CAP'N Crunch's OOPs! All Berries	1 cup	0.20
Honey Graham OH'S	1 cup	0.18
Puffed Rice	1 cup	0.02

Cereal, Cooked	Amount	Vitamin E (mg)
Oats, regular, unenriched	1 cup	0.19
Farina	1 cup	0.10
White corn grits	1 cup	0.07
CREAM OF WHEAT, regular	1 cup	0.05
Yellow corn grits	1 cup	0.05

Cheese	Amount	Vitamin E (mg)
Ricotta, whole milk	1 cup	0.27
Cottage cheese, creamed, small curd	1 cup	0.18
Ricotta, part skim milk	1 cup	0.17
Cottage cheese, low fat, 2%	1 cup	0.09
Cottage cheese, low fat, 1%	1 cup	0.02
Cottage cheese, non fat, uncreamed	1 cup	0.01

Cheese	Amount	Vitamin E (mg)
American, pasteurized process, imitation	1 oz	0.61
American, pasteurized process, fortified	1 oz	0.23
Swiss	1 oz	0.11
Mozzarella, part skim milk, low moisture	1 oz	0.10
Goat cheese, hard type	1 oz	0.09
American, pasteurized process, low fat	1 oz	0.08
Cheddar	1 oz	0.08

RDA is 15 mg for adults

VITAMIN E

Continued

Colby	1 oz	0.08
Fontina	1 oz	0.08
Gruyere	1 oz	0.08
Blue cheese	1 oz	0.07
Brie	1 oz	0.07
Goat cheese, semisoft type	1 oz	0.07
Gouda	1 oz	0.07
Monterey	1 oz	0.07
Muenster	1 oz	0.07
Parmesan, grated	1 oz	0.07
Provolone	1 oz	0.07
Romano	1 oz	0.07
Feta	1 oz	0.05
Goat cheese, soft type	1 oz	0.05
Monterey, low fat	1 oz	0.05
Mozzarella, whole milk	1 oz	0.05
Cream cheese	1 oz	0.04
Muenster, low fat	1 oz	0.04
Provolone, reduced fat	1 oz	0.04
Cheddar, low fat	1 oz	0.02
Swiss, low fat	1 oz	0.02
Cream cheese, fat free	1 oz	0.01
Mozzarella, non fat	1 oz	0
Cheez Whiz, pasteurized process	1 oz	x
Velveeta, pasteurized process	1 oz	x

Cheese, Mexican	Amount	Vitamin E (mg)
Queso seco	1 oz	0.14
Queso blanco	1 oz	0.13
Queso chihuahua	1 oz	0.10
Queso fresco	1 oz	0.10
Queso anejo	1 oz	0.07
Queso asadero	1 oz	0.07
Mexican, blend	1 oz	0.07
Mexican, blend, reduced fat	1 oz	0.05

Chicken, Cooked	Amount	Vitamin E (mg)
Breast, with skin, fried with flour	1/2 breast	1.48
Breast, no skin, roasted	1/2 breast	0.23
Thigh, no skin, roasted	1 thigh	0.14
Drumstick, no skin, roasted	1 drumstick	0.12

RDA is 15 mg for adults

VITAMIN E

Chicken, Cooked	Amount	Vitamin E (mg)
Breast meat only, no skin, roasted	3 oz	0.23
Breast with skin, roasted	3 oz	0.23
Wing meat only, no skin, roasted	3 oz	0.23
Wing with skin, roasted	3 oz	0.23
Cornish game hens, meat only	3 oz	0.20
Drumstick with skin, roasted	3 oz	0.16
Thigh with skin, roasted	3 oz	0.16
Drumstick meat only, no skin, roasted	3 oz	0.15
Thigh meat only, no skin, roasted	3 oz	0.15
Breast with skin, fried in flour	3 oz	x
Drumstick with skin, fried in flour	3 oz	x
Thigh with skin, fried in flour	3 oz	x
Wing with skin, fried in flour	3 oz	x

Cream	Amount	Vitamin E (mg)
Heavy Cream	1 tbsp	0.16
Light Coffe Cream	1 tbsp	0.08
Half & Half	1 tbsp	0.05
Sour Cream, cultured	1 tbsp	0.05
Sour Cream, reduced fat	1 tbsp	0.05
Whipped Topping, pressurized	1 tbsp	0.02
Half & Half, fat free	1 tbsp	0.005

Eggs	Amount	Vitamin E (mg)
Egg substitute, liquid, fat free	1/4 cup	0.95
Egg whole, scrambled	1 large	0.70
Egg whole, fried	1 large	0.60
Egg whole, hard-boiled	1 large	0.52
Egg whole, poached	1 large	0.52
Egg yolk	1 large	0.43
Egg whites, raw	1 large	0
Egg whites, dried	1 ounce	0
Egg whites, dried powder, stabilized	1 tbsp	0

Fish, Canned	Amount	Vitamin E (mg)
White (albacore) tuna, in oil	3 oz	1.95
Atlantic Sardines, in oil	3 oz	1.74
Light tuna, in oil	3 oz	0.74
White (albacore) tuna, in water	3 oz	0.72
Light tuna, in water	3 oz	0.28

VITAMIN E

Fish, Cooked	Amount	Vitamin E (mg)
Atlantic croaker	3 oz	x
Atlantic mackerel	3 oz	x
Atlantic pollock	3 oz	x
Bluefin tuna	3 oz	x
Carp	3 oz	x
Catfish, breaded & fried	3 oz	x
Catfish, wild	3 oz	x
Chinook salmon	3 oz	x
Coho salmon, farmed	3 oz	x
Florida pompano	3 oz	x
Freshwater bass	3 oz	x
Greenland halibut	3 oz	x
Grouper	3 oz	x
Keta (chum) salmon	3 oz	x
King mackerel	3 oz	x
Northern pike	3 oz	x
Rainbow trout, wild	3 oz	x
Sea bass	3 oz	x
Skipjack (aku) tuna	3 oz	x
Snapper	3 oz	x
Spanish mackerel	3 oz	x
Striped bass	3 oz	x
Walleye pike	3 oz	x
Yellowtail	3 oz	x

Fish, Cooked	Amount	Vitamin E (mg)
Rainbow trout, farmed	3 oz	2.37
Swordfish	3 oz	2.05
Orange roughy	3 oz	1.59
Atlantic herring, pickled	3 oz	1.45
Chinock salmon, smoked	3 oz	1.15
Pacific mackerel	3 oz	1.06
Sockeye salmon	3 oz	0.97
Alaskan halibut	3 oz	0.89
Catfish, farmed	3 oz	0.82
Coho salmon, wild	3 oz	0.78
Atlantic perch	3 oz	0.77
Atlantic cod	3 oz	0.69
Tilapia	3 oz	0.67
Flounder & Sole	3 oz	0.65
Atlantic & Pacific halibut	3 oz	0.63
Pacific cod	3 oz	0.57
Haddock	3 oz	0.47
Pink salmon	3 oz	0.41

RDA is 15 mg for adults

VITAMIN E

Continued

Pacific rockfish	3 oz	0.37
Whiting	3 oz	0.32
Yellowfin tuna	3 oz	0.25
Walleye pollock	3 oz	0.24

Fish, Shellfish, Cooked	Amount	Vitamin E (mg)
Shrimp	3 oz	1.87
Blue crab	3 oz	1.56
Blue crab, canned	3 oz	1.56
Crayfish	3 oz	1.28
Eastern oysters, wild	3 oz	1.12
Shrimp, breaded & fried	3 oz	1.10
Octopus	3 oz	1.02
Clams, canned	3 oz	0.95
Shrimp, canned	3 oz	0.94
Northern lobster	3 oz	0.85
Alaskan king crab, imitation	3 oz	0.14
Abalone	3 oz	x
Clams, breaded & fried	3 oz	x
Eastern oysters, farmed	3 oz	x
Queen crab	3 oz	x
Alaskan king crab	3 oz	x

Fruit, Canned	Amount	Vitamin E (mg)
Apricots	1 cup	1.55
Peaches	1 cup	1.28
Olives, green	5 large	0.51
Applesauce, sweetened	1 cup	0.46
Plums	1 cup	0.46
Applesauce, unsweetened	1 cup	0.39
Olives, black	5 large	0.36
Pears,	1 cup	0.21
Pineapple	1 cup	0.03

Fruit, Dried	Amount	Vitamin E (mg)
Apricots	1 cup	5.63
Cranberries	1 cup	1.30
Figs	1 cup	0.52
Apples	1 cup	0.46
Peaches	1 cup	0.30
Currants	1 cup	0.16
Pears	1 cup	0.11

VITAMIN E

Fruit, Frozen	Amount	Vitamin E (mg)
Raspberries	1 cup	1.80
Blackberries, unthawed	1 cup	1.77
Peaches	1 cup	1.55
Blueberries	1 cup	1.20
Strawberries	1 cup	0.59

Fruit, Raw	Amount	Vitamin E (mg)
Avocado, Florida	1 cup	6.12
Avocado, California	1 cup	4.53
Kiwi	1 cup	2.63
Blackberries	1 cup	1.68
Mango	1 cup	1.48
Apricots	1 cup	1.47
Mulberries	1 cup	1.22
Cranberries	1 cup	1.20
Black currants	1 cup	1.12
Peachs	1 cup	1.12
Nectarine	1 cup	1.10
Raspberries	1 cup	1.07
Pomegranates	1 cup	1.04
Blueberries	1 cup	0.83
Prunes, uncooked	1 cup	0.75
Jicama	1 cup	0.55
Strawberries	1 cup	0.48
Stewed prunes	1 cup	0.47
Papayas	1 cup	0.44
Plums	1 cup	0.43
Tangerine mandarin	1 cup	0.39
Florida Oranges	1 cup	0.33
Grapefruit, pink & red, sections	1 cup	0.30
Grapes	1 cup	0.30
Apples	1 cup	0.25
Naval Oranges	1 cup	0.25
Plantains	1 cup	0.21
Pears	1 cup	0.20
Raisins	1 cup	0.17
Cherries	1 cup	0.11
Cantaloupe	1 cup	0.08
Water mellon	1 cup	0.08
Dates	1 cup	0.07
Honeydew	1 cup	0.03

RDA is 15 mg for adults

VITAMIN E

Continued

Kumquats	1 cup	0.03
Pineapple	1 cup	0.03
Pomelo	1 cup	x
Valencias Oranges	1 cup	x

Fruit, Raw	Amount	Vitamin E (mg)
Avocado, Florida	1 fruit	8.09
Avocado, California	1 fruit	2.68
Pomegranates	1 fruit	1.69
Persimmons, Japanese	1 fruit	1.23
Kiwi	1 fruit	1.01
Nectarine	1 fruit	0.99
Peaches	1 fruit	0.72
Cherimoya	1 fruit	0.63
Olives, green	5 large	0.51
Papayas, small	1 fruit	0.47
Olives, black	5 large	0.36
Apricots	1 fruit	0.31
Florida Oranges	1 fruit	0.25
Plantains	1 fruit	0.25
Chayote	1 fruit	0.24
Apples	1 fruit	0.22
Naval Oranges	1 fruit	0.21
Pears	1 fruit	0.20
Prunes, uncooked	5 prunes	0.20
Tangerine	1 fruit	0.18
Plums	1 fruit	0.17
Strawberries	5 fruit	0.17
Grapefruit, pink or red	1/2 fruit	0.16
Star fruit, Carambola	1 fruit	0.14
Banana	1 fruit	0.12
Pineapple guava, Feijoa	1 fruit	0.07
Cherries	10 fruit	0.06
Raisins	1 small box	0.05
Figs, dried	1 fruit	0.03
Kumquats	1 fruit	0.03
Dates	5 dates	0.02
Raisins	1 packet	0.02
Pineapple	1/2" x 3" slice	0.01
Persimmons, small native	1 fruit	x
Pummelo	1 fruit	x
Valencias Oranges	1 fruit	x

VITAMIN E

Game Meat, Cooked	Amount	Vitamin E (mg)
Duck	3 oz	0.60
Deer, ground	3 oz	0.58
Buffalo, steak, free range	3 oz	0.50
Elk, ground, pan-fried	3 oz	0.48
Rabbit	3 oz	0.35
Caribou	3 oz	0.34
Squirrel	3 oz	0.34
Wild boar	3 oz	0.32
Bison, ground	3 oz	0.20
Antelope	3 oz	x
Deer, roasted	3 oz	x
Elk, roasted	3 oz	x

Grains, Cooked	Amount	Vitamin E (mg)
Quinoa	1 cup	1.20
Egg & Spinach noodles	1 cup	0.88
Spelt	1 cup	0.50
Amaranth	1 cup	0.47
Whole-Wheat spaghetti	1 cup	0.42
Wild rice	1 cup	0.39
Egg noodles	1 cup	0.27
Couscous	1 cup	0.20
White rice	1 cup	0.20
Buckwheat	1 cup	0.15
Macaroni	1 cup	0.08
Spaghetti	1 cup	0.08
Brown rice	1 cup	0.06
Pearled barley	1 cup	0.02
Bulgur	1 cup	0.02
Instant white rice	1 cup	0.02
Millet	1 cup	0

Herbs & Spices	Amount	Vitamin E (mg)
Paprika	1 tsp	1.80
Chili powder	1 tsp	0.99
Curry powder	1 tsp	0.44
Ginger, ground	1 tsp	0.30
Oregano	1 tsp	0.27
Cloves, dried	1 tsp	0.20
Basil, dried & ground	1 tsp	0.15
Thyme, dried	1 tsp	0.10

RDA is 15 mg for adults

VITAMIN E

Basil, fresh, chopped	1 tsp	0.07
Turmeric, ground	1 tsp	0.07
Caraway seeds	1 tsp	0.05
Cinnamon powder	1 tsp	0.05
Sage, ground	1 tsp	0.05
Parsley, dried	1 tsp	0.04
Celery seeds	1 tsp	0.02
Garlic powder	1 tsp	0.02
Pepper, black	1 tsp	0.02
Onion powder	1 tsp	0.01

Juice	Amount	Vitamin E (mg)
Carrot	1 cup	2.74
Pomegranate	1 cup	0.95
Tomato	1 cup	0.78
Vegetable	1 cup	0.77
Cranberry	1 cup	0.56
Grapefruit, raw	1 cup	0.54
Lemon, raw	1 cup	0.37
Prune	1 cup	0.31
Orange, raw	1 cup	0.10
Pineapple	1 cup	0.05
Apple	1 cup	0.02
Grape	1 cup	0

Lamb, Cooked	Amount	Vitamin E (mg)
Cubed for stew or kabob	3 oz	0.17
Rib, lean, trimmed to 1/4" fat	3 oz	0.15
Leg, whole	3 oz	0.13
Ground	3 oz	0.12
Chops, loin, lean, trimmed to 1/4" fat	3 oz	0.08
Foreshank, trimmed to 1/8" fat	3 oz	x

Milk	Amount	Vitamin E (mg)
Canned, condensed, sweetened	1 cup	0.49
Soy milk, original & vanila, unfortified	1 cup	0.27
Human milk	1 cup	0.20
Goat milk	1 cup	0.17
Whole milk, 3.25%	1 cup	0.17
Buttermilk, low fat	1 cup	0.12
Reduced fat, 2%	1 cup	0.07
Low fat, 1%	1 cup	0.02
Non fat, fat free or skim milk	1 cup	0.02
Canned, evaporated, non fat	1 cup	0

VITAMIN E

Dry, instant, non fat	1/3 cup	0
Canned, evaporated	1 cup	x
Sheep milk	1 cup	x

Nuts & Seeds	Amount	Vitamin E (mg)
Sunflower seeds	1 oz	9.97
Almonds	1 oz	7.43
Hazelnuts	1 oz	4.26
Pine nuts	1 oz	2.65
Peanut butter, smooth style	1 oz	2.55
Trail mix, regular with chocolate chips	1 oz	2.38
Peanuts	1 oz	2.36
Brazilnuts	1 oz	1.62
Pistachio	1 oz	0.65
Pumpkin seeds	1 oz	0.62
Black walnuts	1 oz	0.51
Pecans	1 oz	0.40
Cashews	1 oz	0.26
English walnuts	1 oz	0.20
Macadamia	1 oz	0.15
Chia seeds	1 oz	0.14
Flax seeds	1 oz	0.09
Coconut, raw meat	1 oz	0.07
Tahini	1 oz	0.07
Sesame seeds	1 oz	0.07
Trail mix, regular, salted	1 oz	x
Trail mix, tropical	1 oz	x
Mixed nuts, roasted with peanuts, no salt	1 oz	x

Nuts & Seeds	Amount	Vitamin E (mg)
Sunflower seeds	1/4 cup	12.31
Almonds, whole	1/4 cup	9.37
Peanut butter, smooth	1/4 cup	5.80
Hazelnuts, chopped	1/4 cup	4.32
Pine nuts	1/4 cup	3.15
Trail mix, regular with chocolate chips	1/4 cup	3.07
Peanuts	1/4 cup	3.04
Brazilnuts, whole	1/4 cup	1.91
Peanut butter, smooth	1 tbsp	1.44
Pistachio	1/4 cup	0.71
Pumpkin seeds	1/4 cup	0.70
Black walnuts, chopped	1/4 cup	0.56
Pecans, halves	1/4 cup	0.35
English walnuts, chopped	1/4 cup	0.18
Macadamia	1/4 cup	0.18

RDA is 15 mg for adults

VITAMIN E

Continued

Flaxseeds	1/4 cup	0.13
Sesame seeds	1/4 cup	0.09
Coconut meat, shredded	1/4 cup	0.05
Flaxseeds	1 tbsp	0.03
Sesame seeds	1 tbsp	0.02
Cashews	1/4 cup	x
Chia seeds	1/4 cup	x
Trail mix, regular, salted	1/4 cup	x
Trail mix, tropical	1/4 cup	x
Mixed nuts, roasted with peanuts, no salt	1/4 cup	x

Oil	Amount	Vitamin E (mg)
Sunflower oil, high oleic, 70% and over	1 tbsp	5.75
Sunflower oil, high linoleic, 65%	1 tbsp	5.59
Safflower oil, high linoleic acid, over 70%	1 tbsp	4.64
Safflower oil, high oleic	1 tbsp	4.64
Grapeseed oil	1 tbsp	3.92
Canola oil	1 tbsp	2.44
Peanut oil	1 tbsp	2.12
Olive oil	1 tbsp	1.94
Corn oil	1 tbsp	1.94
Soybean oil	1 tbsp	1.11
Soybean lecithin oil	1 tbsp	1.11
Soybean oil, partially hydrogenated	1 tbsp	1.10
Palm kernel oil	1 tbsp	0.52
Sesame oil	1 tbsp	0.19
Flaxseed oil	1 tbsp	0.06
Walnut oil	1 tbsp	0.05
Coconut oil	1 tbsp	0.01
Cod liver oil	1 tbsp	x
Menhaden oil	1 tbsp	x
Salmon fish oil	1 tbsp	x

Pork, Cooked	Amount	Vitamin E (mg)
Sausage	3 oz	0.47
Cured ham	3 oz	0.31
Braunschweiger	3 oz	0.30
Spareribs	3 oz	0.29
Sirloin pork chops	3 oz	0.22
Bratwurst	3 oz	0.22
Cured ham, lean	3 oz	0.22
Backribs	3 oz	0.21
Italian sausage	3 oz	0.21
Chops, lean, pan-fried	3 oz	0.19
Ground pork	3 oz	0.18

RDA is 15 mg for adults

VITAMIN E

Chops, pan-fried	3 oz	0.17
Canadian-style bacon	2 slices	0.16
Sausage	1 patty	0.15
Sausage	2 links	0.14
Center loin pork chops	3 oz	0.09
Tenderloin	3 oz	0.07
Bacon	3 slices	0.06
Polish sausage	3 oz	x
Liverwurst spread	1/4 cup	x

Turkey, Cooked	Amount	Vitamin E (mg)
Turkey bacon	3 oz	0.88
Ground turkey, 93% lean	3 oz	0.11
Ground turkey	3 oz	0.09
Breast meat	3 oz	0.08
Ground turkey, fat free	3 oz	0.08
Dark meat	3 oz	0.06
Ground turkey, 85% lean	3 oz	0.06
Light meat	3 oz	0.05
Turkey sausage, reduced fat	3 oz	0

Veal, Cooked	Amount	Vitamin E (mg)
Leg, top round	3 oz	0.42
Loin	3 oz	0.37
Sirloin	3 oz	0.36
Rib	3 oz	0.30
Ground	3 oz	0.13
Breast	3 oz	x
Foreshank	3 oz	x

Vegetables, Canned	Amount	Vitamin E (mg)
Spinach	1 cup	4.15
Asparagus	1 cup	2.95
Pumpkin	1 cup	2.60
Sweet potato	1 cup	2.25
Stewed tomato	1 cup	2.12
Tomatoes	1 cup	1.63
Carrots	1 cup	1.08
Green peas	1 cup	0.65
Sauerkraut	1 cup	0.33
Yellow sweet corn	1 cup	0.08
Beets	1 cup	0.05
Green beans	1 cup	0.04
Mushrooms	1 cup	0.02

RDA is 15 mg for adults

VITAMIN E

Vegetables, Cooked	Amount	Vitamin E (mg)
Spinach	1 cup	3.74
Swiss chard	1 cup	3.31
Sweet potato, mashed	1 cup	3.08
Turnip greens	1 cup	2.71
Butternut squash	1 cup	2.64
Beet greens	1 cup	2.61
Dandelion greens	1 cup	2.56
Broccoli	1 cup	2.26
Asparagus	1 cup	2.16
Raab broccoli	1 cup	2.15
Collard greens	1 cup	2.13
Pumpkin	1 cup	1.96
Mustard greens	1 cup	1.69
Carrots	1 cup	1.61
Parsnips	1 cup	1.56
Kale	1 cup	1.11
Kohlrabi	1 cup	0.86
Brussels sprouts	1 cup	0.67
Snow peas	1 cup	0.62
Green beans	1 cup	0.56
Rutabagas	1 cup	0.54
Celery	1 cup	0.53
Leeks	1 cup	0.52
Yams, cubes	1 cup	0.46
Okra	1 cup	0.43
Broccolini	1 cup	0.42
Eggplant	1 cup	0.41
Hubbard squash	1 cup	0.41
Artichokes	1 cup	0.32
Summer squash	1 cup	0.25
Winter squash	1 cup	0.25
Crookneck and Straightneck squash	1 cup	0.22
Scallop or Pattypan squash	1 cup	0.22
Zucchini	1 cup	0.22
Cabbage	1 cup	0.21
Spaghetti squash	1 cup	0.19
Bok-Choy	1 cup	0.15
Corn	1 cup	0.13
Cauliflower	1 cup	0.09
Beets	1 cup	0.07
Split Peas	1 cup	0.06
Potatoes, flesh, baked	1 cup	0.05
Onions	1 cup	0.04

RDA is 15 mg for adults

VITAMIN E

Potatoes, mashed with whole milk	1 cup	0.04
Turnips	1 cup	0.03
White mushrooms	1 cup	0.02
Prickley pear cactus pads, nopales	1 cup	0
Shitake mushrooms	1 cup	0
Napa cabbage	1 cup	x

Vegetables, Frozen	Amount	Vitamin E (mg)
Spinach	1 cup	6.73
Turnip greens	1 cup	4.36
Broccoli	1 cup	2.43
Asparagus	1 cup	2.16
Collard greens	1 cup	2.13
Carrots	1 cup	1.47
Kale	1 cup	1.20
Brussels sprouts	1 cup	0.79
Okra	1 cup	0.59
Rhubarb	1 cup	0.46
Cauliflower	1 cup	0.11
Yellow corn	1 cup	0.11
Green beans	1 cup	0.05
Green peas	1 cup	0.05

Vegetables, Raw	Amount	Vitamin E (mg)
Red bell peppers	1 cup	2.35
Butternut squash	1 cup	2.02
Dandelion greens	1 cup	1.89
Tomatoes	1 cup	0.97
Radicchio	1 cup	0.90
Tomatoes, cherry	1 cup	0.80
Carrots	1 cup	0.73
Broccoli	1 cup	0.69
Chicory greens	1 cup	0.66
Raab broccoli	1 cup	0.65
Spinach	1 cup	0.61
Green bell peppers	1 cup	0.55
Green onions & scallions	1 cup	0.55
Tomatillos	1 cup	0.50
Snow peas	1 cup	0.38
Spirulina, dried	1 tbsp	0.35
Celery	1 cup	0.32
Endive	1 cup	0.22
Summer squash	1 cup	0.14
Zucchini	1 cup	0.14

RDA is 15 mg for adults

VITAMIN E

Continued

Green leaf lettuce	1 cup	0.12
Savoy cabbage	1 cup	0.12
Cabbage	1 cup	0.11
Butterhead & boston lettuce	1 cup	0.10
Iceburg lettuce	1 cup	0.10
Arugula	1 cup	0.09
Cauliflower	1 cup	0.08
Red cabbage	1 cup	0.08
Romaine lettuce	1 cup	0.07
Bok-Choy	1 cup	0.06
Red leaf lettuce	1 cup	0.04
Cucumbers	1 cup	0.03
Onions	1 cup	0.03
White mushrooms	1 cup	0.01
Prickley pear cactus pads	1 cup	0
Shiitake mushrooms, dried	1 each	0

Yogurt	Amount	Vitamin E (mg)
Plain yogurt, whole milk	8 oz	0.14
Plain yogurt, low fat	8 oz	0.07
Plain greek yogurt, non fat	8 oz	0.02
Plain yogurt, skim milk	8 oz	0

RDA is 15 mg for adults

Nutrient Data Collection Form

Food	Amount	Book Numbers	Multiply By	Estimated Nutrient Intake
Nutrient:	RDA:	Estimated:	% of RDA:	Total Estimated:

To download additional forms for free, go to www.TopNutrients4U.com

VITAMIN K

Vitamin K is a family of three fat soluble vitamins structurally related, derived from different sources with different potencies. They are necessary for proper blood clotting and bone metabolism and require dietary fat for absorption.

One, known as phylloquinone abbreviated as K1, is considered the primary source of vitamin-K activity in humans and its dominant dietary source is plants. A second known as K2 is bacterially synthesized in the intestine, found in small amounts in only a few foods such as cheese, and contributes a relatively small amount to the total daily requirements. The third known as K3 is the synthetic form not found in nature, has no vitamin-K activity, and may produce potentially damaging reactive oxidants.

Classical deficiency symptoms are excessive bleeding, bruising, and frequent nose-bleeds. Known causes of deficiency are intestinal abnormalities, inadequate dietary intake for long periods, and deficiencies induced by chronic use of anti-coagulant drugs and antibiotics. Historically, clinical vitamin-K deficiency has been diagnosed through hemorrhagic episodes, but there is concern since plasma concentrations of vitamin-K have been reported below normal ranges before observed clinical indications of a deficiency.

Adequate Daily Intakes for Vitamin K1 (phylloquinone) are in micrograms, mcg.

Recommend Adequate Intakes Levels for Vitamin K

Children	Vitamin K mcg
1 to 3 year olds	30
4 to 8 year olds	50

Males	
9 to 13 year olds	60
14 to 18 year olds	75
19 to 30 years	120
31 to 50 years	120
51 to 70 years	120
Over 70	120

Females	
9 to 13 year olds	60
14 to 18 year olds	75
19 to 30 years	90
31 to 50 years	90
51 to 70 years	90
Over 70	90
Pregnancy & Lactation	90

VITAMIN K

Alcohol	Amount	Vitamin K (mcg)
Red Wine	1 glass	0.6
White Wine	1 glass	0.6
Light Beer	1 bottle	0
Regular Beer	1 bottle	0
Gin, Rum, Vodka, Whisky	1 shot	0

Beans, Canned	Amount	Vitamin K (mcg)
Green beans	1 cup	59.5
Yellow beans	1 cup	15.1
Kidney beans	1 cup	10.5
Garbanzo beans	1 cup	8.6
Great Northern	1 cup	7.9
Navy beans	1 cup	7.6
White beans, mature	1 cup	7.6
Refried beans	1 cup	5.5
Pinto beans	1 cup	5.0
Black-eyed peas, commom, mature	1 cup	2.9
Baked beans, plain	1 cup	2.0
Cranberry beans	1 cup	x
Fava beans	1 cup	x
Lima beans, large	1 cup	x

Beans, Cooked	Amount	Vitamin K (mcg)
Black-eyed peas, immature	1 cup	43.9
Edamame	1 cup	41.4
Natto	1 cup	40.0
Soybeans, mature, dry roasted	1 cup	34.4
Soybeans, mature	1 cup	33.0
Green beans	1 cup	20.0
Yellow beans	1 cup	20.0
Kidney beans	1 cup	14.9
Split peas	1 cup	9.8
Garbanzo beans, chickpeas	1 cup	6.6
White beans, matured	1 cup	6.3
Black Turtle beans	1 cup	6.1
Pinto beans	1 cup	6.0
Mung beans	1 cup	5.5
Fava beans	1 cup	4.9
Lima beans, large & mature	1 cup	3.8
Lentils	1 cup	3.4
Navy beans	1 cup	1.1
Adzuki	1 cup	x
Black beans	1 cup	x

Adequate intake is 60 to 120 mcg for adults

VITAMIN K

Continued

Cranberry beans, mature	1 cup	x
Great northern beans	1 cup	x
Hyacinth beans	1 cup	x
Lupinis beans, mature seeds	1 cup	x
Mothbeans	1 cup	x
Pigeon peas	1 cup	x
Soybeans, green	1 cup	x
White beans, small	1 cup	x
Winged beans	1 cup	x
Yardlong	1 cup	x

Beef, Cooked	Amount	Vitamin K (mcg)
Ground beef, 75%	3 oz	1.90
Chuck roast, trim to 1/8" fat	3 oz	1.70
Ground beef, 80%	3 oz	1.40
London Broil, trim to 0" fat	3 oz	1.40
Brisket, lean, trim to 0" fat	3 oz	1.30
Filet Mignon, trim to 0"	3 oz	1.40
Ribeye steak, lean, trim 0" fat	3 oz	1.30
Top sirloin, lean, trim to 1/8" fat	3 oz	1.20
Flank steak, lean, trim to 0" fat	3 oz	1.10
Ground beef, 95%	3 oz	1.10
Ground beef, 85%	3 oz	1.00
Ground beef, 90%	3 oz	0.90
Tri Tip steak, lean, trim to 0" fat	3 oz	x

Beef, Cooked	Amount	Vitamin K (mcg)
Chuck roast, trim to 1/8" fat	1 lb cooked	9.10
Top Sirloin, trim to 1/8" fat	1 lb cooked	7.30
Brisket, lean, trim to 0" fat	1 lb cooked	6.80
Flank steak, lean, trim to 0" fat	1 lb cooked	5.90
Flank steak, lean, trim to 0" fat	1 steak	5.00
Ribeye steak, boneless, trim to 0" fat	1 steak	3.30
Ribeye filet, lean, trim to 0" fat	1 filet	2.10
Top Sirloin, choice filet, trim to 0" fat	1 filet	2.00
Filet Mignon, tenderloin, trim to 0" fat	1 steak	1.90
Beef ribs, trim to 1/8" fat	1 lb cooked	x
Porterhouse steak, trim to 0" fat	1 lb cooked	x
Skirt steak, trim to 0" fat	1 lb cooked	x
T-bone steak, trim to 0" fat	1 lb cooked	x
Tri Tip steak, lean, trim to 0" fat	1 lb cooked	x

Adequate intake is 60 to 120 mcg for adults

VITAMIN K

Beef, Cooked	Amount	Vitamin K (mcg)
Ground beef, 75%	1/4 lb patty	1.50
Ground beef, 80%	1/4 lb patty	1.20
Ground beef, 95%	1/4 lb patty	1.10
Ground beef, 85%	1/4 lb patty	0.90
Ground beef, 90%	1/4 lb patty	0.90

Bread	Amount	Vitamin K (mcg)
Mexican roll, bollilo	1 roll	10.7
Indian bread, Naan, whole wheat	1 piece	3.5
Dinner Rolls, brown & serve	1 roll	3.0
Potato bread	1 slice	2.2
White	1 slice	2.2
Bagel, wheat	4" bagel	1.5
Hamburger & Hotdog buns, plain	1 bun	1.3
Tortillas, flour	1 tortilla	1.1
Bagel plain	4" bagel	1.0
Croissants, butter	1 medium	1.0
Rye bread	1 slice	0.9
Wheat	1 slice	0.8
English Muffin, plain	1 muffin	0.7
Bagel, cinnamon & raisins	4" bagel	0.6
Bagel, oat bran	4" bagel	0.4
Egg bread	1 slice	0.4
Multi-Grain, and Whole-Grain	1 slice	0.4
Oatmeal bread	1 slice	0.4
Raisin bread	1 slice	0.4
Kaiser rolls	1 roll	0.3
Pumpernickle	1 slice	0.3
French, italian, sourdough	1 slice	0.2
Whole-Wheat	1 slice	0.2
Pita, white	6" pita	0.1
Reduced calorie rye	1 slice	0.1
Reduced calorie white	1 slice	0.1
Reduced calorie wheat	1 slice	0
Tortillas, corn	1 tortilla	0
Indian bread, Naan, plain	1 piece	x

Butter	Amount	Vitamin K (mcg)
Regular dairy butter, salted	1 tbsp	1.0
Regular dairy whipped butter, salted	1 tbsp	0.7

Adequate intake is 60 to 120 mcg for adults

VITAMIN K

Cereal, General Mills®	Amount	Vitamin K (mcg)
Cinnamon Toast Crunch	1 cup	3.2
Cinnamon Chex	1 cup	2.1
Raisin Nut Bran	1 cup	1.4
Oatmeal Crisp, Hearty Raisin	1 cup	1.2
Dora The Explorer	1 cup	1.1
Wheat Chex	1 cup	1.1
Basic 4	1 cup	1.0
Oatmeal Crisp, Crunchy Almond	1 cup	1.0
Total Raisin Bran	1 cup	1.0
Total Cranberry Crunch	1 cup	0.9
Cocoa Puffs	1 cup	0.8
Golden Grams	1 cup	0.8
Reese's Puffs	1 cup	0.7
Honey Nut Clusters	1 cup	0.6
Trix	1 cup	0.6
Wheaties	1 cup	0.6
Cookie Crisp	1 cup	0.5
Lucky Charms	1 cup	0.5
Rice Chex	1 cup	0.5
Berry Berry Kix	1 cup	0.3
Honey Nut Chex	1 cup	0.3
Multi-Bran CHEX	1 cup	0.2
Total Whole Grain	1 cup	0.2
Corn Chex	1 cup	0.1
Kix	1 cup	0.0
Chocolate Chex	1 cup	x

Cereal, General Mills Cheerios®	Amount	Vitamin K (mcg)
Apple Cinnamon	1 cup	1.9
Original	1 cup	0.9
Berry Burst	1 cup	0.8
Honey Nut	1 cup	0.8
Frosted	1 cup	0.7
Yogurt Burst	1 cup	0.7
Fruity	1 cup	0.5
Multi Grain	1 cup	0.4

Cereal, Kashi®	Amount	Vitamin K (mcg)
Go Lean Crunch	1 cup	3.40
Good Friends	1 cup	1.50
Go Lean	1 cup	1.10
Good Friends, Cinna-Raisin Crunch	1 cup	1.00

Adequate intake is 60 to 120 mcg for adults

VITAMIN K

Continued

Heart to Heart, Honey Toasted Oat	1 cup	1.00
Organic Promise, Autumn Wheat	1 cup	1.00
7-Whole Grain Honey Puffs	1 cup	0.60
7-Whole Grain Puffs	1 cup	0.60
Go Lean Crunch, Honey Almond Flax	1 cup	0.60

Cereal, Kellogg's®	Amount	Vitamin K (mcg)
All-Bran Original	1 cup	3.2
MUESLIX	1 cup	2.4
Cracklin' Oat Bran	1 cup	2.0
Raisin Bran	1 cup	1.2
Honey Smacks	1 cup	1.0
All-Bran Bran Buds	1 cup	0.8
Frosted MINI-Wheat's, Big-Bite	1 cup	0.7
Raisin Bran Crunch	1 cup	0.7
Smart Start, Strong Heart, Antioxidants	1 cup	0.6
All-Bran Complete Wheat Flakes	1 cup	0.5
Smorz	1 cup	0.5
Rice Krispies Treats	1 cup	0.4
Apple Jacks	1 cup	0.1
Froot Loops	1 cup	0.1
Frosted Flakes	1 cup	0.1
Honey Crunch Corn Flakes	1 cup	0.1
Product 19	1 cup	0.1
Cocoa Krispies	1 cup	0
Corn Flakes	1 cup	0
Corn Pops	1 cup	0
Crispix	1 cup	0
Frosted Rice Krispies	1 cup	0
Rice Krispies	1 cup	0
Cinnabon	1 cup	x
Crunchy Nut, Golden Honey Nut Flakes	1 cup	x
Crunchy Nut, Roasted Nut and Honey O's	1 cup	x
Fiberplus Berry Yogurt Crunch	1 cup	x
Fiberplus Cinnamon Oat Crunch	1 cup	x
Krave Chocolate	1 cup	x

Cereal, Kellogg's Special-K®	Amount	Vitamin K (mcg)
Blueberry	1 cup	2.10
Chocolately Delight	1 cup	0.70
Fruit & Yogurt	1 cup	0.50
Cinnamon Pecan	1 cup	0.40
Red Berries	1 cup	0.30
Vanilla Almond	1 cup	0.30
Original	1 cup	0.10

Adequate intake is 60 to 120 mcg for adults

VITAMIN K

Continued

Low Fat Granolia	1 cup	x
Multigrain Oats & Honey	1 cup	x
Protein Plus	1 cup	x

Cereal, Post®	Amount	Vitamin K, mcg
Blueberry Morning	1 cup	5.6
Great Grains, Banana Nut Crunch	1 cup	2.7
Grape-Nuts Cereal	1 cup	2.2
Great Grains, Raisin, Date & Pecan	1 cup	1.9
Great Grains, Crunchy Pecan	1 cup	1.5
Great Grains, Cranberry Almond Crunch	1 cup	1.3
Raisin Bran	1 cup	1.1
Grape-Nuts Flakes	1 cup	1.0
Honey Nut Shredded Wheat	1 cup	0.9
Shredded Wheat n' Bran, spoon-size	1 cup	0.9
Shredded Wheat, Original, spoon-size	1 cup	0.7
Bran Flakes	1 cup	0.6
Cocoa Pebbles	1 cup	0.5
Fruity Pebbles	1 cup	0.5
Shredded Wheat, frosted, spoon-size	1 cup	0.5
Alpha-Bits	1 cup	0.4
Shredded Wheat, Original, big biscuit	1 biscuit	0.4
Golden Crisp	1 cup	0.3
Honeycomb Cereal	1 cup	0.1

Post® Honey Bunches of Oats®	Amount	Vitamin K (mcg)
Just Bunches Honey Roasted	1 cup	6.3
With Vanilla Bunches	1 cup	1.8
With Almonds	1 cup	1.3
Honey Roasted	1 cup	1.2
Pecan Bunches	1 cup	0.5
With Cinnamon Bunches	1 cup	x
With Strawberries	1 cup	x

Cereal, Quaker®	Amount	Vitamin K (mcg)
Toasted Multigrain Crisp	1 cup	1.0
Oatmeal Squares	1 cup	0.9
Oatmeal Squares, Cinnamon	1 cup	0.9
LIFE Cereal, Cinnamon	1 cup	0.5
LIFE Cereal, Original	1 cup	0.5
Puffed Wheat	1 cup	0.3
CAP'N Crunch	1 cup	0.2
CAP'N Crunch & Crunchberries	1 cup	0.2
CAP'N Crunch's Peanut Butter Crunch	1 cup	0.1

Adequate intake is 60 to 120 mcg for adults

VITAMIN K

Continued

Corn Bran Crunch	1 cup	0.1
Honey Graham OH'S	1 cup	0.1
Puffed Rice	1 cup	0
CAP'N Crunch's OOPs! All Berries	1 cup	x
Granola, Apple, Cranberry, & Almond	1 cup	x
LIFE Cereal, Maple & Brown Sugar	1 cup	x
Oatmeal Squares, Golden Maple	1 cup	x

Cereal, Cooked	Amount	Vitamin K (mcg)
Instant Oatmeal, Maple & Brown Sugar	1 packet	0.8
Oats, regular, unenriched	1 cup	0.7
Instant Oatmeal, Apple & Cinnamon	1 packet	0.7
CREAM OF WHEAT	1 cup	0.3
Farina	1 cup	0
White corn grits	1 cup	0
Yellow corn grits	1 cup	0

Cheese	Amount	Vitamin K (mcg)
Ricotta, whole milk	1 cup	2.7
Ricotta, part skim milk	1 cup	1.7
Cottage cheese, lowfat, 1 %	1 cup	0.2
Cottage cheese, nonfat, uncreamed	1 cup	0
Cottage cheese, creamed, small curd	1 cup	0
Cottage cheese, lowfat, 2 %	1 cup	0

Cheese	Amount	Vitamin K (mcg)
American, pasteurized process, imitation	1 oz	10.40
American, pasteurized process, fortified	1 oz	1.00
Goat cheese, hard type	1 oz	0.90
American, pasteurized process, low fat	1 oz	0.80
Cheddar	1 oz	0.80
Colby	1 oz	0.80
Cream cheese	1 oz	0.80
Gruyere	1 oz	0.80
Blue cheese	1 oz	0.70
Fontina	1 oz	0.70
Goat cheese, semisoft type	1 oz	0.70
Gouda	1 oz	0.70
Monterey	1 oz	0.70
Mozzarella, whole milk	1 oz	0.70
Muenster	1 oz	0.70
Swiss	1 oz	0.70
Provolone	1 oz	0.60
Romano	1 oz	0.60

Adequate intake is 60 to 120 mcg for adults

VITAMIN K

Continued

Cheese	Amount	Vitamin K (mcg)
Feta	1 oz	0.50
Goat cheese, soft type	1 oz	0.50
Monterey, low fat	1 oz	0.50
Mozzarella, nonfat	1 oz	0.50
Parmesan, grated	1 oz	0.50
Mozzarella, part skim, low moisture	1 oz	0.40
Muenster, low fat	1 oz	0.40
Provolone, reduced fat	1 oz	0.40
Cheddar, lowfat	1 oz	0.20
Cream cheese, fat free	1 oz	0.10
Swiss, low fat	1 oz	0.10
Brie	1 oz	0.07
Cheez Whiz, pasteurized process	1 oz	x
Velveeta, pasteurized process	1 oz	x

Cheese, Mexican	Amount	Vitamin K (mcg)
Mexican, blend	1 oz	0.7
Queso anejo	1 oz	0.7
Queso asadero	1 oz	0.7
Queso chihuahua	1 oz	0.7
Mexican, blend, reduced fat	1 oz	0.5
Queso fresco	1 oz	0.3

Chicken, Cooked	Amount	Vitamin K (mcg)
Thigh, no skin, roasted	1 thigh	2.0
Drumstick, no skin, roasted	1 drumstick	1.5
Breast, no skin, roasted	1/2 breast	0.3

Chicken, Cooked	Amount	Vitamin K (mcg)
Thigh meat only, no skin, roasted	3 oz	3.3
Drumstick meat only, roasted	3 oz	3.0
Thigh with skin, roasted	3 oz	2.8
Drumstick with skin, roasted	3 oz	2.7
Cornish game hens, meat only	3 oz	2.0
Breast meat only, no skin, roasted	3 oz	0.3
Breast with skin, roasted	3 oz	0.3
Wing meat only, no skin, roasted	3 oz	0.3
Wing with skin, roasted	3 oz	0.3
Breast with skin, fried in flour	3 oz	x
Drumstick with skin, fried in flour	3 oz	x
Thigh with skin, fried in flour	3 oz	x
Wing with skin, fried in flour	3 oz	x

Adequate intake is 60 to 120 mcg for adults

VITAMIN K

Cream	Amount	Vitamin K (mcg)
Heavy Whipping	1 tbsp	0.5
Whipped topping, pressurized	1 tbsp	0.4
Light Coffe cream	1 tbsp	0.3
Half & Half	1 tbsp	0.2
Sour cream, cultured	1 tbsp	0.2
Sour cream, reduced fat	1 tbsp	0.1

Eggs	Amount	Vitamin K (mcg)
Egg whole, scrambled	1 large	2.4
Egg whole, hard boiled	1 large	0.2
Egg yolk	1 large	0.1
Egg substitute, liquid, fat free	1/4 cup	0.1
Egg whites	1 large	0
Egg whites, dried	1 ounce	0
Egg whites, dried powder, stabilized	1 tbsp	0

Fish, Canned	Amount	Vitamin K (mcg)
Light tuna, in oil	3 oz	37.4
White (albacore) tuna, in oil	3 oz	5.9
Atlantic Sardines	3 oz	2.2
White (albacore) tuna, in water	3 oz	2.1
Light tuna, in water	3 oz	0.2

Fish, Cooked	Amount	Vitamin K (mcg)
Catfish, farmed	3 oz	2.1
Orange roughy	3 oz	0.9
Tilapia	3 oz	0.8
Pink salmon	3 oz	0.4
Atlantic herring	3 oz	0.2
Atlantic perch	3 oz	0.1
Chinock salmon, smoked	3 oz	0.1
Coho, wild	3 oz	0.1
Flounder and Sole	3 oz	0.1
Haddock	3 oz	0.1
Pacific mackerel	3 oz	0.1
Perch	3 oz	0.1
Pollock	3 oz	0.1
Rainbow trout, farmed	3 oz	0.1
Sockeye salmon	3 oz	0.1
Swordfish	3 oz	0.1
Walleye pollock	3 oz	0.1
Whiting	3 oz	0.1
Yellowfin tuna	3 oz	0.1

Adequate intake is 60 to 120 mcg for adults

VITAMIN K

Alaskan halibut	3 oz	0
Pacifc cod	3 oz	0
Rockfish	3 oz	0
Atlantic croaker	3 oz	x
Atlantic mackerel	3 oz	x
Atlantic pollock	3 oz	x
Atlantic salmon, farmed	3 oz	x
Atlantic salmon, wild	3 oz	x
Bluefin tuna	3 oz	x
Carp	3 oz	x
Catfish, breaded & fried	3 oz	x
Catfish, wild	3 oz	x
Chinook salmon	3 oz	x
Coho, farmed	3 oz	x
Florida pompano	3 oz	x
Freshwater bass	3 oz	x
Greenland halibut	3 oz	x
Grouper	3 oz	x
Keta, (chum) salmon	3 oz	x
King mackerel	3 oz	x
Northern pike	3 oz	x
Rainbow trout, wild	3 oz	x
Sea bass	3 oz	x
Skipjack, (aku) tuna	3 oz	x
Snapper	3 oz	x
Spanish mackerel	3 oz	x
Striped bass	3 oz	x
Walleye pike	3 oz	x
Yellowtail	3 oz	x

Fish, Shellfish, Cooked	Amount	Vitamin K (mcg)
Eastern oysters, wild	3 oz	1.3
Shrimp, breaded & fried	3 oz	0.8
Shrimp, breaded & fried	6 large	0.5
Alaska king crab, imitation	3 oz	0.3
Blue crab	3 oz	0.3
Blue crab, canned	3 oz	0.3
Clams, canned	3 oz	0.3
Shrimp	3 oz	0.3
Crayfish	3 oz	0.1
Octopus	3 oz	0.1
Northern lobster	3 oz	0
Shrimp, canned	3 oz	0
Abalone	3 oz	x
Alaska king crab	3 oz	x

Adequate intake is 60 to 120 mcg for adults

VITAMIN K

Clams, breaded & fried	3 oz	x
Crab cakes	3 oz	x
Eastern oysters, farmed	3 oz	x
Queen crab	3 oz	x
Scallops, breaded & fried	3 oz	x
Squid, fried	3 oz	x

Fruit, Canned	Amount	Vitamin K (mcg)
Plums	1 cup	11.1
Apricots	1 cup	5.7
Peaches	1 cup	4.5
Applesauce, sweetened	1 cup	1.5
Applesauce, unsweetened	1 cup	1.2
Pears	1 cup	0.8
Pineapple	1 cup	0.8
Olives, black	5 large	0.3
Olives, green	5 large	0.2

Fruit, Dried	Amount	Vitamin K (mcg)
Pears	1 cup	36.7
Peaches	1 cup	25.1
Figs	1 cup	23.2
Currants	1 cup	4.8
Cranberries	1 cup	4.6
Apricots	1 cup	4.0
Apples	1 cup	2.6

Fruit, Frozen	Amount	Vitamin K (mcg)
Blueberries	1 cup	41
Blackberries	1 cup	30
Raspberries	1 cup	16
Peaches	1 cup	6
Strawberries	1 cup	4

Fruit, Raw	Amount	Vitamin K (mcg)
Avocado, Florida	1 cup	x
Valencia Oranges	1 cup	x
Prunes, uncooked	1 cup	103.5
Kiwi	1 cup	73.0
Stewed prunes	1 cup	64.7
Avocado, California	1 cup	48.3
Blackberries	1 cup	28.5

Adequate intake is 60 to 120 mcg for adults

VITAMIN K

Pomegrenates	1 cup	28.5
Blueberries	1 cup	28.0
Grapes, red & green	1 cup	23.4
Plums	1 cup	10.6
Raspberries	1 cup	9.6
Pears	1 cup	7.2
Mango	1 cup	6.9
Apricots	1 cup	5.4
Cranberries	1 cup	5.1
Raisins	1 cup	5.1
Honeydew	1 cup	4.9
Cantaloupe	1 cup	4.0
Dates	1 cup	4.0
Peachs	1 cup	4.0
Papayas	1 cup	3.8
Strawberries	1 cup	3.7
Cherries, without pits	1 cup	3.2
Nectarine	1 cup	3.1
Apples	1 cup	2.8
Mulberries	1 cup	1.4
Pineapple	1 cup	1.2
Plantains	1 cup	1.0
Jicama	1 cup	0.4
Water mellon	1 cup	0.2
Elderberries	1 cup	0
Florida Oranges	1 cup	0
Naval Oranges	1 cup	0
Tangerine	1 cup	0

Fruit, Raw	Amount	Vitamin K (mcg)
Pomegranates	1 fruit	46.3
Avocado, California	1 fruit	28.6
Kiwi	1 fruit	28
Prunes, uncooked	5 prunes	28
Chayote	1 fruit	8.3
Pears	1 fruit	7.5
Persimmons, Japanese	1 fruit	4.4
Plums	1 fruit	4.2
Papayas, small	1 fruit	4.1
Peaches	1 fruit	4.0
Apples	1 fruit	3.0
Nectarine	1 fruit	2.8
Cherries	10 fruit	1.7

Adequate intake is 60 to 120 mcg for adults

VITAMIN K

Pineapple guava, Feijoa	1 fruit	1.5
Raisins	1 small box	1.5
Figs, dried	1 fruit	1.3
Plantains	1 fruit	1.3
Strawberries	5 fruit	1.3
Apricots	1 fruit	1.2
Dates	5 fruit	1.1
Banana	1 fruit	0.6
Raisins	1 packet	0.5
Pineapple	1/2" x 3" slice	0.3
Star fruit, Carambola	1 fruit	0
Florida Oranges	1 fruit	0
Kumquats	1 fruit	0
Naval Oranges	1 fruit	0
Tangerine	1 fruit	0
Avocado, Florida	1 fruit	x
Cherimoya	1 fruit	x
Persimmons, small native	1 fruit	x
Pummello	1 fruit	x
Valencias Oranges	1 fruit	x

Game Meat, Cooked	Amount	Vitamin K (mcg)
Duck	3 oz	3.2
Rabbit	3 oz	1.3
Caribou	3 oz	1.2
Deer, ground	3 oz	1.2
Squirrel	3 oz	1.2
Wild boar	3 oz	1.2
Antelope	3 oz	x
Bison, ground	3 oz	x
Buffalo, steak, free range	3 oz	x
Elk, ground	3 oz	x
Elk, roasted	3 oz	x

Grains, Cooked	Amount	Vitamin K (mcg)
Egg & Spinach noodles	1 cup	162.0
Buckwheat	1 cup	3.2
Chow mein noodles	1 cup	3.0
Pearled barley	1 cup	1.3
Brown rice	1 cup	1.2
Whole-Wheat spaghetti	1 cup	1.0
Bulgur	1 cup	0.9
Wild rice	1 cup	0.8
Millet	1 cup	0.5
Couscous	1 cup	0.2

Adequate intake is 60 to 120 mcg for adults

915

VITAMIN K

Continued

Macaroni	1 cup	0
Egg noodles	1 cup	0
Instant white rice	1 cup	0
White rice	1 cup	0
Spaghetti	1 cup	0

Herbs & Spices	Amount	Vitamin K (mcg)
Basil, dried & ground	1 tsp	24
Thyme, dried, ground	1 tsp	24
Thyme, dried leaves	1 tsp	17
Sage, ground	1 tsp	12
Coriander, dried	1 tsp	8
Parsley, dried	1 tsp	7
Oregano	1 tsp	6
Marjoram	1 tsp	4
Basil, fresh, chopped	1 tsp	4
Pepper, black	1 tsp	3
Cloves, dried	1 tsp	3
Chili powder	1 tsp	3
Chives, raw	1 tsp	2
Curry powder	1 tsp	2
Paprika	1 tsp	1.7
Cinnamon powder	1 tsp	0.7
Onion powder	1 tsp	0.1
Caraway seeds	1 tsp	0
Celery seeds	1 tsp	0
Garlic powder	1 tsp	0
Ginger	1 tsp	0
Nutmeg	1 tsp	0

Juice	Amount	Vitamin K (mcg)
Carrot	1 cup	36.6
Pomegranate	1 cup	25.9
Vegetable	1 cup	12.8
Prune	1 cup	8.7
Tomato	1 cup	5.6
Cranberry	1 cup	2.5
Grape	1 cup	1.0
Pineapple	1 cup	0.8
Orange, raw	1 cup	0.2
Apple	1 cup	0
Grapefruit, raw	1 cup	0
Lemon, raw	1 cup	0

Adequate intake is 60 to 120 mcg for adults

VITAMIN K

Lamb, Cooked	Amount	Vitamin K (mcg)
Ground	3 oz	4.5
Chops, loin, lean, trim to 1/4" fat	3 oz	4.1
Leg, whole, trim to 1/4" fat	3 oz	3.6
Rib, lean, trim to 1/4" fat	3 oz	3.5
Cubed for stew or kabob	3 oz	x
Foreshank, trim to 1/8" fat	3 oz	x

Milk	Amount	Vitamin K (mcg)
Soy milk, original, unfortified	1 cup	7.4
Canned, condensed, sweet	1 cup	1.8
Canned, evaporated	1 cup	1.3
Whole milk, 3.25%	1 cup	0.7
Lowfat, 2%	1 cup	0.5
Goat milk	1 cup	0.7
Human milk	1 cup	0.7
Buttermilk, lowfat	1 cup	0.2
Lowfat, 1%	1 cup	0.2
Canned, evaporated, nonfat	1 cup	0
Dry, instant, nonfat	1/3 cup	0
Nonfat, fat free or skim milk	1 cup	0

Nuts & Seeds	Amount	Vitamin K (mcg)
Pine nuts	1 ounce	15.3
Cashews	1 ounce	9.7
Hazelnuts	1 ounce	4.0
Trail mix, regular with chocolate chips	1/4 cup	2.4
Pumpkin seeds	1 ounce	2.1
Flax seeds	1 ounce	1.2
Pecans	1 ounce	1.0
Black walnuts	1 ounce	0.8
English walnuts	1 ounce	0.8
Peanut butter, smooth style	1 ounce	0.2
Coconut, raw meat	1 ounce	0.1
Almonds	1 ounce	0
Brazilnuts	1 ounce	0
Peanuts	1 ounce	0
Sesame seeds	1 ounce	0
Sunflower seeds	1 ounce	0
Tahini	1 ounce	0
Chia	1 ounce	x
Macadamia	1 ounce	x
Pistacho	1 ounce	x
Trail mix, regular, salted	1/4 cup	x

Adequate intake is 60 to 120 mcg for adults

VITAMIN K

Continued

Trail mix, tropical	1/4 cup	x
Mixed nuts, roasted with peanuts, no salt	1/4 cup	x

Nuts & Seeds	Amount	Vitamin K (mcg)
Pine nuts	1/4 cup	18.2
Hazelnuts	1/4 cup	4.1
Pumpkin seeds	1/4 cup	2.4
Flax seeds	1/4 cup	1.8
Pecans	1/4 cup	0.9
Black walnuts	1/4 cup	0.8
English walnuts	1/4 cup	0.7
Peanut butter, smooth style	1/4 cup	0.4
Peanut butter, smooth style	1 tbsp	0.1
Almonds	1/4 cup	0
Brazilnuts	1/4 cup	0
Coconut, raw meat	1/4 cup	0
Peanuts	1/4 cup	0
Sesame seeds	1 ybsp	0
Sunflower seeds	1/4 cup	0
Tahini	1/4 cup	0
Cashews	1/4 cup	x
Chia	1/4 cup	x
Macadamia	1/4 cup	x
Pistacho	1/4 cup	x

Oils	Amount	Vitamin K (mcg)
Soybean lecithin oil	1 tbsp	25.0
Soybean oil	1 tbsp	25.0
Canola oil	1 tbsp	10.0
Canola oil, partially hydrogenated	1 tbsp	9.7
Olive oil	1 tbsp	8.1
Cottonseed oil	1 tbsp	3.4
Palm kernal vegetable oil	1 tbsp	3.4
Soybean oil, partially hydrogenated	1 tbsp	3.4
Walnut oil	1 tbsp	2.0
Sesame oil	1 tbsp	1.8
Flaxseed oil	1 tbsp	1.3
Safflower oil, high linoleic acid	1 tbsp	1.0
Safflower oil, high oleic acid	1 tbsp	1.0
Sunflower, high oleic acid	1 tbsp	0.8
Sunflower, high linoleic acid	1 tbsp	0.7
Corn oil	1 tbsp	0.3
Coconut oil	1 tbsp	0.1
Peanut oil	1 tbsp	0.1
Code liver fish oil	1 tbsp	x

Adequate intake is 60 to 120 mcg for adults

VITAMIN K

Continued

Grapeseed oil	1 tbsp	x
Menhaden fish oil	1 tbsp	x
Salmon fish oil	1 tbsp	x

Pork, Cooked	Amount	Vitamin K (mcg)
Sausage	1 patty	0.1
Sausage	2 links	0.1
Backribs	3 oz	0
Ground pork	3 oz	0
Bacon	3 slices	0
Canadian-style bacon	2 slices	0
Chops, boned	3 oz	0
Cured ham	3 oz	0

Turkey, Cooked	Amount	Vitamin K (mcg)
Turkey bacon	3 oz	6.0
Liver	3 oz	1
Dark meat	3 oz	0
Light meat	3 oz	0
Breast meat	3 oz	0
Ground turkey	3 oz	0
Ground turkey, 93% lean	3 oz	0
Ground turkey, 85% lean	3 oz	0
Turkey sausage, reduced fat	3 oz	0
Ground turkey, fat free	3 oz	0

Veal, Cooked	Amount	Vitamin K (mcg)
Leg, top round	3 oz	6.0
Sirloin	3 oz	5.6
Loin	3 oz	4.7
Ground	3 oz	1
Breast	3 oz	x
Foreshank	3 oz	x
Rib	3 oz	x

Vegetables, Canned	Amount	Vitamin K (mcg)
Spinach	1 cup	988
Asparagus	1 cup	100
Green peas	1 cup	63
Green beans	1 cup	53
Pumpkin	1 cup	39
Sauerkraut	1 cup	31
Tomato paste	1 cup	30
Carrots	1 cup	14

Adequate intake is 60 to 120 mcg for adults

Continued

Tomato pure	1 cup	9
Tomatoes	1 cup	7
Tomato sauce	1 cup	7
Stewed tomato	1 cup	6
Sweet potato	1 cup	5
Beets	1 cup	0
Corn	1 cup	0
Mushrooms	1 cup	0

Vegetables, Cooked	Amount	Vitamin K (mcg)
Kale	1 cup	1062
Lambsquarters	1 cup	889
Spinach	1 cup	889
Collard greens	1 cup	836
Beet greens	1 cup	697
Dandelion greens	1 cup	579
Swiss Chard	1 cup	572
Turnip greens	1 cup	529
Mustard greens	1 cup	419
Broccoli	1 cup	220
Brussels sprouts	1 cup	219
Cabbage	1 cup	163
Asparagus	1 cup	144
Cabbage, Red	1 cup	71
Okra	1 cup	64
Cabbage, Chinese, Bok-Choy	1 cup	58
Celery	1 cup	57
Snow Peas	1 cup	40
Leeks	1 cup	26
Artichokes	1 cup	25
Carrots	1 cup	21
Green beans	1 cup	20
Cauliflower	1 cup	17
Split peas	1 cup	9.8
Winter Squash	1 cup	9.0
Crookneck and Straightneck squash	1 cup	8.0
Zucchini	1 cup	7.6
Sweet potato, mashed	1 cup	6.9
Scallop or Pattypan squash	1 cup	6.3
Summer squash, all varieties averaged	1 cup	6.3
Potatoes, mashed with whole milk	1 cup	3.8
Hubbard squash, baked	1 cup	3.3
Yams, cubes	1 cup	3.1
Eggplant	1 cup	2.9
Butternut squash, baked	1 cup	2.0

VITAMIN K

Continued

Pumpkin	1 cup	2.0
Parsnips	1 cup	1.6
Spaghetti squash	1 cup	1.2
Onions	1 cup	1.1
Rutabagas	1 cup	0.5
Potatoes, flesh, baked	1 cup	0.4
Beets	1 cup	0
Corn	1 ear	0
Kohlrabi	1 cup	0
Turnips	1 cup	0
Shitake mushrooms	1 cup	0
White mushrooms	1 cup	0
Acorn squash, baked	1 cup	x
Cabbage, Chinese, Pe-Tsai	1 cup	x
Cabbage, Napa	1 cup	x
Cabbage, Savoy	1 cup	x
Mustatrd Spinach	1 cup	x

Vegetables, Frozen	Amount	Vitamin K (mcg)
Kale	1 cup	1147
Collard Greens	1 cup	1059
Spinach	1 cup	1027
Turnip Greens	1 cup	851
Spinach	1 cup	300
Broccoli	1 cup	162
Asparagus	1 cup	144
Okra	1 cup	88
Rhubarb	1 cup	51
Green Peas	1 cup	38
Cauliflower	1 cup	21
Carrots	1 cup	20
Green Beans	1 cup	17
Corn	1 cup	0.5
Butternut Squash	1 cup	x

Vegetables, Raw	Amount	Vitamin K (mcg)
Kale	1 cup	547
Dandelion greens	1 cup	428
Swiss chard	1 cup	298
Green onions & scallions	1 cup	207
Cabbage, Mustard	1 cup	148
Spinach	1 cup	145
Endive	1 cup	116
Radicchio	1 cup	102
Raab broccoli	1 cup	90

Adequate intake is 60 to 120 mcg for adults

VITAMIN K

Broccoli	1 cup	89
Chicory greens	1 cup	86
Green leaf lettuce	1 cup	71
Romaine lettuce	1 cup	57
Butterhead & boston lettuce	1 cup	56
Cabbage	1 cup	53
Cabbage, Savoy	1 cup	48
Red leaf lettuce	1 cup	39
Celery	1 cup	35
Cabbage, Chinese, Pe-Tsai	1 cup	32
Cabbage, Chinese, Bok-Choy	1 cup	32
Cabbage, Red	1 cup	27
Snow peas	1 cup	25
Arugula	1 cup	22
Cucumbers	1 cup	17
Cauliflower	1 cup	16
Carrots	1 cup	15
Tomatoes	1 cup	14
Iceburg lettuce	1 cup	13
Tomatillos	1 cup	13
Tomatoes, cherry	1 cup	12
Green bell peppers	1 cup	11
Red bell peppers	1 cup	7
Zucchini	1 cup	5
Prickley pear cactus pads, Nopales	1 cup	5
Summer squash	1 cup	3
Spirulina, dried	1 tbsp	2
Butternut squash	1 cup	2
Onions	1 cup	0.6
Yellow sweet corn	1 cup	0.5
Shiitake mushrooms, dried	1 each	0
White mushrooms	1 cup	0
Belgian endive	1 cup	X
Cabbage, Danish	1 cup	X

Adequate intake is 60 to 120 mcg for adults

Nutrient Data Collection Form

Food	Amount	Book Numbers	Multiply By	Estimated Nutrient Intake
Nutrient::	RDA:	Estimated:	% of RDA:	Total Estimated:

To download additional forms for free, go to www.TopNutrients4U.com

ZINC

Zinc is a mineral needed for protein and DNA synthesis, for building and maintaining the immune system, for enzyme activity, wound healing, and spermatogenesis. At the sub-cellular level zinc is an essential component of at least one enzyme in every classification of enzymes, which number into the hundreds.

Because of this, it is plausible that constant low dietary zinc deficiency over time may result in a generalized metabolic impairment in all tissues of the body. Deficiency is associated with: dermatitis, stunted and retarded growth, hypogonadism in males, diarrhea in children, slow wound healing, frequent common colds, high rates of infections, and pneumonia.

Deficiencies are related to insufficient dietary intake for long periods, malabsorption, excessive excretion from the body, a restricted diet, and renal insufficiency. However, the most common cause may be from the inhibition of zinc absorption by phosphorus compounds found in beans, seeds, nuts, and all grains, including corn, cereals, rice and flours.

Concerning toxicity, excess zinc is known to induce a copper deficiency in animals and humans and if untreated will result in neurological damage. Please see the chapter on copper.

The recommended daily allowance, RDA, for zinc is in milligram, mg, quantities. Never take any zinc supplements without first consulting with a physician.

ZINC

Recommend Daily Intakes Levels for Zinc

Children	Zinc mg
1 to 3 year olds	3
4 to 8 year olds	5

Males	
9 to 13 year olds	8
14 to 18 year olds	11
19 to 30 years	11
31 to 50 years	11
51 to 70 years	11
Over 70	11

Females	
9 to 13 year olds	8
14 to 18 year olds	9
19 to 30 years	8
31 to 50 years	8
51 to 70 years	8
Over 70	8
Pregnancy	11
Lactation	12

ZINC

Alcohol	Amount	Zinc (mg)
Red Wine	1 glass	0.21
White Wine	1 glass	0.18
Light Beer	1 bottle	0.04
Regular Beer	1 bottle	0.04
Gin, Rum, Vodka, Whisky	1 shot	0.02

Beans, Canned	Amount	Zinc (mg)
Baked beans, plain	1 cup	5.79
White beans	1 cup	2.93
Cranberry beans	1 cup	2.18
Navy beans	1 cup	2.02
Great Northern	1 cup	1.70
Black-eyed peas	1 cup	1.68
Garbanzo beans	1 cup	1.66
Fava beans	1 cup	1.59
Kidney	1 cup	1.59
Lima beans	1 cup	1.57
Refried beans	1 cup	1.55
Pinto beans	1 cup	1.34
Yellow beans	1 cup	0.44
Green beans	1 cup	0.32

Beans, Cooked	Amount	Zinc (mg)
Hyacinth beans	1 cup	5.53
Natto	1 cup	5.30
Soybeans, mature, dry roasted	1 cup	4.44
Adzuki	1 cup	4.07
Garbanzo beans	1 cup	2.51
Lentils	1 cup	2.51
Winged beans	1 cup	2.48
White beans, mature	1 cup	2.47
Lupini beans	1 cup	2.29
Black-eyed	1 cup	2.21
Edamame	1 cup	2.12
Cranberry beans	1 cup	2.02
Soybeans, mature	1 cup	1.98
Split peas	1 cup	1.96
White beans, small	1 cup	1.95
Black beans	1 cup	1.93
Kidney beans	1 cup	1.89
Navy beans	1 cup	1.87
Lima beans	1 cup	1.79
Fava beans	1 cup	1.72

RDA for adults 11 mg for females, and 8 mg for males

ZINC

Continued

Mung beans, mature seeds	1 cup	1.70
Pinto beans	1 cup	1.68
Soybeans, green	1 cup	1.64
Great Northern	1 cup	1.56
Pigeon peas	1 cup	1.51
Black Turtle beans, mature	1 cup	1.41
Mothbeans	1 cup	1.04
Yellow beans	1 cup	0.45
Yardlong beans, Chinese long beans	1 cup	0.37
Green beans	1 cup	0.31

Beef, Cooked	Amount	Zinc (mg)
Ribeye steak, lean, trim 0" fat	3 oz	8
Chuck roast, trim to 1/8" fat	3 oz	7
Brisket, lean, trim to 0" fat	3 oz	7
Tri Tip steak, lean, trim to 0" fat	3 oz	6
Skirt steak, trim to 0" fat	3 oz	6
Ground beef, 95%	3 oz	5
Ground beef, 90%	3 oz	5
Ground beef, 85%	3 oz	5
Ground beef, 80%	3 oz	5
Ground beef, 75%	3 oz	5
Top Sirloin, trim to 1/8" fat	3 oz	5
Beef ribs, trim to 1/8" fat	3 oz	5
Flank steak, lean, trim to 0" fat	3 oz	4
Londom Broil, top round	3 oz	4
Filet Mignon, trim to 0" fat	3 oz	4
T-bone steak, trim 0" fat	3 oz	4
Porterhouse steak, trim to 0" fat	3 oz	4

Beef, Cooked	Amount	Zinc (mg)
Chuck roast, trim to 1/8" fat	1 cooked lb	37
Brisket, lean, trim to 0" fat	1 cooked lb	36
Tri Tip steak, lean, trim to 0" fat	1 cooked lb	33
Skirt steak, trim to 0" fat	1 cooked lb	33
Beef ribs, trim to 1/8" fat	1 cooked lb	25
Flank steak, lean, trim to 0" fat	1 cooked lb	23
Top Sirloin, trim to 1/8" fat	1 cooked lb	22
T-bone steak, trim to 0" fat	1 cooked lb	21
Porterhouse steak, trim to 0" fat	1 cooked lb	21
Ribeye steak, boneless, trim to 0" fat	1 steak	20
Flank steak, lean, trim to 0" fat	1 steak	19
Ribeye filet, lean, trim to 0" fat	1 filet	14
Top Sirloin, choice filet, trim to 0" fat	1 filet	9
Filet Mignon, tenderloin, trim to 0" fat	1 steak	5

     RDA for adults 11 mg for females, and 8 mg for males

ZINC

Beef, Cooked	Amount	Zinc (mg)
Ground beef, 95%	1/4 lb patty	5.27
Ground beef, 90%	1/4 lb patty	5.22
Ground beef, 85%	1/4 lb patty	4.86
Ground beef, 80%	1/4 lb patty	4.81
Ground beef, 75%	1/4 lb patty	4.33

Bread	Amount	Zinc (mg)
Bagel plain	4" bagel	1.69
Indian bread, Naan, whole wheat	1 piece	1.31
Bagel, wheat	4" bagel	1.08
Bagel, cinnamon & raisins	4" bagel	1.01
Bagel, oat bran	4" bagel	0.94
Mexican roll, bollilo	1 roll	0.86
Indian bread, Naan, plain	1 piece	0.73
English Muffin, plain	1 muffin	0.73
Kaiser rolls	1 roll	0.54
Pita, white	6" pita	0.50
Whole-Wheat	1 slice	0.50
Pumpernickle	1 slice	0.47
Potato bread	1 slice	0.46
Multi-Grain, and whole-Grain	1 slice	0.44
Croissants, butter	1 medium	0.43
Rye bread	1 slice	0.36
Tortillas, corn	1 tortilla	0.34
Egg bread	1 slice	0.32
Reduced calorie white	1 slice	0.31
Wheat	1 slice	0.30
Dinner Rolls, brown & serve	1 roll	0.28
Hamburger & Hotdog buns, plain	1 bun	0.28
Oatmeal bread	1 slice	0.28
Reduced calorie wheat	1 slice	0.26
French or sourdough	1 slice	0.23
Raisin bread	1 slice	0.19
White	1 slice	0.19
Tortillas, flour	1 tortilla	0.17
Reduced calorie rye	1 slice	0.15

Butter	Amount	Zinc (mg)
Regular dairy butter, salted	1 tbsp	0.01
Regular dairy whipped butter, salted	1 tbsp	0

ZINC

Cereal, General Mills®	Amount	Zinc (mg)
Total Whole Grain	1 cup	20.00
Total Raisin Bran	1 cup	15.00
Total Cranberry Crunch	1 cup	12.00
Wheaties	1 cup	10.01
Wheaties Raisin Bran	1 cup	7.48
Wheat Chex	1 cup	7.02
Lucky Charms	1 cup	6.70
Chocolate Chex	1 cup	5.33
Raisin Nut Bran	1 cup	5.03
Multi-Bran CHEX	1 cup	5.01
Cinnamon Chex	1 cup	5.00
Dora The Explorer	1 cup	5.00
Golden Grams	1 cup	5.00
Honey Nut Chex	1 cup	5.00
Cookie Crisp	1 cup	4.99
Reese's Puffs	1 cup	4.99
Cinnamon Toast Crunch	1 cup	4.42
Kix	1 cup	4.18
Cocoa Puffs	1 cup	4.17
Honey Nut Clusters	1 cup	3.76
Corn Chex	1 cup	3.75
Rice Chex	1 cup	3.75
Basic 4	1 cup	3.74
Trix	1 cup	3.74
Berry Berry Kix	1 cup	3.01
Oatmeal Crisp, Hearty Raisin	1 cup	0.93
Oatmeal Crisp, Crunchy Almond	1 cup	0.82

Cereal, General Mills Cheerios®	Amount	Zinc (mg)
Frosted	1 cup	5.19
Apple Cinnamon	1 cup	5.00
Banana Nut	1 cup	5.00
Berry Burst, Triple Berry	1 cup	5.00
Chocolate	1 cup	5.00
Dulce De Leche Cherrios	1 cup	5.00
Fruity	1 cup	5.00
Honey Nut	1 cup	5.00
Oat Clusters Cherrios Crunch	1 cup	5.00
Yogurt Burst, Strawberry	1 cup	5.00
Honey Nut , Medley Crunch	1 cup	4.84
Original	1 cup	4.68
Cinnamon Burst	1 cup	3.74
Multi Grain	1 cup	3.74

RDA for adults 11 mg for females, and 8 mg for males

ZINC

Cereal, General Mills Fiber One®	Amount	Zinc (mg)
Honey Clusters	1 cup	7.8
Original Bran	1 cup	7.6
80 Calorie Chocolate Squares	1 cup	5.0
80 Calorie Honey Squares	1 cup	5.0
Caramel Delight	1 cup	3.8
Nutty Clusters & almonds	1 cup	3.7
Raisin Bran Clusters	1 cup	3.7
Frosted Shredded Wheat	1 cup	1.5

Cereal, Kashi®	Amount	Zinc (mg)
Heart to Heart, Warm Cinnamon	1 cup	2.38
Heart to Heart, Honey Toasted Oat	1 cup	1.98
Heart to Heart, Oat Flakes & Blueberry Clusters	1 cup	1.48
Island Vanilla	27 biscuits	1.43
Good Friends	1 cup	1.40
Berry Fruitful	29 biscuits	1.21
Go Lean Crisp, Toasted Berry Crumble	1 cup	1.09
Go Lean Crisp, Cinnamon Crumble	1 cup	0.88
Autum Wheat	29 biscuits	0.81
7-Whole Grain Flakes	1 cup	0.75
7-Whole Grain Honey Puffs	1 cup	0.75
Go Lean Crunch	1 cup	0.69
Indigo Morning	1 cup	0.65
Simply Maize	1 cup	0.65
7-Whole Grain Puffs	1 cup	0.59
Strawberry Fields	1 cup	0.50
Berry Blossom	1 cup	0.48
Go Lean Crunch, Honey Almond Flax	1 cup	0.42
Go Lean	1 cup	0.36
Honey Sunshine	1 cup	0.36
7-Whole Grain Nuggets	1 cup	x
Blackberry Hills	1 cup	x
Cinnamon Harvest	28 biscuits	x
Go Lean Vanilla Graham	1 cup	x
Heart to Heart, Nutty Chia Flax	1 cup	x

Cereal, Kellogg's®	Amount	Zinc (mg)
All-Bran Complete Wheat Flakes	1 cup	19.99
Product 19	1 cup	15.00
Smart Start, Strong Heart, Antioxidants	1 cup	15.00
All-Bran Original	1 cup	7.69
MUESLIX	1 cup	5.58
All-Bran Bran Buds	1 cup	4.50

ZINC

Cocoa Krispies	1 cup	2.07
Krave Chocolate	1 cup	2.07
Cracklin' Oat Bran	1 cup	2.03
Crunchy Nut, Roasted Nut and Honey O's	1 cup	2.02
Fiberplus Cinnamon Oat Crunch	1 cup	2.01
Raisin Bran	1 cup	2.00
Frosted MINI-Wheat's, Bit-Size	1 cup	1.76
CINNABON	1 cup	1.68
Apple Jacks	1 cup	1.51
Crispix	1 cup	1.51
Froot Loops	1 cup	1.51
Corn Pops	1 cup	1.50
Smorz	1 cup	1.50
Raisin Bran Crunch	1 cup	1.48
Frosted MINI-Wheat's, Big-Bite	1 cup	1.12
Fiberplus Berry Yogurt Crunch	1 cup	0.90
Honey Smacks	1 cup	0.61
Rice Krispies	1 cup	0.40
Frosted Rice Krispies	1 cup	0.32
Rice Krispies Treats	1 cup	0.32
Corn Flakes	1 cup	0.28
Crunchy Nut, Golden Honey Nut Flakes	1 cup	0.25
Honey Crunch Corn Flakes	1 cup	0.12
Frosted Flakes	1 cup	0.06

Cereal, Kellogg's Special-K®	Amount	Zinc (mg)
Low Fat Granolia	1 cup	1.66
Protein Plus	1 cup	1.41
Multigrain Oats & Honey	1 cup	0.83
Cinnamon Pecan	1 cup	0.60
Vanilla Almond	1 cup	0.60
Chocolately Delight	1 cup	0.58
Blueberry	1 cup	0.52
Fruit & Yogurt	1 cup	0.51
Original	1cup	0.40
Red Berries	1 cup	0.37

Cereal, Post®	Amount	Zinc, mg
Grape-Nuts Cereal	1 cup	6.44
Grape-Nuts Flakes	1 cup	3.02
Raisin Bran	1 cup	2.24
Fruity Pebbles	1 cup	2.02
Golden Crisp	1 cup	2.02
Cocoa Pebbles	1 cup	2.01
Bran Flakes	1 cup	2.00

RDA for adults 11 mg for females, and 8 mg for males

Continued

Great Grains, Cranberry Almond Crunch	1 cup	1.98
Great Grains, Raisin, Date & Pecan	1 cup	1.61
Great Grains, Crunchy Pecan Cereal	1 cup	1.59
Alpha-Bits	1 cup	1.50
Honey Nut Shredded Wheat	1 cup	1.50
Shredded Wheat, Frosted, spoon-size	1 cup	1.50
Shredded Wheat, Original, spoon-size	1 cup	1.49
Great Grains, Banana Nut Crunch	1 cup	1.48
Shredded Wheat n' Bran, spoon-size	1 cup	1.48
Honeycomb Cereal	1 cup	1.00
Shredded Wheat, Original, big-biscuit	1 biscuit	0.75
Blueberry Morning	1 cup	0.70

Post® Honey Bunches of Oats®	Amount	Zinc (mg)
Just Bunches Honey Roasted	1 cup	2.21
Honey Roasted	1 cup	2.01
With Strawberries	1 cup	0.41
With Cinnamon Bunches	1 cup	0.40
Pecan Bunches	1 cup	0.39
With Almonds	1 cup	0.38
With Vanilla Bunches	1 cup	0.28

Cereal, Quaker®	Amount	Zinc (mg)
Honey Graham OH'S	1 cup	6.60
LIFE Cereal, Cinnamon	1 cup	5.88
CAP'N Crunch	1 cup	5.82
CAP'N Crunch's OOPs! All Berries	1 cup	5.75
LIFE Cereal, Maple & Brown Sugar	1 cup	5.75
CAP'N Crunch & Crunchberries	1 cup	5.73
Corn Bran Crunch	1 cup	5.51
CAP'N Crunch's Peanut Butter Crunch	1 cup	5.50
LIFE Cereal, Original	1 cup	4.80
Oatmeal Squares, Cinnamon	1 cup	4.21
Oatmeal Squares	1 cup	4.04
Toasted Multigrain Crisp	1 cup	3.17
Oatmeal Squares, Golden Maple	1 cup	2.46
Puffed Wheat	1 cup	0.46
Puffed Rice	1 cup	0.21
Granola, Apple, Cranberry, & Almond	1 cup	x

ZINC

Cereal, Cooked	Amount	Zinc (mg)
Oats, regular, unenriched	1 cup	2.34
WHEATENA	1 cup	1.68
Farina	1 cup	0.55
White corn grits	1 cup	0.44
Yellow corn grits	1 cup	0.34
CREAM OF WHEAT, regular	1 cup	0.33
Malt-o-Meal, plain	1-serving	0.19

Cheese	Amount	Zinc (mg)
Ricotta, part skim milk	1 cup	3.30
Ricotta, whole milk	1 cup	2.85
Cottage cheese, lowfat, 2 %	1 cup	0.93
Cottage cheese, creamed, small curd	1 cup	0.90
Cottage cheese, lowfat, 1 %	1 cup	0.86
Cottage cheese, nonfat, uncreamed	1 cup	0.68

Cheese	Amount	Zinc (mg)
Swiss	1 oz	1.24
Gouda	1 oz	1.11
Gruyere	1 oz	1.11
Mozzarella, nonfat	1 oz	1.11
Parmesan, grated	1 oz	1.10
Swiss, low fat	1 oz	1.09
Fontina	1 oz	0.99
American, pasteurized process, low fat	1 oz	0.93
Provolone	1 oz	0.92
Provolone, reduced fat	1 oz	0.90
Mozzarella, part skim milk, low moisture	1 oz	0.89
Cheddar	1 oz	0.88
Colby	1 oz	0.87
Monterey	1 oz	0.85
Monterey, low fat	1 oz	0.84
Mozzarella, whole milk	1 oz	0.83
Feta	1 oz	0.82
Muenster	1 oz	0.80
Muenster, low fat	1 oz	0.79
Blue cheese	1 oz	0.75
Romano	1 oz	0.73
American, pasteurized process, fortified	1 oz	0.71
Brie	1 oz	0.67
Roquefort	1 oz	0.59

RDA for adults 11 mg for females, and 8 mg for males

ZINC

Cheddar, lowfat	1 oz	0.52
Velveeta, pasteurized process	1 oz	0.52
Cheez Whiz, pasteurized process	1 oz	0.46
Goat cheese, hard type	1 oz	0.45
Cream cheese, fat free	1 oz	0.43
Goat cheese, soft type	1 oz	0.26
Goat cheese, semisoft type	1 oz	0.19
Cream cheese	1 oz	0.14
American, pasteurized process, imitation	1 oz	0.06

Cheese, Mexican	Amount	Zinc (mg)
Mexican, blend, reduced fat	1 oz	1.22
Queso chihuahua	1 oz	0.99
Quesco seco	1 oz	0.93
Quesco blanco	1 oz	0.87
Queso asadero	1 oz	0.86
Mexican, blend	1 oz	0.85
Queso anejo	1 oz	0.83
Queso fresco	1 oz	0.73

Chicken, Cooked	Amount	Zinc (mg)
Thigh, with skin, fried in batter	1 thigh	1.75
Drumstick, with skin, fried in flour	1 drumstick	1.42
Drumstick, no skin, roasted	1 drumstick	1.40
Thigh, no skin, roasted	1 thigh	1.34
Breast, with skin, fried in flour	1/2 breast	1.08
Breast, no skin, roasted	1/2 breast	0.86

Chicken, Cooked	Amount	Zinc (mg)
Drumstick with skin, fried in flour	3 oz	2.46
Thigh with skin, fried in flour	3 oz	2.14
Drumstick meat only, no skin, roasted	3 oz	2.06
Drumstick with skin, roasted	3 oz	1.90
Wing meat only, no skin, roasted	3 oz	1.82
Thigh meat only, no skin, roasted	3 oz	1.52
Wing with skin, fried in flour	3 oz	1.50
Wing with skin, roasted	3 oz	1.50
Thigh with skin, roasted	3 oz	1.38
Cornish game hens, meat only	3 oz	1.30
Breast with skin, fried in flour	3 oz	0.94
Breast with skin, roasted	3 oz	0.87
Breast meat only, no skin, roasted	3 oz	0.85

RDA for adults 11 mg for females, and 8 mg for males

ZINC

Cream	Amount	Zinc (mg)
Half & Half	1 tbsp	0.08
Sour Cream, reduced fat	1 tbsp	0.08
Sour cream, cultured	1 tbsp	0.05
Light Coffe Cream	1 tbsp	0.04
Heavy Cream	1 tbsp	0.03
Whipped Topping, pressurized	1 tbsp	0.01

Eggs	Amount	Zinc (mg)
Egg whole, poached	1 large	0.64
Egg whole, fried	1 large	0.64
Egg whole, scrambled	1 large	0.63
Egg substitute, liquid, fat free	1/4 cup	0.59
Egg whole, hard-boiled	1 large	0.53
Egg yolk	1 large	0.38
Egg whites, dried	1 ounce	0.03
Egg whites, raw	1 large	0.01
Egg whites, dried powder, stabilized	1 tbsp	0.01

Fish, Canned	Amount	Zinc (mg)
Atlantic sardines, in oil	3 oz	1.11
Light tuna, in oil	3 oz	0.77
Light tuna, in water	3 oz	0.59
White (albacore) tuna, in water	3 oz	0.41
White (albacore) tuna, in oil	3 oz	0.40

Fish, Cooked	Amount	Zinc (mg)
Carp	3 oz	1.62
Skipjack (aku) tuna	3 oz	0.89
Atlantic mackerel	3 oz	0.80
Catfish, breaded & fried	3 oz	0.73
Northern pike	3 oz	0.73
Pacific & Jack mackerel	3 oz	0.73
Freshwater bass	3 oz	0.71
Atlantic salmon, wild	3 oz	0.70
Walleye pike	3 oz	0.67
Swordfish	3 oz	0.66
Bluefin tuna	3 oz	0.65
Alaskan halibut	3 oz	0.64
King mackerel	3 oz	0.61
Florida pompano	3 oz	0.59
Yellowtail	3 oz	0.57
Spanish mackerel	3 oz	0.53
Catfish, wild	3 oz	0.52

RDA for adults 11 mg for females, and 8 mg for males

ZINC

Continued

Atlantic pollock	3 oz	0.51
Keta (chum) salmon	3 oz	0.51
Atlantic cod	3 oz	0.49
Catfish, farmed	3 oz	0.49
King, chinook salmon	3 oz	0.48
Coho salmon, wild	3 oz	0.48
Walleye pollock	3 oz	0.48
Rainbow trout, farmed	3 oz	0.46
Atlantic herring, pickled	3 oz	0.45
Whiting	3 oz	0.45
Atlantic croaker	3 oz	0.44
Sea bass	3 oz	0.44
Greenland halibut	3 oz	0.43
Grouper	3 oz	0.43
Rainbow trout, wild	3 oz	0.43
Stripped bass	3 oz	0.43
Sockeye salmon	3 oz	0.42
Coho salmon, farmed	3 oz	0.40
Pink salmon	3 oz	0.39
Yellowfin tuna	3 oz	0.38
Atlantic & Pacific halibut	3 oz	0.37
Atlantic salmon, farmed	3 oz	0.37
Snapper	3 oz	0.37
Tilapia	3 oz	0.35
Haddock	3 oz	0.34
Flounder and Sole	3 oz	0.33
Pacific cod	3 oz	0.33
Atlantic perch	3 oz	0.30
Orange roughy	3 oz	0.27
Chinook salmon, smoked	3 oz	0.26

Fish, Shellfish, Cooked	Amount	Zinc (mg)
Oysters, breaded & fried	3 oz	74.06
Eastern oysters, wild	3 oz	51.88
Eastern oysters, farmed	3 oz	38.38
Alaskan king crab	3 oz	6.48
Crab cakes	3 oz	3.48
Northern lobster	3 oz	3.44
Blue crab	3 oz	3.24
Blue crab, canned	3 oz	3.24
Queen crab	3 oz	3.05
Octopus	3 oz	2.86

ZINC

Shrimp, canned	3 oz	1.67
Crayfish	3 oz	1.50
Squid	3 oz	1.48
Shrimp	3 oz	1.39
Clams, breaded & fried	3 oz	1.24
Shrimp, breaded & fried	3 oz	1.17
Scallops, breaded & fried	3 oz	0.90
Abalone	3 oz	0.81
Clams, canned	3 oz	0.71
Alaskan king crab, imitation	3 oz	0.28

Fruit, Canned	Amount	Zinc (mg)
Pineapple	1 cup	0.30
Apricots	1 cup	0.28
Peaches	1 cup	0.24
Pears	1 cup	0.21
Plums	1 cup	0.18
Applesauce, sweetened	1 cup	0.08
Applesauce, unsweetened	1 cup	0.07
Olives, black	5 large	0.05
Olives, green	5 large	0.01

Fruit, Dried	Amount	Zinc (mg)
Currants	1 cup	0.95
Peaches	1 cup	0.91
Figs	1 cup	0.82
Pears	1 cup	0.70
Apricots	1 cup	0.51
Apples	1 cup	0.17
Cranberries	1 cup	0.13

Fruit, Frozen	Amount	Zinc (mg)
Raspberries	1 cup	0.45
Blackberries	1 cup	0.38
Strawberries	1 cup	0.15
Blueberries	1 cup	0.14
Peaches	1 cup	0.13

Fruit, Raw	Amount	Zinc (mg)
Avocado, California	1 cup	1.56
Chayote, 1" pieces"	1 cup	0.98
Avocado, Florida	1 cup	0.92
Prunes, uncooked	1 cup	0.77
Blackberries	1 cup	0.76

RDA for adults 11 mg for females, and 8 mg for males

ZINC

Pomegrenates	1 cup	0.61
Raspberries	1 cup	0.52
Stewed prunes	1 cup	0.47
Dates	1 cup	0.43
Apricots	1 cup	0.33
Raisins	1 cup	0.32
Black currants	1 cup	0.30
Cataloupe	1 cup	0.29
Cherimoya, pieces	1 cup	0.26
Peachs	1 cup	0.26
Kiwi	1 cup	0.25
Nectarine	1 cup	0.24
Blueberries	1 cup	0.23
Strawberries	1 cup	0.23
Jicama	1 cup	0.21
Plantains	1 cup	0.21
Pineapple	1 cup	0.20
Mulberries	1 cup	0.17
Elderberries	1 cup	0.16
Grapefruit, pink & red, sections	1 cup	0.16
Pears	1 cup	0.16
Plums	1 cup	0.16
Florida Oranges	1 cup	0.15
Honeydew	1 cup	0.15
Mango	1 cup	0.15
Pummelo. sections	1 cup	0.15
Water mellon	1 cup	0.15
Tangerine	1 cup	0.14
Naval Oranges	1 cup	0.13
Oranges	1 cup	0.13
Papayas	1 cup	0.12
Cherries, without pits	1 cup	0.11
Grapes, red & green	1 cup	0.11
Valencias oranges	1 cup	0.11
Cranberries	1 cup	0.10
Apples	1 cup	0.05

Fruit, Raw	Amount	Zinc (mg)
Persimmons, small native	1 fruit	x
Chayote, 1" pieces"	1 fruit	1.50
Avocado, Florida	1 fruit	1.22
Pomegranates	1 fruit	0.99
Avocado, California	1 fruit	0.95
Pummelo	1 fruit	0.49
Cherimoya, pieces	1 fruit	0.38

RDA for adults 11 mg for females, and 8 mg for males

Continued

Nectarine	1 fruit	0.23
Plantains	1 fruit	0.21
Banana	1 fruit	0.18
Persimmons, Japanese	1 fruit	0.18
Prunes, uncooked	5 fruit	0.18
Peaches	1 fruit	0.17
Pears	1 fruit	0.17
Papayas, small	1 fruit	0.13
Dates	5 fruit	0.12
Star fruit, Carambola	1 fruit	0.11
Florida Oranges	1 fruit	0.11
Kiwi	1 fruit	0.11
Naval Oranges	1 fruit	0.11
Grapefruit, pink & red	1/2 fruit	0.09
Raisins	1 small box	0.09
Strawberries	5 fruit	0.08
Apricots	1 fruit	0.07
Valencias Oranges	1 fruit	0.07
Apples	1 fruit	0.06
Cherries	10 fruit	0.06
Pineapple	1/2" x 3" slice"	0.06
Plums	1 fruit	0.06
Tangerine	1 fruit	0.06
Figs, dried	1 fruit	0.05
Olives, green	5 large	0.05
Pineapple guava, Feijoa	1 fruit	0.03
Kumquats	1 fruit	0.03
Olives, black	5 large	0.01

Game Meat, Cooked	Amount	Zinc (mg)
Deer, ground	3 oz	5.58
Elk, ground	3 oz	5.58
Caribou	3 oz	4.47
Bison, ground	3 oz	4.37
Buffalo, steak, free range	3 oz	4.30
Elk, roasted	3 oz	2.69
Wild boar	3 oz	2.56
Deer	3 oz	2.34
Duck, meat only	3 oz	2.21
Rabbit, wild, stewed	3 oz	2.02
Squirrel	3 oz	1.51
Antelope	3 oz	1.43

ZINC

Grains, Cooked	Amount	Zinc (mg)
Kamut	1 cup	3.04
Spelt	1 cup	2.42
Oats, regular, unenriched	1 cup	2.34
Wild rice	1cup	2.20
Amaranth	1 cup	2.12
Quinoa	1 cup	2.02
Millet	1 cup	1.58
Spaghetti, spinach	1 cup	1.51
Barley, pearled	1 cup	1.29
Brown rice	1 cup	1.23
Oat bran	1 cup	1.16
Macaroni, Whole-Wheat	1 cup	1.13
Spaghetti, Whole-Wheat	1 cup	1.13
Bulgur	1 cup	1.04
Egg noodles	1 cup	1.04
Buckwheat, groats	1 cup	1.02
Egg & Spinach noodles	1 cup	1.01
White rice, instant	1 cup	0.81
White rice, regular	1 cup	0.77
Macaroni	1 cup	0.71
Spaghetti, enriched	1 cup	0.71
White rice, paraboiled	1 cup	0.58
Rice noodles	1 cup	0.44
Couscous	1 cup	0.41
Soba noodles	1 cup	0.14

Herbs & Spices	Amount	Zinc (mg)
Celery seeds	1 tsp	0.14
Anise seed, whole	1 tsp	0.11
Chili powder	1 tsp	0.11
Basil, dried & ground	1 tsp	0.10
Paprika, powder	1 tsp	0.10
Turmeric, ground	1 tsp	0.10
Onion powder	1 tsp	0.09
Thyme, dried	1 tsp	0.09
Coriander, seed	1 tsp	0.08
Curry powder	1 tsp	0.08
Garlic powder	1 tsp	0.08
Caraway seeds	1 tsp	0.07
Ginger, ground	1 tsp	0.07
Tarragon, dried	1 tsp	0.06
Basil, fresh, chopped	1 tsp	0.05
Chervil, dried	1 tsp	0.05
Cloves, dried	1 tsp	0.05

RDA for adults 11 mg for females, and 8 mg for males

ZINC

Cinnamon powder	1 tsp	0.04
Oregano	1 tsp	0.04
Rosemary, dried	1 tsp	0.04
Coriander, dried	1 tsp	0.03
Parsley, dried	1 tsp	0.03
Sage, ground	1 tsp	0.03
All spice	1 tsp	0.02
Marjoram, dried	1 tsp	0.02
Pepper, black	1 tsp	0.02
Chives, raw	1 tsp	0.01
Saffron	1 tsp	0.01

Juice	Amount	Zinc (mg)
Prune juice	1 cup	0.54
Vegetable juice	1 cup	0.48
Carrot juice	1 cup	0.42
Tomato juice	1 cup	0.36
Pineapple, unsweetened	1 cup	0.28
Pomegranate	1 cup	0.22
Grape juice, unsweetened	1 cup	0.18
Grapefruit juice, raw	1 cup	0.12
Lemon juice, raw	1 cup	0.12
Orange juice, raw	1 cup	0.12
Cranberry juice	1 cup	0.08
Apple juice	1 cup	0.05

Lamb, Cooked	Amount	Zinc (mg)
Foreshank, trim to 1/8" fat	3 oz	6.54
Cubed for stew or kabob	3 oz	4.90
Rib, lean, trim to 1/4" fat	3 oz	4.48
Ground	3 oz	3.97
Leg, whole, trim to 1/4" fat	3 oz	3.74
Chops, loin, lean, trim to 1/4" fat	3 oz	2.96

Milk	Amount	Zinc (mg)
Canned, condensed, sweetened	1 cup	2.88
Canned, evaporated, nonfat	1 cup	2.30
Canned, evaporated	1 cup	1.94
Sheep milk	1 cup	1.32
Coconut milk, canned	1 cup	1.27
Reduced fat, 2%	1 cup	1.17
Buttermilk, lowfat	1 cup	1.03
Nonfat, fat free or skim liquid milk	1 cup	1.03

RDA for adults 11 mg for females, and 8 mg for males

ZINC

Lowfat, 1%	1 cup	1.02
Dry, instant, nonfat	1/3 cup	1.01
Whole milk, 3.25%	1 cup	0.90
Goat milk	1 cup	0.73
Human milk	1 cup	0.42
Soy milk, original, unfortified	1 cup	0.29

Nuts & Seeds	Amount	Zinc (mg)
Pumpkin seeds	1 oz	2.21
Sesame seeds	1 oz	2.20
Pine nuts	1 oz	1.83
Cashews	1 oz	1.64
Sunflower seeds	1 oz	1.42
Tahini	1 oz	1.31
Chia seeds	1 oz	1.30
Pecans	1 oz	1.28
Flaxseeds	1 oz	1.23
Brazil nuts	1 oz	1.15
Mixed nuts, roasted with peanuts, no salt	1 oz	1.08
Black walnuts	1 oz	0.96
Peanuts	1 oz	0.93
Trail mix, regular, salted	1 oz	0.91
Trail mix, regular with chocolate chips	1 oz	0.89
English walnuts	1 oz	0.88
Almonds	1 oz	0.87
Peanut butter, smooth	1 oz	0.82
Hazelnuts	1 oz	0.69
Pistachio	1 oz	0.62
Macadamia	1 oz	0.37
Trail mix, tropical	1 oz	0.33
Coconut, raw meat	1 oz	0.31

Nuts & Seeds	Amount	Zinc (mg)
Sesame seeds	1/4 cup	2.79
Pumpkin seeds	1/4 cup	2.52
Pine nuts	1/4 cup	2.18
Peanut butter, smooth	1/4 cup	1.88
Flaxseeds	1/4 cup	1.82
Sunflower seeds	1/4 cup	1.75
Brazilnuts, whole	1/4 cup	1.35
Mixed nuts, roasted with peanuts, no salt	1/4 cup	1.30
Trail mix, regular, salted	1/4 cup	1.21
Peanuts	1/4 cup	1.19

ZINC

Continued

Trail mix, regular with chocolate chips	1/4 cup	1.15
Pecans, halves	1/4 cup	1.12
Almonds	1/4 cup	1.10
Black walnuts, chopped	1/4 cup	1.05
English walnuts, chopped	1/4 cup	0.77
Hazelnuts	1/4 cup	0.70
Pistachio	1/4 cup	0.68
Peanut butter, smooth	1 tbsp	0.47
Macadamia	1/4 cup	0.44
Trail mix, tropical	1/4 cup	0.41
Coconut meat, shredded	1/4 cup	0.22
Cashews	1/4 cup	x
Chia seeds	1/4 cup	x

Pork, Cooked	Amount	Zinc (mg)
Spareribs	3 oz	3.91
Bacon	3 oz	2.98
Chops, lean, pan-fried	3 oz	2.91
Bratwurst	3 oz	2.76
Ground pork	3 oz	2.73
Chops, pan-fried	3 oz	2.72
Backribs	3 oz	2.61
Braunschweiger	3 oz	2.39
Cured ham, lean	3 oz	2.18
Tenderloin	3 oz	2.05
Italian sausage	3 oz	2.03
Cured ham	3 oz	1.97
Sirloin chops	3 oz	1.83
Center loin chops	3 oz	1.82
Chops, broiled	3 oz	1.82
Sausage	3 oz	1.77
Polish sausage	3 oz	1.64
Canadian-style bacon	3 oz	1.44
Liverwurst spread	1/4 cup	1.26
Canadian-style bacon	2 slices	0.79
Bacon	3 slices	0.67
Sausage	1 patty	0.56
Sausage	2 links	0.49

Turkey, Cooked	Amount	Zinc (mg)
Ground turkey, 93% lean	3 oz	3.15
Dark meat	3 oz	2.98
Ground turkey, 85% lean	3 oz	2.76
Ground turkey	3 oz	2.64
Turkey bacon	3 oz	2.55

RDA for adults 11 mg for females, and 8 mg for males

ZINC

Turkey sausage, Reduced Fat	3 oz	1.96
Ground turkey, Fat-Free	3 oz	1.86
Breast meat	3 oz	1.48
Light meat	3 oz	1.46

Veal, Cooked	Amount	Zinc (mg)
Foreshank	3 oz	5.64
Breast	3 oz	3.56
Rib	3 oz	3.48
Leg, top round	3 oz	3.37
Ground	3 oz	3.29
Sirloin	3 oz	2.85
Loin	3 oz	2.58

Vegetables, Canned	Amount	Zinc (mg)
Mushrooms	1 cup	1.12
Green peas	1 cup	1.07
Spinach	1 cup	0.98
Yellow sweet corn	1 cup	0.97
Asparagus	1 cup	0.97
Tomato pure	1 cup	0.90
Tomato sauce	1 cup	0.49
Sauerkraut	1 cup	0.45
Stewed tomato	1 cup	0.43
Pumpkin	1 cup	0.42
Carrots	1 cup	0.38
Green beans	1 cup	0.38
Beets	1 cup	0.36
Tomatoes	1 cup	0.34
Sweet potato	1 cup	0.31

Vegetables, Cooked	Amount	Zinc (mg)
Split peas	1 cup	1.96
Shitake mushrooms	1 cup	1.93
Spinach	1 cup	1.37
White mushrooms	1 cup	1.36
Asparagus	1 cup	1.08
Corn	1 cup	0.92
Beet greens	1 cup	0.72
Broccoli	1 cup	0.70
Summer squash	1 cup	0.70
Okra	1 cup	0.69
Artichokes	1 cup	0.67
Sweet potato, mashed	1 cup	0.66

RDA for adults 11 mg for females, and 8 mg for males

ZINC

Beets	1 cup	0.60
Rutabagas	1 cup	0.60
Potatoes, mashed with whole milk	1 cup	0.59
Snow Peas	1 cup	0.59
Zucchini	1 cup	0.59
Swiss chard	1 cup	0.58
Pumpkin	1 cup	0.56
Lambsquarters	1 cup	0.54
Brussels sprouts	1 cup	0.51
Kohlrabi	1 cup	0.51
Raab broccoli	1 cup	0.46
Winter squash	1 cup	0.45
Collard greens	1 cup	0.44
Onions	1 cup	0.44
Scallop and Pattypan squash	1 cup	0.43
Parsnips	1 cup	0.41
Crookneck and Straightneck squash	1 cup	0.40
Cabbage, Red	1 cup	0.38
Acorn squash	1 cup	0.35
Potatoes, flesh, baked	1 cup	0.35
Broccolini	1 cup	0.34
Cabbage, Savoy	1 cup	0.33
Cactus pads, Nopales	1 cup	0.31
Carrots	1 cup	0.31
Green beans	1 cup	0.31
Hubbard squash	1 cup	0.31
Kale	1 cup	0.31
Spaghetti squash	1 cup	0.31
Cabbage	1 cup	0.30
Bok-Choy	1 cup	0.29
Dandelion greens	1 cup	0.29
Butternut squash	1 cup	0.27
Yams, cubes	1 cup	0.27
Cauliflower	1 cup	0.21
Celery	1 cup	0.21
Mustard Spinach	1 cup	0.20
Turnip greens	1 cup	0.20
Turnips	1 cup	0.19
Cabbage, Napa	1 cup	0.15
Mustard greens	1 cup	0.15
Eggplant	1 cup	0.12
Leeks	1 cup	0.06

RDA for adults 11 mg for females, and 8 mg for males

ZINC

Vegetables, Frozen	Amount	Zinc (mg)
Green peas	1 cup	1.07
Corn	1 cup	1.03
Spinach	1 cup	0.93
Okra	1 cup	0.90
Asparagus	1 cup	0.74
Turnip greens	1 cup	0.67
Broccoli	1 cup	0.52
Carrots	1 cup	0.51
Collard greens	1 cup	0.46
Brussels sprouts	1 cup	0.37
Green beans	1 cup	0.32
Butternut squash	1 cup	0.29
Cauliflower	1 cup	0.23
Kale	1 cup	0.23
Rhubarb	1 cup	0.19

Vegetables, Raw	Amount	Zinc (mg)
Crimini mushrooms	1 cup	0.79
Oyster mushrooms, sliced	1 cup	0.66
Portabella mushrooms	1 cup	0.46
Enoki mushrooms	1 cup	0.42
Endive	1 cup	0.40
Green onions & scallions	1 cup	0.39
Red bell peppers, sliced	1 cup	0.37
Broccoli	1 cup	0.36
White Mushrooms	1 cup	0.36
Zucchini	1 cup	0.36
Summer squash	1 cup	0.33
Raab broccoli	1 cup	0.31
Tomatoes	1 cup	0.31
Kale	1 cup	0.29
Tomatillos	1 cup	0.29
Shiitake mushrooms, dried	1 each	0.28
Cauliflower	1 cup	0.27
Onions	1 cup	0.27
Carrots	1 cup	0.26
Snow peas	1 cup	0.26
Mustard spinach	1 cup	0.26
Radicchio	1 cup	0.25
Tomatoes, cherry	1 cup	0.25
Yellow bell pepper	1 cup	0.25

RDA for adults 11 mg for females, and 8 mg for males

ZINC

Continued

Dandelion greens	1 cup	0.23
Prickley pear cactus pads	1 cup	0.22
Butternut squash	1 cup	0.21
Cucumbers	1 cup	0.21
Green bell peppers	1 cup	0.19
Savoy cabbage	1 cup	0.19
Celery	1 cup	0.16
Spinach	1 cup	0.16
Red cabbage	1 cup	0.15
Belgian endive	1 cup	0.14
Spirulina, dried	1 tbsp	0.14
Bok-Choy	1 cup	0.13
Cabbage	1 cup	0.13
Romaine lettuce	1 cup	0.13
Swiss chard	1 cup	0.13
Chicory greens	1 cup	0.12
Butterhead & Boston lettuce	1 cup	0.11
Green leaf lettuce	1 cup	0.10
Arugula	1 cup	0.09
Iceburg lettuce	1 cup	0.08
Watercress	1 cup	0.04

Yogurt	Amount	Zinc (mg)
Plain, greek, nonfat	8 ounces	1.70
Plain, skim milk and nonfat	8 ounces	1.38
Plain, low fat	8 ounces	1.27
Plain, whole milk	8 ounces	0.84

RDA for adults 11 mg for females, and 8 mg for males

Nutrient Data Collection Form

Food	Amount	Book Numbers	Multiply By	Estimated Nutrient Intake
Nutrient::	RDA:	Estimated:	% of RDA:	Total Estimated:

To download additional forms for free, go to www.TopNutrients4U.com

NOTES

REFERENCES

CALCIUM REFERENCES

1969 Importance of dietary calcium / phosphorus ratios on skeletal, calcium, magnesium, and phosphorus metabolism. *Irwin Clark. American Journal of Physiology. September 1969, Vol. 217, No. 3, 865-80.*

1986 Relationships between unusual nutrient intake and bone-mineral content of women 35-65 years of age: longitudinal and cross-sectional analysis. *Jo. L. Freudenheim, MS., Nancy E. Johnson, PhD., Everett L. Smith, PhD. American Journal of Clinical Nutrition. December 1986, Vol. 44, No. 6, 863- 876.*

1987 Influence of nutritional factors on calcium-regulating hormones and bone loss. *Luket BP, Carey M, McCarty B, Tiemann S, Goodnight L, Helm M, Hassanein R, Stevenson C, Stoskopf M, Doolan L. Calcified Tissues International. March 1987, Vol. 4, No. 3, 119-125*

1988 Elevated secretion and action of parathyroid hormones in young women assembled from ordinary foods. *Calvo MS, Kumar R, Heath H 3rd. Journal of Clinical Endocrinology & Metabolism. April 1988, Vol. 66, No. 4, 823-829.*

1990 Persistently elevated parathyroid hormone secretion and action in young women after four weeks of ingesting high phosphorus, low calcium diets. *Mona S. Calvco, Rajiv Kumar, Hunter Heath . Journal of Clinical Endocrinology & Metabolism. May 1990, Vol. 70, 1334-1340.*

1992 Effects of a short course of oral phosphate treatment on serum parathyroid hormone and biochemical markers of bone turnover: A Dose-Response Study. *Kim Brixan, Henning K. Nielsen, Peder Charles, Leif Mosekilde. Calcified Tissues International. 1992, Vol.51, 276-281.*

1993 Dietary phosphorus, calcium metabolism, and bone. *Mona Schiess Calvo. Journal of Nutrition. 1993, Vol.123, 1627-1633.*

1996 Changing phosphorus content of the U.S. *diet: potential for adverse effects on bone. Mona S. Calvo, Youngmee K. Park. Journal of*

Nutrition. April 1996, Vol. 126(4Supp), 1168s-1180s.

1996 **Calcium, Phosphorus and Human Bone Development.** *John J.B. Anderson. Journal of Nutrition. 1996, Vol. 126(4Supp), 1153s-1158s.*

1998 **Dietary calcium, protein, and phosphorus are related to bone mineral density and content in young women.** *Dorothy Teegarden, Roseann M Lyle, George P McCabe, Linda D Mcabe, William R Proulx, Kathryn Michon, Ada P Knight, C Conrad Johnson, and Connie M Weaver. American Journal of Clinical Nutrition. September 1998, Vol.68, No.3, 749-754.*

1999 **Relationship between bone mineral density, serum vitamin D metabolites and calcium / phosphorus intake in healthy perimenopausal women.** *C. Brot, N. Jorgensen, O.R. Madsen, L.B. Jensen, O.H. Sorensen. Journal of Internal Medicine. May 1999, Vol. 245, Issue 5, 509-516.*

2004 **Positive association between 25-hydroxyvitamin D levels and bone mineral density: a population based study of young and older adults.** *Bischoff-Ferrari H.A., Dietrich T., Orav E.J. Dawson-Hughes B., American Journal of Medicine. 2004, Vol. 116, 634-639.*

2006 **High phosphorus intakes acutely and negatively affect calcium and bone metabolism in a dose-dependent manner in healthy young women.** *Kemi VE, Karkkainen MU, Lamberg-Allardt CJ. British Journal of Nutrition. 2006, Vol. 96, 545-552.*

2009 **Dietary calcium and serum 25-hydroxyvitamin D status in relation to BMD among U.S.** *adults. Bischoff-Ferrari H.A., Kiel D.P., Dawson-Hughes B. Journal Bone Mineral Research. 2009, Vol. 24, 935-942.*

2010 **Low calcium / phosphorus ratio in habitual diets affects serum parathyroid hormone concentration and calcium metabolism in healthy women with adequate calcium intake.** *Virpi E. Kemi, Merja U.M. Karkkainen, Hannu J. Rita, Marika M.L. Laaksonen, Terhi A. Outila, Christel J.E. Lamberg-Allardt. British Journal of Nutrition. 2010, Vol. 103, 561-568.*

REFERENCES

CHOLESTEROL REFERENCES

1965 Quantitative effects of dietary fat on serum cholesterol in man. *D.M. Hegsted Ph.D., R.B. McGandy M.D., M.L. Myers S.M., F.J. Stare, M.D. American Journal of Clinical Nutrition. November 1965, Vol.17, No.5, 281-295.*

1966 Serum–cholesterol response to changes in dietary lipids. **Ancel Keys Ph.D.,** *R. Willis Parlin, B.A., American Journal of Clinical Nutrition. September 1966, Vol.19, No.3, 175-181.*

1971 Effects of dietary cholesterol on the regulation of total body cholesterol in man. *Eder Quintao, Scott M. Grundy, E.H. Ahrens, J.R. Journal of Lipid Research. 1971, Vol.12, 233-247.*

1972 Effect of dietary cholesterol on serum cholesterol in man. *F.H. Mattson, Ph.D., B.A. Erickson, Ph.D., A.M. Kligman, M.D. American Journal of Clinical Nutrition. June 1972, Vol.25, No.6, 589-594.*

1976 Independence of the effects of cholesterol and degree of saturation of the fat in the diet on serum cholesterol in man. *Joseph T. Anderson, Ph.D., Francisco Grande, M.D., Ancel Keys, Ph.D. American Journal of Clinical Nutrition. November 1976, Vol.29, No.11, 1184-1189.*

1978 The influence of a wide range of absorbed cholesterol on plasma cholesterol levels in man. *L.A. Simons, J.C. Gibson, C. Paino, M. Hosking, J. Bullock, J. Trim. American Journal of Clinical Nutrition. August 1978, Vol.31, No. 8, 1334-1339.*

1986 Serum-cholesterol response to dietary cholesterol: a re-evaluation. *D. Mark Hegsted, Ph.D. American Journal of Clinical Nutrition. August 1986,   Vol.44, No.2, 299-305.*

1988 Plasma cholesterol responsiveness to saturated fatty acids. *Scott M. Grundy, M.D., Ph.D., Gloria Lena Vega, Ph. D. American Journal of Clinical Nutrition. May 1988, Vol. 47, No.5, 822-824.*

1989 Serum lipid response to dietary cholesterol in subjects fed a low-fat, high-fiber diet. *Jacqueline D. Edington, Moira Geekie, Robin*

Carter, Lisa Benfield, Madeleine Ball, Jim Mann. American Journal of Clinical Nutrition. July 1989, Vol. 50, No.1, 58-62.

1990 **Cholesterol-lowering effect of a low-fat diet containing lean beef is reversed by the addition of beef fat.** *Kerin O'Dea, Kathy Traianedes, Kerry Chrishol, Helen Leyden, Andrew J. Sinclair. American Journal of Clinical Nutrition. September 1990, Vol.52, No.3, 491-494.*

1992 **Reducing total dietary fat without reducing saturated fatty acids does not significantly lower total plasma cholesterol concentrations in normal males.** *Susan Learner Barr, R. Ramakrishnan, Colleen Johnson, Steve Holleran, Ralph B. Dell, Henry N. Ginsberg. American Journal of Clinical Nutrition. March 1992, Vol. 55, No.3, 675-681.*

1992 **Saturated and unsaturated fatty acids independently regulate low density lipoprotein receptor activity and production rate.** *Laura A. Woollett, David K. Spady, John M. Dietschy. Journal of Lipid Research. 1992, Vol. 33, 77-88.*

1993 **Dietary fat and serum lipids: an evaluation of the experimental data.** *D. Mark Hegsted, Ph.D., Lynne M. Ausman, Julia A. Johnson, Gerald E. Dallal. American Journal of Clinical Nutrition. June 1993, Vol. 57, No.6, 875-883.*

1994 **Relationships between serum saturated fatty acids and serum total cholesterol and HDL-Cholesterol in humans.** *Teruo Nagaya, Ken-Ichi Nakaya, Akemi Takahashi, Yoshinari Okamoto. Annuals of Clinical Biochemistry. May 1994, Vol. 31, No. 3, 240-244.*

2004 **Dietary fat and cholesterol and the risk of cardiovascular disease among women with type 2 diabetes.** *Mihaela Tanasescu, Eunyoung Cho, JoAnn E. Manson, Frank B Hu. American Journal of Clinical Nutrition. June, 2004, Vol. 79, No. 6, 999-1005.*

2005 **Maternal cholesterol in fetal development: transport of**

cholesterol from the maternal to the fetal circulation. *Laura A Woollett. American Journal of Clinical Nutrition. December 2005, Vol. 82, No. 6, 1155-1161.*

2005   **Mechanism by which dietary fatty acids modulate plasma lipids.** *Maria Luz Fernandez, Kristy L. West. Journal of Nurtrition. September 1, 2005, Vol. 135, No. 9, 2075-2078.*

COPPER REFERENCES
&
REPORTED CASES OF COPPER DEFICIENCY

A nine year old boy was diagnosed with Wilsons disease, based on a laboratory test, and was prescribed zinc supplements to assist in controlling the disease. After four years of a daily zinc intake of approximately 280 mg the child developed neurological abnormalities. At the age of thirteen the boy was admitted to a hospital with difficulty holding objects, using his hands, and slurring while he talked. The child's copper level on admission was 16 mcg / dL (milligrams per deciliter) much lower than the normal range of 80 to 120 mcg / dL. Treatment with copper supplements stabilized the patient, but neurological functions did not improve.

A forty seven year old man was hospitalized because of progressive numbness and weakness in his lower extremities. Initial laboratory tests detected severe anemia and low serum levels of B-12. Therefore, it was believed the symptoms were due to a B-12 deficiency. Despite continued B-12 treatment, eight months later, the patient was unable to walk and was confined to a wheelchair. Only after a bone marrow biopsy was copper suspected. A further test revealed dangerously low levels in copper, reduced activity of copper-bound enzymes, low concentrations of copper-bound proteins, a low white cell count, lowered hemoglobin concentrations, and unusual elevated serum zinc concentrations. Two months after copper treatment, blood counts returned to normal. However, no improvement in his peripheral neuropathy or loss of strength was observed. The cause of excessive zinc was never determined.

REFERENCES

A young female ingested approximately 2000 mg of zinc gluconate daily for 12 months. She subsequently developed anemia and severe nephrosis. After cessation of zinc ingestion, her anemia and nephrosis resolved.

A forty two year old man was admitted to an emergency room for tingling and numbness of his lower extremities, finger tips, and difficulty walking and holding objects. His serum copper levels could not be detected. An investigation revealed the man had been consuming an entire tube of denture cream daily for the past 4-5 years containing zinc salts. Three weeks after copper treatment, his serum copper and blood levels returned to normal, but there was no improvement in his neuropathic conditions.

COPPER REFERENCES

1956 **Copper deficiency in infants a syndrome characterized by hypocupremia and iron deficiency anemia.** *Phillip Sturgeon, M.D., Charles Brubaker, M.D. Am J Dis Child. September 1956, Vol. 92, No.3, 254-265.*

1978 **Hypocupremia induced by zinc therapy in adults.** *Ananda S. Prasad, M.D., Ph.D., George J. Brewer, M.D., Eric B. Schoomaker, M.D., Parviz Rabbani, Ph.D. Journal American Medical Association. November 10, 1978, Vol. 240, No.20, 2166-2168.*

1978 **Zinc interference with copper metabolism.** *Harold H. Sandstead, M.D. Journal American Medical Association. November 10, 1978, Vol. 240, No. 20, 2188-2189.*

1985 **Dietary intake of zinc associated with a reduction in copper.** *M.D. Festa, H.L. Anderson, R.P. Dowdy, M.R. Ellersieck. American Journal of Clinical Nutrition. February 1985, Vol. 41, No. 2, 285-292.*

1990 **Zinc toxicity.** *Gary J. Fosmire. American Journal of Clinical Nutrition. February 1990, Vol. 51, No.2, 225-227.*

REFERENCES

1990 Excessive zinc ingestion a reversible cause of sideroblastic anemia and bone marrow depression. *E. Randolph Broun, M.D., Anne Greist, M.D., Guido Tricot, M.D., Ph.D., Ronald Hoffman, M.D. Journal American Medical Association September 19, 1990, Vol. 264, No. 11, 1441-1443.*

1991 Zinc supplementation and anemia. *Donald A Frambach, M.D., Rick E. Bendel. Journal American Medical Association. February 20, 1991, Vol. 265, No. 8, 869.*

1995 Requirements and toxicity of essential trace elements, illustrated by zinc and copper. *Harold H. Sandstead. American Journal of Clinical Nutrition. March 1995, Vol. 61, No.3, 621s-624s.*

1998 Clinical conditions altering copper metabolism in humans. *D. Beshgetoor M.D., M. Hambidge, M.D. American Journal of Clinical Nutrition. May 1998, Vol.67, No.5, 1017s-1021s.*

2003 Copper deficiency anemia and nephrosis in zinc-toxicity: a case report. *M.S. Hein. South Dakota Journal of Medicine. April 2003, Vol. 56, No. 4, 143-147.*

2005 Zinc-induced copper deficiency: a report of three cases initially recognized on bone marrow examination. *Monte S. Willis, M.D., Ph.D., Sara A. Monagham, M.D., Michael L. Miller, DO., Robert W. McKenna, M.D., Wiley D. Perkins, M.D., Barry S. Levinson, M.D., Vikas Bhushan, M.D., Steven H. Kroft, M.D. American Journal of Clinical Pathology. 2005, Vol. 123, 125-131.*

2006 CNS demyelination due to hypocupremia in Wilson's disease from overzealous treatment with zinc. *Sunil K. Narayan, Nandigam Kaveer. NEUROIMAGE. 2006, Vol. 54, No. 1, 110-111.*

2013 Hypocupremia associated cytopenia and myelopathy: a national retrospective review. *Alemayehu A. Gabreyes, Hina Naz Abbasi, Kirsten P. Forbes, Grant McQuaker, Andrew Duncan, Ian Morrison. European Journal of Haematology. January 2013, Vol. 90, Issue 1, pages 1-9.*

REFERENCES

ESSENTIAL FATTY ACIDS

1958 **Essential fatty acids in infant nutrition.** *Arild E. Hansen, Mary Ellen Haggard, Arr Nell Boelsche, Doris J.D. Adam, Hilda F. Wiese. Journal of Nutrition. 1958, Vol. 66, No. 4, 565-576.*

1972 **Essential fatty acid deficiency in infants induced by fat-free intravenous feeding.** *John R Paulsrud, Leslie Pensler, Charles F. Whitten, Sheila Stewart, Ralph T. Holman. American Journal of Clinical Nutrition. September 1972, Vol. 25, No. 9, 897-904.*

1975 **Essential fatty acid deficiency in four adult patients during total parenteral nutrition.** *T.J. Richardson, D. Sgoutas. American Journal of Clinical Nutrition. March 1975, Vol. 28, No. 3, 258-263.*

1975 **Development of essential fatty acid deficiency in healthy men fed fat-free diets...** *Jamie D. Wene, William E. Connor, Lawrence DenBesten. Journal Clinical Investigation. 1975, Vol. 56, 127-134.*

1989 **Ingestion of fish oil increases susceptibility of cellular membranes to induction of oxidative stresses.** *Argelia Garrido, Fernando Garrido, Ricardo Guerra, Alfonso Valenzuela. Lipids. 1989; Vol. 24, No. 9, 833-835.*

1990 **Effect of long-term fish oil supplementation on vitamin E status and lipid peroxidation in women.** *M. Meydani., F. Natiello., B. Goldin., N. Free., M. Woods., E. Schaefer., J.B. Blumberg., S.L. Gorbach. Journal of Nutrition. 1990, Vol. 121, 484-491.*

1991 **Lipid, lipoprotein, and hemostatic effects of fish vs fish-oil n-3 fatty acids in mildly hyperlipidemic males.** *Lynne Cobiac., Peter M. Clifton., Mavis Abbey., G. Bryan Belling., Paul J. Nestel. American Journal of Clinical Nutrition. May 1991, Vol. 53, No. 5, 1210-1216.*

1993 **Increased oxidative stress after ingestion of high doses of fish oil.** *Garrido, A., Garate, M., Campos R., Villa A., Nieto, S., Valenzuela, A. The Journal of Nutrition Biochemistry. February 1993, Vol. 4, No.2, 118-122.*

REFERENCES

1996 n-3 fatty acids induce oxidative modifications in human erythrocytes depending on dose and duration of dietary supplementation. *Paola Palozza., Elisabetta Sgarlata., Chiara Luberto., Elisabetta Piccioni, Marcello Anti., Giancarlo Marra., Franco Armelao., Piergiorgio Franceschelli., Gianna Maria Bartoli. American Journal of Clinical Nutrition. September 1996, Vol. 64, No.3, 297-304.*

1997 Lipid peroxidation during n-3 fatty acid and vitamin E supplementation in humans. *Johane P. Allard., Regina Kurian, Elaheh Aghdassi., Reto Muggli., Dawna Royall. Lipids. 1997, Vol. 32, No.5, 535-541.*

1998 Effect of n-3 fatty acid supplementation on lipid peroxidation and protein aggregation in rat erythrocyte membranes. *K. Ando, K. Nagata, M. Beppu, T. Kikugawa, T. Kawabata, K. Hasegawa, M. Suzuki. Lipids 1998, Vol. 33, 505-512.*

1999 Dietary docosahexaenoic acid enhances ferric nitrilotriacetate induced oxidative damage in mice but not when additional alpha-tocopherol is supplemented. *Free Radical Research. 1999, Vol. 30, 260-274.*

1999 Susceptibility to hepatic oxidative stress in rabbits fed different animal and plant fats. *Journal of American College of Nutrition. June 1999, Vol. 15, No. 3, 289-294.*

2001 Enhanced level of n-3 fatty acid in membrane phospholipids induces lipid peroxidation in rats fed dietary docosahexaenoic acid oil. *H.J. Song, T. Miyazawa. Atherosclerosis. 2001, Vol. 155 9-18.*

2005 Ratio of n-6 to n-3 fatty acids and bone mineral density in older adults: the Rancho Bernardo Study. *Lauren A. Weiss, Elizabeth Barrett-Connor, Denise Von Muhlen. American Journal of Clinical Nutrition. April 2005, Vol. 81, No. 4, 934-938.*

2010 Mercury Levels in Commercial Fish and Shellfish. *(1990-2010). U.S. Food and Drug Administration Mercury Update: Impact of Fish Advisories. U.S. Environmental Protection Agency. EPA 823-F-01-011. June 2001.*

REFERENCES

2012 **A diet enriched in docosahexaenoic acid exacerbates brain parenchymal extravasation of Apo B lipoproteins...** Menuka M. *Pallebage-Gamarallage., Virginie Lam., Ryusuke Takechi., Susan Galloway., John C. L. Mamo.*

International Journal of Vascular Medicine. *Volume 2012, Article ID 647689, 8 pages.*

FAT REFERENCES

1929 **A new deficiency disease produced by rigid exclusion of fat from the diet.** *George O. Burr., Mildred M. Burr. Journal of Biological Chemistry. 1929, Vol. 82, 345-367.*

1956 **Vitamin E deficiency in man.** *Calvin W. Woodruff, M.D., American Journal of Clinical Nutrition. November 1956, Vol. 14, No. 6, 597-602.*

1958 **Essential fatty acids in infant nutrition: clinical manifestations of linoleic acid deficiency.** *Arild E. Hansen, Mary Ellen Haggard, Hilda F. Wiese. Journal of Nutrition. December 1958, Vol. 66, No. 4, 656-576.*

1963 **Influence of bile acids on digestion and absorption of lipids.** *Henry Danielsson. American Journal of Clinical Nutrition. March 1963, Vol. 12, No. 3, 214-219.*

1972 **Essential fatty acid deficiency in infants induced by fat-free intravenous feeding.** *John R. Paulsrud, Leslie Pensler, Charles F. Whitten, Sheila Stewart, Ralph T. Holman. American Journal of Clinical Nutrition. September 1972, Vol. 25, No. 9, 897-904.*

1975 **Essential fatty acid deficiency in four adult patients during total parenteral nutrition.** *Timothy J. Richardson, Demetrios Sgoutas. American Journal of Clinical Nutrition. March 1975, Vol. 28, No. 3, 258-263.*

1975 **Development of essential fatty acid deficiency in healthy men fed fat-free diets.** *Jamie D. Wene., William E. Connor., Lawrence BenBesten. Journal of Clinical Investigation. July 1975, Vol. 56, No. 1,*

127-134.

1988 **Essential fatty acid deficiency in premature infants.**

Philip M. *Farrell, M.D., Ph.D., Gary R. Gutcher, M.D., Mari Palta, Ph.D., David DeMets, Ph.D. American Journal of Clinical Nutrition. August 1988, Vol.48, No.2, 220-229.*

1994 **Role of essential fatty acids: dangers in the USDA pyramid and in low-fat diets.** *Edward N. Siguel, Robert H. Lerman. American Journal of Clinical Nutrition. December 1994, Vol.6, No.6, 973-974.*

1996 **Considerations about dietary fat restrictions for children.** *Fima Lifshitz., Omer Tarim., Journal of Nutrition. 1996, Vol. 126, 1031s-1041s.*

1999 **A very low fat diet is not associated with improved lipid profiles in men with a predominance of large, low-density lipoproteins.** *Karin Nilausen, Hans Meinertz. American Journal of Clinical Nutrition. March 1999, Vol.69, No.3, 411-418.*

2000 **Deficiencies of essential fatty acids, vitamin A and E and changes in plasma lipoproteins in patients with reduced fat absorption...** *P.B. Jeppesen., C-E Hoy., P.B. Mortenson. European Journal Clinical Nutrition. 2000, Vol.54, 632-642.*

2004 **Low-Fat...Diets decrease primary bile acid synthesis in humans.** *Peter H. Bisschop, Robert HJ Bandsma, Frans Stekkaard, Anke ter Harmsel, Alfred J Meijer, Hans P. Sauerwein, Folkert Kuipers, Johannes A. Romijn. American Journal of Clinical Nutrition. April 2004, Vol.79, No.4, 570-576.*

2005 **Carotenoid absorption from salad and salsa by humans is enhanced by the addition of avocado or avocado oil.** *Nuray Z. Unlu, Torsten Bohn, Steven K. Clinton, Steven J. Schwartz. Journal of Nutrition. March 2005, Vol. 134, No. 3, 431-436.*

REFERENCES

2007　Carotene rich plant foods ingested with minimal fat enhance total body vitamin A pool size in Filipino schoolchildren as assessed by stable-isotope-dilution methodology. *Judy D. Ribaya-Mercado, Cherry C. Maramag, Lorena W. Tengco, Gregory G Dolnikowski, Jeffrey B. Blumberg, Florentio S. Solon. American Journal of Clinical Nutrition. April 2007, Vol. 85, No.4, 1041-1049.*

PHOSPHORUS REFERENCES

1968　Bone mineral metabolism and osteodystrophy in uremia. *Shaul G. Massry, Jack W. Corburn, Charles R. Kleeman. American Journal of Clinical Nutrition. May 1968, Vol. 21, No.5, 457-466.*

1972　On the prevention of secondary hyperparathyroidism in experimental chronic renal disease using "proportional reduction" of dietary phosphorus intake. *Eduardo Slatopolsky, Sali Caglar, Liliana Gradowska, Janet Canterbury, Eric Reiss, Neal S. Bricker.Kidney International. 1972, Vol. 2, 147-151.*

1973　The role of phosphorus restriction in the prevention of secondary hyperparathyroidism in chronic renal disease. *Eduardo Slatopolskym, Neal S. Bricker. Kidney International. 1973, Vol. 4, 141-145.*

1978　Preservation of function in experimental renal disease by dietary restriction of phosphate. *Lloyd S.Ibeis, Allen C. Alfrey M.D., Lewis Haut M.D. William E. Huffer M.D. New England Journal of Medicine. 1978, Vol. 298, 122-126.*

1980　Early dietary phosphorus restriction and calcium supplementation in the prevention of renal osteodystrophy. *Giuseppe Maschio, M.D., Nicola Tessitore, M.D., Angela D' Angelo, M.D., Ermanno Bonucci, M.D., Antonio Lupo, M.D., Enrico Valvo, M.D., Carmelo Loschiavo, M.D. Antonia Fabris, M.D., Paolo Morachiello, M.D., Guido Previato, M.D., Ernico Fiaschi, M.D. American Journal of Clinical Nutrition. July 1980, Vol.33, No.7, 1546-1554.*

REFERENCES

1982 Effect of dietary protein and phosphorus restriction on the progression of early renal failure. *Giuseppe Maschio, Lamberto Oldrizzi, Nicola Tessitore, Angela D' Angelo, Antonio Lupo, Enrico Valvo, M.D., Carmelo Loschiavo, M.D. Antonia Fabris, Linda Gammero, Carlo Rugiu, Giovanni Panzetta. Kidney International. 1982, Vol. 22, 371-376.*

1983 Role of dietary factors in the progression of chronic renal disease. *Saulo Klahr, John Buerkert, Mabel L. Purkerson. Kidney Internationl. 1983, Vol.24, 579-587.*

1984 Phosphate deprivation increases serum 1,25-(OH)2-vitamin D concentrations in healthy men. *William J. Maierhofer, Richard W. Gray, Jacob Lemann Jr. Kidney International. 1984, Vol. 25, 571-575.*

1986 Oral intake of phosphorus can determine the serum concentration of 1,25-dihydroxyvitamin D by determining its production rate in humans. *A.A. Portale, B.P. Halloran, M.M. Murphy, R.C. Morris. Journal of Clinical Investigation. 1986, Vol. 77, No. 1, 7-12.*

1988 Effect of dietary phosphate restriction on renal function and deterioration. *Allen C. Alfrey, M.D., American Journal of Clinical Nutrition. January 1988, Vol. 47, No. 1, 153-156.*

1989 Physiologic regulation of the serum concentration of 1,25-dihydroxyvitamin D by phosphorus in normal men. *Portale AA, Halloran BP, Morris RC Jr. Journal Clinical Investigation. May 1989, Vol. 83, No.5, 1494-1499.*

1990 Persistently elevated parathyroid hormone secretion and action in young women after four weeks of ingesting high phosphorus, low calcium diets. *Mona S. Calvco, Rajiv Kumar, Hunter Heath . Journal of Clinical Endocrinology & Metabolism. May 1990, Vol. 70, 1334-1340.*

1993 Dietary phosphorus, calcium metabolism, and bone. *Mona Schiess Calvo. Journal of Nutrition. 1993, Vol. 123, 1627-1633.*

1996 Calcium, Phosphorus and Human Bone Development. *John B. Anderson. Journal of Nutrition. 1996, Vol. 126(4Supp), 1153s-1158s.*

REFERENCES

1996 **Changing phosphorus content of the U.S.** *diet: potential for adverse effects on bone. Mona S. Calvo, Youngmee K. Park. Journal of Nutrition. April 1996, Vol. 126(4Supp), 1168s-1180s.*

1996 **Phosphorus restriction prevents parathyroid gland growth.** *High phosphorus directly stimulates PTH secretion in vitro. E. Slatopolsky, J. Finch, M. Dendra, C. Ritter, M. Zhong, A. Dusso, P.N. MacDonald, A.J. Brown. The Journal of Clinical Investigation. June 1996, Vol.97, No. 11, 2534-2540.*

1997 **Reversibility of experimental secondary hyperparathyroidism.** *Ewa Lewin, Wanmei Wang, Klaus Olgaard. Kidney International. 1997, Vol.52, 1232-1241.*

1998 **Dietary calcium, protein and phosphorus are related to bone mineral density and content in young women.** *D. Teegarden, R.M. Lyle, G.P. McCabe, L.D. McCabe, W.R. Proulx, K. Michon, A.P. Knight, C.C. Johnston, C.M. Weaver. American Journal of Clinical Nutrition. September 1998, Vol. 68, No.3, 749-754.*

1999 **Relationship between bone mineral density, serum vitamin D metabolites and calcium / phosphorus intake in healthy perimenopausal women.** *C. Brot, N. Jorgensen, O.R. Madsen, L.B. Jensen, O.H. Sorensen. Journal of Internal Medicine. May 1999, Vol. 245, Issue 5, 509-516.*

2000 **Phosphate regulation of vascular smooth muscle cell calcification.** *Shuichi Jono, Marc D. McKee, Charles E. Murry, Atsushi Shioi, Yoshiki Nishizawa, Katshuito Mori, Hirotoshi Morii, Cecilia M. Giachelli. Circulation Research. 2000, Vol. 87, e10-e17.*

2001 **Vascular calcification and inorganic phosphate.** *Celcilia M. Giachelli, PhD., Shuichi Jono, M.D., Atshushi Shioi, M.D., Yoshiki Nishizawa, M.D., Katshuhito Mono, M.D., Hirotoshi Morii, M.D. American Journal of Kidney Disease. October 2001, Vol. 38, Issue 4, s34-s37.*

REFERENCES

2003 Hyperphosphatemia aggravates cardiac fibrosis and microvascular disease in experimental uremia. *Kerstin Amann, Johannes Tornig, Birgit Kugel, Marie-Luise Gross, Karen Tyralla, Abdussalam El-Shakmak, Andras Szabo, Eberhard Ritz. Kidney International. 2003, Vol. 63, 1296-1301.*

2004 The role of abnormal phosphorus metabolism in the progression of chronic kidney disease and metastatic calcification. *Allen C. Alfrey. Kidney International. 2004, Vol. 66, S13-S17.*

2005 Hidden phosphorus in popular beverages: Part 1. *Lisa Murphy Gutekunst. Journal of Renal Nutrition. April 2005, Vol.15, Issue 2, e1-e6.*

2005 Serum phosphorus levels are associated with mortality risk in people with chronic kidney disease. *Journal of the American Society of Nephrology. 2005, Vol.16, No.2, 520-528.*

2005 Relation between serum phosphate level and cardiovascular events in people with coronary disease. *Marcello Tonelli, M.D., Frank Sacks, M.D., Marc Pfeffer, M.D., PhD, Zhiwei Gao, MSc., Gary Curhan, M.D., Circulation. 2005, Vol. 112, 2627-2633.*

2006 Hyperphosphatemia and related mortality. *Guillaume Jean, Charles Chazot, Bernard Charra. Nephrology Dialysis Transplantation. February 2006, Vol.21, No.2, 273-280.*

2006 Association of disorders in mineral metabolism with progression of chronic kidney disease. *Stephan Schwarz, Bhairvi K. Trivedi, Kamyar Kalantar-Zadeh, Csaba P. Kovesdy. Clinical Journal of the American Society of Nephrology. July 2006, Vol.1, No.4, 825-831.*

2006 Vascular calcification in chronic kidney disease. *Jono, S., Shioa, A., Ikari, Y., Nishizawa, Y. Journal Bone Mineral Metabolism 2006, Vol.24, No.2, 176-181.*

2006 High phosphorus intakes acutely and negatively affect Ca and bone metabolism in a dose-dependent manner in healthy young females. *Kemi VE, Karkkainen MU, Lamberg-Allardt CJ. British Journal Nutrition. September 2006, Vol. 96, No.3, 545-552.*

REFERENCES

2007   **Relations of serum phosphorus and calcium levels to the incidence of cardiovascular disease in the community.** *Dhingra R M.D., Lisa M. Sullivan, PhD., Caroline S. Fox, M.D., Thomas J. Wang. M.D., Ralph B. D'Agostino, PhD., J. Michael Gaziano, M.D., Ramachanandran S. Vasan, M.D. Archive Internal Medicine. May 14, 2007, Vol.167, No.9, 879-885.*

2007   **High plasma phosphate as a risk factor for decline in renal function and mortality in pre-dialysis patients.** *Nora Voormolen, Marlies Noordzij, Diana C. Grootendorst, Ivo Beetz, Yvo W. Sijpkens, Jeannette G. van Manen, Elisabeth W. Boeschoten, Roel M. Huisman, Raymond T. Krediet, Friedo W. Dekker. Nephrology Dialysis Transplantation. May 2007, Vol.22, No.10, 2909-2916.*

2007   **Vascular calcification: Contribution of parathyroid hormone in renal failure.** *K.R. Neves, F.G. Graciolli, L.M. dos Reis, R.G. Graciolla, C.L. Neves, A.O. Magalhaes, M.R. Custodio, D.G. Batista, V. Jorgetti, RM A Moyses. Kidney International. 2007, Vol.71, 1262-1270.*

2007   **Transient severe metastatic calcification in acute renal failure.** *Daniel Landau, Hanna Krymko, Hanna Shalev, Svetlana Agronovich. Pediatric Nephrology. April 2007, Vol. 22, No.4, 607-611.*

2008   **Mechanism of vascular calcification in chronic kidney disease.** *Sharon M. Moe, Neal X. Chen. Journal of the American Society of Nephrology. February 2008, Vol. 19, No.2, 213-216.*

2008   **Hyperphosphatemia of chronic kidney disease.** *Keith A Hruska, Suresh Mathew, Richard Lund, Ping Qiu, Raymond Pratt. Kidney International. 2008, Vol.74, 148-157.*

2008   **Increased inorganic phosphate induces human endothelial cell apoptosis in vitro.** *G.S. Di Marco, M. Hausberg, U. Hillebrand, W. Wittkowski, D. Lang, H. Pavenstadt. American Journal of Physiology June 2008, Vol. 294, No. F1381-1387.*

2008   **Phosphorus levels are associated with subclinical atherosclerosis in the general population.** *Stephan J. Onufrak, Antono Bellasi, Leslee J. Shaw, Charles H. Herzog, Francesca Cardarelli, Peter W. Wilson, Viola Vaccarino, Paolo Raggi. Atherosclerosis. August 2008, Vol. 199, Issue. 2, 424-431.*

2008 Basic science for clinicians: Vascular calcification. *Linda L. Dimer, MD, PhD., Yin Tintut, PhD. 2008, Circulation, Vol. 117, 2938-2948.*

2009 Association of serum phosphate with vascular and valvular calcification in moderate chronic kidney disease. *Kathryn L. Adeney, Siscovick D.S., Ix J.H., Seliger S.L., Shlipak M.G., Jenny N.S., Kestenbaum B.R. Journal of the American Society Nephrology. February 2009, Vol. 20, No. 2, 381-387.*

2009 Association of serum phosphorus concentration with cardiovascular risk. *Vincenzo Savica, MD, Guido Bellinghieri, MD, Lorenzo A. Calo, MD, PhD. American Journal of Kidney Diseases. August 2009, Vol. 54, Issue. 2, Page 389.*

2009 Serum phosphorus concentrations and arterial stiffness among individuals with normal kidney function to moderate kidney disease in MESA. *Joachim H. Ix, Ian H. De Boer, Carmen A. Peralta, Kathryn L. Adeney, Daniel Duprez, Nancy S. Jenny, David S. Sisovick, Bryan R. Kestenbaum. Clinical Journal American Society Nephrology. March 2009, Vol.4, No.3, 609-615.*

2009 Serum phosphorus levels associate with coronary atherosclerosis in young adults. *Robert F. Foley, Allan J. Collins, Charles A. Herzog, Areef Ishani, Philip A. Kalra. Journal of the American Society of Nephrology. February 2009, Vol.20, No.2, 397-404.*

2009 Phosphate levels and cardiovascular disease in the general population. *Robert N. Foley. Clinical Journal of the American Society of Nephrology. June 2009, Vol. 4, No. 6, 1136-1139.*

2009 Vascular calcification: The killer of patients with chronic kidney disease. *Masahid Mizobuchi, Dwight Towler, Eduardo Slatopolsky. Journal of the American Society of Nephrology. July 2009, Vol.20, No.7, 1453-1464.*

2009 Dietary phosphorus acutely impairs endothelial function. *Emi Shuto, Yutaka Taketani, Rieko Tanaka, Nagakatsu Harada, Masashi Isshiki, Minako Sato, Kunitaka Nashiki, Kikuko Amo, Hironori Yamamoto, Yukihito Higashi, Yutaka Nakaya, Eiji Takeda. Journal of the American Society of Nephrology. July 2009, Vol.20, No.7, 1504-1512.*

REFERENCES

2009 In vivo genetic evidence for suppressing vascular and soft-tissue calcification through the reduction of serum phosphate levels, even in the presence of high serum calcium and 1,25-Dihydroxyvitamin D levels. *Mutsuko Ohnishi, M.D., PhD, Teruyo Nakatani, PhD., Beate Lanske, PhD., M.Shawkat Rannaque, M.D., PhD. Circulation: Cardovascular Genetics. September 2009, Vol.2, 583-590.*

2009 Relationship between alkaline phosphatase, serum phosphate, and all-cause or cardiovascular mortality. *Marcello Tonelli, MD, SM., Gary Curham, MD, ScD., Marc Pfeffer, MD, PhD., Frank Sacks, MD., Ravi Thadhani, MD, MPH., Michal L. Melamed, MD, MHS., Natasha Wiebe, MMath, Psat, Paul Muntner, PhD. Circulation 2009, Vol. 120, 1784-1792.*

2010 Understanding sources of dietary phosphorus in the treatment of patients with chronic kidney disease. *Kamyar Kalantar-Zadeh, Lisa Gutekunst, Rajnish Mehrotra, Csaba P. Kovesdy, Rachelle Bross, Christian S. Shinaberger, Nazanin Noori, Raimund Hirschberg, Debbie Benner, Allen R. Nissenson, Joel D. Kopple. Clinical Journal of the American Society of Nephrology. March 2010, Vol. 5, No. 3, 519-530.*

2010 Organic and inorganic dietary phosphorus and its management in chronic kidney disease. *Nazanin Noori, John J. Sims, Joel D. Kopple, Anuja Shah, Sara Colman, Christian S. Shinaberger, Rachelle Bross, Rajinish Mehrota, Csaba P Kovesdy, Kamyar Kalantar-Zadeh. Iranian Journal of Kidney Disease. April 2010, Vol. 4, No.2, 89-100.*

2010 Association of dietary phosphorus intake and phosphorus to protein ratio with mortality in hemodialysis patients. *Nazanin Noori, Kamyar Kalantar-Zadeh, Csaba P. Kovesdy, Rachel Bross, Debbie Benner, Joel D. Kopple. Clinical Journal of the American Society of Nephrology. April 2010, Vol. 5, No. 4, 683-692.*

REFERENCES

2010 Low calcium / phosphorus ratio in habitual diets affects serum parathyroid hormone concentration and calcium metabolism in healthy women with adequate calcium intake. *Virpi E. Kemi, Merja U.M. Karkkainen, Hannu J. Rita, Marika M.L. Laaksonen, Terhi A. Outila, Christel J.E. Lamberg-Allardt. British Journal of Nutrition. 2010, Vol. 103, 561-568.*

2011 Phosphorus and nutrition in chronic kidney disease. *Emilio Gonzalez-Parra, Carolina Gracia-Iguacel, Jesus Egido, Albero Ortiz. International Journal of Nephrology. Volume 2012, Article ID 597605, 5 pages.*

2011 The role of phosphorus in the development and progression of vascular calcification. *Jessica Kendrick, M.D., Michel Chonchol, M.D. American Journal of Kidney Disease. November 2011, Vol. 58, Issue 5, 826-834.*

2011 Lower concentrations of serum phosphorus within the normal range could be associated with less calcification of the coronary artery in Koreans with normal renal function. *Kyung Sun Park, Jai Won Chang, Tae Young Kim, Hyun Woo Kim, Eun Kyoung Lee, Hyun-Sook Kim, Won Seok Yang, Soon Bae Kim, Su-Kil Park, Sang Koo Lee, Jung Sik Park. American Journal of Clinical Nutrition. December 2011, Vol. 94, No. 6, 1465-1470.*

2012 Severe hyperphosphatemia after administration of sodium-phosphate containing laxatives in children: case series and systemic review of literature. *H.N. Ladenhauf, O. Stunder, F. Spreitzhofer, S. Deluggi. Pediat Surg Int. August 2012, Vol. 28, No. 8, 805-814.*

2013 Mechanistic insights into vascular calcification in CKD. *Rukshana Shroff, David A. Long, Catherine Shanahan. Journal of the American Society of Nephrology. February 2013, Vol. 24, No. 2, 179-189.*

2013 Dietary phosphorus is associated with greater left ventricular mass. *Kalani T. Yamamoto, Cassianne Robinson-Cohn, Marcia Cde Oliveira, Alina Kosti, Jennifer A. Nettleton, Joachim H. Ix, Ha Nguyen, John Eng, Joal A.C. Lima, David S. Siscovick, Noel S. Weiss, Bryan Kestenbaum. Kidney International. April 2013, Vol.83, 707-714.*

REFERENCES

2013   **Public health impact of dietary phosphorus excess on bone and cardiovascular health in the general population.** *Mona S. Calvo, Jaime Uribarri. American Journal of Clinical Nutrition. July 2013, Vol.98, No.1, 6-15.*

2013   **High dietary phosphorus intake is associated with all-cause mortality: results from NHANESIII.** *Alex R. Chang, Mariana Lazo, Lawrence J. Appeal, Orlando M. Gutierrez, Morgan E. Crams. American Journal of Clinical Nutrition. July 2013, Vol.99, No.2, 320-327.*

2013   **The connection between dietary phosphorus, cardiovascular disease, and mortality: where we stand and what we need to know.** *Orlando M. Gutierrez. Advances in Nutrition. November 2013, Vol.4, 723-729.*

2013   **Hyperphosphatemia is a combined function of high serum PTH and high dietary protein intake in dialysis patients.** *Elani Streja, Wei Ling Lau, Leanne Goldstein, John J. Slim, Miklos Z. Molna, Allen R. Nissenson, Csab P. Kovesdy, Kamyar Kalantar-Zadeh. Kidney International Supplements. December 2013, Vol.3, 462-468.*

2014   **Assessing the health impact of phosphorus in the food supply: Issues and consideration.** *Mona S. Calvo, Alanna J. Moshfegh, Katherine L. Tucker. Advances in Nutrition. January 2014. Vol. 5, 104-113.*

2014   **Phosphate overload directly induces systemic inflammation and malnutrition as well as vascular calcification in uremia.** *Shunsuke Yamada, Masanori Tokumoto, Narihito Tatsumoto, Masatomo Taniguchi, Hideko Noguchi, Toshiaki Nakano, Kosuke Masutani, Hiroaki Ooboshi, Kazuhiko Tsuruya, Takanari Kitazono. American Journal of Physiology. Renal Physiology. June 2014, Vol. 306, No. F1418-F1428.*

REFERENCES

PROTEIN REFERENCES

1978 Human protein requirements: nitrogen balance response to graded levels of egg protein in elderly men and women. *Ricardo Uauy, M.D., Ph.D., Nevin S. Scrimshaw, Ph.D., M.D., Vernon R. Young, Ph.D. American Journal of Clinical Nutrition. May 1978, Vol.31, No.5, 779-785.*

1981 Urinary calcium and calcium balance in young men as affected by level of protein and phosphorus intake. *Maren Hegsted, Sally A. Schuette, Michael B. Zemel, Hellen M. Linkswiler. Journal Nutrition. 1981, Vol. 111, 553-562.*

1981 Calcium metabolism in postmenopausal and osteoporotic women consuming two levels of dietary protein. *Josephine Lutz, Ph.D., Hellen M. Linkswiler, Ph.D. American Journal of Clinical Nutrition. October 1981, Vol. 34, No.10, 2178-2186.*

1995 Elderly women accommodate to a low-protein diet with losses of body cell mass, muscle function, and immune response. *Carmen Castaneda, Jacqueline M. Charnley, William J. Evans, Marilyn C. Crim. American Journal of Clinical Nutrition. July 1995, Vol. 62, No.1, 30-39.*

1995 Protein turnover and energy metabolism of elderly women fed a low-protein diet. *Carmen Castaneda, Gregory G. Dolnikowski, Gerald E. Dallal, William J. Evans, Marilyn C. Crim. American Journal of Clinical Nutrition. July 1995, Vol.62, No.1, 40-48.*

1997 Increased circulating concentrations of parathyroid hormone in healthy, young women consuming a protein-restricted diet. *Jane E. Kerstetter, Donna M. Caseria, MaryAnn E. Mitnick, Alice F. Ellison, Linda F. Gay, Tara AP Liskov, Thomas O Carpenter, Karl L. Insogna. American Journal of Clinical Nutrition. November 1997, Vol. 66, No. 5, 1188-1196.*

1998 Dietary protein affects intestinal calcium absorption. *Jane E. Kerstetter, Kimberly O. O'Brien, Karl L. Insogna. American Journal of Clinical Nutrition. October 1998, Vol. 68, No.4, 859-865.*

REFERENCES

1999 Prospective study of dietary protein intake and risk of hip fracture in postmenopausal women. *Ronald G. Munger, James R. Cerhan, Brian C-H Chiu. American Journal of Clinical Nutrition. January 1999 Vol. 69, No.1, 147-152.*

2000 Effect of dietary protein on bone loss in elderly men and women: the Framingham Osteoporosis Study. *Hannan MT, Tucker KL, Dawson-Hughes B, Cupples LA, Felson DT, Kiel DP. Journal of Bone Mineral Research. December 2000, Vol. 15, No.12, 2504-2512.*

2001 The recommended dietary allowance for protein may not be adequate for older people to maintain skeletal muscle. *Wayne W. Campbell, Todd A. Trappe, Robert R. Wolfe, William J. Evans. The Journals of Gerontology Series A: Biological Sciences and Medical Sciences. 2001, Vol. 56, No .6, m373-m380.*

2003 Protein intake: effects on bone mineral density and the rate of bone loss in elderly women. *Prema B. Rapuri, J. Christopher Gallagher, Ver Haynatzka. American Journal of Clinical Nutrition. June 2003, Vol. 77, No.6, 1517-1525.*

2003 Dietary protein, calcium metabolism, and skeletal homeostasis revisited. *Jane E. Kerstetter, Kimbly O O'Brien, Karl L. Insogna. American Journal of Clinical Nutrition. September 2003, Vol.78, No.3, 584s-592s.*

2005 The impact of dietary protein on calcium absorption and kinetic measures of bone turnover in women. *Jane E. Kerstetter, Kimberly O. O'Brien, Donna M. Caseria, Diane E. Wall, Karl L. Insogna. Journal of Clinical Endocrinology & Metabolism. January 2005, Vol.90, No.1, 26-31.*

2005 Protein consumption is an important predictor of lower limb bone mass in elderly women. *Amanda Devine, Ian M. Dick, Amirul FM Islam, Satvinder S. Dhaliwal, Richard L. Prince. American Journal of Clinical Nutrition. June 2005, Vol.81, No.6, 1423-1428.*

REFERENCES

2005 Dietary protein: an essential nutrient for bone health. *Jean-Philippe Bonjour, M.D. Journal of the American College of Nutrition. December 2005, Vol. 24, 526s-536s.*

2007 Inadequate protein intake affects skeletal muscle transcript profiles in older humans. *Anna E. Thalacker-Mercer., James C. Fleet, Bruce A Craig, Nadine S. Carnell, Wayne W. Campbell. American Journal of Clinical Nutrition. May 2007, Vol.85, No.5, 1344-1352.*

2008 Dietary protein intake is associated with lean mass change in older, community-dwellng adults: the Health, Aging, and Body Composition Study. *(Health ABC). Denise K. Houston, Barbara J. Nicklas, Jingzhong Ding, Tamara B. Harris, Frances A Tylavsky, Anne B. Newman, Jung Sun Lee, Nadrine R. Sahyoun, Majolein Visser, Stephen B. Kritchevsky, American Journal of Clinical Nutrition. January 2008, Vol. 87, No.1, 150-155.*

2008 Amount and type of protein influences bone health. *Robert P. Heaney, Donald K. Laymen. American Journal of Clinical Nutrition. May 2008, Vol.87, No.5, 1567s-1570s.*

2008 Protein quality assessment: impact of expanding understanding of protein and amino acid needs for optimal health. *D. J. Millward, Donald K. Layman, Daniel Tome, Gertjan Schaafsma. American Journal of Clinical Nutrition. May 2008, Vol. 87, No. 5, 1576s-1581s.*

2009 Dietary protein and calcium interact to influence calcium retention: a controlled feeding trial. *Janet R. Hunt, LuAnn K. Johnson, and ZK Fariba Roughead. American Journal of Clinical Nutrition. May 2009, Vol. 89, No. 5, 1357-1365.*

2009 Dietary protein and bone health: a systematic review and meta-analysis. *Andrew L Darling, Joe D. Millward, David J. Torgerson, Csatherine E Hewitt, Susan A. Lanham. American Journal of Clinical Nutrition. December 2009, Vol.90, No.6, 1674-1692.*

2010   Is protein intake associated with bone mineral density in young women? *Jeannette M. Beasley, Laura E. Ichikawa, Brett A. Ange, Leslie Spangler, Andrea Z. LaCroix, Susan M. Ott, and Dela Scholes. American Journal of Clinical Nutrition. May 2010, Vol.91, No.5, 1311-1316.*

2011 Dietary acid load is not associated with lower bone mineral density except in older men. *Robert R. McLean,Ning Qiao, Kerry E. Broe, Katherine L. Tucker, Virginia Casey, Adrienne L. Cupples, Douglas P. Kiel, Marian T. Hannan. Journal of Nutrition. April1, 2011, Vol. 141, No.4, 588-594.*

2011   Hypercalciuria associated with high dietary protein Intake is not due to acid load. *Naim M. Maalouf, Orson W. Moe, Beverly Adams-Huet, Khashayar Sakhaee. Journal of Clinical Endocrinology & Metabolism. December 1, 2011, Vol. 96, No.12, 3733-3740.*

VITAMIN A REFERENCES
&
REPORTED CASES OF VITAMIN A TOXICITY

One study reported 579 cases of acute toxicity. Twenty two percent resulted from excess retinol consumption from animal liver. Twenty five percent resulted from accidental overdosing of children with supplements by overly zealous parents and grandparents. The remaining resulted from misuse of supplements.

In one case a fifteen-year old male soccer player in anticipation of increasing his performance consumed what he was told to be a healthy diet. For four weeks prior to hospitalization he experienced painful muscular fatigue and stiffness after exercise. On admission he had aching pain in both legs and was lethargic and weak. A dietary investigation revealed 6 capsules of cod liver oil and two multivitamin capsules a day while maintaining a strict diet of liver, milk products, and yellow vegetables. A dietary analysis estimated the boy consumed 20-times the RDA for at least two months.

Many cases of chronic toxicity have resulted in persons who over committed to bizarre and faddish types of diets. One case described vitamin A toxicity in a two-year old boy and his six-year old brother from ingestion of excessive amounts of chicken liver spread. Another case reported sever toxicity in a forty eight year old man who every day for years consumed large quantities of carrot juice along with supplements. The coroner listed the cause of death as an addiction to carrot juice.

A sixty-two year old woman was admitted to Saint Luke's Hospital with skin lesions on the lower part of both legs. For three years she suffered from dry scaly skin, daily shoulder and back pain, persistent dull headaches, and loss of body hair including her eyebrows. A dietary investigation disclosed she was a food faddist who adhered to a lactovegetarian diet for 20-years. A dietary analysis revealed her vitamin A intake was 8-times greater than the RDA. Intake of all supplements stopped, and over the ensuing two months there was a striking improvement. Her skin cleared, leg lesions were healing, body hair increased, headaches ceased, and her serum vitamin A levels returned to normal.

A fifty-seven year old house wife was referred to the Liver Clinic at the Royal Brisbane Hospital for an unexplainable liver problem and complaining of joint pain, dry skin, and a loss of body hair. Her eyebrows were nonexistent. During a dietary investigation she admitted to partaking in many "health diets" believing they would improve her hair, and skin conditions. A dietary analysis revealed a vitamin A intake 19-times greater than the RDA for four years. She was advised to stop all supplements and to avoid items in her diet such as carrots, pumpkin, and cheese which contain large amounts of retinol and beta-carotenes. Four months later her liver functions and tests returned to normal, but it took one-year to see hair and skin improvements.

A 6-year old autistic boy was hospitalized because of vomiting, abdominal pain, and constipation with mild dehydration. Two days later, he developed hives and dry lips, and on the fifth day he was experiencing a loss of body hair and weight. His calcium and vitamin A levels were above normal, and had all the symptoms of a condition known as hypercalcemia. After all known possible causes for hypercalcemia were ruled out a dietary investigation was begun and revealed the following. Four weeks earlier the child was placed on a casein-and-gluten-free diet in an attempt to manage his behavior. Four months earlier the child was placed on a variety of vitamin supplements as part of the management of his autism. The diet consisted of egg-protein shakes with fruits and vegetables. The supplements included six vitamin A drops / day along with weekly vitamin B12 shots, and a "custom-made" multivitamin containing vitamin E, Coenzyme Q, and Omega-3 fatty acids. A dietary analysis showed a four month vitamin A daily intake 10-times greater than the RDA. Thirty days after discontinuation of vitamin A intake, the body's vitamin A and calcium levels returned to normal, and symptoms subsided. The investigators concluded that in cases of hypercalcemia it is important to obtain a careful dietary history to assist in identifying the underlying cause.

Acute toxicity is characterized with nausea, vomiting, headaches, vertigo, and blurred vision and usually associated with mega doses of supplements. Chronic toxicity is more closely associated with long-term abuse of supplements while consuming a vitamin A rich diet. Conditions in children include skin problems, cracks at lip corners, bone tenderness, and anorexia. Noticed conditions in adults include weight loss, pain in bone and joint areas, brittle nails, persistent headaches, scaly dry skin, facial dermatitis, body hair loss, and fatigue.

VITAMIN A REFERENCES

1956 **Hypervitaminosis A: experimental induction in the human subject.** *Robert W. Hillman, American Journal of Clinical Nutrition. November 1956, Vol.4, No.6, 603-608.*

1965 **Hypervitaminosis A, Report of a Case.** *Stanley S. Bergen, Jr., M.D., Oswald A. Roels, Ph. D. American Journal of Clinical Nutrition. February 1965, Vol.16, No.2, 265-269.*

REFERENCES

1965 Liver lipids in a case of hypervitaminosis A. Krause, RF. American Journal of Clinical Nutrition. *June 1965, Vol.16, No.3, 455-457.*

1975 Fatal self-medication with retinol and carrot juice. *Z.A. Leitzer, T. Moor, IM Sharman. Proc Nutr Soc. September 1975, Vol. 34, No. 2, 44A-45A.*

1976 Vitamin A transport in human vitamin A toxicity. *Smith F.R., Goodman D.S. New England Journal of Medicine. 1976, Vol. 294, 805-808.*

1977 Abnormal liver function in chronic hypervitaminosis A. *G.C. Farrell, MB, P.S. Bhathal, PhD, L.W. Powell, PhD, MD. American Journal of Digestive Disease. 1977, Vol. 22, issue 8, pp 724-728.*

1980 Chronic vitamin A intoxication in infants fed chicken liver. *Mahoney, C., Margolis, M., Knauss, T. & Labbe, R. Pedriatric 1980, Vol.65, 893-897.*

1981 The luxus vitamins – A and B12. *Donald S. McLaren, M.C. Ph.D., M.R.C.P.E. American Journal of Clinical Nutrition. August 1981, Vol. 34, 1611-1616.*

1987 Sever Hypervitaminosis A in Siblings: evidence of variable tolerance to retinol intake. *Carpenter T.O., Pettifor J.M., Russell R.M., Pitha J., Mobarhan S., Ossip M.S., Wainer S., Anast C.S. Journal of Pediatrics. October 1987, Vol. 111, No. 4, 507-512.*

1990 Evaluation of vitamin A toxicity. *John N. Hathcock, David G Hattan, Mamie Y Jenkins, Janet T. McDonald, P. Ramnathan Sundaresan, Virgina L. Wilkening. American Journal of Clinical Nutrition. August 1990, Vol. 52, No. 2, 183-202.*

1990 Excess vitamin A injures the liver. *H. Baker., W ten Hove., N. Kanagasundaram., G. Zaki., C.B. Leevy., O. Frank., C.M. Leevy. Journal of the American College of Nutrition. October 1990, Vol.9, No.5, 503-509.*

1991 Liver damage caused by therapeutic vitamin A administration: estimate of dose-related toxicity in 41 cases. *Geubel A.P., De Galocsy C., Alves N., Rahier J., Dive C. Gastroenterology. June 1991, Vol. 100, No.6, 1701-1709.*

REFERENCES

1994 Vitamin A hepatotoxicity: a cautionary note regarding 25,000 IU supplements. *Kowaiski T.E., Falestiny M., Furth E. Malet P.F. American Journal of Medicine. December 1994, Vol. 97, No.6, 523-528.*

1997 Role of Ito cells in the liver. *Flisiak R. Pol J. Pathol. 1997, Vol. 48, No. 3, 139-145.*

1998 Excessive dietary intake of Vitamin A is associated with reduced bone mineral density and increased risk of hip fracture. *Melhus H, Michaelsson K, Kindmark A. Ann Intern Med 1998, Vol. 129, 770-778.*

2003 Water-miscible, emulsified, and solid forms of retinol supplements are more toxic than oil-based preparations. *Anne M. Myhre, Monica H. Carlsen, Siv K Bohn, Heidi L. Wold, Petter Laake, Rune Blomhoff. American Journal of Clinical Nutrition. December 2003, Vol.78, No.6, 1152-1159.*

2006 Acute and chronic toxic effects of vitamin A. *Kristina L. Penniston., Sherry A. Tanumihardjo. American Journal of Clinical Nutrition. February 2006, Vol.83, No. 2, 191-201.*

2006 Risk of vitamin A toxicity from candy-like chewable vitamin supplements for children. *Hugh Simon Lam, MRCPCH, Chung Mo Chow, MRCPCH, Wing Tat Poon, MBChB, Chi Kong Lai, MSc, Kwan Chee Allen Chan, FRCPA, Wai Lan Yeung, MRCP, Joannie Hui, MRCP, Albert Yan WoChan, MD, Park Cheung Ng, MD. August 2006, Pediatrics. Vol. 118, No. 2, 820-824.*

2011 Reported Case of Hypercalcemia Secondary to Hypervitaminosis A in a 6-Year Old Boy with Autism. *Case Reports in Endocrinology. Volume 2011, Article ID 424712, 5 pages.*

VITAMIN D REFERENCES
&
REPORTED CASES of VITAMIN D DEFICIENCY

A 10-day-old boy born in September is admitted to an emergency ward for uncontrollable seizures. Upon admission his left sided arm and leg are twitching, and lip smacking with right-sided head turning. Episodes lasted approximately 30 seconds and were occurring up to 7 times an hour. Laboratory test of the infant revealed calcium and vitamin D levels below acceptable ranges with elevated parathyroid hormone levels. An investigation noted, the baby had been breast feed, the mother had a diet low in calcium, she reported not taking any prenatal vitamins, and always wearing sunscreen when outdoors. Laboratory test of the mother revealed although her calcium levels were within an acceptable range her vitamin D and parathyroid hormones levels were abnormal confirming a vitamin D deficiency in both the mother and child.

The baby was managed with intravenous calcium gluconate infusion and oral intake of calcium and vitamin D. The seizures resolved within 48 hours and the infant was discharged home with oral calcium and vitamin D. Two weeks after discharge the infant was seizure free with normal laboratory test. Attending physicians conclude a vitamin D deficiency in infants and mothers is a re-emerging public health issue and sunscreen with a sun protection of 8 reduces the skins production of vitamin D by 98%.

A 67 year-old man with no past medial history was found in a coma during winter and admitted to the intensive care unit. Physical exam showed constricted pupils, irregular heartbeat, and spastic lower extremities. Laboratory data included low calcium and phosphorus levels, high thyroid stimulus hormone levels with normal renal and liver functions. He was diagnosed with stroke, atrial fibrillation, hypothyroidism and hypocalcemia. He was given intravenous calcium gluconate 1000 mg (elementary calcium 90 mg) and regained consciousness in 7 days. Further work-up for hypocalcemia revealed low vitamin D levels and parathyroid hormone levels were 891.6 pg/ml with normal being below 72 pg/ml. On day 9 he was started on

50,000 IU of vitamin D daily for two weeks in conjunction with oral 500 mg of elemental calcium plus vitamin D three times daily. It took 28 days for all laboratory test to return to normal. This patient who was critically ill had hypocalcemia, hyperparathyroidism, and a vitamin D deficiency. Attending physicains reported the patients response to treatment with vitamin D supported a vitamin D deficiency as the most plausible cause for hypocalcemia.

VITAMIN D REFERENCES

1975 Studies of vitamin D deficiency in man. *M.A. Preece, S. Tomlinson, C.A. Ribot, J. Pietrek, H. T. Korn, D.M. Davis, J. A. Ford, M.G. Dunnigan, J.L.H. O'Riordan. October 1975, Quarterly Journal of Mediciene. New Series XLIV, No. 176, 575-589.*

1976 Advances in vitamin D metabolism as they pertain to chronic renal disease. *Jack W. Coburn, M.D., David L. Hartenbower, M.D., Arnold S. Brickman,M.D. American Journal Clinical Nutrition. November 1976, Vol. 29, No.11, 1283-1289.*

1980 Requirements of vitamin D metabolites in patients with renal disease. *Shaul G. Massry. American Journal Clinical Nutrition. July 1980, Vol. 33, No. 7, 1530-1535.*

1984 Ultraviolet irradiation increases serum 1,25-dihydroxyvitamin D in vitamin-D-repleted adults. *E.B. Mawer, J.L. Berry, Tsilenis E. Sommer, W. Beykirch, A. Kuhlwein, B.T. Rohde. Mineral Electrolyte Metabolism. 1984, Vol. 10, No, 2, 117-121.*

1986 Oral intake of phosphorus can determine the serum concentrations of 1,25-dihyrdoxyvitamin D by determining the production rate in humans. *Anthony A. Portael, Bernard P.Halloran, Margaret M. Murphy, R. Curtis Morris Jr. Journal of Clinical Investigation. January 1986, Vol. 77, 7-12.*

REFERENCES

1996 Lower serum 25-hydroxyvitamin D is associated with increased bone resorption markers and lower bone density at the proximal femur in normal females: a population-based study. *Scharia SH, Scheidt-Nave C, Leidg G, Wusteer C, Seibel MJ, Ziegler R. Exp Clin Endocrinol Diabetes. 1996, Vol. 104, No. 3, 289-292.*

1998 Ultraviolet irradiation corrects vitamin D deficiency and suppresses secondary hyperparathyroidism in the elderly. *V.G Chell, M.E Ooms, C. Popp-Snijders, S. Pavel, A.A. Schothorst, C.C. Meulemans, P. Lips. Journal Bone Mineral Research. August 1998, Vol. 13, No. 8, 1238-1242.*

1998 Hypervitaminosis D: Report on Three Patients. *Raimundo G. Pinto, Amal Al Essa, Khunder Al Nagdy. Annuals of Saudia Medicine 1998, Vol. 18, No. 3, 244-246.*

2004 Nutritional rickets among children in the United States: review of cases reported between 1986 and 2003. *American Journal Clinical Nutrition. December 2004, Vol. 80, No. 6, 1697s-1705s.*

2007 Vitamin D deficiency. *Michael F. Hollock, M.D. Ph.D., New England Journal of Medicine. July 2007, Vol. 357: 266-281.*

2007 Hypovitaminosis D in British adults and age 45 years: nationwide cohort study of dietary and lifestyle predictors. *Elina Hypponen., Chris Power. American Journal Clinical Nutrition. March 2007, Vol. 85, No. 3, 860-868.*

2009 Prevalence and associations of 25-hydroxyvitamin D deficiency in U.S. *children: NHANES 2001-2004. Juhi Kumar, M.D., MPH, Paul Munter, PhD, Frederick J. Kaskel, M.D., PhD., Susan M. Hailpern PhD, MS., Michael L. Melamed, M.D., MHS. Pediatrics September 1, 2009, Vol. 24, No. 3, e362-e370.*

2009 Vitamin D deficiency as an ignored cause of hypocalcemia in acute illness: Report of 2 Cases and Review of Literature. *Hiroshi Noto, Howard J. Heller. The Open Endocronlgy Journal. 2009, Vol. 3, 1-4.*

REFERENCES

VITAMIN E REFERENCES

1960 Vitamin E and lipid metabolism in man. *M. K. Horwitt, Ph.D. American Journal of Clinical Nutrition. July 1960, Vol. 8, 451-461.*

1962 Interrelations between vitamin E and polyunsaturated fatty acids in adult men. *M.K. Horwitt. Vitamins & Hormones. 1962, Vol.20, 541-568.*

1963 Quantitative consideration of the effect of polunsaturated fatty acid content of the diet upon the requirements for vitamin E. *Philip L. Harris, Ph.D., Norris D. Embree, Ph.D. American Journal of Clinical Nutrition. December 1963, Vol. 13, 384-392.*

1967 Tocopherol deficiency in Man. *Henry J. Binder, M.D., Howard M. Spiro,M.D. American Journal of Clinical Nutrition. June 1967, Vol.20, N.6, 594-601.*

1968 Tocopherol in infants fed diets rich in polyunsaturated fatty acids. *Sami A. Hashim, M.D., Raja H. Asfour, M.D. American Journal of Clinical Nutrition. January 1968, Vol.21, N.1, 7-14.*

ZINC REFERENCES

1978 Zinc interference with copper metabolism. *Harold H. Sandstead, M.D. Journal American Medical Association. November 10, 1978, Vol. 240, No. 20, 2188-2189.*

1984 Effect of zinc supplementation on copper status in adult man. *Fisher PW, Giroux A, L'Abbe MR, American Journal of Clinical Nutrition. October 1984, Vol. 40, No.4 , 743-746.*

1985 Clinical and biochemical manifestation of zinc deficiency in human subjects. *Anandan S. Prasad. Journal of the American College of Nutrition. 1985, Vol. 4, No.1, 65-72.*

REFERENCES

1990 **Excessive zinc ingestion a reversible cause of sideroblastic anemia and bone marrow depression.** *E. Randolph Broun, M.D., Anne Greist, M.D., Guido Tricot, M.D., Ph.D., Ronald Hoffman, M.D. Journal American Medical Association. September 19, 1990, Vol. 264, No. 11, 1441-1443.*

1990 **Zinc toxicity.** *Gary F. Fosmire. American Journal of Clinical Nutrition. February 1990, Vol.51, No.2, 225-227.*

1991 **Zinc supplementation and anemia.** *Donald A. Framback, M.D., Rick E. Bendel. Journal American Medical Association 1991, Volume 265, Issue 7, 869.*

2003 **Copper deficiency anemia and nephrosis in zinc-toxicity: a case report.** *M.S. Hein. South Dakota Journal of Medicine. April 2003, Vol. 56, No. 4, 143-147.*

2005 **Zinc-induced copper deficiency: A Report of Three Cases Initially Recognized on Bone Marrow Examination.** *Monte S. Willis, M.D., Ph.D., Sara A. Monagham, M.D., Michael L. Miller, DO., Robert W. McKenna, M.D., Wiley D. Perkins, M.D., Barry S. Levinson, M.D., Vikas Bhushan, M.D., Steven H. Kroft, M.D. American Journal of Clinical Pathology. 2005, Vol. 123, 125-131.*